Comprehensive
Casebook of
Cognitive Therapy

Comprehensive Casebook of Cognitive Therapy

Edited by

Arthur Freeman

Cooper Hospital/University Medical Center
Robert Wood Johnson Medical School at Camden
University of Medicine and Dentistry of New Jersey
Camden, New Jersey

and

Frank M. Dattilio

University of Pennsylvania School of Medicine
Philadelphia, Pennsylvania

Plenum Press • **New York and London**

Library of Congress Cataloging-in-Publication Data

Comprehensive casebook of cognitive therapy / edited by Arthur Freeman
  and Frank Dattilio.
      p.   cm.
   Includes bibliographical references and index.
   ISBN 0-306-44069-5 (hardbound). -- ISBN 0-306-44070-9 (paperbound)
   1. Cognitive therapy--Case studies.   I. Freeman, Arthur M.
II. Dattilio, Frank M.
   [DNLM: 1. Cognitive Therapy.   WM 425 C7365]
   RC489.C63C658 1992
   616.89'14--dc20
   DNLM/DLC
   for Library of Congress   92-49299
                                                                     CIP

ISBN 0-306-44069-5 (hardbound)

ISBN 0-306-44070-9 (paperbound)

©1992 Plenum Press, New York
A Division of Plenum Publishing Corporation
233 Spring Street, New York, N.Y. 10013

Printed in the United States of America

Contributors

Aaron T. Beck
Center for Cognitive Therapy
Department of Psychiatry
University of Pennsylvania School of Medicine
Philadelphia, Pennsylvania 19104

Robert Becker
Psychological Services Group, Inc.
Fort Washington, Pennsylvania 19034

Robert J. Berchick
Center for Cognitive Therapy
Department of Psychiatry
University of Pennsylvania School of Medicine
Philadelphia, Pennsylvania 19104

Thomas D. Borkovec
The Stress and Anxiety Disorders Institute
Department of Psychology
Pennsylvania State University
University Park, Pennsylvania 16802

Donald A. Bux
Department of Mental Health Sciences
Hahnemann University
Philadelphia, Pennsylvania 19102

Ellen Costello
Butler Hospital
Providence, Rhode Island 02906

Constance V. Dancu
Department of Psychiatry
Center for the Treatment and Study of Anxiety
Medical College of Pennsylvania/EPPI
Philadelphia, Pennsylvania 19129

Frank M. Dattilio
Center for Cognitive Therapy
Department of Psychiatry
University of Pennsylvania School of Medicine
Philadelphia, Pennsylvania 19104

Mary Helen Davis
Department of Psychiatry and Behavioral Sciences
University of Louisville School of Medicine
Louisville, Kentucky 40292
and Norton Psychiatric Clinic
200 East Chestnut Street
Louisville, Kentucky 40232

Esther Deblinger
Center for Children's Support
University of Medicine and Dentistry of
    New Jersey
School of Osteopathic Medicine
Stratford, New Jersey 08084-1505

E. Thomas Dowd
Department of Educational Psychology
Kent State University
Kent, Ohio 44242-0001

Bruce N. Eimer
The Behavior Therapy Center
Jenkintown, Pennsylvania 19046

Norman Epstein
Department of Family and Community
    Development
University of Maryland
College Park, Maryland 20742

Catherine G. Fine
The Institute of Pennsylvania Hospital
Philadelphia, Pennsylvania 19139

Edna B. Foa
Department of Psychiatry
Center for the Treatment and Study of Anxiety
Medical College of Pennsylvania/EPPI
Philadelphia, Pennsylvania 19129

Arthur Freeman
Department of Psychiatry
Cooper Hospital/University Medical Center
and Robert Wood Johnson Medical School at Camden
Camden, New Jersey 08103

Michael B. Frisch
Department of Psychology
P.O. Box 97334
Baylor University
Waco, Texas 76798-7334

Dolores Gallagher-Thompson
Older Adult and Family Research and Resource Center
Division of Gerontology
Stanford University School of Medicine
 and Gerontology
Stanford, California 94305
and Geriatric Research, Education, and Clinical Center
 Veterans Affairs Medical Center
Palo Alto, California 94304

Frank E. Gantz
Psychology Service
Veterans Affairs Medical Center
Salisbury, North Carolina 28144

David Garner
Department of Psychiatry
Michigan State University
East Lansing, Michigan 48824-1316

Mark Gilson
Atlanta Center for Cognitive Therapy
1772 Century Boulevard
Atlanta, Georgia 30345

Wayne A. Gordon
Department of Rehabilitation Medicine
The Mount Sinai Medical Center
New York, New York 10029-6574

Ruth L. Greenberg
Center for Cognitive Therapy
Department of Psychiatry
University of Pennsylvania School of Medicine
Philadelphia, Pennsylvania 19104

Dennis Greenberger
Private Practice
1851 East First Street
Santa Ana, California 92705

Susan E. Grober
Section of Physical Medicine and Rehabilitation
Norwalk Hospital
Norwalk, Connecticut 06856

Mary R. Hibbard
Department of Rehabilitation Medicine
The Mount Sinai Medical Center
New York, New York 10029-6574

Andrea Karfgin
Dissociative Disorders Program
Sheppard Pratt Hospital
Towson, Maryland 21204

Kevin T. Kuehlwein
Center for Cognitive Therapy
Department of Psychiatry
University of Pennsylvania School of Medicine
Philadelphia, Pennsylvania 19104

Cory F. Newman
Center for Cognitive Therapy
Department of Psychiatry
University of Pennsylvania School of Medicine
Philadelphia, Pennsylvania 19104

Gullan Nordstrom
Ersboda Cognitive Treatment Center
Stävgränd 73
S-902 63 Umeå, Sweden

Carlo Perris
Department of Psychiatry
Umeå University Hospital
and WHO Collaboration Center for Research
and Training in Mental Health
Umeå University
S-901 85 Umeå, Sweden

Jacqueline B. Persons
Department of Psychiatry
University of California, San Francisco
San Francisco, California 94143

Mark A. Reinecke
Center for Cognitive Therapy
Department of Psychiatry
University of Chicago
Chicago, Illinois 60637

John L. Rodman
Department of Psychiatry
The Ramsey Clinic
St. Paul, Minnesota 55101-2595

David Roth
Inpatient and Outpatient Eating Disorders
    Program
Sheppard Pratt Hospital
Towson, Maryland 21204

Paul Salmon
Arts in Medicine Program
Departments of Psychology and Psychiatry
University of Louisville
Louisville, Kentucky 40292

G. Randolph Schrodt, Jr.
Department of Psychiatry and Behavioral
    Sciences
University of Louisville School of Medicine
Louisville, Kentucky 40292
and Norton Psychiatric Clinic
200 East Chestnut Street
Louisville, Kentucky 40232

Paula N. Stein
Department of Rehabilitation Medicine
The Mount Sinai Medical Center
New York, New York 10029-6574

Yona Teichman
Department of Psychology
Tel-Aviv University
Ramat-Aviv, Tel-Aviv 69978
Israel

Larry W. Thompson
Older Adult and Family Research and Resource Center
Division of Gerontology
Stanford University School of Medicine
    and Gerontology
Stanford, California 94304
and Geriatric Research, Education, and Clinical Center
    Veterans Affairs Medical Center
Palo Alto, California 94304

Louise Troeng
Ersboda Cognitive Treatment Center
Stävgränd 73
S-902 63 Umeå, Sweden

Ralph M. Turner
Adolescents and Families Treatment Research Center
Department of Psychiatry
Temple University School of Medicine
Philadelphia, Pennsylvania 19140

Adrian Wells
Department of Psychiatry
University of Oxford
Warneford Hospital
Oxford OX3 7JX, England

Janet L. Wolfe
Institute for Rational-Emotive Therapy
45 East 65th Street
New York, New York 10021

Fred D. Wright
Center for Cognitive Therapy
Department of Psychiatry
University of Pennsylvania School of Medicine
Philadelphia, Pennsylvania 19104

Jesse H. Wright
Department of Psychiatry and Behavioral Sciences
University of Louisville School of Medicine
Louisville, Kentucky 40292
and Norton Psychiatric Clinic
200 East Chestnut Street
Louisville, Kentucky 40232

M. Jane Yates
Atlanta Center for Cognitive Therapy
1772 Century Boulevard
Atlanta, Georgia 30345

Foreword

This is the golden age of cognitive therapy. Its popularity among society and the professional community is growing by leaps and bounds. What is it and what are its limits?

What is the fundamental nature of cognitive therapy? It is, to my way of thinking, simple but profound. To understand it, it is useful to think back to the history of behavior therapy, to the basic development made by Joseph Wolpe. In the 1950s, Wolpe astounded the therapeutic world and infuriated his colleagues by finding a simple cure for phobias. The psychoanalytic establishment held that phobias—irrational and intense fear of certain objects, such as cats—were just surface manifestations of deeper, underlying disorders. The psychoanalysts said their source was the buried fear in male children of castration by the father in retaliation for the son's lust for his mother. For females, this fear is directed toward the opposite sex parent. The biomedical theorists, on the other hand, claimed that some as yet undiscovered disorder in brain chemistry must be the underlying problem. Both groups insisted that to treat only the patient's fear of cats would do no more good than it would to put rouge over measles.

Wolpe, however, reasoned that irrational fear of something isn't just a symptom of a phobia; it is the whole phobia. If the fear could be removed (and it could, through various Pavlovian extinction procedures), it would extinguish the phobia. If you could get rid of your fear of cats, the problem would be solved.

In the 1960s, Tim Beck and Albert Ellis drew exactly the same conclusions about depression that Wolpe had drawn about phobias. Depression is nothing more than one of the key symptoms of key symptoms; it is caused by conscious negative thoughts. There is less to depression than meets the eye. There is no deep, underlying disorder to be rooted out: not unresolved childhood conflicts, not unconscious anger, and not even faulty brain chemistry. Emotion comes directly from what we think: Think "I am in danger" and you feel anxiety. Think "I am being trespassed against" and you feel anger. Think "loss" and you feel sadness. Depression results from lifelong habits of conscious thought. If we change these habits of thought, we will cure depression. Let us make a direct assault on conscious thought, Beck and Ellis reasoned, using everything we know to change the way our patients think about bad events. Out of this came the new approach, which Beck called "cognitive therapy." It changes the way the depressed patient consciously thinks about failure, defeat, loss, and helplessness. The National Institute of Mental Health has spent millions of dollars testing whether the therapy works on depression. It does.

What is the domain of cognitive therapy? This illuminating casebook begins to answer this question. It is written in the spirit of an expanding, imperialistic new therapy. Cognitive therapy is applied to an excitingly broad range of clinical problems: post-traumatic stress disorder, bulimia, childhood depression, obesity, cocaine abuse, schizotypy (even schizophrenia and multiple personality), and chronic pain. From this work, we as therapists will begin to determine the limits of cognitive therapy. What does it work on and, more important, what doesn't it work on? This is the adventure that awaits the reader of this important casebook.

Martin E. P. Seligman

Department of Psychology
University of Pennsylvania
Philadelphia, Pennsylvania

Preface

In the past dozen years, a number of books have been published that have attempted to define and describe the historical, empirical, and philosophical underpinnings of the cognitive therapy model of psychotherapy. Other volumes have addressed the technical and clinical aspects of the model and described how to do cognitive therapy. Far fewer volumes have been made available that offer the clinician the types of step-by-step treatment procedures offered in a casebook.

We have found in our educational work—whether in structured university classroom settings, short-term workshops, or longer-term training programs—that by far the best educational experience is a product of our ability to communicate to participants the assessment, conceptual framework, strategic focus, and technical details of how therapy is conducted. Rather than simply discussing what needs to be accomplished in therapy, we have found that a clinical case approach that involves either direct demonstration by instructors or direct supervision of the participants is the most effective manner for teaching the process of therapy.

It is for this reason that we decided to compile this casebook as an adjunct in our educational work and to complement Plenum's successful *Comprehensive Handbook of Cognitive Therapy* (1989). When we first discussed the idea, we envisioned a volume of 12 to 15 cases. But as we developed a list of the types of cases we thought would be important to include in a clinical casebook, we found that the list kept growing and growing. Some of the chapters were invited by us. Others were the result of an author's learning of our project from a colleague and calling to offer his or her ideas and work. Still others were the result of our serendipitously discovering a particular work and inviting the author to join the project. The present volume of 37 chapters is the result of those efforts.

Despite the length of the volume and the number of cases presented, we recognize that there are still gaps within the text. There are clinical syndromes we have not addressed and clinical populations we have not included. This is due to several factors. First, we had to select disorders that were representative of types of particular conditions, inasmuch as we could not present a treatment protocol for every DSM-III-R disorder. We therefore have chosen to present the case discussions for certain anxiety or depression cases, but not all. Second, we have tried to present representative treatment models out of all the variants on the theme. Recognizing that there may be several styles or types of therapy for a particular disorder, we had to choose one style that would help the reader see how a cognitive-behavioral approach to therapy is conducted, including the assessment, conceptualization, and implementation of treatment. For this reason we did not choose a "standard" or parochial theoretical position; rather, we have tried to include representative therapists from a broad range of cognitive-behavioral practice. Some of the authors present their cases from a more cognitive and others a more behavioral perspective. Third, there is a limit to how much can be included in one volume without the volume becoming too heavy to carry, too expensive to purchase, and too unwieldy to use. Fourth, the press of work and other commitments kept several potential contributors from meeting the deadline that had to be met to allow the volume to come to a close and go to press. For what we have omitted or neglected, we apologize. We are, however, very pleased with the final product as comprehensive and representative of how to do cognitive therapy.

Because of the potential unevenness that is inherent in any edited volume, we have asked our contributors to follow a standard outline. Each chapter starts with a brief introduction, an overview of the problem to be discussed, and a brief review of the literature. We specifically asked the authors not to use their limited space to offer the reader extensive reviews of the literature. These reviews are available by scanning the authors' reference lists and recommended readings.

The authors then address issues of assessment and problem definition. The patient is then introduced and the details of the therapy presented, along with a conceptualization of the problem, the treatment approach, and the goals of therapy. The authors were asked to present and illustrate how the therapy was performed through the use of verbatim transcripts of one or more sessions. Finally, a discussion of the session(s) and the overall course of therapy is offered to serve to integrate theory and practice. We edited the manuscripts to keep the chapters of approximately the same length; the reader will notice some disparity in length, though not in quality or content.

The casebook is divided into three main parts. Part I offers an introduction to the volume. Part II is the "meat" of the volume, representing the main discussions of clinical interventions. We have attempted to group similar cases together to allow the reader to compare and contrast the similarities and differences in treatments. Part III includes several more extensive case studies. Our goal in including these extensive cases—along with the relatively briefer case reports in Part II—is to give a flavor of the therapy work in even greater detail. In all instances, the authors were asked to disguise the identity of the patients sufficiently to maintain the necessary confidentiality. In some cases where there might have been any hint of identifying data, we took the editorial prerogative and disguised the patient's identity further.

A book of this kind cannot exist without the cooperation and collaboration of many people. The first person we must thank is Eliot Werner, Medical and Social Sciences Editor at Plenum. Eliot is, without a doubt, one of the best psychology editors in the business. Aaron T. Beck has provided training, moral support, and encouragement to both of us over the years. Our contributors have offered the reader the product of their extensive experience and clinical skill. Because of their ability to translate what they do into their case reports, we have the rare opportunity to "listen in" as master therapists work.

The burden of the secretarial work has fallen on the shoulders of Lisa Golba (F.M.D.) and Donna Battista (A.F.); they have helped to make this volume a reality. Maryann Dattilio and Karen M. Simon have been supportive of our work; they have put up with our long, late phone calls and the weekend consultations necessary to coordinate the work of this volume. Martin E. P. Seligman, colleague and friend, agreed to write the foreword to this volume, and we are most grateful for his support. A special thank you is due to Thomas A. Seay for his early support and training in case conceptualization (F.M.D.). Finally, we dedicate this book to you, the reader. We hope that you will profit from our work and be better able to help those patients with whom you work.

Contents

III. EXTENDED CASE STUDIES

IV. EPILOGUE

I

Introduction

1

Introduction to Cognitive Therapy

Frank M. Dattilio and Arthur Freeman

Cognitive therapy has had a tremendous impact on the mental health field within the past decade as a result of its demonstrated effectiveness in understanding and treating the broad ranges of emotional and behavioral disorders (DeRubeis, Hollon, Evans, & Bemis, 1982; Dobson, in press; Epstein, 1982; Foreyt & Rathjen, 1979; Freeman, Simon, Beutler, & Arkowitz, 1989; Hollon & Beck, 1986; Holroyd & Andrasik, 1982; Jacobson, 1984), including medical disorders (Freeman & Greenwood, 1987; Hibbert, Gordon, Egelko, & Langer, 1986; Horan, Hackett, Buchanan, Stone, & Demchik-Stone, 1977; Kendall & Hollon, 1979; Weisman & Worden, 1979), the control of obesity and eating disorders (Clark & Bemis, 1982; Dunkel & Garlos, 1978), and group therapy for depression (Yost, Beutler, Corbishley, & Allender, 1986). Most recently, cognitive therapy has been applied to resolving marital discord (Beck, 1988; Dattilio, 1989; Dattilio and Padesky, 1990; Epstein, 1982; Margolis & Weiss, 1978); family problems (Epstein, Schlesinger, & Dryden, 1988; Dattillio, in press); and personality disorders (Beck, Free-

man, & Associates, 1990; Young, 1990). The literature had indicated that recent surveys document cognitive therapy as also being one of the most influential modalities among mental health practitioners today (Ritter, 1985).

The purpose of this chapter is to provide practitioners with a broad overview of cognitive therapy theory and procedures. Cognitive therapy is a "system of psychotherapy based on a theory which maintains that how an individual structures his or her experiences largely determines how he or she feels and behaves" (Beck & Weishaar, 1986). Psychopathology, from this perspective, is viewed as an exaggeration of normal adaptive responses. For example, anxiety is a normal survival reaction to threat; however, anxiety disorders, such as panic, are considered to be excessive dysfunctional reactions to misperceived threats.

Cognitive therapy differs from traditional modes of psychotherapy. "It is a collaborative process of empirical investigation, reality testing, and problem solving between the therapist and patient" (Beck & Weishaar, 1986, p. 43) and can clearly be differentiated as a system of psychotherapy as opposed to simply a cluster of techniques. It provides a format for understanding the psychological disorders that it proposes to treat, as well as a clear blueprint of the general principles and specific procedures of treatment (Beck, 1976, p. 15).

The theoretical underpinnings of cognitive therapy have been developed and shaped by a variety of approaches, including the phenomenological approach, structural theory, and cognitive psychology. The phenomenological approach contends that the individual's views

Frank M. Dattilio • Center for Cognitive Therapy, Department of Psychiatry, University of Pennsylvania School of Medicine, Philadelphia, Pennsylvania 19104.   Arthur Freeman • Department of Psychiatry, Cooper Hospital/University Medical Center and Robert Wood Johnson Medical School at Camden, Camden, New Jersey 08103.

Comprehensive Casebook of Cognitive Therapy, edited by Arthur Freeman and Frank M. Dattilio. Plenum Press, New York, 1992.

of the self and the personal world are central to the determination of behavior (Adler, 1936; Horney, 1950). Structural theory, on the other hand, promotes the concept of hierarchical structuring of cognitive processes, with an emphasis on the division into primary and secondary process thinking. Integrating aspects of both theories, cognitive psychology stresses the importance of cognition in information processing and behavioral change. As a result then, cognitive therapy combines features of the more traditional systems of therapy within its own conceptual framework.

Cognitive therapy began in the early 1960s as a result of Beck's (1963, 1964, 1967) research on depression, evolving from his earlier attempts to validate Freud's theory of depression as the result of anger turned toward the self. In his attempt to substantiate this theory, Beck made clinical observations of depressed patients and investigated their treatment under traditional psychoanalysis. Rather than finding retroflected anger in the content of their thoughts and dreams, he observed a negative bias in the cognitive processing of depressed individuals. As a result of much clinical observation and experimental testing, he developed the cognitive theory of emotional disorders and, in particular, the cognitive model of depression (Beck, 1976).

Contemporary cognitive therapy also grew out of the work of a number of earlier writers. George Kelly (1955) developed a model of personal constructs and beliefs in behavioral change. Kelly viewed a construct as an individual's way of construing or interpreting the world; he was interested in observing how the individual places structure and meaning on these constructs. Cognitive theories of emotion, such as those developed by Magda Arnold (1960) and Richard Lazarus (1966) proposed that cognition had a primary role in emotional and behavioral change.

The work of Albert Ellis (1962) in rational-emotive therapy (RET) has also provided support to the principles of cognitive therapy and impetus to the development of what is now known as cognitive-behavior therapy. The theories of rational-emotive therapy and cognitive therapy both contend that individuals consciously adopt reasoning patterns and possess control over their thoughts and actions. Both approaches view the individuals' underlying assumptions, which generate these thoughts, as targets of interventions in therapy. The cognitive therapist works to obtain the *specific content* of the patients' cognitions and/or beliefs. Patients are taught to obtain and report in detail their dysfunctional cognitions, including when they occur and their impact on the patients' feelings.

According to Ellis (1973, 1980), RET therapists would work to persuade the individuals that the beliefs they have are irrational, offering to teach them a more adaptive philosophy of living. Beck, on the other hand, attempts to collaborate with the clients in testing the validity of their cognitions (Beck, Kovacs, & Weissman, 1979).

A number of contemporary behaviorists have also made an indelible impact on the growth and development of cognitive therapy. The social learning theory of Albert Bandura (1977), which involves the conceptualization of new behavior patterns (observational learning), has contributed to the cognitive model and serves as a guide for action in participant modeling. This theory formed the basis for the shift in behavior therapy to the cognitive domain. Mahoney's (1974) early work on cognitive control of behavior and Meichenbaum's (1977) on cognitive behavior modification made important theoretical contributions.

Cognitive therapy gained recognition initially as a mode of treatment for depression (Beck, 1970, 1976). Research has provided empirical support for the model and its effectiveness in cases of unipolar depression (Beck & Rush, 1978). Studies comparing cognitive therapy and antidepressant medications have also been conducted (Beck, 1986; Hollon, et al., 1985; Murphy, Simmons, Wetzel, & Lustman, 1984). In several outcome comparisons, cognitive therapy was shown to be equal in effectiveness to antidepressant medication in treating depression. Still more impressively, the double blind study of Rush, Beck, Kovacs, and Hollon (1977) demonstrated that cognitive psychotherapy was more effective than medication in the alleviation of depression. The research of Kovacs, Rush, Beck, and Hollon (1981) suggested that cognitive therapy tends to produce longer-lasting effects, and other studies have supported this finding (Blackburn, Bishop, Glen, Whalley, & Christie, 1981; Murphy, Simmons, Wetzel, & Lustman, 1984).

As an offshoot to the work on depression, the development of theoretical concepts of treatment for suicidal clients has gained attention (Beck, Weissman, Lester, & Trexler, 1974). A major finding of that work was that hopelessness was a key component of suicidal intent and outcome. Resulting from his work on suicide, Beck generated a number of assessment scales for depression and suicidality, such as the Beck Depression Inventory (Beck, Ward, Mendelson, Mock, & Erbaugh, 1961), the Scale for Suicide Ideation (Beck, Kovacs, & Weissman, 1979), the Suicide Intent Scale (Beck, Schuyler, & Herman, 1974), the Hopelessness Scale (Beck, Weissman, et al., 1974), and the Beck Anxiety Inventory (Beck, Epstein, Brown, & Steer, 1985).

Cognitive therapy has also devoted research to the study of anxiety disorders (Alford, Beck, Freeman, & Wright, 1990; Beck & Emery, 1979; Beck, Emery, & Greenberg, 1985; Beck, Laude, & Bohnert, 1974; Dattilio, 1986, 1987, 1988, 1990 in press; Ottaviani & Beck,

1987; Sokol, Beck, Greenberg, Wright, & Berchick, 1989), as well as marital discord (Baucom & Epstein, 1990; Beck, 1988; Dattilio, 1989, 1990b, 1992; Dattilio & Padesky, 1990; Epstein, 1986; Schlesinger & Epstein, 1986), and personality disorders (Beck, Freeman, & Associates, 1990; Pretzer, 1983; Young, 1990).

THEORY OF PERSONALITY

Cognitive therapy views personality as being shaped by central values (or core beliefs) that develop early in life as a result of factors in one's environment. These schemas constitute the basis for coding, categorizing, and evaluating experiences and stimuli that an individual encounters in his or her world.

Psychological problems are perceived as stemming from commonplace processes such as faulty learning, making incorrect inferences on the basis of inadequate or incorrect information, and not distinguishing adequately between imagination and reality (Kovacs & Beck, 1979). Individuals often formulate rules or standards that are excessively rigid and absolutist, based on erroneous assumptions. Such standards are derived from what Beck terms *schemas*, or complex patterns of thoughts that determine how experiences will be perceived and conceptualized. These schemas or thought patterns are usually employed even in the absence of environmental data and may serve as a type of transformation mechanism that shapes the incoming data so as to fit and reinforce preconceived notions (Beck & Emery, 1979). This distortion of experience is maintained through the operation of characteristic errors in information processing. It has also been proposed that several types of fallacious thinking contribute to the feedback loops that support psychological disorders; for example, systematic errors in reasoning, which are termed *cognitive distortions*, are present during psychological distress and include the following:

- *Arbitrary inferences*—Conclusions that are made in absence of supporting substantiating evidence (e.g., the working executive who after a busy day in the office concludes, "I'm a lazy employee"
- *Selective abstraction*—Conceptualizing a situation on the basis of a detail taken out of context, ignoring other information (e.g., a man who becomes jealous upon seeing his fiance tilt her head toward another man in a conversation in order to hear him better during a noisy outing)
- *Overgeneralization*—Allowing an isolated incident or two to serve as a representation of similar situations everywhere, related or unrelated (e.g.,

after a skeptical meeting an author concludes, "All editors are alike; I'll always be rejected"
- *Magnification and minimization*—Perceiving a case or situation in a greater or lesser light than it truly deserves (e.g., a professor worries, "If I appear the slightest bit disorganized while lecturing, my class will think I am inept"; or, less significant, "I did okay with my lecture this time, but I was lucky; next time may not be so good")
- *Personalization*—Attributing external events to oneself when insufficient evidence exists to render a conclusion (e.g., a woman says hello to a neighbor and, failing to receive a return greeting, assumes, "I must have done something to anger her")
- *Labeling and mislabeling*—Portraying one's identity on the basis of imperfections and mistakes made in the past and allowing these to define one's true self (e.g., subsequent to making a mistake an individual states, "I am worthless," as opposed to recognizing his errors as being human)
- *Dichotomous thinking*—Codifying experiences as being black or white; for example, as a complete success or total failure (a researcher presenting a paper states, "Unless I render one of the best presentations my colleagues have ever seen, I am a failure as a scientist")

COGNITIVE MODELS FOR DEPRESSION AND ANXIETY

In the cognitive model of depression, Beck (1967) emphasizes the *cognitive triad* to characterize depression. Depressed individuals maintain a negative view of themselves, the world and experiences, and the future. They perceive themselves as inadequate, deserted, and worthless. Their negative view of the world is apparent in their beliefs that they have been burdened with enormous demands and impenetrable barriers that exist between them and their goals. The world appears devoid of pleasure or gratification and the future is viewed pessimistically, reflecting the belief that their current problems will only become worse.

As a reality-based intervention, cognitive therapy accepts the life situation of individuals and focuses on altering only the biased views of themselves, their situations, and the impoverished resources that limit their response repertoires and prevent them from generating solutions. Cognitive therapy is therefore an active, structured, and usually time-limited approach to the treatment of depression. It teaches clients to take a number of steps in combating depression, including: monitoring negative automatic thoughts; recognizing connections among cognition, affect, and behavior; critically examining their underlying thoughts; substituting more objective interpretations for negative cognitions; and learning to identify and alter the higher-order dysfunctional beliefs that predispose individuals to distortions in interpreting experience (Beck & Rush, 1978).

The collaborative empiricism that occurs between client and therapist is what ties these strategies together in a system that consists of identification of the problem, design and execution of tests of specific hypotheses, and reanalysis of certain beliefs. With mild to moderate depression (scores of 15 to 22 on the Beck Depression Inventory [BDI]), it is possible to begin immediately to examine the clients' misinterpretations and negative beliefs about themselves, their personal worlds, and the future.

In the most severe cases of depression (scores of 22 and higher on the BDI), it is often important to start out with behavioral assignments such as designing a daily activity schedule with the client to monitor day-to-day tasks (e.g., getting out of bed when not sleeping, tending to essential hygiene details, and attempting to be more active overall). Specific objectives may be agreed upon and worked into the graded task assignment, the rationale of which is to start with easily mastered assignments and then work up to the more difficult ones. Often, specific cognitions can be set up as hypotheses that the patient can then test as part of the graded task assignment.

Once the client is active, the more purely cognitive procedures may then be used, and the client can track his or her automatic thoughts, particularly when they precede or accompany a negative feeling. Clients are instructed to fill out a daily record of dysfunctional thoughts and are trained to give alternative or rational responses to their negative automatic thoughts. As the client progresses through treatment, more attention is focused on the his or her underlying assumptions. These assumptions are examined in the same manner as automatic thoughts, that is, by scrutinizing the evidence or the logic that upholds them and testing them empirically as a method for validation.

ANXIETY DISORDERS

Anxiety disorders are mainly the result of overactive survival strategies. When there is a cognitive appraisal of danger, the body prepares itself for fight, flight, freeze, or faint by activation of the autonomic nervous system. This is followed by such responses as rapid heartbeat to increase oxygen flow to the body, sweating to cool down the body, muscle tension to prepare for action, and so forth.

These sensations are considered normal when one is faced with an actual threat (e.g., someone holding a gun to one's head).

The anxious person experiences anxiety and has the accompanying psychological responses even when there is no objective threat. For example, the anxiety disorder client perceives certain innocuous situations as threatening. Once in such a dreaded situation, the individual dwells fearfully on the outcome and underestimates his or her own ability to perform. The images created are often strong enough to induce the physiological symptoms of anxiety. As the attacks of anxiety persist, the individual dreads the unpleasant symptoms as strongly as the precipitating cause. The experience of fear is linked not only to the actual situations but to images and symbols representing the past and the future (Beck & Emery, 1979; Beck, Emery, & Greenberg, 1985).

The anxiety symptoms often inhibit or interfere with the client's coping strategies. Once this inhibition occurs, the feedback mechanism that normally helps an individual cope breaks down. The anxious individual then distorts innocuous events, exaggerates the potential for harm, and experiences recurrent thoughts or images about being physically or psychologically injured. The assessment of his or her inability to cope may cause the individual to perceive the external situation as being more dangerous than it truly is (Dattilio, 1986). The result is a loop in which anxiety reinforces fear and, in turn, further anxiety.

When working with the anxious client, it is often important to delay the behavioral tasks until a certain amount of groundwork has been laid. Emphasis is placed on an understanding of the individual's cognitive set or schema. This allows the therapist to develop a comprehensive conceptualization of how clients view themselves and their anxiety. It is the manner in which these individuals interpret stressful or potentially stressful events that contributes to the feelings of anxiety. With respect to alleviating anxiety, the initial work involves aiding clients in reducing the amount of catastrophizing that they engage in regarding negative outcomes (Beck & Emery, 1979; Dattilio, 1990). Additional coping techniques are also taught in order to improve the chance of a positive outcome and to deal with any negative outcome that might occur.

THE PRACTICE OF COGNITIVE THERAPY

As with most other modalities of therapy, one of the initial goals of treatment is to develop rapport with the client. This is particularly important in light of the fact that cognitive therapy involves a collaboration between client and therapist that is essential in the change process.

Providing a rational and effective structure is also a key issue in therapy for both the course of treatment and the individual therapy session itself. This assures continuity and focus on the issues at hand and also makes the best use of time and effort. Once a structure has been established, the collaborative process is first employed to aid the therapist and client in developing a list of specific problems to address in therapy.

Once this has been established, the therapist may begin to narrow the focus in therapy and, in collaboration with the client, to develop an agenda for the proceeding sessions. Often this involves a review of the past week's events. In addition, prior homework assignments are discussed, along with any difficulty experienced while completing them. It is understood that some flexibility will be maintained in the structure of the sessions should the client wish to focus on a more immediate or urgent problem. The specific interventions or strategies will be contingent on the skill level of the client, as well as the nature of the presenting problem.

The last stage of the session is devoted to collaborative assessment and evaluation of homework from the previous session. Any homework assignment for the subsequent session are discussed at this time as well. This period is also set aside for receiving feedback from the client in evaluation of what he or she has learned from the current session. As a result of this format, a gradual yet structured termination occurs that also sets the stage for the succeeding session.

TREATMENT STRATEGIES

There are a number of strategies within the armamentarium of cognitive therapy that were designed specifically to aid clients in testing the reality of their cognitions. These strategies can be classified as either cognitive or behavioral in approach, but some overlap may occur. The following are adapted from Freeman and Greenwood (1987).

Cognitive Techniques

Downward Arrow

This term, first coined by Beck et al. (1979), is phrased because of its actual use of downward-pointing arrows to aid clients in understanding the logic and sequencing of their reasoning. The therapist follows a client's statement by asking, "If so, then what?" This elicits a sequence of thoughts and beliefs, which aids in uncovering the client's underlying assumptions.

Idiosyncratic Meaning

This is the process or clarifying a term of statement made by the client so that the therapist may have a high level of understanding of the client's perceived reality.

Labeling of Distortions

By labeling distortions, clients are able to identify automatically any dysfunctional thoughts and monitor their cognitive patterns. Through this type of monitoring a more accurate route toward change occurs. For a more detailed description, see Burns (1980) and (1989).

Questioning the Evidence

Once the client learns to question the actual evidence, the process of substantiation is initiated and becomes an automatic procedure following any irrational thought statement. This allows clients to decide whether their statements are based on erroneous information.

Examining Options and Alternatives

This entails going back over all of the possible options and alternatives that exist in attempts to avoid the trap of seeing "no way out" of a circumstance or situation. The specific task is to work until the individual is generating new options.

Reattribution

Placing all of the blame on oneself is a common occurrence seen with patients, particularly in the guilt-ridden or depressed cases. Reattribution merely involves the individual appropriately distributing responsibility to the rightful parties and dispelling the notion that any single individual is responsible for everything.

Decatastrophizing

Those who engage in catastrophic thinking are individuals who choose to focus on the most extreme negative outcome of any given situation. Decatastrophizing involves aiding in balancing out their focus on the worst anticipated state by reestimating the situation and asking, "So what's the worst thing that might occur? And if so, would this be so horrible?"

Advantages and Disadvantages

In attempts to have patients sway away from dichotomous thought patterns, instructing them to list advantages and disadvantages of a situation allows them to change their perspective and balance out the alternatives.

Paradox or Exaggeration

This technique may be viewed as the inverse of decatastrophizing. It involves the therapist taking an issue or idea to the extreme for the patient, allowing the latter to view the absurdity of an overinflated viewpoint. This often aids the patient in developing a more balanced perspective on the issue.

Turning Adversity to Advantage

Taking an unfortunate situation and using it as an advantage can be very helpful. For example, being rejected by the school of your choice may be an indirect route toward a more promising alternative.

Replacement Imagery

Freeman (1986) describes a more detailed account of how this is used. In essence, the fact that many individuals experience negative dreams and images does indicate that the power of imagery is strong. Patients can therefore be helped to change the direction of these dreams and images to positive, more successful coping scenes.

Cognitive Rehearsal

Many of the target behaviors for change rely on the strength of visualizing in the mind the desired outcome. The use of cognitive rehearsal may aid individuals in practicing assertiveness, overcoming the awkwardness in confronting others, and so forth.

Behavioral Techniques

While the mechanics involved with cognitive therapy involve the primary use of cognitive techniques such as those stated above, behavioral techniques are also used as supportive measures and as means for collecting information in facilitating change. The following behavioral techniques are the ones most frequently used in cognitive therapy.

Assertiveness Training

A large component of assertiveness training involves both cognitive processes and behavioral practice. The latter, in essence, consists of the therapist teaching or modeling for the patient desired behaviors in social situa-

tions. This is used particularly often for anxiety disorders such as social phobias or agoraphobia. The term *in vivo* is used to indicate that the behaviors are acted out in real life.

Behavioral Rehearsal

This is the behavioral counterpart to cognitive rehearsal. The difference lies with the actual behaviors themselves being the subjects rehearsed (e.g., asserting oneself in public, or getting up and going to work). Feedback from the therapist to the patient is then given as a means of guidance and development of effective responses and styles. This also involves the reinforcing of existing skills.

Graded Task Assignments

This is the process of establishing a hierarchy of events that involve the target behaviors, whether approaching a parent or overcoming a fear of meeting new people. The specific tasks are arranged in steps from least anxiety producing or threatening to most anxiety producing. This allows for a gradual approach to facing the threatening object/event.

Bibliotherapy

The prescription of reading assignments has always been a strong characteristic of cognitive therapy. Readings frequently assigned to patients are books designed for the general public such as *Love is Never Enough* (Beck, 1988), *Feeling Good* or the *Feeling Good Handbook* (Burns, 1980, 1989), *Cognitive Therapy and the Emotional Disorders* (Beck, 1976), *Own Your Own Life* (Emery, 1984), *Talk Sense to Yourself* (McMullin & Casey, 1975), and *Woulda, Coulda, Shoulda* (Freeman & DeWolf, 1990). These readings are assigned as an adjunct to therapy and are primarily to serve as a supportive and educational tool to the actual therapeutic process.

Relaxation and Meditation

The use of programs including relaxation, meditation, and focused breathing has proven to be helpful to anxiety patients in learning to distract themselves and gain control over their anxiety.

Overbreathing and the encouragement of hyperventilation is an effective technique for helping patients learn that they can master breathing control and regulate symptoms.

Social Skills Training

This involves reviewing and instructing the patient in behaviors that are necessary to social interaction (e.g., maintaining conversations with others, posture, eye contact, and assertiveness skills; in addition, developing techniques for self-expression and conveying individual thoughts and opinions).

Shame-Attacking Exercises

An exercise promoted most by RET therapists involves having the patient engage in activities that emphasize their concern for what others may think of them. A typical example might be to have the patient announce out loud each stop that a public bus makes while it is en route and carrying a full load of passengers. The point is to aid the patient in seeing how people really react and that their thoughts really do not matter.

Homework

One of the most important features of cognitive therapy is the use of homework assignments. Because the actual therapy sessions are limited to only one or two hours per week in the office, it is imperative that activities in support of the treatment continue outside of the sessions. The emphasis is placed on self-help assignments that serve as a continuation of what was addressed in the preceding session. This is also an integral part of the collaborative process between the patient and the therapist. Assignments typically include those techniques listed above. The assignments are tailored according to the specific problem and are a result of the collaborative process that occurs during treatment.

DISCUSSION

Because it is a relative newcomer to the field of psychotherapy models, cognitive therapy has been subject to misunderstanding and misinterpretation concerning its principles and practice. In an introductory chapter, Freeman (Freeman & Greenwood, 1987) discusses several popular myths of cognitive therapy. In summary, cognitive therapy is not simplistic, nor is it just the power of positive thinking. It does not promote a Band-Aid or surface model approach to psychotherapy that avoids working on the deep problems or getting to the core issues. The focus is not so much on what was but rather on what is and what maintains or reinforces dysfunctional behavior.

Although cognitive therapy is a time-limited approach, the cognitive therapist would not generally set a specific limit on the number of sessions that a patient may have for treatment. Research studies (Blackburn, Bishop, Glen, Wholley, & Christie, 1981; Murphy, Simmons, Wetzel, & Lustman, 1984; Rush, Kovacs, Beck, & Hollon, 1977) have clearly demonstrated that there is a major amelioration of symptoms by the end of 12 to 20 sessions over 16 weeks. Unless the patient is participating in an outcome study, the amount of time that the patient spends in therapy is dependent on the nature of the problems being confronted, the level of motivation, that patient's availability for sessions, and the number of presenting life issues.

Although cognitive therapy has been found to be as effective as pharmacotherapy in the treatment of unipolar depression (Murphy, Simmons, Wetzel, & Lustman, 1984), medication is nonetheless recommended as an adjunct with certain patients, for example, bipolar depressives, psychotics, and those patients whose depression has made them vegetative and unable to respond fully to cognitive therapy.

For an optimum outcome, the therapist must be mindful of the importance of a number of nonspecific factors over and above the techniques employed, including the therapists's abilities to establish and maintain a working relationship, to demonstrate empathy and caring, to engage in active listening, and the like. The reality of the patient's having a specific response to the individual therapist cannot be denied, and the cognitive therapist must deal with these reactions directly by having the patient examine the cognitions that are generating the response.

The model's usefulness in conceptualizing patient problems within the cognitive-behavioral framework and generating additional strategies as needed is an essential benefit of the cognitive approach. Particular emphasis is placed on developing a detailed case conceptualization in order to understand clearly how the client views his or her world (Persons, 1989).

In summary, cognitive therapy is effective in treating a broad range of disorders commonly encountered in the mental health field. This chapter is intended to offer a review of the fundamental theory and techniques of cognitive therapy in order to utilize fully the cases that follow.

REFERENCES

Adler, A. (1936). The neurotic's picture of the world. *International Journal of Individual Psychology*, 2, 3–10.

Alford, B., Beck, A. T., Freeman, A., & Wright, F. (1990). Brief focused cognitive therapy of panic disorder. *Psychotherapy*, 27(2), 230–234.

Arnold, M. (1960). *Emotions and personality* (Vol. 1). New York: Columbia University Press.

Bandura, A. (1977). *Social learning theory.* Englewood Cliffs, NJ: Prentice-Hall.

Baucom, D., and Epstein, N. (1990). *Cognitive–behavioral marital therapy.* New York: Brunner/Mazel.

Beck, A. T. (1963). Thinking and depression: 1. Idiosyncratic content and cognitive distortions. *Archives of General Psychiatry, 9,* 324–333.

Beck, A. T. (1964). Thinking and depression: 2. Theory and therapy. *Archives of General Psychiatry, 10,* 561–571.

Beck, A. T. (1967). *Depression: Clinical, experimental, and theoretical aspects.* New York: Hoeber. (Republished as *Depression: Causes and treatment.* Philadelphia: University of Pennsylvania Press, 1972)

Beck, A. T. (1970). Cognitive therapy: Nature and relation to behavior therapy. *Behavior Therapy, 1,* 184–200.

Beck, A. T. (1976). *Cognitive therapy and the emotional disorders.* New York: International Universities Press.

Beck, A. T. (1986, June 28). Treating depression: Can we talk? [Letter to the editor.] *Science News, 129*(6), 12.

Beck, A. T. (1988). *Love is never enough.* New York: Harper and Row.

Beck, A. T., & Emery, G. (1979). *Cognitive therapy of anxiety and phobic disorders.* Philadelphia: Center for Cognitive Therapy.

Beck, A. T., Emery, G., & Greenberg, R. (1985). *Anxiety and phobias: A cognitive approach.* New York: Basic Books.

Beck, A. T., Epstein, N., Brown, G., & Steer, R. A. (1985, November). *An inventory for measuring clinical anxiety.* Paper presented at the annual meeting of the Association for Advancement of Behavior Therapy, Houston, TX.

Beck, A. T., Freeman, A., and Associates (1990). *Cognitive therapy of personality disorders.* New York: Guilford.

Beck, A. T., Kovacs, M., & Weissman, A. (1979). Assessment of suicidal intention: The Scale for Suicidal Ideation. *Journal of Consulting and Clinical Psychology, 47,* 343–352.

Beck, A. T., Laude, R., & Bohnert, M. (1974). Ideational components of anxiety neurosis. *Archives of General Psychiatry, 31,* 319–325.

Beck, A. T., & Rush, A. J. (1978). Cognitive approaches to depression and suicide. In G. Serban (Ed.), *Cognitive defects in the development of mental illness* (pp. 235–257). New York: Brunner/Mazel (published under the auspices of the Kittay Scientific Foundation).

Beck, A. T., Schuyler, D., & Herman, I. (1974). Development of the suicidal intent scales. In A. T. Beck, H. L. P. Resnik, & D. J. Lettieri (Eds.), *The prediction of suicide* (pp. 45–56). Bowie, MD: Charles.

Beck, A. T., Ward, C. H., Mendelson, M., Mock, J. E., & Erbaugh, J. K. (1961). An inventory for measuring depression. *Archives of General Psychiatry, 4,* 561–571.

Beck, A. T., & Weishaar, M. E. (1986). *Cognitive therapy.* (Available from the Center for Cognitive Therapy, 133 South 36th Street, Philadelphia, PA 19104)

Beck, A. T., Weisman, A., Lester, D., & Trexler, L. (1974). The measurement of pessimism: The hopelessness scale. *Journal of Consulting and Clinical Psychology, 42,* 861–865.

Blackburn, I. M., Bishop, S., Glen, A. M., Whalley, L. J., & Christie, J. E. (1981). The efficacy of cognitive therapy in depression: A treatment trial using cognitive therapy and psy-

chotherapy, each alone and in combination. *British Journal of Psychiatry, 139,* 181–189.

Burns, D. (1980). *Feeling good: The new mood therapy.* New York: Signet.

Burns, D. (1989). *The feeling good handbook.* New York: William Morrow.

Clark, D. M., & Bemis, K. M. (1982). A cognitive-behavioral approach to anorexia nervosa. *Cognitive Therapy and Research, 6,* 123–150.

Dattilio, F. M. (1986). Differences in cognitive responses to fear among individuals diagnosed as panic disorder, generalized anxiety disorder, agoraphobia with panic attacks, and simple phobia. *University Microfilms International,* Pub. No. 8711320, p. 216.

Dattilio, F. M. (1987). The use of paradoxical intention in the treatment of panic attacks. *Journal of Counseling and Development, 66,* 102–103.

Dattilio, F. M. (1988). Relation of experiences in sex and panic: A preliminary note. *The Cognitive-Behaviorist, 10*(3), 3–4.

Dattilio, F. M. (1989). A guide to cognitive marital therapy. In P. A. Keller & S. R. Heyman (Eds.), *Innovations in clinical practice: A source book* (Vol. 8, pp. 27–42). Sarasota, FL: Professional Resource Exchange.

Dattilio, F. M. (1990a). Symptom induction and de-escalation in the treatment of panic attacks. *Journal of Mental Health Counseling, 12*(4), 515–519.

Dattilio, F. M. (1990b) Una guida Alla teràpia di coppia àd orientàsmento cognitivistà, *terapia familiare* 33 (Luglio) 17–34.

Dattilio, F. M., & Padesky, C. A. (1990). *Cognitive therapy with couples.* Sarasota, FL: Professional Resource Exchange.

Dattilio, F. M. (1992) Les thérapies cognitives de couple, *Journal De Thérapie Comportmentale et Cognitive,* May, Vol. 2(2), 17–25.

Dattilio, F. M. Cognitive Techniques with Couples and Families. *The Family Journal* (in press).

DeRubeis, R. J., Hollon, S. D., Evans, M. D., & Bemis, K. M. (1982). Can psychotherapies for depression be discriminated? A systematic investigation of cognitive therapy and interpersonal therapy. *Journal of Consulting and Clinical Psychology, 50,* 794–756.

Dobson, K. (in press). A meta-analysis of the efficacy of cognitive therapy for depression. *Journal of Consulting and Clinical Psychology.*

Dunkel, L. D., & Garlos, A. G. (1978). Comparison of self instructional and stimulus control treatments for obesity. *Cognitive Therapy and Research, 2,* 75–78.

Ellis, A. (1962). *Reason and emotion in psychotherapy.* New York: Lyle Stuart.

Ellis, A. (1973). Are cognitive behavior and rational therapy synonymous? *Rational Living, 8,* 8–11.

Ellis, A. (1980). Rational-emotive therapy and cognitive-behavior therapy: Similarities and differences. *Cognitive Therapy and Research, 4,* 325–340.

Emery, G. (1984). *Own your own life.* New York: Signet.

Epstein, N. (1982). Cognitive therapy with couples. *American Journal of Family Therapy, 10,* 5–16.

Epstein, N. (1986, Spring/Summer). Cognitive marital therapy. *Journal of Rational-Emotive Therapy, 4*(1), 68–81.

Epstein, N., Schlesinger, S. E., & Dryden, W. (1988). *Cognitive-behavior therapy with families.* New York: Brunner/Mazel.

Foreyt, J., & Rathjen, D. (Eds.). (1979). *Cognitive behavior therapy: Research and applications.* New York: Plenum.

Freeman, A. (1986). Understanding personal cultural and family schemata in psychotherapy. *Journal of Psychotherapy and the Family*, 2(3/4), 79–99.

Freeman, A., & Greenwood, V. (Eds.). (1987). *Cognitive therapy: Applications in psychiatric and medical settings.* New York: Human Sciences Press.

Freeman, A., Simon, K. A., Beutler, L. E., & Arkowitz, H. (Eds.). (1989). *Comprehensive handbook of cognitive therapy.* New York: Plenum.

Freeman, A., & DeWolf, R. (1990). *Woulda, coulda, shoulda.* New York: William Morrow.

Hibbert, M. R., Gordon, W. A., Egelko, S., & Langer, K. (1986). Issues in the diagnosis and cognitive therapy of depression in brain damaged individuals. In A. Freeman & V. Greenwood (Eds.), *Cognitive therapy: Applications in psychiatric and medical settings* (pp. 62–76). New York: Human Sciences Press.

Hollon, S. D., & Beck, A. T. (1986). Cognitive and cognitive-behavioral therapies. In S. L. Garfield & A. E. Bergin (Eds.), *Handbook of psychotherapy and behavior change* (3rd ed.). New York: Wiley.

Hollon, S. D., DeRubeis, R. J., Evans, M. D., Tauson, V. B., Weimer, M. J., & Garvey, M. J. (1985). *Combined cognitive-pharmacotherapy versus cognitive therapy alone in the treatment of depressed outpatients: Differential treatment outcomes in the CPT project.* Unpublished manuscript, University of Minnesota and St. Paul-Ramsey Medical Center, Minneapolis-St. Paul, MN.

Holroyd, K. A., & Andrasik, F. (1982). Do the effects of cognitive therapy endure? A two-year followup of tension headache sufferers treated with cognitive therapy or biofeedback. *Cognitive Therapy and Research*, 6, 325–334.

Horan, J. J., Hackett, G., Buchanan, J. D., Stone, C. I., & Demchik-Stone, D. (1977). Coping with pain: A component analysis of stress inoculation. *Cognitive Therapy and Research*, 1, 211–222.

Horney, K. (1950). *Neurosis and human growth: The struggle toward self-realization.* New York: Norton.

Jacobson, N. S. (1984). The modification of cognitive processes in behavioral marital therapy, integrating cognitive and behavioral intervention strategies. In K. Hahlweg & N. S. Jacobson (Eds.), *Marital interaction: Analysis and modification.* New York: Guilford.

Kelly, G. (1955). *The psychology of personal constructs.* New York: Norton.

Kendall, P. C., & Hollon, S. D. (Eds.). (1979). *Cognitive-behavioral interventions: Theory, research and procedures.* New York: Academic Press.

Kovacs, M., & Beck, A. T. (1979). Cognitive-affective processes in depression. In C. E. Izard (Ed.), *Emotions in personality and psychopathology* (pp. 417–442). New York: Plenum.

Kovacs, M., Rush, A. J., Beck, A. T., & Hollon, S. D. (1981).

Depressed outpatients treated with cognitive therapy or pharmacotherapy: A one-year followup. *Archives of General Psychiatry, 38,* 33–39.

Lazarus, R. (1966). *Psychological stress and the coping process.* New York: McGraw-Hill.

Mahoney, M. J. (1974). *Cognition and behavior modification.* Cambridge, MA: Ballinger.

Margolis, G., & Weiss, R. L. (1978). A comparative evaluation of therapeutic components associated with behavioral marital treatment. *Journal of Consulting and Clinical Psychology, 46,* 1476–1486.

McMullin, R. E., & Casey, B. (1975). *Talk sense to yourself: A guide to cognitive restructuring therapy.* New York: Counseling Research Press.

Meichenbaum, D. (1977). *Cognitive-behavior modification: An integrative approach.* New York: Plenum.

Murphy, G. E., Simmons, A. D., Wetzel, R. D., & Lustman, P. J. (1984). Cognitive therapy versus tricyclic antidepressants in major depression. *Archives of General Psychiatry, 41,* 33–41.

Ottaviani, R., & Beck, A. T. (1987). Cognitive aspects of panic disorder. *Journal of Anxiety Disorders, 1*(1), 15–28.

Persons, J. (1989). *Cognitive therapy in practice: A case formulation approach.* New York: Norton.

Pretzer, J. L. (1983, August). *Borderline personality disorder: Too complex for cognitive therapy?* Paper presented at the annual meeting of the American Psychological Association, Anaheim, CA.

Ritter, K. Y. (1985). The cognitive therapies: An overview for counselors. *Journal of Counseling and Development, 64,* 42–46.

Rush, A. J., Beck, A. T., Kovacs, M., & Hollon, S. D. (1977). Comparative efficacy of cognitive therapy and pharmacotherapy in the treatment of depressed outpatients. *Cognitive Therapy and Research, 1,* 17–37.

Schlesinger, S. E., & Epstein, N. B. (1986). Cognitive-behavioral techniques in marital therapy. In P. A. Keller and L. G. Ritt (Eds.), *Innovations in clinical practice: A source book* (Vol. 5, pp. 137–156). Sarasota, FL: Professional Resource Exchange.

Sokol, L., Beck, A. T., Greenberg, R. L., Wright, F., & Berchick, R. J. (1989). Cognitive therapy of panic disorder: A nonpharmacological alternative. *Journal of Nervous & Mental Disease, 177,* 711–716.

Weisman, A. D., & Worden, J. W. (1979). *Coping and vulnerability in cancer patients: A research report.* Boston: Massachusetts General Hospital.

Yost, E. B., Beutler, L. E., Corbishley, M. A., & Allender, J. R. (1986). *Group cognitive therapy: A treatment approach for older adults* [Psychology Practitioners Guidebook]. New York: Pergamon.

Young, J. E. (1990). *Cognitive therapy for personality disorders: A schema-focused approach.* Sarasota, FL: Professional Research Exchange.

2

The Development of Treatment Conceptualizations in Cognitive Therapy

Arthur Freeman

INTRODUCTION

As a young child, I recall watching my mother bake a cake. It appeared that she took a pinch of this, a handful of that, two eggs, and mixed it all together. When I asked her about her recipe, she told me that she had no written recipe, that the only recipe that she had was in her head. When I asked her how she knew how much of each ingredient to use, she shrugged, and replied, "After a while, you just know." When I asked her how and from whom she learned these recipes, she responded that she learned them from her mother by watching quietly, and not asking so many questions. Despite the apparent lack of a written recipe or formula, my mother's food always came out tasting just as good each time as it was the time before. How could that be, I wondered, if she had no written recipe? That mystery persists to this day. When I ask her

for the recipe for a favorite food, she replies, "I'll cook it for you. You just watch and see what I do." Watching her is easy. The process looks so astoundingly simple that I wonder why I couldn't do it myself. After watching and carefully writing down what I see, I go home and try the recipe. On some intermittent schedule, the recipe works. Yet, there is something missing, and I am not sure what it is.

As a supervisor of therapists, I have often had my supervisees observe my work with patients, either in vivo or on videotape. I have been told that I make therapy look easy. A question that supervisees often ask is, "How do you know what interventions have the greatest utility factor with a specific patient? How do you recognize the best time to use a particular strategy or specific intervention? How far do you press a particular strategy or intervention until you either revise it or abandon it? The simplest response would be to use the old cliche, "therapy is an art form, not a science." They just have to study the art and, if they are talented, they will one day magically "understand." I could also tell them what my mother told me. "Keep quiet and watch." Hopefully, if they use a pinch of this and a scoop of that, all based on having a "sense" of the patient's dynamics, a positive outcome will ensue. If, however, we believe that the therapuetic process needs to be more scientific, then we need to examine the

Arthur Freeman • Department of Psychiatry, Cooper Hospital/ University Medical Center and Robert Wood Johnson Medical School at Camden, Camden, New Jersey 08103.

Comprehensive Casebook of Cognitive Therapy, edited by Arthur Freeman and Frank M. Dattilio. Plenum Press, New York, 1992.

process, identify the elements that combine for successful therapy, and evaluate therapy outcome.

One way of operationalizing and understanding what to do with a patient in therapy can be understood in terms of the cooking metaphor described above. To be an effective and successful cook, my mother had to start with an idea of where she was going—that is, she had to have a cognitive representation of the end-product that she sought. She had to decide how much to make and when it needed to be ready. She then had to assess her skills and equipment and check for the availability of the ingredients. When she had everything in place, she could begin. In fact, if an ingredient was missing, she often would substitute another ingredient, without substantially changing the product. At other times, she made alterations with a specific, desired effect in mind. In the final evaluation, it is clear that my mother had a working conceptualization of her desired outcome in mind all along. That conceptualization included the desired taste, presentation, and appearance. By having an overall conceptualization of where she had to go, the ingredients available to her, the final goal, and the limits of time, she was able to bake cakes that are still memorable almost fifty years later.

As therapists, we need to have an effective conceptualization of our patient's problems. We need to develop an agreement with our patient about the goals and time-parameters of therapy, taking into account the patient's skills, our skills, the patient's response to previous therapies, and the extent of the pathology. With these in mind, we can begin to develop a conceptualization of the problem and of the therapeutic interventions that we might utilize with the greatest efficacy.

The highest-order clinical skill is the ability to develop treatment conceptualizations. We can identify five types of therapists (or styles of therapy) that transcend any particular theoretical background, training, and practice. They are the theoretician, the technician, the magician, the politician, and the clinician.

The *theoretician* is well grounded in the theory and research of therapy, but does not believe that one has to gain skills in therapy to do therapy. They operate on the assumption that if the theory is correct then the implementation is a mere technical maneuver that anyone of normal intelligence can effect. These individuals spend their time teaching about therapy, discoursing about therapy, theorizing about therapy, and researching therapy, but never doing therapy.

The *technician* is the therapist who acquires specific skills, regardless of the model. They can do therapy "by the book." That is, they do a little bit of this and a little bit of that. They go to conferences and attend numerous skills-workshops so that they can enhance their bag of technical tricks. They do Gestalt work, behavioral work,

analytic work, etc. These individuals often term what they do as "eclectic." What they lack, however, is a unifying theory of development, behavior, or therapy. They try to do what they believe works, without regard for its effectiveness, why it works—if it does, or how it might work better. They avoid philosophical or theoretical discussions as distracting and boring.

The *magician* doesn't need skills. They are charismatic, so that an hour a week in their aura is, by itself, therapeutic. Like the theoretician, they would not think of lowering themselves by learning mundane technique. They may label themselves "supportive" in their work. They often pride themselves on having avoided extensive therapeutic training, and focus on their ability to discuss esoteric therapeutic issues in obscure journals. In the view of the magician, the mental "laying on of hands" is enough to effect a therapeutic change. They believe that therapy will just happen by force of their ability to establish a positive relationship with the patient.

The *politician* practices what is most popular at the moment. Whether Primal Scream, EST, or cognitive-behavior therapy is used, the politician is on the cutting edge of popularity. They are presently waiting to see what will be next on the horizon.

The fifth type of therapist is the *clinician*, and is a combination of all of the above types. The clinician has a theoretical understanding of development and behavior, and what works within that framework in terms of therapeutic techniques, and is able to develop and maintain a strong working relationship with the patient. This type of therapist is far more likely to attend both theoretical meetings and skills sessions at a conference. These therapists are far more willing to combine modalities, e.g. behavioral marital therapy, and to try to develop models further in depth and scope. Safran and Segal (1990) sum it up quite well:

> "The assertion that therapy is fundamentally a human encounter does not mean that there is no theory for therapists to learn and no skills for them to acquire. It does mean, however, that the relevant theory must clarify the process through which this human encounter brings about change, and that the relevant skills must include the ability to use one's own humanity as a therapeutic instrument" (p. 5).

Therapy has been taught and practiced as a reactive experience, that is, the therapist responds to what the patient brings into the therapy or the specific session. The conceptual model demands that the therapeutic encounter be far more proactive. The proactive stance first involves a careful evaluation of the patient's problems based on the relevant historical data typically collected in a structured interview format. The therapist then develops hypotheses about why patients respond the way they do, what were probable formative elements in the style, what are the operative schema, and the best possible points of entry into the system. Many of these hypotheses will be shared with the patients to include their reaction, and redirection, in the process. The ability to develop conceptualizations and to transform them into therapeutic interventions can be viewed in a hierarchical manner (Freeman, Pretzer, Fleming, and Simon, 1990). At the lowest skill level, the therapist does not appear to have developed a conceptualization of the case. The session would appear to have a "shotgun" approach without a theme or focus. The session has no agenda or structure, and the direction is dictated by the patient's last statement. If the therapist has begun to develop a conceptualization, the interventions would have a greater focus and direction. At the highest level, there would be a clear treatment conceptualization that eventuates in a series of organized and focused treatment interventions.

The therapist uses the conceptual framework to elicit specific thoughts, assumptions, images, meanings, or beliefs. It assists the therapist to develop questions for the guided discovery process. Without the treatment conceptualization, the focus of the cognitive therapy work might be vague, or irrelevant, even when the basic tools of cognitive therapy, e.g. the dysfunctional thought record or the simpler double or triple column technique to collect thoughts are used. The development of conceptualization skills is the focus of this chapter.

The oversimplified ideas of cognitive therapy have thoughts and feelings in a direct linear relationship. According to this overly simple model, all emotional reactions are the result of a thought, or image, held by the individual. Simple mood induction techniques can easily demonstrate that 30 seconds of imaging a sad or depressing experience can significantly increase an individual's level of depression. It would follow then, that if the thoughts can be changed, the feelings will also change. In many cases this is what occurs clinically. Individuals can be helped to test their automatic thoughts, develop more adaptive responses, and experience a significant change in levels of depression or anxiety. These patients are the easiest to treat.

With many other patients, however, the relationship between thoughts and feelings is a far more complex one, requiring an exploration of thoughts, feelings, behavior, and the underlying schemas that generate and fuel the thoughts and actions. The misunderstandings of the cognitive model are many. Hammer (1990), a psychoanalyst writing on the therapeutic goal of dealing with affective issues in psychotherapy, states,

"Even the last bastion of the emphasis on the rational in interpretation, Albert Ellis' theory has moved toward the affect and signals this in its name change from Rational Therapy to Rational Emotive Therapy. Ellis, too, lately joins the view that illumination offered the patient, even if it is valid, is not nearly enough" (p. 19).

It is, unfortunately, Hammer who is late on the scene. The first discussion of the importance of emotion in therapy and hence the addition of the "E" to RET took place over 30 years ago (Ellis and Harper, 1961).

Crowley (1985), in discussing the work of Harry Stack Sullivan states, "Sullivan . . . was explicit in his view that affect, cognition, and conation . . . were inseparable" (p. 291–292). In seeking to alter a particular belief that has endured for a long period of time, it would be necessary to help the individual to deal with the belief from as many different perspectives as possible. A purely cognitive strategy would leave the behavioral and affective untouched. The purely affective strategy is similarly limited and, of course, the strict behavioral approach is limited by its disregard for cognitive-affective elements. To focus on any one area to the exclusion of the other two is to provide a therapeutic context that would allow, at best, partial change. It would seem far more reasonable to structure a therapeutic program that takes into account all three areas, and provides both opportunities and direction for change in these three areas.

Particular schemas may engender a great deal of emotion and be emotionally bound by both the individual's past experience and by the sheer weight of the time in which that belief has been held. In addition, the perceived importance and credibility of the source from whom the schemas were acquired must also be addressed. There is a cognitive element to the schemas which pervades the individual's thoughts and images. With the proper training, individuals can be helped to describe schemas in great detail or to deduce them from behavior, or automatic thoughts. Finally, there is a behavioral component which involves the way the belief system governs the individual's responses to a particular stimulus or set of stimuli. For some patients the sequence may be cognitive-affective-behavioral, for another patient the therapeutic sequence would be behavioral-cognitive-affective.

DEVELOPING A TREATMENT CONCEPTUALIZATION

The focus of cognitive therapy is on the automatic thoughts and behaviors, first. It is from the automatic thoughts and behavior that the therapist can begin to structure a conceptualization regarding a particular schema and the relevance of that schema to the patient's behavior. An understanding of the role of schemas in the therapeutic process is essential, whether for problems coded on Axis I or on Axis II (Beck, Freeman, et al., 1990;

Freeman, 1988; Freeman and Leaf, 1989; Freeman, et al., 1990).

Inasmuch as the schemas become, in effect, how one defines oneself, both individually, and as part of a group, they are important to understand and factor into the treatment conceptualization. They may be said to be unconscious, using a definition of the unconscious as "ideas we are unaware of," or "ideas that we are not aware of simply because they are not in the focus of attention but in the fringe of consciousness" (Campbell, 1989).

Inactive schemas are called into play to control behavior in times of stress. Stressors will evoke the inactive schemas, which become active and govern behavior. When the stressor is removed, the schemas will return to their previously dormant state. Conceptually, understanding the activity-inactivity continuum explains two related clinical phenomena. The first involves the rapid, though transient, positive changes often evidenced in therapy, the so-called transference cure or flight into health. The result of this phenomenon is that a patient with clinical symptoms seems to have a partial or full recovery in a surprisingly brief period of time, and will then seek to terminate therapy as no longer needed. What we are seeing is the patient, under stress, responding to several dormant schemas made active. They may direct the patient's behavior in a number of dysfunctional and self-destructive ways. Upon entering therapy and experiencing the acceptance and support of the therapist, the stress may be lowered, and the individual is once again operating on the more functionally active schema. If, however, the patient leaves therapy without gaining the skills for coping with stress, the problem may emerge again when, and if, the stressor returns. If the individual develops effective coping strategies, they may be able to deal with stress throughout their lives and rarely have the dormant schema activated.

The second clinical phenomenon is the arousal of dormant schema that cause the patient to appear, upon intake or admission to the hospital, to be extremely disturbed. After brief psychotherapy, pharmacotherapy, or combination, the patient appears far better integrated, far more attentive, and far "healthier." In fact, after the stress is removed, the therapist may question the existence of the psychopathology.

The particular extent of effect that a schema has on an individual's life depends on several factors: (a) how strongly held is the schema?, (b) how essential individuals see that schema to be to their safety, well being or existence, (c) the lack of disputation that individuals engage in when a particular schema is activated, (d) previous learning vis-a-vis the importance and essential nature of a particular schema, and (e) how early a particular schema was internalized.

Beck, Wright and Newman (1992) identify eight steps in establishing a treatment plan: (1) conceptualization of the problem, (2) developing a collaborative relationship, (3) motivation for treatment, (4) patient formulation of the problem, (5) setting goals, (6) socializing the patient into the cognitive model, (7) cognitive/behavioral interventions, and (8) relapse prevention. The initial step involves the therapist in developing a conceptualization of the problem. This conceptualization will, of necessity, be based on family and developmental histories, test data, interview material, and reports of previous therapists, or other professionals. This conceptualization must meet several criteria. It must be (a) useful, (b) simple, (c) theoretically coherent, (d) explain past behavior, (e) make sense of present behavior, and (f) be able to predict future behavior.

The first part of the conceptualization process is the compilation of a problem list. This list can then be prioritized in terms of identifying a sequence of problems to be dealt with in therapy. The reasons for choosing one problem as opposed to another as the primary, secondary or tertiary focus of the therapy depends on many factors. A particular problem may be the primary focus of therapy because of its debilitating effect on the individual. In another case, there may be no debilitating problems. The focus may be on the simplest problem, thereby giving a family, for example, practice in problem solving and some measure of success. In a third case, the choice of a primary focus might be on a "keystone" problem, that is, a problem whose solution will cause a ripple effect in solving other problems.

Having set out the treatment goals, the therapist can begin to develop strategies and the interventions that will help effect the strategies. The conceptualization also suggests strategies for intervention, and the most potentially promising interventions to be tried to effect the strategy. For maximum impact and effectiveness, the therapist will need a range of skills and techniques in order to implement the treatment strategy. The techniques or combinations of techniques are selected to suit the purpose and goals of therapy, the therapist's conceptualization of the problem, the needs of the patient at the specific point in therapy, the resources available in the patient's environment, and the therapist's skill and style.

While the available techniques are broadly categorized as cognitive (focused primarily on modifying thoughts, images and beliefs) and behavioral (focused primarily on modifying overt behavior) they are not mutually exclusive. A "behavioral" technique such as assertiveness training has many cognitive aspects. Assertiveness-training techniques can be used to accomplish cognitive changes, such as adjustment in expectancies regarding the consequences of assertion as well as changes in interpersonal behavior.

The treatment conceptualization is a picture, or model, of the patient's problems. Like the model used by an architect, the conceptual model allows a more thorough examination of the size, shape, and overall mass of the patient's problems. If the problems are well conceptualized, the patient becomes more understandable and predictable in thought and action. By developing hypotheses about the patient's operant schema based on the patient's own verbalizations, behavior, and developmental information, the therapist can, by direct questioning, work toward validating, modifying, or rejecting the original hypotheses. The following example illustrates the development of the conceptualization.

Example 1

A 44-year-old married male was referred for therapy by his family physician afer having ingested approximately 100 aspirin. He was hopeless about his perceived business failures. He came for his initial therapy appointment accompanied by his mother. She refused to remain in the waiting room and demanded to sit in on the session, he quietly agreed.

THERAPIST: (Entering the waiting room) Mr. Smith, please come in.
MOTHER: (Getting out of her chair)
THERAPIST: I would like to meet with Mr. Smith alone at first.
MOTHER: James, do you not want me with you?
PATIENT: (Quietly) It's okay, you can come in.

In the consulting room, the patient directed his mother to the chair closest to the therapist.
THERAPIST: Can we begin with why you are here?
MOTHER: He's here because no one really cares for what happens to him . . . His boss, doesn't care. He keeps giving him impossible work. His wife doesn't care. What would you expect? He's only human.

After several more questions were answered by the mother, the therapist questioned the pattern.

THERAPIST: I'd now like to hear from James.
MOTHER: Why are you putting pressure on him? That's what's wrong! Everyone does it to him. Do you mind my being here with you, honey?
PATIENT: (Looking down) No, no mom.
THERAPIST: Was your wife not able to be here?
PATIENT: Well . . .

MOTHER: That woman doesn't care about anything but herself. She didn't even care that Alan took the pills. He could have killed himself. All she cares about is what she can buy. Spend, spend, spend.
PATIENT: Mom . . . That's not fair . . .
THERAPIST: Was your wife not able to be here?
PATIENT: It's hard for her . . .
MOTHER: I told you about what bothers him most . . .

Alan's passivity, his mother's assertiveness, and the hostility toward Alan's wife are quite clear.

Given the available data, several hypotheses immediately come to mind as we begin to build a conceptualization. The therapist can begin, quite quickly, to gather the data necessary to confirm or refute any or all of the initial hypothetical alternatives. The hypotheses might include, but are not limited to,

- He is dependent (he brought his mother and easily acceded to her demand).
- He is having marital difficulties (his wife did not accompany him).
- He is feeling helpless or weak (he brought someone with him).
- Mother is overbearing (she may have accompanied him against his will; she demands to be in the session).
- Mother is very concerned (she has accompanied him and demands to be in the session).
- Wife is unavailable or unconcerned (she is absent).

The treatment can be focused on any, or all, of the following with the agreement of the patient: reducing hopelessness, developing motivation for treatment, marital therapy, assertiveness training, building self-esteem and personal efficacy, separating from his mother. The model that is initially constructed is open for revision as additional data is collected and processed.

In the next example, the same conceptualization-building strategy is used.

Example 2

A call came in at 3:00 p.m. on a Thursday from a prospective patient requesting an appointment.

PATIENT: Hello, Dr. Freeman?
THERAPIST: Yes.
PATIENT: You don't know me, but I was referred by Dr. Smith here in Smalltown. He is a former classmate of my GP, Dr. White. I would like to set up an appointment to see you as soon as possible. What would be the earliest you could see me?

THERAPIST: I have two openings. How about Monday at 1:00 P.M. or Wednesday at 11:00?

PATIENT: Is that the earliest appointments that you have? How about Saturday? I could come in on Saturday.

THERAPIST: I'm sorry, but I'm not in the office on Saturday.

PATIENT: Well . . . Let me see. Monday at 1:00 or Wednesday at 11:00. Could you make it Monday at 11:00?

THERAPIST: I'm sorry, but that time is filled.

PATIENT: The 1:00 is late. I'll take the Wednesday at 11:00. Wait, wait, could you make it Wednesday at 11:30?

THERAPIST: No, the 11:00 is the available time. I could make it Friday at 11:30.

PATIENT: That's too far away. I'll take the Wednesday . . . No, make it the Monday. Yes, the Monday. I have to get my hair cut. Besides, Friday I play tennis. Wait, do you think that the later, I mean earlier, time will open up? Oh never mind.

One hour later the patient calls back.

PATIENT: Dr. Freeman, is the Wednesday still open?

We can generate many hypotheses from this initial interaction:

- The patient has difficulty making decisions.
- The patient expects the therapist to change to accommodate her wishes and needs.
- Her needs and wishes supersede the needs of all others.
- Therapy may be difficult in terms of setting and keeping appointments.

In terms of treatment, the therapy must include limit-setting for the protection of the therapist and to offer structure to the therapy. The therapist must be prepared for the general demands that will undoubtedly be part of the therapeutic work.

Critical Incident

One sampling technique that is useful in the conceptualization process is the "critical incident" technique. The patient (family member, significant other, or teacher) is asked to describe a situation or incident that they see as indicative of the patient's problems, or descriptive of the problem's that they have in coping with the patient. It can be of any circumstance and any length.

For example, a husband described an incident that typified, in his eyes, his wife, her problem, and the difficulty in their marriage.

"She's always late. If we have to be somewhere at 2:00 p.m., we'll get there at 3:00. It can be to my folks or hers, friends, or even a play. When I say something, she just tells me that she's going as fast as she can and to leave her alone. She knows that it bugs me, and whenever I bring it up, she begins to cry and tells me that I don't care for her. If I did, I wouldn't keep bugging her for something so small.

One time we were invited to my sister's house for a surprise party for my dad's 65th birthday. We had to be there early so that we could all jump up and shout 'surprise.' I told my wife that the party was set for 12 noon when we were really expected between 1:00 and 1:30. Of course, we got there at 1:15, just in time for everything. When she walked in and saw that my dad wasn't there yet, and that we were on time, she exploded. She demanded to know why I had lied to her, why I had tricked her, and made a fool of her. She still hasn't forgiven me."

By looking at the critical incident, we can begin to generate hypotheses about the nature of the marital relationship; the possibility of the wife's behavior being passive-aggressive, the husband's behavior being passive-aggressive, the contribution of each of them to the problem, and the lack of communication between them.

A second example of the critical incident involves information gathered from an observer of a patient's behavior. The receptionist in a counseling center was asked by the therapist to report a critical incident regarding a patient at the center.

"She comes in for her weekly appointment about 2 to 3 minutes before the appointment time. One time I saw her out in the hall waiting to come in. She generally walks in, announces her name, drops her check on my desk without a further word, and sits down. She never talks to anyone in the waiting room even though there are pretty much the same people there each week and they are all talking to each other. She'll sometimes turn off the radio in the waiting room, and then she then sits and looks at her watch. If the therapist isn't down at the exact second of the appointment, she begins to look upset."

The patient's social skills, fear of abandonment, dependence, obsessive-compulsive characteristics, and demanding behavior may all be part of the picture that can be used to develop the conceptualization and then become part of the problem list that can be offered as grist for the therapeutic mill.

SHARING THE CONCEPTUALIZATION WITH THE PATIENT

Given that the conceptualization is an essential part of the therapy progress, the working hypotheses can be shared with the patient using the questioning format of the Socratic dialogue. Rather than interpreting the patient's thoughts or actions, the therapist can raise questions about the thoughts, actions, and feelings. In fact, if the therapist verbally communicates evolving hypotheses *as* interpretations, he or she runs the risk of appearing to be "mind-reading" the patient's thoughts and intentions. Further, offering an interpretation, e.g., "you seem angry," may evoke agreement from the patients when they really are more annoyed than angry. It may seem simpler to accept the therapist's statement than try to disagree, and seem ungrateful or contrary. The questioning format allows the patient to maintain integrity and allows the therapist to gather the most accurate data.

Sharing working hypotheses can sometimes be problematic for the therapist. If a depressed patient asks, "Doctor, what's wrong with me?", we may have no difficulty in offering a statement about their depression or using the term with the patient. After all, they can read about depression in any of a number of popular books and magazines. We may have no difficulty in discussing or describing diagnoses of anxiety, panic, or phobia. The difficulty in discussing or describing diagnoses of anxiety, panic, or phobia. The difficulty occurs when the problem is more serious, such as an Axis II problem. What can the clinician say when the working diagnosis and conceptualization are of Borderline Personality Disorder? Or, for that matter, any of the personality disorders? These categories are less well known to the general public and filled with many pitfalls. Is the problem easily solved? Can it be treated with medication? Will it last forever? Can cognitive therapy (or any therapy) cure this disorder? What motivation is necessary to cure or help this problem? How long will it take? These are all reasonable questions.

We can, of course, be evasive and take the position that these questions can only be answered over the long term of the therapy. If, however, we are conceptualizing the patient's problems as Axis II, we know that the problem is generally more difficult to work with, motivation is low, medication is not generally useful, and so on (Beck, Freeman, et al, 1990; Freeman, et al. 1990). It is probably of less value to share the label with the patient because of the problems in definition among professionals. It is essential for the therapist to share the conceptualization, however, with the patient so that the patient can know what the therapist is seeing and the direction of the therapy.

Using reframing, the therapist can share the conceptualization that will be the basis for the therapy. For example, in working with the schizoid patient, the therapist can highlight the patient's autonomy: "You tend to like doing things on your own." For the dependent patient, the therapist can say "You prefer to have lots of others around you", or "You generally try to arrange your life to have consultants or people you can call upon to help you make decisions." The patient can then be asked whether this is congruent with their personal view. If the patient disagrees, the therapist can obtain the patient's own clarification to sharpen the conceptualization.

The working hypotheses can be shared with the patients to allow them to understand what the therapist understands of their problems, and to have the patients and the therapists collaborate on building the most useful conceptualizations. One technique for sharing hypotheses is for the therapist to make sketches of how they "see" the patient. These sketches force the therapist to graphically and concretely look at their conceptualization, and to share that model with the patient. The following examples will serve to illustrate the process.

Example 1

Don, a 52-year-old attorney came for therapy with diagnoses of avoidant personality disorder, obsessive-compulsive personality disorder, and generalized anxiety disorder. He would spend great blocks of time in activities that he recognized as wasted effort, yet necessary, in his view. The therapist drew the following sketch with an explanation (Figure 2-1).

THERAPIST: What you describe is a life where you want to cross the road. But you're afraid that a car will come racing down and run you over. So to avoid that situation, you run a mile to your left to see if there are any cars coming. If there are none you return to your starting point. But you cannot cross yet, because there may be cars coming from your left. So you run a mile to your left and if there are no cars coming, you return to your starting point. But, you still cannot cross the road because while you were off to the left, a car may be coming from the right. So you spend your life running miles, but never crossing the 20 feet of road.

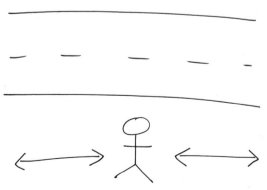

Figure 2-1. Don, 52-year-old attorney.

PATIENT: In a way you're right, but you don't understand. You've drawn the road as only two lanes. I see it as 100 lanes wide, with cars coming from every direction.

It was important to get the patient's modification. Conceptually, however, the issue is the same. The treatment might take several directions. The patient can be helped (or taught) to cross the road one lane at a time. Other examples of treatment interventions might include his searching for someone who can assist him in crossing the road (the therapist), his looking for a safe place to cross such as a bridge or tunnel, and his not crossing at an area where visibility is poor.

Example 2

Alex was a 32-year-old certified public accountant. He reported that he had suffered from anxiety for his entire life. Relaxation strategies had been unsuccessful because every time that Alex started to relax he experienced an increase in anxiety. He could not give up control. He feared a total loss of control in every aspect of his life. The therapist drew the following sketch with explanation (Figure 2-2).

THERAPIST: It appears that you carry your anxiety around like a scuba tank. Wherever you are you can get

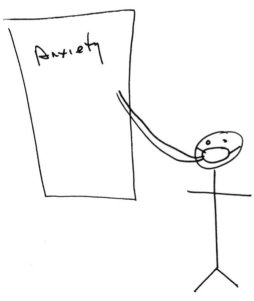

Figure 2-2. Alex, 32-year-old accountant.

a good healthy whiff of anxiety. If you were disconnected, you fear suffocating.

PATIENT: Yeah. If I lose my connection, I don't know what will happen to me. I'll probably die. If I didn't try to watch out for everything, I could die.

THERAPIST: While a scuba tank helps the diver underwater, what good does it do above the water?

PATIENT: Well, no good.

THERAPIST: It's heavy, cumbersome, and, most of all, unnecessary.

PATIENT: Except if the atmosphere is filled with poisonous gas. Then it could save my, I mean, his life.

The danger that he saw as inherent in the world was to be the main focus of the therapy.

Example 3

A third example was Sam. He came into therapy with the complaint of loneliness. He wanted a relationship, but could never find a partner who met his standards. His statement was that, "every time that I meet a woman we have a brief, passionate affair, and then it ends abruptly. I get bored with her and just end up dropping her." The following sketch was offered as a model of what I saw as the problem (Figure 2-3).

THERAPIST: You're here all alone. There are lots of people around, but all of them are down here beneath you.

PATIENT: I've been trying to have someone up here with me.

THERAPIST: But there's only room at the top for one. What are you going to do?

PATIENT: I guess I need to find a mountain big enough for two.

THERAPIST: How about a lower mountain? That might allow you to be on top, but still reach down to the others.

By accepting the patient's narcissistic style as a starting point, the therapy can proceed without generating anxiety based on trying to totally change the patient's style. It is clear that the only way that a partner can stay up at the peak with Sam was for him to clutch her to him. After a while he fatigues and then "drops her." Some of the therapeutic work could include building steps, or a ladder, to the top allowing for greater access for others to reach him, and for him to reach others. What might be quite important would be to prepare Sam for the possibility of some individual trying to share the space (a family member, parent, or a child). This will cause difficulty in that there is room for *two*.

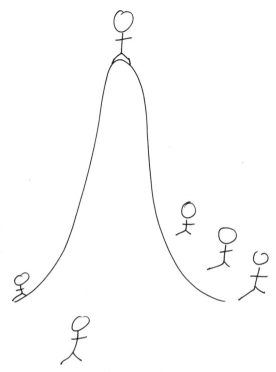

Figure 2-3. Sam.

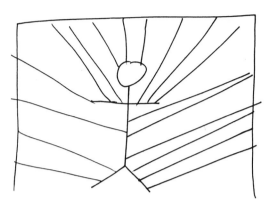

Figure 2-4. 36-year-old woman.

Example 4

The final example is of a 36-year-old woman who was beset by numerous obsessive rituals. She had rules for everything she did. She followed an Orhtodox Jewish tradition although she had been raised in a Reform tradition. She like the orthodoxy because, "It tells me what I can and cannot do." Unfortunately, she never thought that she properly followed the rules, so was always guilty. The therapist offered the following sketch (Figure 2-4).

THERAPIST: It's almost as if you have no skeleton. Nothing inside to hold you up. What would that mean?
PATIENT: I feel just like that. I have no backbone.
THERAPIST: If there is no skeleton, you would just be a mass of protoplasm on the floor. What you depend on is lots and lots of external rules to support you.
PATIENT: Even then it doesn't work.
THERAPIST: With all of those rules it's hard to know what to do. Some of these rules contradict each other. What I've drawn shows that there are several rules to run your legs, several to run your arms, several more to run your head. What would happen if we could elimi-

nate just one of these supports on your right leg, one on your left leg, one on each of your arms . . . Would you collapse?
PATIENT: Well I might be able to give one up . . . But which one?

The sketch not only identifies the plethora of rules, but the possibility of therapy, i.e. removing only one or two—thereby having fewer rules, and still maintaining her external supports. The therapy can focus on first, helping her to see that she *has* an endoskeleton, and that she can survive with fewer supports.

By concretizing the conceptualization and then sharing the conceptualization with the patient, the therapist can positively affect the collaborative set. The patient's input can guide the therapist to sharpen and focus his or her understanding of the patient's problems, and the patient's schema.

Finally, the conceptualization would be basic to the use of the homework assignments in therapy. Homework must be used within the context of the therapy, not merely an addendum to the therapy. The therapist must review the previously developed homework. The future homework is carefully and collaboratively agreed upon. Homework drawn directly from session material to allow the patient to test ideas, try new experiences, experiment with new ways of responding.

CONCEPTUALIZING THERAPEUTIC CHANGE

There are several possibilities for change (Beck, Freeman and Asociates, 1990; Freeman, 1988; Freeman and Leaf, 1989) which can be viewed as a change continuum from the greatest schematic changes to the least schematic change.

The first possibility is *schematic reconstruction*. Reconstruction—the ultimate goal of psychoanalytic psychotherapy—involves removing, rebuilding, or reconstructing old schemas. For example, it would involve reconstructing or removing the dependency schema, "I must always have other people around for me to survive," that is so typical of the dependent personality disorder, so that they are no longer dependent. The data regarding these cures is sparse (Beck, Freeman and Associates, 1990).

The second point on the change continuum is *schematic modification*. This may involve greater or lesser modification. The modification goal is, ideally, to attempt to effect the smallest modification as part of a series of small modifications. The schema, "I must always have other people around for me to survive" can be modified to, "I must *almost* always have other people around for me to survive." If this is successful, the next change might be, "I must *generally* have other people around for me to survive."

The third point is *schematic reinterpretation*. This involves using the schema in a more effective manner. Most people interpret their schema through their relationships or vocational choices. The individual who chooses a career in medicine but who dislikes being with other people might be most interested in specialties of pathology, radiology, or animal research. Sir Francis Chichester, famous as a trans-oceanic sailor commented, "Somehow, I never seemed to enjoy so much doing things with other people. I know I don't do a thing nearly as well when with someone. It makes me think I was cut out for solo jobs, and any attempt to diverge from that lot only makes me half a person." Chichester further said that, "I quite understand why people used to, and still do, go into retreat. During a month alone I think at last you become a real person and are concerned with the real value of life."

The final point on the continuum is schematic camouflage. This involves "doing the right thing." The patient can be helped to acquire skills to cover the schematic problems. For example, the schizoid individual can be encouraged to act in a more socially appropriate manner.

Overall, the change goals are a series of small sequential steps that approximate the final goals. The greatest hindrance to therapeutic progress is often the impatience of the therapist who tries to move the patient along far too quickly.

SUMMARY

The highest order skill in psychotherapy is the ability to develop treatment conceptualizations. Too often, therapy becomes a reactive experience; the therapist responds to what the patient brings into the therapy or the specific session—therapy is seen as proactive. Treatment involves a careful evaluation of the patient's problems based on a collection of the relevant historical data typically collected in a structured interview format. The therapist then develops hypotheses about why the patients respond the way they do, what were probable formative elements in the style, what are the operative schema, and the best possible points of entry into the system. There are eight steps in establishing a treatment plan: (1) conceptualization of the problem, (2) developing a collaborative relationship (3) motivation for treatment, (4) patient formulation of the problem, (5) setting goals, (6) socializing the patient into the cognitive model, (7) cognitive/behavioral interventions, and (8) relapse prevention. The conceptualization becomes the guide for the therapist in determining direction and targets for therapy. The cognitive therapist develops hypotheses about the reasons for the patients' behavior, and about what maintains the patients' thinking and acting the way that they do. The conceptualization also suggests strategies for intervention and the most promising interventions to be tried to effect the strategy.

In seeking to alter a particular belief that has endured for a long period of time, it would be necessary to help the individual to deal with the belief from as many different perspectives as possible: cognitive, affective, and behavioral. The conceptualizations often revolve around understanding the patient's schemas. The schemas are the organizing factors around which perception is built. There are many schemas that occur in complex combinations and permutations. The schemas may be personal, family, religious, cultural, age-related, or gender-related, or any combination of the above. The schemas become, in effect, how one defines oneself, both individually, and as part of a group. The two most prominent issues in understanding schemas are whether which schemas are active or inactive and whether the particular schema are non-compelling or compelling. Inactive schemas are called into play to control behavior in times of stress. Stressors of a variety of types will evoke the inactive schemas—which become active, govern behavior, and when the stressor is removed will return to their previously dormant state.

Understanding the activity-inactivity continuum explains two related clinical phenomena: the rapid, though transient, positive changes often evidenced in therapy and the so-called transference cure. The particular extent of effect that a schema has on an individual's life depends on several factors: (a) how strongly held is the schema, (b) how essential the individual sees that schema to their safety, well-being or existence, (c) the lack of disputation that the individual engages in when a particular schema is activated, (d) previous learning vis-a-vis the importance and essential nature of a particular schema, and (e) how early a particular schema was internalized. Schemas are in a constant state of change and evolution. From the child's earliest years there is a need to alter old schemas and develop new schemas to meet the different and increasingly complex demands of the world. Schemas are not maladaptive, no matter how they are stated. It is, rather, the expression of the schema in the person's life, and the goodness of fit with the personal goals and skills, and with societal expectations and demands.

A useful tool in the conceptualization process is the "critical incident" technique. The patient (family member, significant other, or teacher) is asked to describe a situation or incident that they see as indicative of the patient's problems.

The working hypotheses can be shared with the patient to allow the patient to understand what the therapist understands of their problem, and to have the patient and the therapist collaborate on building the most useful conceptualization. One technique for sharing the working hypotheses is for the therapist to sketch how the therapist perceives the patient's problems.

Finally, the conceptualization is not only the backbone of the therapy, but the clinician will find that the intervention techniques are more easily derived and implemented when part of an overall treatment program.

REFERENCES

Beck, A. T., Freeman, A., and Associates. (1990). *Cognitive therapy of personality disorders*. New York: Guilford.

Beck, A. T., Wright, F., and Newman, C. (1992). Taking the kick out of the habit. In A. Freeman and F. Dattilio (Eds.), *The comprehensive casebook of cognitive therapy*. New York: Plenum.

Campbell, R. J. (1989). *Psychiatric dictionary* (6th ed.). New York: Oxford University Press.

Crowley, R. M. (1985). Cognitiion in interpersonal theory and practice. In M. Mahoney and A. Freeman (Eds.), *Cognition and psychotherapy*. New York: Plenum.

Freeman, A. (1988). Cognitive therapy of personality disorders. In C. Perris, H. Perris, and I. Blackburn (Eds.), *The theory and practice of cognitive therapy*. Heidelberg: Springer Verlag.

Freeman, A. and Leaf, R. (1989). Cognitive therapy of personality disorders. In A. Freeman, K. M. Simon, L. E. Beutler, and H. Arkowitz (Eds.), *The comprehensive handbook of cognitive therapy*. New York: Plenum.

Freeman, A., Pretzer, J., Fleming, B. and Simon, K. M. (1990). *Clinical applications of cognitive therapy*. New York: Plenum.

Hammer, E. F. (1990). *Reaching for the affect*. New York: Lawrence Erlbaum.

Rosen, H. (1985). *Piagetian dimensions of clinical relevance*. New York: Columbia University Press.

Rosen, H. (1989). Piagetian dimensions of clinical relevance. In A. Freeman, K. M. Simon, L. E. Beutler, and H. Arkowitz (Eds.), *The comprehensive handbook of cognitive therapy*. New York: Plenum.

Safran, J. D. and Segal, Z. V. (1990). *Interpersonal process in cognitive therapy*. New York: Basic Books, Inc.

Young, J. E. (1990). *Cognitive therapy for personality disorders: A schema-focused approach*. Sarasota, FL: Professional Resource Exchange.

II

Treatment of Clinical Problems

3

Use of the Quality of Life Inventory in Problem Assessment and Treatment Planning for Cognitive Therapy of Depression

Michael B. Frisch

PROBLEM SOLVING AND ASSESSMENT IN COGNITIVE THERAPY

Cognitive therapy procedures involve the self-monitoring of thoughts and assumptions, logical analysis in which dysfunctional thoughts are disputed through logical argument, and hypothesis testing in which negative assumptions are challenged through real-world experiments aimed at testing their veracity (Jarrett & Nelson, 1987). Problem solving may constitute a little-recognized fourth component of cognitive therapy, one that is repeatedly mentioned in both the treatment manual (called "the manual") (Beck, Rush, Shaw, & Emery, 1979) and more recent works (DeRubeis & Beck, 1988). According to Beck et al. (1979), "external," "situational," or "practi-

Michael B. Frisch • Department of Psychology, P.O. Box 97334, Baylor University, Waco, Texas 76798-7334.

Comprehensive Casebook of Cognitive Therapy, edited by Arthur Freeman and Frank M. Dattilio. Plenum Press, New York, 1992.

cal" problems or "precipitants" related to depression usually involve perceived losses at home, work, or school such as divorce or a business failure. The resolution of even simple and circumscribed problems—through consultation with either the therapist or an appropriate "medical, legal, financial, or vocational" expert—can in itself alleviate depressive symptoms (Beck et al., 1979). For example, the manual describes the case of a beleaguered homemaker whose "symptoms quickly disappeared" (p. 204) once she secured help with household chores.

According to the manual, the focus of cognitive therapy at any given time is either a "target symptom" of depression (such as passivity, sadness, or negative thoughts) or an external problem situation that seems to cause, maintain, or intensify depressive symptoms. Initially, the focus is on specific depressive symptoms targeted for treatment (Beck et al., 1979). With less severe depressions, or once acute symptoms have been relieved, the focus is on external problems related to the depression. In the more recent works (Young & Beck, 1982; DeRubeis & Beck, 1988) and videotapes of Dr. Beck, problem solving with regard to external problems seems characteristic of cognitive therapy throughout the course of treatment, even when clients are suicidal (Beck et al., 1979). Empirical studies have also pointed to the need for comprehensive problem assessment and treatment in dealing with depressed patients, suggesting that different problems and skill deficits can cause depression and that treatment should be aimed at the particular problems of a particular client in order to be effective (McKnight, Nelson, Hayes, & Jarrett, 1984).

Despite frequent allusions to the importance of problem solving as it concerns difficulties related to a client's depression, the cognitive therapy literature offers little guidance in comprehensive problem assessment and resolution. This may reflect an undue emphasis on internal, "cognitive" factors to the neglect of external "behavioral" factors even though cognitive therapy is clearly cognitive-behavioral in technique (Hollon & Beck, 1986). Recent theoretical formulations—such as Abramson, Metalsky, and Alloy's (1989) hopelessness theory of depression—persuasively argue for a balanced consideration of internal and external causes of depression, reiterating the importance of cognitive, behavioral, and environmental change in alleviating depression. Frisch's Quality of Life Inventory (QOLI) (Frisch, 1988, 1989, 1992; Frisch, Cornell, Villanueva, & Retzlaff, 1992; Frisch, Villanueva, Cornell, & Retzlaff, 1990) may meet the need in cognitive therapy for a comprehensive scheme of problem assessment that may prove useful in fostering external and environmental (as well as internal and cognitive) therapeutic change.

The absence of comprehensive problem assessment in cognitive therapy may be part of a larger problem for most cognitive-behavioral approaches in which treatment is begun before adequate assessment and treatment planning has taken place (Morganstern, 1988). For example, Lazarus (1971) discusses a "typical" case in which systematic desensitization for a "simple bridge phobia" (p. 33) seemed indicated. More thorough assessment, however, revealed that the client also feared failure at a new job, which required travel over a bridge in order to get to work. The bridge phobia "vanished" when the client's performance anxiety was effectively dispelled.

The complex, subjective process of assessment and treatment planning, or *macroanalysis* (Emmelkamp, 1982), involves at least three steps (Emmelkamp, 1982; Frisch, 1989; Turkat & Wolpe, 1985):

1. An accurate and complete assessment of a client's problems. This overall assessment should precede any "microanalysis" or functional analysis of a particular problem.
2. A conceptualization of how a client's problems developed, are maintained, and interrelate. Often individual problems are part of a larger integrated system, requiring intervention at a more basic level in order to impact the particular problems of an individual (Evans, 1985).
3. The establishment of treatment goals and priorities based on steps 1 and 2.

Some cognitive-behavioral therapists may give short shrift to the process of assessment and treatment planning, because the process is complex, subjective, and hence not amenable to easy "rules of thumb" (Morganstern, 1988). The cognitive therapy manual (Beck et al., 1979) briefly discusses the establishment of treatment priorities without giving any specific guidelines for a complete problem assessment or for conceptualizing problems and their interrelationships; the symptoms or problems given priority for treatment are those viewed by the therapist and client as most urgent, distressing, and amenable to change. Cognitive therapists assume a "snowball effect" in which improvement of one problem or symptom will somehow lead to changes in other areas. This may not be true in every case, especially for problems not related to the client's depression. In addition, the absence of a comprehensive problem assessment scheme or device, as recommended by Morganstern (1988), makes it possible to ignore, altogether, key symptoms or problems that may be maintaining or intensifying the client's depression. Once again, the use of the QOLI may be invaluable in this regard.

DEVELOPMENT AND PSYCHOMETRICS OF THE QOLI

The abundant literature on subjective well-being and life satisfaction has direct implications for (a) assessing the outcome of psychotherapy, pharmacotherapy, and behavioral medicine treatments; (b) defining "mental health" and positive adjustment; and (c) understanding numerous psychological disorders, including depression (Frisch, 1989; Frisch et al., 1990, 1992). For example, authors from diverse traditions have argued for the development of nonpathology-oriented measures of subjective well-being to augment those that focus on negative affect and symptoms (Blau, 1977; Bigelow, Brodsky, Stewart, & Olson, 1982; Frisch & Froberg, 1987; Hollandsworth, 1987, 1988; Lehman, Ward, & Linn, 1982; Rogers, 1951; Strupp & Hadley, 1977; Wolf, 1978). For example, some behavioral and psychodynamic theorists agree that a client's happiness or satisfaction with life is an essential criterion of "mental health" and positive outcome in psychotherapy that should be routinely assessed by researchers and clinicians alike (Hollandsworth, 1987, 1988; Strupp & Hadley, 1977). These theorists and others (Beiser, 1971; Bigelow et al., 1982; Coan, 1977; Diamond, 1985; Jahoda, 1958; Seeman, 1989; Taylor & Brown, 1988) wish to broaden the criteria for "mental health" and adjustment to include personal happiness and life satisfaction, as well as the mere absence of "disease" or psychiatric symptoms. Frisch (1989) reviews research linking depression with the constructs of life satisfaction and subjective well-being and then uses these constructs to integrate existing cognitive-behavioral theories of depression. (In like fashion, Watson, Clark, & Carey, 1988, related depression to a "generalized sense of well being" or positive affectivity as well as to negative affects.) According to Frisch (1989), "dissatisfaction depression," an etiologically distinct subtype of clinical depression, is immediately caused by the combination of a negative self-evaluation and hopelessness, which, in turn, are based on repeated failures to fulfill aspirations and meet personal standards in highly valued areas of life (i.e., life dissatisfaction).

Current measures of subjective well-being and life satisfaction can be characterized in general as conceptually vague and inconsistent in terminology, psychometrically weak due to a preponderance of single-item measures that are rarely externally validated, and nonapplicable to clinical populations because of a reliance on "normal" and specialized (e.g., geriatric) samples for validation purposes (for reviews, see Diener, 1984; Hollandsworth, 1988; Kane & Kane, 1981; Mulhern et al., 1989; Mulhern, Fairclough, Friedman, & Leigh, 1990; and Salamon, 1988). The QOLI (Frisch, 1988, 1992; Frisch et al., 1990, 1992) is the only clinically oriented, domain-based (nonglobal) measure of life satisfaction available; unfortunately, related scales confound affect (Salamon, 1988) or performance (Bigelow et al., 1982) items with satisfaction items.

The QOLI improves upon existing measures of life satisfaction and subjective well-being by its (a) basis in an explicit theoretical framework called Quality-of-Life Therapy (Frisch, 1989; Hollandsworth, 1988); (b) specific applicability to psychiatric or clinical populations; (c) multi-item format that bases overall satisfaction on satisfaction within 17 "domains" or areas of life (such as "work" and "health") that are explicitly defined for the first time in the literature; and (d) weighted satisfaction scoring scheme that considers both a respondent's satisfaction with an area of life and the value or importance of that area to the individual's overall well-being (Diener, Emmons, Larsen, & Griffin, 1985). The QOLI has been described as a unique, comprehensive, and much-needed measure of life satisfaction and "positive functioning" that may complement symptom- or pathology-oriented

measures of psychological functioning (Hans H. Strupp, personal communication, October 14, 1989).

The QOLI is based on an empirically validated, linear, additive model of life satisfaction called Quality-of-Life Therapy (Frisch, 1989; Frisch et al., 1992) that assumes that an individual's overall life satisfaction consists largely of the sum of satisfactions in particular "domains" or areas of life deemed important.* The model further assumes that a person's satisfaction with a particular area of life is weighted according to its importance or value before it enters into the "equation" of overall life satisfaction; thus, it is assumed that satisfaction in highly valued areas of life has a greater influence on evaluations of overall life satisfaction than areas of equal satisfaction judged of lesser importance. The scoring scheme of the QOLI reflects both of these theoretical assumptions. According to Frisch (1989), *life satisfaction* or *quality of life* refers to an individual's subjective evaluation of the degree to which his or her most important needs, goals, and wishes have been fulfilled. Life satisfaction along with negative and positive affect are viewed as components of the broader construct of subjective well-being or happiness (Andrews & Withey, 1976; Diener, 1984; Veenhoven, 1984). It is further assumed that the affective correlates of subjective well-being stem largely from cognitively based satisfaction judgments of valued areas of life.

Finally, the present theory of life satisfaction assumes that a finite number of areas of human aspiration and fulfillment may be identified that are applicable to both psychiatric and nonpsychiatric populations. Based upon an exhaustive review of the literature, especially "cognitive mapping" studies of human concerns (Andrews & Inglehart, 1979; Andrews & Withey, 1976) and studies identifying particular areas of life associated with overall life satisfaction and happiness (Andrews & Withey, 1976; Campbell, Converse, & Rogers, 1976; Cantril, 1965; Diener, 1984; Flanagan, 1978; Veenhoven, 1984), a comprehensive list of 17 human concerns, "domains," or areas of life was developed for inclusion in the QOLI. An effort was made to be comprehensive but to limit the areas of life to those empirically associated with overall satisfaction and happiness. The 17 areas of life included in the QOLI are listed in Table 3-1.

The QOLI consists of 17 items (see Figure 3-1 for an example of a completed QOLI answer sheet). Each of the 17 areas of life deemed as potentially relevant to overall

---

*Copies of the QOLI, QOLI answer sheets, and the QOLI test manual and treatment guide are available from Michael B. Frisch, Ph.D., Psychology Department, P. O. Box 97334, Baylor University, Waco, TX 76798-7334.

TABLE 3-1   The 17 Areas of Life Assessed by the QOLI

1. *Health* refers to being physically fit and free from sickness, pain, or disability.
2. *Self-regard* refers to liking and respecting yourself in light of your assets and limitations, successes and failures, and your ability to cope with problems.
3. *Philosophy of life* refers to having a set of guiding values, goals, and beliefs which give your life meaning or a sense of purpose, help you plan and make decisions about how to live your life, help you cope with day-to-day problems, and help you decide on the best way to act in a given situation. This personal system of ethics and values may or may not be based on religious beliefs.
4. *Standard of living* refers to your income, the things you have, such as a car or furniture, and the expectation that you will have what you need financially in the future.
5. *Work* refers to your occupation or how you spend most of your time—whether it be at a job, in school (if you are a student), or in the home (if you are a homemaker or conduct a business based in your home). "Work" consists of the work itself, pay (if applicable), surroundings, job security, relationships with co-workers, and the availability of needed equipment and supervision.
6. *Recreation* refers to non-work-related, spare-time activities aimed at entertainment, relaxation, or self-improvement. Such activities include watching movies or football games, visiting friends, or pursuing hobbies like gardening, fishing, and jogging.
7. *Learning* refers to gaining knowledge, skill, or understanding in an area of interest through study, experience, or instruction. The area of study may be mainly intellectual, such as history or art appreciation, or it may be practical, such as home improvement or car repair. These learning experiences may take place either in or outside of a school setting.
8. *Creativity* involves expressing what is unique and special about you by being original, imaginative, and inventive in your approach to a hobby (like playing a musical instrument or photography), to work-related situations, or to everyday activities like home decorating or repair.
9. *Social service* consists of helping, encouraging, and promoting the welfare of others. It involves helping adults or children who are neither relatives or close friends. Such service may be done on your own or as a member of an organization such as a church, club, or volunteer group.
10. *Civic action* refers to activities related to being a citizen of a community, state, and nation. It may include involvement in government (local, state, or national) or community affairs. Activities such as voting, keeping informed of local or national news, supporting a political cause or candidate, or efforts to make one's community a better place to live are examples of civic action.
11. *Love relationship* refers to an intimate, romantic relationship with a spouse, boyfriend, or girlfriend. Such relationships usually involve sexual attraction, companionship, understanding, and deep feelings of affection.
12. *Friendships* refer to the number and quality of close friends (who are not relatives) that you have. "Close friends" are people you like and know well who have interests and viewpoints similar to yours. Friendships involve a mutual give and take of companionship, acceptance, trust, and support.
13. *Relationships with children* refers to how you get along with your child (or children). These relationships involve helping, teaching, and caring for your child (or children) as well as watching their development and enjoying their companionship.
14. *Relationships with relatives* consist of your relationships with parents, brothers, sisters, and in-laws. These relationships may involve visiting, shared activities, mutual understanding, and assistance.
15. *Home* refers to the house or apartment where you live, including the attractiveness, space, layout, physical structure, and cost of your home as well as the yard and surrounding area.
16. *Neighborhood* refers to the immediate area where you live and includes the area's attractiveness, the people and their values, the natural surroundings (such as the air, land, and water), safety from crime, and the cost and quality of goods and services like fire and police protection, garbage collection, street maintenance, recreational facilities (like parks, playing fields, and bowling alleys), schools, medical care, and shopping centers.
17. *Community* refers to the city, town, or rural area in which you live, including the area's attractiveness, safety from crime, the people and their values, the natural surroundings, the cost and quality of goods and services, the local government, taxes, court and transportation systems, the climate, recreational facilities, and available entertainment such as local events and places to visit, restaurants, movies, concerts, plays, newspapers, radio, and television.

Source: Copyright 1988 by Michael B. Frisch. Reprinted by permission.

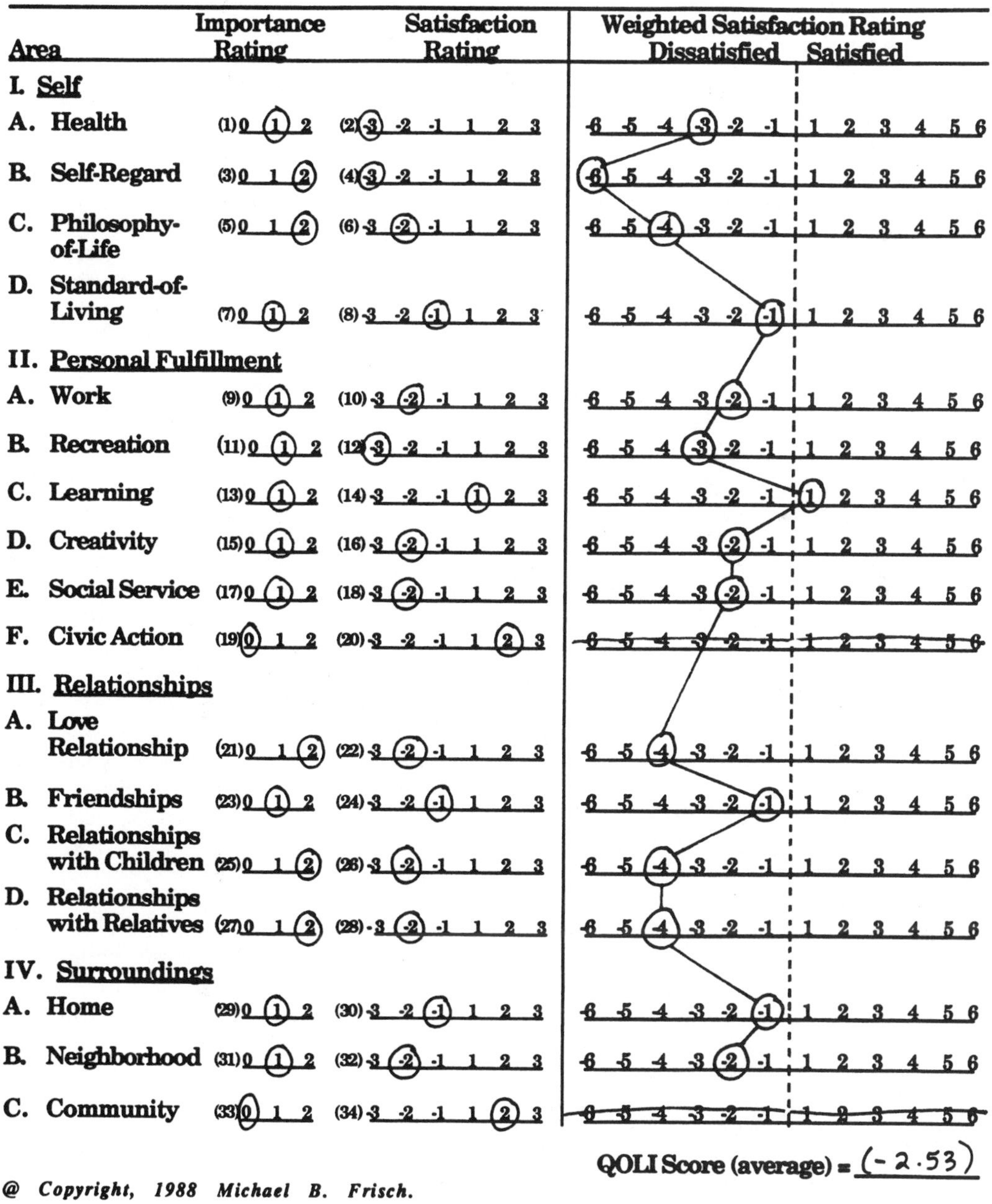

Area	Importance Rating	Satisfaction Rating	Weighted Satisfaction Rating Dissatisfied — Satisfied
I. Self			
A. Health	(1) 0 ① 2	(2) ③ -2 -1 1 2 3	-6 -5 -4 ③ -2 -1 ¦ 1 2 3 4 5 6
B. Self-Regard	(3) 0 1 ②	(4) ③ -2 -1 1 2 3	⊘ -5 -4 -3 -2 -1 ¦ 1 2 3 4 5 6
C. Philosophy-of-Life	(5) 0 1 ②	(6) -3 ② -1 1 2 3	-6 -5 ④ -3 -2 -1 ¦ 1 2 3 4 5 6
D. Standard-of-Living	(7) 0 ① 2	(8) -3 -2 ① 1 2 3	-6 -5 -4 -3 -2 ① ¦ 1 2 3 4 5 6
II. Personal Fulfillment			
A. Work	(9) 0 ① 2	(10) -3 ② -1 1 2 3	-6 -5 -4 -3 ② -1 ¦ 1 2 3 4 5 6
B. Recreation	(11) 0 ① 2	(12) ③ -2 -1 1 2 3	-6 -5 -4 ③ -2 -1 ¦ 1 2 3 4 5 6
C. Learning	(13) 0 ① 2	(14) -3 -2 -1 ① 2 3	-6 -5 -4 -3 -2 -1 ①¦ 2 3 4 5 6
D. Creativity	(15) 0 ① 2	(16) -3 ② -1 1 2 3	-6 -5 -4 -3 ② -1 ¦ 1 2 3 4 5 6
E. Social Service	(17) 0 ① 2	(18) -3 ② -1 1 2 3	-6 -5 -4 -3 ② -1 ¦ 1 2 3 4 5 6
F. Civic Action	(19) ⓪ 1 2	(20) -3 -2 -1 1 ② 3	-6 -5 -4 -3 -2 -1 ¦ 1 2 3 4 5 6
III. Relationships			
A. Love Relationship	(21) 0 1 ②	(22) -3 ② -1 1 2 3	-6 -5 ④ -3 -2 -1 ¦ 1 2 3 4 5 6
B. Friendships	(23) 0 ① 2	(24) -3 -2 ① 1 2 3	-6 -5 -4 -3 -2 ① ¦ 1 2 3 4 5 6
C. Relationships with Children	(25) 0 1 ②	(26) -3 ② -1 1 2 3	-6 -5 ④ -3 -2 -1 ¦ 1 2 3 4 5 6
D. Relationships with Relatives	(27) 0 1 ②	(28) -3 ② -1 1 2 3	-6 -5 ④ -3 -2 -1 ¦ 1 2 3 4 5 6
IV. Surroundings			
A. Home	(29) 0 ① 2	(30) -3 -2 ① 1 2 3	-6 -5 -4 -3 -2 ① ¦ 1 2 3 4 5 6
B. Neighborhood	(31) 0 ① 2	(32) -3 ② -1 1 2 3	-6 -5 -4 -3 ② -1 ¦ 1 2 3 4 5 6
C. Community	(33) ⓪ 1 2	(34) -3 -2 -1 1 ② 3	-6 -5 -4 -3 -2 -1 ¦ 1 2 3 4 5 6

QOLI Score (average) = (-2.53)

@ Copyright, 1988 Michael B. Frisch.

Figure 3-1. Clinical example of completed QOLI answer sheet (page 1).

life satisfaction is rated by respondents in terms of its importance to their overall happiness and satisfaction (0 = not at all important; 1 = important; 2 = extremely important) and in terms of their satisfaction with the area (ranging from −3 = very dissatisfied to 3 = very satisfied). The inventory's scoring scheme reflects the assumption that a person's overall life satisfaction is a composite of the satisfactions in particular areas of life weighted by their relative importance to the individual. Thus, the products of the satisfaction and importance ratings for each area of life are computed (these weighted satisfactions ratings range from −6 to 6). Next, the overall life satisfaction or QOLI score is obtained by averaging all weighted satisfaction ratings that have nonzero importance ratings. This essentially allows items or areas to be omitted by individuals who deem them as irrelevant to their overall happiness, allowing for a subjective measure with both normative and ipsative features, as recommended by Lazarus and Folkman (1984). The QOLI takes about 10 minutes to complete and can be administered via interview to illiterate clients.

Test-retest coefficients for the QOLI range from .80 to .91 and internal consistency coefficients range from .77 to .89, based on a study of three clinical and three nonclinical samples (Frisch et al., 1990, 1992). QOLI item-total correlations are adequate and the QOLI correlates with related measures of subjective well-being, including a peer rating and clinical interview measure. As expected, the QOLI correlates negatively and moderately with measures of general psychopathology, anxiety, and depression. The QOLI does not correlate substantially with measures of social desirability. Analyses of variance and discriminant function analyses show that clinical and nonclinical criterion groups differ both in mean QOLI scores and in their item response patterns on the QOLI (Frisch et al., 1990, 1992). Factor analysis of the QOLI has yielded a two-factor solution which, according to a subsequent oblique multiple groups confirmatory factor analysis, fits four different samples (Frisch et al., 1990).

The psychometric soundness of the QOLI exceeds that of most related measures, making it one of the best available measures of life satisfaction (for reviews of related measures see Diener, 1984; Hollandsworth, 1988; Kane & Kane, 1981; Mulhern et al., 1989; and Salamon, 1988). In fact, few (if any) measures of subjective well-being designed for clinical use have been evaluated as extensively as the QOLI for reliability, internal consistency, and criterion-related and construct validity. It is especially rare for a measure to be evaluated against external nonself-report criteria such as peer ratings and clinical ratings of interviews and to demonstrate a consistent ability to distinguish clinical from nonclinical criter-

ion groups (Diener, 1984; Mulhern et al., 1989; Veenhoven, 1984). In light of these results, the QOLI seems to meet the requirements for a useful measure of satisfaction or perceived quality of life (see Diener, 1984; Hollandsworth, 1988; Mulhern et al., 1989), including sufficient reliability, internal consistency and item-total correlations, sufficient construct (including convergent, discriminative, and nomological) and criterion-related (both external and "known-group") validity, relative freedom from social-desirability response bias, focus on respondent's subjective experience rather than objective circumstances, validation on clinical samples for whom the measure is primarily intended, availability of norms, and convenience (the QOLI takes only ten minutes to complete, is easily scored, and is interpretable by nonpsychologists as suggested by Mulhern et al., 1989.)

CASE EXAMPLE

The QOLI has numerous potential research and clinical applications. It may be fruitfully applied as a measure of positive outcome both on a routine clinical basis and in studies of psychotherapeutic, pharmacological, and social interventions aimed at alleviating psychological disorders, physical illnesses, and communitywide social problems. With respect to psychotherapy, the QOLI may meet the need for a measure of individual contentment—cited by Strupp and Hadley (1977) as the primary criterion of positive outcome and "mental health" from the perspective of a client—that goes beyond measures of symptoms and negative affect. The QOLI also appears useful in treatment planning for psychotherapy clients, in general, and for cognitive therapy clients, in particular. Its "treatment utility" (Hayes, Nelson, & Jarrett, 1987) has been demonstrated informally with several hundred clients from a variety of inpatient, outpatient, community mental health, private practice, and mood disorder clinics both in the United States and abroad. It is currently being used in training cognitive therapists at the University of Texas Southwestern Medical Center in Dallas and the psychology service of the Adult Probation Department in Waco, Texas. The QOLI, like Lazarus's (1981) BASIC ID assessment scheme, fills the need for a broad-spectrum, multifaceted assessment device that provides a comprehensive overview of clients' problems and strengths (Morganstern, 1988). It goes beyond Lazarus's scheme by inquiring about 17 areas rather than 7 (Lazarus, 1981). The QOLI profile of a client's weighted satisfaction ratings for each area of life—which is akin to an MMPI profile (see Figure 3-1) and ranges from −6 (extreme dissatisfaction) to 6 (extreme satisfaction)—is supplemented by a narrative section of the QOLI answer sheet, which asks respondents to list problems that interfere with their satisfaction in the 17 areas of life assessed by the QOLI. This information has been invaluable to clinicians in conducting a "macro-analysis" (Emmelkamp, 1982; Frisch, 1989) in which clients' problems are comprehensively assessed, conceptualized, and prioritized for treatment. This macroanalytic overview can be followed by a "microanalysis" or functional analysis of a problem area in which the specific parameters of and reasons for dissatisfaction can be explicated. Often dissatisfactions can be traced to difficult circumstances, misconceptions about an area of life, unrealistic standards of fulfillment, the overvaluing of an area, or a neglect of other potential sources of satisfaction (Frisch, 1989).

The use of the QOLI in problem assessment and treatment planning for cognitive therapy is illustrated in the following case. A 34-year-old white, married homemaker with a high school education and a 5-month-old infant born with a severe heart deformity scored well below average or "very low" on the QOLI (-2.53) and easily met the DSM-III-R criteria for major depression. In the first session of treatment, the weighted satisfaction "profile" (see Figure 3-1 for this client's responses) and the problem narrative section of her QOLI revealed dissatisfaction in the following areas:

1. *Work*. She described her work as a homemaker as "thankless, lonely, and always there." Her new infant was at serious risk of further disability or death and required constant care and monitoring. Her husband worked long hours and was uninvolved with child care when home. The client was unable to find a baby sitter with requisite CPR training, and she also cared for an 8-year-old daughter from a previous relationship.
2. *Love relationship*. On the QOLI She indicated "a lack of intimate, romantic time" as well as feelings of being "taken for granted or not appealing to spouse" and "scared to air true feelings—afraid of rejection." She mistakenly assumed that her husband was uncommitted to the marriage, unappreciative of her efforts at home, and unwilling to help with child care. She withdrew from her husband in silence, assuming that, like her father and ex-boyfriend, her husband would critically reject and even leave her if she shared her thoughts of desperation and hopelessness.
3. *Relationships with children*. In regard to her jealous and defiant older daughter, the client said, "I can't seem to relate anymore to my 8-year-old. I lose patience quickly." She mistakenly believed

that her husband was unwilling to discipline the child or back her up in her own efforts to do so.
4. *Relationships with relatives*. The client described her family as "too judgmental"—especially her father, who was often irritable and depressed, himself, and who constantly criticized his daughter for being overweight and for making "mistakes" in how she cared for her children.

Dissatisfaction was also expressed with respect to recreation ("There never seems to be time for it. It's very limited because of a lack of time, money, and preparations."), friendships (she had few friends and would not share her concerns with them), health ("weight gain problem since 13 years old"), self-regard ("Hard to cope with problems. I'm scared to air my true feelings. I'm afraid of rejection."), philosophy of life ("Hard to cope. I've never had a good way to solve problems."), standard of living ("I'm tired of barely making ends meet."), home ("not big enough for our needs"), neighborhood ("do not feel safe . . . never go out . . . fear my child not safe to play outside . . . want to live in the country"), creativity ("I have no time to myself to explore this"), and social service ("Hard to share with others on a personal basis. Don't know what to say."). "Learning" constituted an area of relative strength in so far as this was the only area of any importance with which the client felt fairly satisfied (as opposed to dissatisfied). The client felt that "civic action" and "community" were "not at all important" to her overall happiness and life satisfaction.

In keeping with both cognitive (Beck et al., 1979) and hopelessness theories (Abramson et al., 1989), the client's depression was conceptualized in diathesis-stress terms. The stressor of caring for an infant with severe congenital heart disease activated negative schemas that prompted the client to withdraw resentfully from all sources of social support, fearing rejection if she shared her concerns and assertively expressed her needs to those around her, including her husband, friends, and family. Several cognitive-behavioral vulnerabilities seemed to predispose the client to depression, including tendencies for shyness, social isolation, unassertiveness, self-denigration, and low self-efficacy in the face of adversity. The client admitted these tendencies, attributing them to her father's treatment of her both as a child and as an adult. She perceived her father (who had a history of several "nervous breakdowns") as viciously critical, rejecting, depressed, and bitter. He apparently predicted failure for his children and would withdraw emotionally and even physically when he disapproved of their behavior. This experience of being "disowned," as the client describes it, included physical absences from the home for days, time. The client was similarly "disowned" by a boyfriend who left her once she became pregnant. The client also recalls being overprotected, isolated, and "parentified" as a child and young adult, an experience that clearly retarded her social development and poise.

The client's depression seemed to be precipitated by the stressor of caring for her disabled infant, which made her feel inadequate as a mother, estranged from her husband, and unable to pursue any recreational or social pursuits. Her lack of assertion prevented her from "burdening" her friends and family with her distress or with requests for assistance. The perceived lack of commitment and support from her husband seemed especially depressogenic, as the client concluded that she had failed as a wife in securing her husband's affection and sympathy. Another contributing stressor was her relationship with her father, which deteriorated once her infant was born and he began to criticize her handling of the baby (to some extent, she held out hope for a complete reconciliation with and unconditional support from her father as she had received at the hands of her grandfather while growing up). Finally, the client's efficacy as a mother was further challenged by the hostile reaction of her 8-year-old daughter to her disabled infant sister. At one point the older daughter announced her intentions to be oppositional by saying to her mother, "I want to make you hate me, 'cause I don't want you to have a baby besides me!" Each of these contributing factors were addressed in the treatment plan designed for the client.

Once the problem assessment and conceptualization phases were complete, treatment goals, priorities, and strategies were established and carried out in the following three consecutive phases of treatment:

1. *Cognitive therapy*—including use of the Daily Record of Dysfunctional Thoughts (Beck et al., 1979), activity schedule, bibliotherapy (e.g., Jakubowski & Lange, 1978; Burns, 1980), treatment of insomnia (Beck et al., 1979), and assertion training (Beck et al., 1979; Frisch, 1989; Frisch, Elliot, Atsaides, Salva, & Denney, 1982) in relation to the client's best friend, church acquaintances, husband, father, and 8 year old daughter— was instituted in the first six sessions in order to quickly relieve her acute symptoms of depression and to begin to resolve the key problems maintaining the depression (e.g., dissatisfaction in work, relationships, recreation, philosophy of life, and self-regard) by engineering small initial success experiences in problem solving and coping with the most pressing, immediate problems.

The client gained some confidence in this initial phase of treatment by assertively and successfully asking for assistance from her best friend, husband, church acquaintances, and doctors (in clarifying her daughter's di-

agnosis and in finding parents in similar circumstances for purposes of mutual support). She memorized the cognitive distortions listed in Burns (1980) and felt that the cognitive model fit her closely. Numerous automatic thoughts were disputed in sessions and in homework, such as "I'm a big girl and shouldn't need help," "needing help proves I'm a worthless mother and wife," "you shouldn't burden others with your problems if they have any of their own," "it's my fault if the baby catches cold and dies from heart failure," "my husband doesn't love or appreciate me and wants a divorce," "it's terribly wrong for me to 'recharge my batteries' with recreation and leave the baby for a minute, even with a nurse," "I must continue to help my parents as I did before I was married," "I can make my dad as loving as my granddad even after 34 years of failure," and "it's never worth the risk to trust someone enough to share your true feelings and ask for help; you're bound to be let down."

2. *Couples cognitive therapy* (Beck, 1988; Beck et al., 1979; Dattilio & Podesky, 1990; Epstein, 1983; Frisch, 1989), including relationship enhancement exercises (or "positive behavior exchange"; Jacobson & Margolin, 1979), logical analysis and "reality testing" of erroneous beliefs about the relationship, and skills training in communication and problem solving, took place during sessions 7 through 13 (each session lasted 90 minutes). Relationship enhancement activities included homework in listing and performing acts "pleasing" to the partner, reviewing the perceived strengths of each partner both in the past and present, the scheduling of a weekly "date" in which the couple went out by themselves as they did in their courtship, and sexual enrichment exercises (Beck, 1988). The couples therapy was aimed at effecting a lasting solution to the factor judged to be primary in maintaining the client's depression (i.e., her marital distress). The client also continued her efforts in individual cognitive therapy during this phase of the treatment, especially her bibliotherapy, the use of the Daily Record of Dysfunctional Thoughts (DRDT), and "reality testing" of negative automatic thoughts and schemata.

It was clear from the start of this phase that the couple experienced a recurring pattern in which resentments grew and a brief fight or argument took place, followed by a period of complete silence on the topic of concern. Thus, problems were never fully discussed or resolved. Misunderstandings were common, as each spouse made false attributions to and interpretations of the other's behavior (Beck, 1988). In the context of communication skills training it quickly became clear, for example, that the client's husband was very committed to the relationship and increased his working hours to help pay for the infant's medical bills and not in an effort to withdraw from the family (as alleged by the client). In the context of problem-solving training, the couple gradually learned to discuss problems fully and to reach a workable compromise (Beck, 1988; Frisch, 1989) in order to deal with the problems at hand. Problems discussed here included managing family finances, disciplining the eldest daughter, providing respite and housekeeping help for the client, increasing the size of the family, socializing with the husband's "drinking buddies" with the children present, and the division of labor for child care and household tasks.

3. *Cognitive therapy (in general) and assertion training (in particular)* were instituted with the client alone in sessions 14 through 22 in order to help her resolve problems with her father which, at this point in treatment, were the most pressing to the client and seemed to be the primary "external" difficulty contributing to her depression. In addition, the client was assisted through graded task assignments in setting up a *support group* for parents of children with coronary heart disease (the first of its kind in central Texas), and in solidifying and extending the previous gains made in cognitive individual and couples therapy. The establishment of the support group represented the culmination of problem solving and numerous graded task assignments aimed at establishing ties with parents in a similar situation.

The client's thoughts and feelings (e.g., extreme guilt and anger) toward her father were clarified in a homework assignment to write an uncensored letter to the father that would never be sent but would nonetheless discuss the client's feelings and specific requests for behavior change (Frisch, 1989). Problem solving was pursued by choosing three general strategies for life satisfaction enhancement from Quality-Of-Life Therapy (Frisch, 1989). The client decided to try and improve her relationship with her father by sharing her concerns with him in an assertive but respectful way, even though the possibility of ostracism and rejection could not be ruled out. She also decided to boost her overall satisfaction by lessening the importance of her relationship to her father to her overall well-being and by concentrating more on gaining satisfaction from her husband (who was receptive to change). A second letter was carefully constructed and delivered to the client's father who shocked the client by admitting his errors and by consistently changing his behavior in his daughter's presence.

By the end of therapy (session 22), the client's depression remitted completely, as evidenced by both a DSM-III-R interview and a reduction in her Beck Depression Inventory scores from 22 to 4. Her overall life satisfaction score on the QOLI changed markedly from -2.53 to 2.88, indicating a move from very low satisfaction to satisfaction in the normal range for a general, nonclinical

adult sample of 509 participants (Frisch, 1992). While the client's initial QOLI indicated dissatisfaction (negative ratings) in 14 of 17 areas, the reverse was true of her QOLI at the end of treatment, which consisted of 14 positive ratings. These improvements were echoed by the client's husband, who at the conclusion of therapy remarked, "Our house is like a different world. I've got my wife back. She's no longer moody, depressed, and moping around the house!" These gains over the course of therapy are particularly striking in light of the stressors impinging upon the client at the time of her second assessment—that is, the serious illness and imminent major heart surgery of her infant daughter, and the loss of her husband's job (which burdened an already-poor family). A four-month follow-up assessment showed that the client had continued to improve.

Hayes, Nelson, and Jarrett (1987) define the treatment utility of assessment as the degree to which assessment is shown to contribute to beneficial treatment outcome. While it is impossible to conclusively demonstrate the QOLI's utility with a single case, use of the QOLI appeared to enhance the therapeutic outcome of the present case by quickly identifying all major problem areas related to the client's depression before her first interview with the therapist and by providing normative information on the client's overall level of life satisfaction. No other assessment device or interview procedure seems as comprehensive as the QOLI in assessing life problems and strengths. In addition, use of the QOLI may have enhanced the outcome of this case by orientating the client to the rationale and procedures of cognitive therapy; the simplicity of the QOLI and its scoring scheme helped the client see how external problems and her attitudes about these directly contributed to her dissatisfaction and depression. Life satisfaction is a subjective, cognitive construct that fits nicely with cognitive therapy. Since life satisfaction is defined in the QOLI as the extent to which a person believes that his or her most important needs, wishes, and goals have been fulfilled, many clients (including the one discussed here) can readily see how their happiness can be a function of both external circumstances and cognitions such as their perception and interpretation of life circumstances, the importance assigned to particular areas of life, and the standards of fulfillment or goals that they set for themselves in valued areas of life (Frisch, 1989).

To the extent that the QOLI helps clients to understand the rationale of cognitive therapy and to see a direct relationship between assessment and treatment, it also enhances the therapist's credibility and facilitates the development of a collaborative therapeutic relationship. This may be another mechanism through which use of the

QOLI may contribute to beneficial treatment outcome. It also points up the potential value of the QOLI as a cognitive therapy treatment tool in its own right and not just an assessment device. The QOLI has aided treatment in ways besides making the rationale for treatment more understandable. For example, many clients react to their QOLI rating profiles with surprise at recognizing the many areas of satisfaction in their lives and the moderate (as opposed to severe) level of dissatisfaction in some valued areas. The reaction is akin to what cognitive therapists observe in clients who express surprise in seeing high pleasure and mastery ratings in their completed activity schedules. Some clients also benefit by using the narrative portion of the QOLI to generate solutions to the problems that hinder their satisfaction in valued areas of life. Finally, overextended clients can establish priorities by ranking areas of life in terms of their importance.

PROBLEMS AND COGNITIVE THERAPY TREATMENTS ASSOCIATED WITH QOLI'S 17 AREAS OF LIFE

An examination of problems expressed about each area of life assessed by the QOLI reveals (a) key specific problems associated with the client's depression and other difficulties; (b) important information about the client's thoughts, schemas, and cognitive distortions; and (c) important information about the client's life circumstances and life-style. Often this information is not revealed by initial interviews because of time constraints limiting the number of life areas that can be discussed, ignorance on the part of the clients as to how life problems may contribute to their distress, and their reticence to reveal information in a face-to-face encounter with a relative stranger. Examples of client concerns associated with various areas of life reported in the narrative portion of the QOLI under the rubric "Problems Interfering with Satisfaction" are presented in Table 3-2. In addition, the results of an informal content analysis of problems associated with each area of life are presented below, along with associated cognitive and quality-of-life therapy techniques.

The content analysis of the narrative portion of the QOLI is based on five samples of 281 psychotherapy outpatients (92%) and inpatients (8%) who completed the QOLI at the start of treatment. In order to represent the concerns of typical psychotherapy outpatients, the content analysis was based primarily on a sample of 20 depressed outpatients referred to the author by primary care physicians and a sample of 127 counselees seeking treatment at the Baylor University Psychological Services and Health Center (see Frisch et al., 1992, for a full description of the

sample). All of the depressed outpatients displayed prominent symptoms of depression, with half of these meeting the full DSM-III-R criteria for major depression. The remaining three samples included inpatients residing in a chemical dependency unit of a private psychiatric hospital ($N = 22$), residents of the Waco Family Abuse Center ($N = 14$) who were involved in either group or individual psychotherapy, and outpatients referred by the McLennan County Adult Probation Department ($N = 98$).

The problems enumerated by depressed outpatients and Baylor counselees with respect to *health* (see Table 3-1 for definitions of each area of life) fall within the following four categories:

1. *Poor fitness and health habits.* Typically, the problems of being overweight and "out of shape" (i.e., in need of exercise) were seen as impediments to satisfaction in the area of "health." Some respondents also cited problems with alcohol, drug, and cigarette use.
2. *Chronic illness or disability.* These included back problems, impaired hearing and eyesight in the elderly, coronary heart disease, and allergies (a common problem in central Texas).
3. *Recent illness, injury, and surgery.* Among the reported problems were ulcers, kidney stones, and pain from an automobile accident.
4. *Symptoms of psychological disturbance.* Symptoms included those of depression (e.g., tired, irritable, poor appetite, insomnia), anxiety (e.g., dizzy spells, upset stomach, faintness, fear of panic or anxiety attacks), anger, bulimia, and headaches.

Clinical examples of problems associated with health and other areas of life can be found in Table 3-2.

Problem solving and other cognitive therapy interventions can be effective in ameliorating clients' depression by boosting their satisfaction in the area of health. One client felt significantly less depressed after changing her shift work schedule and being referred to an allergist for the treatment of debilitating allergies. This case illustrates what Beck (1976) calls the "speck in the eye syndrome" (p. 227), in which an unresolved practical problem contributes significantly to psychological distress and depression.

Cognitive therapy techniques aimed at alleviating "target" symptoms (Beck et al., 1979) of depression such as sadness, anger, passivity, and sleep disturbance can also effectively boost satisfaction in the area of health by giving clients some measure of control over their symptoms of distress. For example, one depressed client

TABLE 3-2 Clinical Examples of Problems Listed in the Narrative Portion of the QOLI ($N = 281$)

Health-Related Concerns

I have AIDS.

The stomach and sleep problems, fatigue, headaches, and aching joints for over a month have been very frustrating.

I suffer from excessive birthdays. They've given me a bad back and a touch of arthritis, which keeps me from doing the things I'd like to do.

I'm overweight and need to exercise more. I have terrible allergies. My arthritis and bad hearing make it hard to do things like drive.

I have fibercitis nuisance pain, and my eyesight isn't good. Can't read as much as I'd like without pain, and reading's a big part of my job (teacher).

Increasing problems with "PMS". I'm angry and irritable all the time. I smoke, drink, do drugs, and eat poorly.

I suffer from mental and physical exhaustion from my weekly rotating-shift work. Lots of stress, very bad back problems, teeth need work, body needs exercise. Frequent headaches, insomnia, and upset stomach.

My bouts of fainting spells scare me. I have ulcers, chest pain, and get out of breath easily.

I'm always getting sick due to stress. My allergies are killing me! Bulimia.

I'm afraid these anxiety attacks will cut my life short. Polio in my right leg keeps me from doing the things I'd like to do, like exercise.

Self-Regard Concerns

I feel worthless and inferior to the "gracious" ladies I know in society. They've got college degrees, faithful husbands, and perfect poise in groups. I'm a loon, a loser, and a kook.

I feel very inadequate. I'm no good at anything.

I've lost confidence in myself, in my looks, job, car, bank account, and my ability to hold on to the people most dear to me.

My main problem here is my failure to maintain the moral standards I set for myself by having an affair and wanting to leave my wife.

I'm dumb and unattractive.

I don't feel consistently good about me as a person or a professional. I often feel like I'm inadequate, lazy, and don't work enough. It's like I don't have the right to live and be happy.

I am too critical of myself and expect too much of myself. I expect myself to be perfect. I'm fat and weird. I don't like the way I handle stress. I only feel good about me when other people say good things about me.

Sometimes I really don't like or care about myself and I don't want to live.

I have a tendency to believe it's my fault when things go wrong.

I always feel like a failure. I can't make decisions and feel comfortable about them.

I have no willpower over life's temptations, especially drugs and alcohol. I'm tempted to hide from responsibilities and not commit myself to anything.

The way I cope with my problems is by drinking and using drugs, therefore I have little respect for myself when I'm sober.

My self-regard is very low at present due to my divorce and use of drugs.

I would like to think of myself as a good person, but I hate myself for leaving my husband even though he beat me up. I wish I could quit blaming myself whenever things go wrong.

I think I'm stupid for not knowing what to do with my life. I can't seem to get my priorities straight. I wish people wouldn't take advantage of me so much. That's how I got in trouble with the law.

I'd feel better about myself if I could control my temper more.

I feel like I've had more failures than successes.

I'm working at a job where you're likely to get criticized a lot. Nurses are such bitches.

Philosophy of Life Concerns

I never set goals for myself. I just live one day at a time.

I need to define my personal goals more clearly and achieve them in a more gradual stepwise fashion. I don't know what my priorities should be.

I have no idea what career to pursue and I'm about to graduate.

(Continued)

TABLE 3-2   *(Continued)*

I'd like to be a good wife, mother, and teacher. I'd like to start going to church and meet people.

I'm afraid to be hopeful or excited about the future because, if I do, I'll get "zapped" for sure.

I forsake my goals and values when upset. I second-guess all my goals, values, and decisions. This makes it impossible to enjoy what I'm doing, since I wonder if I should be doing something else or should get more out a situation, like my marriage.

I'm confused about religion, something that's important to me. My family and their church think it's a sin to be lesbian. I wonder if that's why I'm depressed. It's God's punishment for my life-style.

I'm not sure what's right or how to act in a situation. I'm tired of following the crowd or just following my parents' advice.

I get "wasted" on drugs and daydream about how good things are going but really all it is, is a dream, because I really have nothing under control in my life.

I've lost all direction and wandered out of my moral bounds. I'm trying to "grow up" and find my own direction.

I wish I could control my temper and not give up on life because of tough situations.

My only philosophy was to make money, but no matter how much I make, it just seems to disappear.

I would like a better set of values. Something to help me cope with everyday hassles.

My standards and goals are too high. I never feel satisfied, like I accomplished something.

I can't really speak for myself. I almost always ask someone else to make decisions for me.

The challenge here is to accept myself as not perfect, and to learn to live one day at a time instead of trying to get everything done at once.

I have no philosophy. I wish someone would help me so I'd have something to go by. I don't know what to believe anymore.

I want to be a good father and husband and a good provider. It's most important to be respected by people and by my family.

I still haven't achieved the goals I set for myself as a teenager.

I get stressed out easily due to being raised religious and straying from this rearing. I have no basic core of values or beliefs to work from.

Being honest and hardworking doesn't work when you've got five patients to please and someone gets left out or thinks the service is lousy while you're working yourself to death!

Abortion is murder. I aborted a child and can't live with it. My husband threatened to leave and take the kids if I didn't get rid of the baby [he wasn't the father].

Standard of Living Concerns

I'm broke and overspent on my credit cards. Financial problems constantly burden me. I feel inferior to friends with more money.

I don't have enough money to buy the things I want, live in a better place, pay for school, and be more independent of my parents.

I need help in planning for retirement and a secure income.

Texas real estate is in a recession. Can't keep my standard of living or predict what the economy will be in the future.

My husband and I don't budget money very well. When we get bored or depressed, we spend more than we have. Always buying things for the kids to make 'em happy and make up for our crazy life on drugs.

I'm very materialistic, with expensive taste.

Bettering myself through promotions or education and a better job would help.

I want to get my own place and get on with my life.

Trying to find a job. Don't have a car or furniture right now.

I wish my husband had a job so we didn't have to scrape to pay for gas and diapers.

I have a problem budgeting out money.

I wish I had a two-story brick house on 100 acres of land with Jags [Jaguars], Mercedes, and Caddies [Cadillacs] in the garage and no rent houses in the neighborhood.

Tired of being broke and owing everybody in the country money.

We live on a very strict budget, and I feel a whole lot of pressure to help out with the finances by working. I'd much rather be home with the kids.

(Continued)

TABLE 3-2 (*Continued*)

Work-Related Concerns

My job [as a homemaker] is thankless, lonely, and always there.

Unemployed.

I hate my new boss and my new job at the bank.

I would like to teach and not just be a teacher's aide.

One must be able to take care of material needs. I can't and haven't proved myself adequate to find a job or make a living. Pitiful!

The economy makes my job uncertain. Could lose it any time, and that scares me.

My wife's professional job conflicts with mine and takes me away from my work.

My job doesn't use my potential. It's high stress, with 10 talky people working in the same room.

My job is boring and I'm not appreciated.

Work and school take too much time. I have no time for myself.

My grades are lousy. I procrastinate and study at the last minute. I feel dumb compared with my friends.

I don't enjoy what I'm doing anymore and want to change jobs.

I need a job outside of the home so I can learn to deal with people. But I really don't want one just yet. I'm still afraid of people.

I'm not sure what type of occupation I want. I've been a housewife and a "druggie." Can't decide what kind of schooling I want.

My work performance has been halfhearted at best.

Work is very important, but I just don't seem to get the results the way I wanted or the way someone else like my boss wants.

My job is the only thing I could come up with at the time. It is in no way satisfying. It's just a paycheck.

I'm stuck on one step of the ladder to the top.

Need to learn to try not to control others working under me—to accept them as they are and trust them with responsibility. Need to lower my outrageous expectations of myself and others.

I want to be a performing artist in the music industry. I'd be miserable doing anything else.

I would like to learn a new trade as a building contractor once I learn how to manage a business.

Too much pressure. Not enough pay.

I hate work. I can't satisfy all these people—the patients or the other nurses.

Recreation Concerns

I never recreate. I just work, come home, and watch TV.

I seem to spend all my time working or keeping my house in reasonable shape. Wish I had more time for reading and seeing good movies and plays.

I worry about work all the time, which ruins the leisure time I have. I feel guilty for taking time off.

I don't know exactly what to do to enjoy myself.

I don't seem to have the time for this, and when I do have time, I don't seem to have the money.

There is no recreation in my life. I spend all my time away from work getting drugs or trying to figure a way to get them.

My definition of recreation has been to see how high or drunk I can get. That's not fun for my wife or kids.

I need to find some new hobbies.

I like to go dancing and jogging, but there is almost never a babysitter or enough time. I like to watch TV, but my husband always watches what he wants to watch.

I would like to find more things to do that don't involve drinking or drugs.

Learning-Related Concerns

I'd like to go to college, but I'm not smart enough. I always hated school.

I used to be a real student of my profession, but now I've lost interest in keeping up.

I lack formal education or training in my field.

I would like to finish my B.A., but I can't justify the money for this, since our children need to be educated and this is our first priority.

I'd like to take a class in photography or ceramics, but I never get around to it.

My grades are lousy. I can't seem to concentrate or pick up on things like other students do.

(*Continued*)

TABLE 3-2   (*Continued*)

I've been killing off brain cells [with drugs] instead of feeding them with knowledge. Need to find some interest or direction and go for it. Would like to get my GED and maybe some college.

My husband don't want me to go to school or college, but I do.

Afraid I can't cut it in technical school. Tried once, but couldn't get what the books or teacher were saying.

Creativity-Related Concerns

Most of my "creative time" is taken up by my job and family demands.

I'm just not imaginative enough.

I'm bright enough to understand the brilliance of "stars" in my field, but not bright enough to shine equally brilliantly.

My bad attitude has basically killed any creativity I had in business.

I am too shy to share my creative ideas with others.

I'm creative, but have felt "blocked" lately and don't know why.

I'm boring not creative.

My mind thinks of things to do all the time, but if I start to do something, I just get disappointed or bored and quit.

I never really express myself. I used to in school. I played every kind of saxophone and clarinet and even won awards for it!

I used to develop new ways to approach people in telemarketing and introduce the product. I also loved to decorate my home. Now I have no interest or energy for this.

I'm not a very creative person.

Creativity is important to me. You need it to do small jobs around the house and fix things.

I used to collect recipes and stamps, but my husband would get mad and throw them in the trash. He said it wasn't important, but it made me feel good inside knowing that the things I collected were of good use again and again.

I don't have the time or privacy to really be creative in what I like doing, which is art.

I can't concentrate enough on one thing to stay interested.

Need some training and money for equipment to pursue photography. Can't seem to learn to play guitar.

I used to paint in my little travel trailer when my husband and kids were off in the world. I loved it and hours would pass before I noticed it. Something keeps me from it now. I don't know what.

Social Service Concerns

I thought about becoming an AA "buddy" to help out and keep my sobriety going.

I felt better when I used to volunteer at the food bank. I felt useful there.

I'm not making the time. This is an area that used to make me happy, but I put it on the back burner.

I would like to get involved, but I don't know how to help or where to get started.

I'm overcommitted to causes and groups and need to cut back to balance this with other priorities, like family and work.

I'm too wrapped up in myself to see the needs of those around me.

I feel guilt for not doing more, but I don't have the time.

I haven't done this. Drugs made me selfish. I was interested in no one except myself.

No problem if I stay sober.

Two problems with my social service are time and money. I seem to have neither one right now.

I'm new here and don't know any volunteer groups I could join. I don't do anything. I used to be active in my church.

Civic Action Concerns

I can't undo the damage I suffered, but I can help change the laws that make marital rape legal in this state.

I haven't cared about this until now, but I'd like to learn enough about our nation, state, and community to at least vote.

I don't care enough to get informed about what's happening in the world.

I'm interested, but don't know how to get involved.

No time.

I hate politics, 'cause politicians lie all the time. It's just a big game and makes no difference who wins.

(*Continued*)

TABLE 3-2   (*Continued*)

This is important, 'cause I want my son to grow up in a good town.

I should try and expose myself more to local and national information, so I can vote and play my role in society like a respectable citizen.

Need to get more involved.

I always keep up with the news, but I never voted before or supported a political cause or candidate. My husband takes up all my time. I want to vote in the next election.

As a "retired" housewife with no career, I still see caring for kids as my "vocation." We do a lousy job in this town, and I'd like to try and change that.

Love Relationship Concerns

I feel taken for granted and unappealing to my husband. We don't have enough romantic time together.

My wife is the obstacle.

Men in general are assholes.

Screw 'em.

I feel I can't compete with his (my husband's) first wife, so I put up walls to keep from getting hurt.

I have an outstanding relationship with the woman I'm involved with. My marriage is hindering my ability to pursue this relationship.

There's a lack of physical and emotional intimacy. I can't be honest with him.

My sour moods get in the way. She isn't affectionate enough. I make demands, she withdraws.

I'm shy and don't date.

My boyfriend's suicide and memories of us together make it impossible for me to get on with my life. I can't go anywhere or do anything without being reminded of him.

Lost. I feel at my age and as a divorced person, there is no more right or opportunity for a relationship.

We don't understand each other and fight over stupid things. This is the most important thing in my life right now. It's a roller coaster ride that's destroying me.

My wife has been "having" her doctorate for five years, and we've had to defer gratification in several areas of our relationship in order to achieve her professional goals.

I'm separated from my husband, who is selfish and likes to drink, do dope, and smoke. He is violent to me and the kids at times.

I want a lover very badly!

I demand too much.

My husband is irritable, rude, and just wants to "watch the grass grow" now that he's retired. He's driving me crazy now that he's home all the time.

I place too much importance on this.

I've never been in love. I don't know what it is. I think I confuse it with sex. Still, I want a man.

I can't decide if it's worth the pain. It seems like a form of dependency.

I won't let people get close to me.

My husband is overseas in the army with drug and legal problems.

Not happy due to so many hurts. It's just that I'm scared to trust men.

My relationship with my wife and family has suffered. I put drugs before them. I felt I needed no companionship as long as I had drugs.

I seem to hurt everyone who tries to get close to me.

My wife and I get along well and she loves me very much, but I don't consider her needs and give her the love and understanding she gives me. She is being cheated out of what she deserves.

I'm not able to maintain a lasting relationship.

I've shown very little feeling of affection to my wife for the past couple of years. There's hardly any romance left in our relationship.

I'm afraid that my wife won't stay clean and support my sobriety.

It's wonderful if there's no abuse. The violence *must* stop.

I would love to be in love again.

I feel used and deceived. I wanted more from our relationship than he did.

Too many complications. I don't seem to have enough money or hair to get the girls I like.

I need someone to love me. I feel that without that I wouldn't make it sometimes.

Not satisfied. One big problem. I'm 19 and never "did it," but I lie so other people won't make fun of me.

I found out he was unfaithful after he died, and it's tearing me apart.

(*Continued*)

TABLE 3-2   *(Continued)*

I don't know what the big problem is. He's much older than me. Perhaps it's a generation gap.

Friendship-Related Concerns

I have no friends of my own. My only friends are my ex-wife's friends.

Need to find people who won't tempt me to do drugs. Need to develop friendships with equal give-and-take. No schemes or distrust, just open acceptance.

Friendships take time. My time goes to work and family. That troubles me.

I don't put regular time into this like I should. My moods interfere. It's easier to stay to myself. I'm also picky and have trouble accepting friends who seem too boring or conventional. My wife won't socialize as much as I would like, which keeps me home in "solitary confinement."

I used to have friends coming out of the walls. I only have a few now. I just haven't been much of a friend lately.

I feel inferior to my friends, so I put up walls to keep from being hurt.

My wife and I withdraw socially when under stress and haven't developed the close friends that could give us support in these hard [economic] times.

Don't really trust them. Afraid they'll dump me eventually.

I have no friends now. My best friend ran off with my son's father.

I'd like a girlfriend I could talk to. My husband said I'd "fool around" if I had friends. What shit! But I believed it and still have the fear myself.

I worry if they like me. They aren't caring enough and seem too moody and preoccupied with their own problems.

I can't get along in groups or with other women.

I expect too much of them.

I should have realized a long time ago the need to nourish and maintain friendships.

It's hard to like others when I dislike myself.

I'm not outgoing enough. My insecurity pushes people away.

I don't stand up for myself, and spend too much time with people I don't like.

I hold back a lot. Don't want to burden them with my problems.

I hurt everyone I come in contact with.

Don't have no friends besides my sister and her husband.

Seems like my friends deceived me, like they weren't real friends. Everyone is so two-faced!

I have acquaintances, but no friends. I also miss my sister terribly.

Concerns About Children

I'm always a taskmaster rather than a friend to my kids. I need freedom from the pressures of making a living so we can do more fun things together.

I feel I let my children down by not being there while they were growing up.

Don't spend enough time with my oldest because of our busy schedules.

My 8-year-old won't mind me now that the baby is here, and my husband doesn't back me up enough when I discipline her.

Our baby has a heart condition and may need a transplant. We have to find a babysitter who knows CPR. A cold or the flu could take her from us.

I'm often impatient with our children, wanting kids of 7 and 19 to think and act like a 47-year-old. Our son is off at school, and I'm not enjoying disengaging.

I'm having maternal urges, but I'm scared to start a family.

I wish our son could see that we're aging and make more time for us.

I want children, but only with the right woman.

I don't know my kids as good as I want to. I hardly ever touch them, much less hug them.

My relationship with my stepkids is strained, to say the least.

Things are great when my wife is around, but I get nervous and I can't handle the responsibility when I'm the only one around to care for them.

I have no children right now, but I really want to.

I've neglected my children in many ways for years. They have problems with drugs because of my influence. I

TABLE 3-2   (*Continued*)

need to provide them a good example and give them support to grow and change.

My eldest two kids stay with their grandmother. It's hard to have one here and two over there. I love 'em all and want us all to be together again.

I'd like to have two kids before I leave this world. This would put something positive in my life instead of being empty.

I can't have kids, but would like very much to have two or three.

I'd like to get custody of my kid.

If I could just figure out where I went wrong and why. They're avoiding me. Everything went wrong with my kids.

Concerns About Relatives

My parents are very judgmental. My dad "needles" me about my weight and tells me how to raise my kids.

In order to keep a "peaceful" atmosphere at home with my wife, I've had to completely turn my back on my relatives.

I have no relationship with my father or brother.

I have disowned my family and have just recently, after 20 months of not speaking, started to communicate again.

It seems there has been more arguments lately, but I'm not sure why.

Most of our relatives have so many personal problems of their own that they aren't in a position to offer us support.

I don't know what to do now that my mother is gone. She was my best friend, and I cared for her for 35 years.

There is an empty space when it comes to my dad.

My parents expect a lot, and I hate to disappoint them. Sometimes I feel I don't measure up. My dad intimidates me.

Bad.

All my relatives have drug or alcohol problems.

I don't know. I love and respect them, but it doesn't seem I can trust them anymore.

I'm too ashamed of myself—my actions, how I look when I'm stoned—to spend time with them, so the relations haven't been good.

I need to open up the channels of communication and show them I care.

My sisters are all crazy. They want me to do everything for them but won't give me any help when I need it. My father always bitches when I go to see him, so we all have bad relations right now.

Can't get along with my mom. We're always fighting. The whole family looks down on me for being arrested three times in one year.

I feel like I always have to prove myself to them, and I'm tired of it. Don't like to be told to act different when I know what I want.

Home-Related Concerns

My home is a mess. It's falling down around me. I let the yard go to hell. It was beautiful when I moved into it. Now it should be condemned. I live in a nice neighborhood. My run-down house and I are the only dark spots in it.

We live on my mother's land. I think if my mobile home was elsewhere, I would feel more like it was mine.

I can't stand living with my in-laws. I do ok with my mother-in-law, but I hate her son with a passion.

My home is an apartment, and I'm not satisfied with this. Would like to build a house for my family. Don't know if I could do the concentration and planning required.

The house needs work, but I can't afford it and I don't feel well enough to do what needs to be done.

Our house is too small and cramped for a family with three kids. I'd like more space and to live in the country.

I hate living at home with my mother. My girlfriend made me leave the house we worked so hard to fix up.

I hate my roommate. He's messy, noisy, and won't give me any privacy!

I hate living alone, and I'm a homebody. Maybe I'll move back home with my family.

I don't have a home right now, but I really want one with plenty of space, nice furniture and a big, well-kept yard.

The psychiatric hospital staff here are too damn bossy and mean. I've got a nice home but can't afford it now that my wife left me.

Neighborhood Concerns

I don't like it. There aren't enough lights. Alcoholics take over the playground from the kids. I don't feel it's even

TABLE 3-2   (*Continued*)

safe enough for my kids to play outside. We'd like to move but can't afford it.

I just want to live in a clean, safe neighborhood with decent people, not druggies, thieves, and prostitutes.

I love living in the country, but I get insecure when my husband is on the road.

This is a bad neighborhood. It's scummy and full of trashy people. Some of them dig through the dumpsters for garbage.

I live in a bad part of town. Lots of crime; rude, noisy people.

Too much concrete. I want to live somewhere with some trees and lakes around.

Too expensive.

My hallmates in the dorm are a pain. It's too loud and there's no privacy.

Baylor is stagnant, nonintellectual, complacent, and conformist. The "Baylor Bubble" is too insulated from the rest of the world.

I have to find one. I've got no place to go when I leave the hospital.

There's nothing here—no parks, ball fields, restaurants, or things to do.

Lots of break-ins. I had one just three months ago.

There's lots of robberies and shootings. There's not really any safety, and the electric bills are very high.

The people next door are slobs. The street is all dirt road, and they never pick up the trash on time.

We're isolated in the country. Not enough neighbors around to make friends with.

Too many drugs and not enough things to do. Seems like everyone around my house is a drinker.

I hate living in the projects. People look down on me, 'cause I'm white in a black neighborhood.

Community Concerns

Waco is hell, a cultural and gourmet wasteland.

I don't like the conservative, Baptist influence and the extreme poverty and segregation. There's not enough entertainment, culture, or decent restaurants.

There are very few single people my age here, except those who are divorced with children.

I live a double life as a gay in a conservative town.

The economy and political climate are antibusiness. My business is dying, and I see no hope or help on the horizon.

The U.S. is hypocritical. It says it's a democracy, but it supports terrorism.

I hate it because the violence is very bad.

Waco is boring.

Not too pretty or crime free.

It's too unsafe. I can't even go jogging and feel OK.

The job market is bad, and I'd prefer a larger city.

The community as a whole is too conservative. It's lacking in culture and open-minded people.

It sucks.

I live in a small community where there is nothing of interest to do.

I want to live closer to my family and relations.

The town seems geared for white-collar folks, with little to offer the working man.

Waco is Baptist! A fundamentalist Baptist is a terror, don't you think?

Other Concerns

Can I ever be "normal" again?

Consistent mood control is elusive.

I'm not taking care of the things I should be as a husband and father. I took all the good things life has to offer for granted. I've been living as if the whole world owes me. My life is a small circle. I go to work and get stoned. My wife takes care of the kids and everything else.

I'm tired! I'm going home to sleep. I have insomnia. I've been taking my husband's sleeping pills when I feel so tired but can't get to sleep.

I can't decide on professional work goals and standards that are reasonable.

I'm concerned about my wife's relationship with my best friend. She also doesn't get along with my older sister.

I'm weak and easily led. My mother, grandfather, and sister give me a hard time. My husband is lazy a lot.

(*Continued*)

TABLE 3-2 (*Continued*)

Fear of craving for alcohol. I also fear being with my wife and kids. My wife drinks and I hope she'll quit. It will help us both.	I'm in debt to my ears. I want to move to Dallas, but I can't afford it and the probation department won't let me.
I have a very serious stomach disorder that drove me to do drugs in the first place.	I have no father, and I have to listen to a stepfather who doesn't give a shit about me and who won't practice what he preaches.
I worry about the urge to do drugs and steal. I avoided the mall, 'cause I found myself in stores thinking about shoplifting.	I worried about the future, my finances, my ability to be successful and happy.

learned to manage sadness through "self-sympathy" and "diversion" techniques in the early stages of treatment, thereby increasing his "health" satisfaction. Another client had a similar positive reaction to techniques for controlling his insomnia. Finally, the cognitive therapy techniques of graded task assignments, bibliotherapy, and problem solving (dubbed "search for alternative solutions" by Beck et al., 1979) can alleviate concerns related to *all* areas of life assessed by the QOLI, including health.

With respect to *self-regard*, both depressed and counseling-center outpatients felt inadequate (i.e., low self-efficacy) and self-disparaging over their failure to meet their own standards of performance and success in key areas of life such as work, school, love relationships, parenthood, weight control and physical appearance, friendships, ethical conduct, coping with life problems, and "psychological self-control" (the ability to manage and control symptoms of psychological disturbance such as depression, anxiety, and substance abuse). Clinical examples of problems associated with self-regard can be found in Table 3-2. Many of the self-regard concerns expressed in Table 3-2 are indicative of "dissatisfaction depression" (Frisch, 1989) and "demoralization" (Franks, 1974) insofar as respondents seem depressed, demoralized, and self-critical about their failures in meeting personal standards of performance and success in valued areas of life. For this reason, the strategy of boosting self-esteem and alleviating dissatisfaction depression by building clients' competencies in valued areas of life and programming success experiences in these areas through homework assignments has been successfully applied in these cases (Beck et al., 1979; Frisch, 1989). Cognitive therapy techniques such as graded task assignments, cognitive rehearsal of task assignments, the scheduling of activities that foster a sense of mastery or accomplishment, and assertion training are also useful in

boosting self-regard through success experiences in valued areas of life.

Cognitive difficulties characteristic of depression were common in concerns related to self-regard, including perfectionism and excessively high standards ("I expect myself to be perfect"), self-blame ("it's my fault when things go wrong"), labeling ("I'm dumb and unattractive"), and overgeneralization ("I'm no good at anything"). Many of these concerns are alleviated by standard cognitive therapy techniques such as reality- or hypothesis-testing of self-disparaging thoughts (e.g., "I'm a lousy mother") and teaching clients to "talk back" to self-critical thoughts with rational replies (e.g., "I do a lot of things right as a mother"), both informally and with the aid of the Daily Record of Dysfunctional Thoughts. Reattribution techniques aimed at reducing self-blame for events beyond a client's control have also been helpful in improving self-regard.

With respect to *philosophy of life*, both depressed outpatients and counselees reported difficulties in formulating, following, and achieving key personal goals and ethical standards (see Table 3-2 for examples). Depressive symptoms of excessive guilt over transgressions and suicidal thoughts were also expressed here. Interventions useful in this area include developing short- and long-term career goals, cognitive rehearsal of tasks needed to achieve long- and short-term goals, graded task assignments and activity scheduling to implement strategies for achieving goals, cognitive restructuring of immediate fears of failure, and referral of clients to ministers, priests, and rabbis known to be tolerant in order to clarify religious questions (e.g., "Is it a sin to be gay?") and alleviate guilt (Beck et al., 1979; Frisch, 1989). The evaluation of depressogenic philosophical assumptions and values by weighing their advantages and disadvantages has also been helpful, as in the case of a client who decided it was not wrong to leave an unhappy marriage of 20 years given his wife's adamant refusal to discuss problems, make changes, or pursue marital therapy. The cognitive therapy manual also offers helpful treatment suggestions for making decisions, establishing priorities in life, and dealing with unfair treatment, guilt, and suicidal thoughts. Such issues are commonly tapped by the philosophy-of-life dimension of the QOLI.

Cognitive techniques must usually be supplemented with behavioral techniques to successfully challenge depressogenic philosophies. For example, a client effectively disputed the assumption that her encopretic child was "lazy" and disobedient though a medical examination that revealed a physical cause of the encopresis (i.e., a bowel obstruction). Similarly, a redheaded adolescent changed her view that redheads looked "gross" to guys after finding redheaded models in teen magazines as part of a "reality-testing" homework assignment. Perfectionist clients benefit from experimenting with less ambitious short-term and intermediate goals. Religious clients often benefit from church involvement in two ways: (a) Church can provide a major recreational and social outlet, buffering the client from the major life stresses usually associated with depression (Abramson et al., 1989); and (b) religious beliefs are often extremely adaptive, comforting, and helpful in encouraging clients either to make change efforts or to accept intractable problems such as physical disabilities or relationship problems that have proved impervious to change. Even the most farfetched religious beliefs may be adaptive rather than disruptive to day-to-day functioning in the "real world" (Lazarus & Folkman, 1984; Taylor, 1989). Of course, some religious beliefs may be psychonoxious to particular clients in particular circumstances (Walen, DiGiuseppe, & Wessler, 1980).

With respect to *standard of living,* clients reported problems in budgeting and a need for greater income to pay for basic necessities, a car, a home, hobbies, retirement, and financial independence from their parents (see Table 3-2 for clinical examples). Clients' satisfaction in this area has been increased through teaching budgeting skills via bibliotherapy, changing expensive "tastes," vocational counseling aimed at securing better jobs, and both problem solving and graded task assignments aimed at experimenting with new budgets and financial arrangements. The cognitive therapy manual suggests referral of clients to financial consultants when therapists lack the expertise to deal with their difficulties. Some clients have also benefited from assertion training aimed at securing needed child support and government assistance (e.g., food stamps).

Depressed outpatients typically cited one of five problems as interfering with their "work" satisfaction: (a) interpersonal conflicts with coworkers, the boss, or upper-level management; (b) the nature of the work itself being unfulfilling; (c) excessive work demands or "pressure"/ stress; (d) feeling inadequate either in finding a job or in doing the work; or (e) job insecurity (see Table 3-2 for examples). Less frequently, unemployment, a lack of necessary skills and education, low salary, and competition from a spouse's career were cited as problems. In contrast, undergraduate counselees typically complained of poor school performance in terms of either grades or the ability to learn, retain material, and show their knowledge on tests. Most often, students attribute their subpar performance to distracting "emotional problems," an internal and stable character flaw that makes learning difficult, a lack of motivation, a lack of career goals and direction, an overload of courses, "procrastination," or poor study habits.

Assertion training including role-playing and/or graded task assignments has been helpful in: (a) resolving conflicts with coworkers or family members who object to the client's career goals; (b) promoting job-finding and interviewing skills; and (c) encouraging clients to request help from professors or employment counselors on ways to improve school performance or to find a job that fits their ability and interests. For example, a depressed nurse felt great relief after assertively requesting that she not be placed on an intensive care unit until she received further job training. The cognitive therapy techniques of problem solving, graded task assignments, and bibliotherapy related to careers have been effectively supplemented with counseling test instruments such as the Career Assessment Inventory that identify potential career paths. Graded task assignments to visit technical, community, and liberal arts colleges have also been valuable in helping clients establish short- and long-term career goals. Such goals by themselves can often resolve academic problems in students who saw no connection between classwork and their intended lifelong careers.

Impediments to *recreational* satisfaction typically involve a perceived lack of time or failure to engage in favorite hobbies or pastimes like golf, reading, or socializing. Those who perceived a lack of time for recreation seemed to let other activities take priority, leading to an impoverished, dull, and routinized life-style dominated by work (see Table 3-2 for examples). Less often, respondents said they could not enjoy available leisure time due to not knowing what to do to relax and enjoy themselves; worry or guilt over taking time away from work or household duties; an overreliance on television for entertainment; an unwilling spouse; or, in the case of an agoraphobic client, fear of recreating alone. Counselees frequently cited loneliness—that is, a lack of friends or a social group—as an obstacle to enjoyable recreation.

Involvement in leisure-time pursuits may alleviate clients' depression by providing efficacy-related success experiences and by reducing self-disparagement and self-preoccupation (Beck et al., 1979; Frisch, 1989). Cognitive therapy techniques of problem solving with the aid of instruments like the Reinforcement Survey Schedule, graded task assignments, time management, and hourly activity scheduling (including some pleasurable activities each day) have been useful in increasing clients' recreational satisfaction. Lonely college students and problem drinkers with alcoholic friends have also benefited from social skills training aimed at making new friends and developing love relationships. Bibliotherapy and classroom instruction in favored hobbies like photography have also proven useful in enhancing clients' satisfaction with leisure (Frisch, 1989). Increasing clients' satisfaction in the areas of learning, creativity, social service, civic action, and relationships also increases recreational satisfaction for some clients who associate all of these areas with leisure. When clients dismiss the value of recreational outlets, "philosophy-of-life" and other cognitive interventions may be necessary. For example, one "workaholic" client would only recreate after proving to himself through activity scheduling and discussions with his therapist and wife that such recreation was essential to his mood control and marital satisfaction. Bibliotherapy and other interventions based on the emerging field of leisure therapy can effectively complement cognitive therapy techniques for increasing satisfaction with recreation (DiLorenzo, Prue, & Scott, 1987).

With respect to *learning*, depressed outpatients saw a need for further education and training in other careers but felt unable to pursue this because of financial constraints, a lack of time, higher priorities such as educating their children, or a lack of intelligence or ability to complete necessary schoolwork (see Table 3-2). Undergraduate counselees typically saw poor school performance as an obstacle to satisfaction. They attributed their poor performance to myriad factors, including a lack of intelligence or ability, distracting "emotional problems," lack of motivation, lack of career goals, an overload of courses, or poor study habits. Occasionally, clients expressed a desire to take courses for recreational purposes, including classes in ceramics or cooking. Many of the cognitive therapy techniques applicable to the areas of "work" and "philosophy of life" are useful in addressing learning-related concerns; these techniques include problem solving, bibliotherapy, graded task assignments, assertion training, and "reality" or hypothesis testing to dispute clients' feelings of inadequacy. With respect to the last

approach, a math-phobic nurse successfully completed a required math course after debunking her assumptions that she was "too dumb" and more intimidated by the subject than her classmates. Specifically, these assumptions were rejected once she successfully completed the arithmetic subtest of the WAIS-R (administered by her therapist) and discovered that her classmates were equally concerned about their performance in the class.

Respondents felt their *creativity* stifled by a lack of time, ability, or confidence (see Table 3-2 for examples). Less often, they attributed their poor creativity to a lack of assertion (some felt too shy or fearful to express creative ideas); an unsupportive spouse, boyfriend, or girlfriend; or a lack of money needed for necessary equipment or instruction. Small success experiences such as the expression of one's emotional pain through a diary, poetry, or a drawing have helped to boost the self-efficacy of depressed clients, thereby helping them to question their beliefs of generalized inadequacy and impotence (Frisch, 1989; see Sarason, 1990) for a discussion of successful programs to treat depression through skill training in creativity). While fostering clients' creative skills through graded task assignments, skill training, problem solving, and bibliotherapy does not constitute a complete treatment plan for depression, such efforts may have a definite "snowball effect" (Beck et al., 1979) that begins the process of debunking the cognitive triad and other depressogenic beliefs. This is especially true when a broad definition of creativity is employed (as in the QOLI) that allows for creative expression in everyday pursuits such as work or home decorating. The cognitive therapy techniques applicable to the area of recreation have also proved useful in addressing client concerns related to creativity, including the use of instruments like the Reinforcement Survey Schedule to identify creative hobbies of interest.

Most clients saw their satisfaction with *social service* stymied by underinvolvement due to a lack of time, interest, or a compelling cause or issue (see Table 3-2 for examples). Some did not know how to get involved, had become cynical about the value of service, or lacked logistical support (e.g., transportation). A few clients felt dissatisfied due to overinvolvement in this area such that other priorities in life (e.g., work, love relationship) were beginning to suffer. For those to whom social service was important, it enhanced satisfaction and alleviated distress in at least four ways. First, it often functioned as a social and recreational outlet (e.g., coaching on a softball team, volunteering at a hospital) that, when neglected, resulted in a noticeable drop in pleasure or fulfillment. Secondly, it could boost clients' self-esteem and sense of efficacy to think that as "down and out" as they were, they could help others in a significant way (Frisch, 1989; Frisch & Gerrard, 1981). When helping others with similar difficulties, as when a problem drinker would serve as an AA "sponsor" or an assault victim would serve as a counselor in a shelter or rape crisis center, clients reinforced their own coping efforts by imparting these to others. Depressed patients also benefited from the lowered self-preoccupation and opportunities for downward social comparisons associated with service pursuits (Frisch, 1989). Problem solving and graded task assignments are especially useful in devising and carrying out social service projects for depressed clients.

Dissatisfaction with *civic action* was usually attributed to underinvolvement in the area due to a lack of time or interest (see Table 3-2). Lack of interest was often attributed to apathy, cynicism, and a sense of hopelessness in being able to effect change, especially for college counselees. A few clients felt dissatisfied due to an overinvolvement in civic affairs. The role of civic action in efforts to alleviate psychological distress seems similar to that of social service activities. While therapists and clients often discount the importance of these areas, involvement in social service and civic action can significantly ameliorate both depression and problems of addiction that are often associated with depression (Lazarus & Folkman, 1984; Peele & Brodsky, 1991). Satisfaction in both areas can be promoted through problem solving and graded task assignments.

Dissatisfaction in the area of *love relationships* was typically attributed to either conflict and communication problems in an existing relationship or to loneliness and the lack of such a relationship (see Table 3-2). Conflict often centered upon feeling misunderstood, alienated, unloved, or sexually dissatisfied. Grief over the end of a relationship or the death of a partner or spouse was a major obstacle to fulfillment cited by a few clients. Relationship interventions in general, and love relationship treatments in particular, focus on either improving relationship skills or cognitive restructuring. Typical cognitive intervention techniques such as use of the Daily Record of Dysfunctional Thoughts and reattribution of blame are useful in cases where a partner either takes too much (e.g., victims of domestic violence) or too little (Jacobson & Margolin, 1979) responsibility for their relationship difficulties. Cognitive techniques are also called for in the case of single clients who feel too unworthy, unlovable, and unattractive to ever find a suitable partner.

Relationship competencies and confidence (or self-efficacy) in the key areas of communication, problem solving, and positive behavior exchange can be increased through the application of social skills and assertion training, role-playing, problem solving, graded task assign-

ments, activity scheduling, bibliotherapy, and other cognitive-behavioral approaches described in the cognitive therapy manual and elsewhere (Beck, 1988; Burns, 1985; Frisch, 1989; Frisch et al., 1982; Frisch & Higgins, 1986; Jacobson & Margolin, 1979; Primakoff, 1983). The need to modify overt interactional patterns as well as internal cognitions has increasingly been acknowledged by cognitive therapists treating relationship difficulties (Beck, 1988; Epstein, 1983). This dual emphasis necessitates the involvement of all parties in a relationship dispute at some point during treatment. Additionally, single clients usually need to develop attitudes and life-styles that promote self-acceptance and the ability to form new relationships (Burns, 1985; Primakoff, 1983).

Conflicts or alienation with existing friends and the lack of close friendships are commonly cited as barriers to satisfaction in the area of *friendships* (see Table 3-2 for examples). Clients typically feel distant from friends and neglectful of these relationships. Those without close friends blame a lack of time or personal problems such as shyness, mistrust, and self-preoccupation for their isolation. The cognitive and skill training techniques useful in treating difficulties in love relationships are also effective in treating relationship difficulties involving clients' friends, children, and relatives. In addition, techniques specifically earmarked for developing and maintaining friendships have proven useful (Burns, 1985; Fensterheim & Baer, 1975; Frisch, 1989; Frisch et al., 1982; Primakoff, 1983).

Typically, clients attributed their dissatisfaction in *relationships to children* to feeling distant or in conflict with their children (see Table 3-2). A few depressed clients and most college counselees (whether single or married) cited the lack of any children as the chief impediment to satisfaction in this area. In addition to the cognitive and skill training approaches discussed with respect to "love relationships," cognitively based family treatments (Bedrosian, 1983) and child behavior management approaches (Clark, 1985; Masters, Burish, Hollon, & Rimm, 1987) have proved useful in this area. Single clients who are desirous of children benefit most from interventions aimed at developing a "love relationship," which they usually view a prerequisite to starting a family.

Most clients saw distance from or conflict with parents or siblings as an obstacle to satisfaction in the area of *relationships with relatives* (see Table 3-2 for examples). College counselees attributed problems with parents—almost always their father—to exorbitant parental expectations and pressure to be "the best in everything." Others cited poor communication, limited autonomy, and parental fighting or emotional problems as the source of their conflict and alienation. A few clients mentioned grief over a lost parent as a significant obstacle to satisfaction. Depressed outpatients often felt at odds with what they saw as parental interference in and criticism of the new families they had started for themselves. In addition to the "love relationship" interventions discussed above, clients' satisfaction in this area has been increased through assertion training, problem solving, and cognitively oriented family therapy (Bedrosian, 1983).

Physical surroundings can be ignored by cognitive therapists preoccupied with client's inner experience, even though surroundings directly impact one's life satisfaction and mood (Andrews & Withey, 1976; Campbell et al., 1976; Frisch, 1989). Problems interfering with satisfaction with one's *home* typically involved problems with the physical structure of the house, the desire for a new home or residence, or interpersonal conflicts with those residing in the home (see Table 3-2). Clients often saw their homes as unattractive, in need of remodeling or repair, or too small, but felt unable to afford the cost of redecorating or moving. A few felt happy with their home but were either unable to afford it or in danger of losing it due to divorce. Many counselees disliked the lack of space, privacy, quiet, and freedom from rules in dormitories. Many counselees and a few depressed outpatients cited interpersonal conflicts with those residing in the home as an obstacle to satisfaction. Counselees typically reported conflicts with roommates over messiness, noise, privacy, and boyfriends or girlfriends. A few counselees who still lived with their family of origin also cited problems with family members. Concerns about surroundings, including one's home, are usually addressed by problem solving with respect to a particular concern, followed by graded task assignments aimed at implementing the problem's solution. For example, a depressed outpatient began to clean and decorate her house for the first time in years after implementing a plan to work as little as 20 minutes a day. Another client began to save money for a new house and to explore more lucrative career options to make a new home affordable. Clients in conflict with housemates have benefited from the above-mentioned interventions geared to relationships. In one case, a client successfully persuaded his wife to no longer allow their toddler to sleep in their bed.

Not feeling safe was the typical obstacle to *neighborhood* satisfaction cited by clients, whether they lived in a high-crime area of the city or in an isolated rural area (see Table 3-2). Counselees, in particular, also saw the inner-city neighborhood surrounding the university as "trashy" and "unattractive" with a lack of natural beauty (e.g., trees) and too many "loud, rude, noisy" or homeless people. Other clients wished to live in a neighborhood closer to work that was less expensive, noisy, and politically conservative. One patient with major depression feared ostracism from his neighbors once they learned of his affair and impending divorce of his wife of 20 years. Problem solving with regard to ways to minimize the danger of, improve, or leave a "bad" neighborhood, followed by graded task assignments aimed at implementing proposed solutions, have proved useful in increasing clients' satisfaction with their neighborhoods (Frisch, 1989). For example, a depressed widow who lived alone alleviated her anxiety and insomnia about a recent burglary by installing a home security system. Some clients find it useful to get involved with neighborhood political associations or police-sponsored "neighborhood watch" programs in order to deal with safety concerns. Others have resolved conflicts with neighbors through assertion training; one client successfully lobbied local government officials to increase the police protection and garbage collection services in her neighborhood after undergoing assertion training. In some cases, clients' exorbitant expectations for their surroundings must be lowered (in keeping with their financial resources and occupation) to boost satisfaction with their neighborhood (Frisch, 1989).

Clients typically cited the conservative climate and the lack of cultural amenities and good restaurants as Waco's major obstacles to *community* satisfaction (see Table 3-2). Others also cited a lack of available singles and recreational outlets, job opportunities, safety from crime, and well-paved roads. Two depressed patients, suffering from an economic recession, who commuted from Austin to Waco for psychotherapy criticized the political and economic climate of Austin as "anti-business." A few counselees criticized the Baylor University community as too conservative and insulated from the "rest of the world." One counselee criticized his community of origin and the United States as a whole! As in the case of neighborhood concerns, problem solving followed by graded task assignments aimed at implementing solutions has proven useful in addressing community concerns. One homosexual client decided to sell his business and move to Dallas in order to pursue a "love relationship" and to find a more active and supportive gay community. Other clients have benefited from aggressively testing their hypothesis that there is "nothing to do" in the community (Frisch, 1989). This assumption often functions as an untested excuse for not taking interpersonal risks. Some clients have created needed community resources where none existed, including a support group for parents of children with congenital heart disease, a singles group, and a group of folk musicians who play monthly at a local nightclub.

The QOLI answer sheet allows for the listing of "additional problems or concerns" on the back page of the inventory. This often elicits new concerns that clients cannot neatly fit into any of the 17 areas of the QOLI, or that come to mind only at the end of the inventory. Often these additional concerns relate to relationship, work, health, standard of living, psychological symptom(s), and substance abuse issues (see Table 3-2). Concerns related to an area of life assessed by the QOLI can be treated in ways suggested above. For example, a 19-year-old client successfully refused to go to summer school and to date a man imposed on her by her parents through the successful application of assertion training and cognitive restructuring techniques. The cognitive therapy manual also describes applicable treatments for problems that do not fit neatly into areas covered by the QOLI. For example, a client who listed insomnia as an "additional" concern on the QOLI responded to techniques for this problem suggested in the manual.

CONCLUSION AND FUTURE DIRECTIONS

The treatment utility of the QOLI may be assessed more formally with the "manipulated assessment strategy" suggested by Hayes, Nelson, and Jarrett (1987), by which the outcome of clients treated with and without information from the QOLI could be compared. Treatment utility may be more broadly defined and assessed by surveying clinicians about the extent to which the ease, efficiency, and pace of assessment, treatment planning, and treatment proper are increased though assessment instruments like the QOLI (Frisch et al., 1992). It may prove unrealistic to expect the use of initial assessment devices to consistently impact gross measures of outcome that are susceptible to numerous other influences (Kazdin, 1980). Even if treatment outcome is not measurably affected by use of the QOLI, its use may be warranted on the grounds that it increases the ease, efficiency, and pace of treatment planning and assessment, as seemed to occur in the cases discussed here. Furthermore, the QOLI's treatment utility may vary for therapists with different levels of experience; novice cognitive therapists may particularly benefit from the timely and comprehensive problem assessment provided by the QOLI. The usefulness of the QOLI may also vary with client characteristics. For example, it seems particularly suited to clients who (a) are unaware of some or all of the life problems contributing to their depression; (b) are unaware of strengths, resources, and areas of satisfaction they can draw upon in coping with their depression; (c) do not readily understand or accept the rationale for cognitive therapy; and (d) feel more comfortable with self-disclosure through a paper-and-pencil questionnaire than through a face-to-face interview with a relative stranger (the therapist) at the start of treatment.

ACKNOWLEDGMENTS. This research was supported, in part, through sabbaticals, Baylor University research committee grants, and release-time fellowships awarded to the author.

REFERENCES

Abramson, L. Y., Metalsky, G. I., & Alloy, L. B. (1989). Hopelessness depression: A theory-based subtype of depression. *Psychological Review, 98*, 358–372.

Andrews, F. M., & Inglehart, R. F. (1979). The structure of well-being in nine Western societies. *Social Indicators Research, 6*, 73–90.

Andrews, F. M., & Withey, S. B. (1976). *Social indicators of well being: Americans' perceptions of life quality*. New York: Plenum.

Beck, A. T. (1976). *Cognitive therapy and the emotional disorders*. New York: Meridian.

Beck, A. T. (1988). *Love is never enough*. New York: Harper & Row.

Beck, A. T., Rush, A. J., Shaw, B. F., & Emery, G. (1979). *Cognitive therapy of depression*. New York: Guilford.

Bedrosian, R. C. (1983). Cognitive therapy in the family system. In A. Freeman (Ed.), *Cognitive therapy with couples and groups* (pp. 107–124). New York: Plenum.

Beiser, M. (1971). A study of personality assets in a rural community. *Archives of General Psychiatry, 24*, 244–254.

Bigelow, D. A., Brodsky, G., Stewart, L., & Olson, M. (1982). The concept and measurement of quality of life as a dependent variable in evaluation of mental health services. In G. J. Stahler & W. R. Tash (Eds.), *Innovative approaches to mental health evaluation* (pp. 345–366). New York: Academic Press.

Blau, T. H. (1977). Quality of life, social indicators, and criteria for change. *Professional Psychology, 8*, 464–473.

Burns, D. D. (1980). *Feeling good: The new mood therapy*. New York: Signet.

Burns, D. D. (1985). *Intimate connections*. New York: Signet.

Campbell, A., Converse, P. E., & Rogers, W. L. (1976). *The quality of American life*. New York: Russell Sage.

Cantril, H. (1965). *The pattern of human concerns*. New Brunswick, NJ: Rutgers University.

Clark, L. (1985). *SOS! Help for parents*. Bowling Green, KY: Parents Press.

Coan, R. W. (1977). *Hero, artist, sage, or saint? A survey of views on what is variously called mental health, normality, maturity, self-actualization and human fulfillment*. New York: Columbia University.

Dattilio, S. M., & Podesky, C. (1990). *Cognitive therapy with couples*. Sarasota, FL: Professional Resource Exchange.

DeRubeis, R. J., & Beck, A. T. (1988). Cognitive therapy. In K. S. Dobson (Ed.), *Handbook of cognitive-behavioral therapies* (pp. 273–306). New York: Guilford.

Diamond, R. (1985). Drugs and the quality of life: The patient's point of view. *Journal of Clinical Psychiatry, 46*, 29–35.

Diener, E. (1984). Subjective well-being. *Psychological Bulletin, 95*, 542–575.

Diener, E., Emmons, R. A., Larsen, R. J., & Griffin, S. (1985). The Satisfaction with Life Scale. *Journal of Personality Assessment, 49,* 71–75.

DiLorenzo, T. M., Prue, D. M., & Scott, R. R. (1987). A conceptual critique of leisure assessment and therapy: An added dimension to behavioral medicine and substance abuse treatment. *Clinical Psychology Review, 7,* 597–609.

Emmelkamp, P. M. (1982). *Phobic and obsessive-compulsive disorders: Theory, research and practice.* New York: Plenum.

Epstein, N. (1983). Cognitive therapy with couples. In A. Freeman (Ed.). *Cognitive therapy with couples and groups* (pp. 107–124). New York: Plenum.

Evans, I. M. (1985). Building systems models as a strategy for target behavior selection in clinical assessment. *Behavioral Assessment, 7,* 21–32.

Fensterheim, H., & Baer, J. (1975). *Don't say "yes" when you want to say "no."* New York: Dell.

Flanagan, J. C. (1978). A research approach to improving our quality of life. *American Psychologist, 33,* 138–147.

Franks, J. C. (1974). *Persuasion and healing* (rev. ed.). New York: Schocken.

Frisch, M. B. (1988). *Quality of life inventory.* Waco, TX: Author.

Frisch, M. B. (1989, June). *Quality of life therapy: An integrative model of etiology, assessment, and treatment of depression and related disorders.* Paper presented at the World Congress of Cognitive Therapy, Oxford, England.

Frisch, M. B. (1992). *Test manual and treatment guide for the Quality of Life Inventory.* Waco, TX: Author.

Frisch, M. B. Cornell, J., Villanueva, M., & Retzlaff, P. J. (1992). Clinical validation of the Quality of Life Inventory: A measure of life satisfaction for use in treatment planning and outcome assessment. *Psychological Assessment: A Journal of Consulting and Clinical Psychology, 4,* 92–101.

Frisch, M. B., Elliot, C. H., Atsaides, J. P., Salva, D. M., & Denney, D. R. (1982). Social skills and stress management training to enhance patients' interpersonal competencies. *Psychotherapy: Theory, Research, & Practice, 19,* 349–358.

Frisch, M. B., & Froberg, W. (1987). Social validation of assertion strategies for handling aggressive criticism: Evidence for consistency across situations. *Behavior Therapy, 2,* 181–191.

Frisch, M. B., & Gerrard, M. (1981). Natural helping systems: A survey of Red Cross volunteers. *Journal of Community Psychology, 9,* 567–579.

Frisch, M. B., & Higgins, R. L. (1986). Instructional demand effects and the correspondence among self-report, naturalistic, and role-play measures of social skill as influenced by instructional demand. *Behavioral Assessment, 8,* 221–236.

Frisch, M. B., Villanueva, M., Cornell, J., & Retzlaff, P. J. (1990, November). *Clinical validation of the Quality of Life Inventory: A measure of life satisfaction for use in treatment planning and outcome assessment.* Paper presented to the annual meeting of the Association for Advancement of Behavior Therapy, San Francisco.

Hayes, S. C., Nelson, R. O., & Jarrett, R. B. (1987). The treatment utility of assessment: A functional approach to evaluating assessment quality. *American Psychologist, 42,* 963–974.

Hollandsworth, J. G. (1987). Subjective well-being and behavior therapy: Challenge, opportunity, or dead end? *Behavior Therapist, 3,* 65–68.

Hollandsworth, J. G. (1988). Evaluating the impact of medical treatment on the quality of life: A 5-year update. *Social Science and Medicine, 4,* 425–434.

Hollon, S., & Beck, A. T. (1986). Research on cognitive therapies. In S. L. Garfield & A. E. Bergin (Eds.), *Handbook of psychotherapy and behavior change* (pp. 443–482). New York: Wiley.

Jacobson, N. S., & Margolin, G. (1979). *Marital therapy.* New York: Brunner/Mazel.

Jahoda, M. (1958). *Current concepts of positive mental health.* New York: Basic Books.

Jakubowski, P., & Lange, A. J. (1978). *The assertive option.* Champaign, IL: Research Press.

Jarrett, R. B., & Nelson, R. O. (1987). Mechanisms of change in cognitive therapy of depression. *Behavior Therapy, 18,* 227–241.

Kane, R. A., & Kane, R. L. (1981). *Assessing the elderly: A practical guide to measurement.* Lexington, MA: Lexington Books.

Kazdin, A. E. (1980). *Research design in clinical psychology.* New York: Harper & Row.

Lazarus, A. A. (1971). *Behavior therapy and beyond.* New York: McGraw-Hill.

Lazarus, A. A. (1981). *The practice of multimodal therapy.* New York: McGraw-Hill.

Lazarus, R. S., & Folkman, S. (1984). *Stress, appraisal, and coping.* New York: Springer.

Lehman, A. F., Ward, N. C., & Linn, L. S. (1982). Chronic mental patients: The quality of life issue. *American Journal of Psychiatry, 139,* 1271–1276.

Masters, J. C., Burish, T. G., Hollon, S. D., & Rimm, D. C. (1987). *Behavior therapy: Techniques and empirical findings* (3rd Ed.). New York: Harcourt Brace Jovanovich.

McKnight, D. L., Nelson, R. O., Hayes, S. C., & Jarrett, R. B. (1984). Importance of treating individually assessed response classes in the amelioration of depression. *Behavior Therapy, 15,* 315–335.

Morganstern, K. P. (1988). Behavioral interviewing. In A. S. Bellack & M. Hersen (Eds.), *Behavioral assessment: A practical handbook* (3rd ed.). New York: Pergamon.

Mulherm, R. K., Horowitz, M. E., Ochs, J., Friedman, A. G., Armstrong, F. D., Copeland, D., & Kun, L. E. (1989). Assessment of quality of life among pediatric patients with cancer. *Psychological Assessment, 1,* 130–138.

Mulhern, R. K., Fairclough, D. L., Friedman, A. G., & Leigh, L. D. (1990). Play performance scale as an index of quality of life of children with cancer. *Psychological Assessment, 2,* 149–155.

Peele, S. & Brodsky, A. (1991). *The truth about addiction and recovery.* New York: Simon & Schuster.

Primakoff, L. (1983). One's company; two's a crowd: Skills in living alone groups. In A. Freeman (Ed.), *Cognitive therapy with couples and groups.* New York: Plenum.

Rogers, C. R. (1951). *Client-centered therapy.* Boston: Houghton Mifflin.

Salamon, M. J. (1988). Clinical use of the Life Satisfaction in the Elderly Scale. *Clinical Gerontologist, 8,* 45–54.

Sarason, S. B. (1990). *The challenge of art to psychology.* New Haven, CT: Yale University.

Seeman, J. (1989). Toward a model of positive health. *American Psychologist, 44,* 1099–1109.

Strupp, H. H., & Hadley, S. W. (1977). A tripartite model of mental health and therapeutic outcomes. *American Psychologist, 32,* 187–196.

Taylor, S. E. (1989). *Positive illusions: Creative self-deception and the healthy mind.* New York: Basic Books.

Taylor, S. E., & Brown, J. D. (1988). Illusion and well-being: A social psychological perspective on mental health. *Psychological Bulletin, 103*, 193–210.

Turkat, I. D., & Wolpe, J. (1985). Behavioral case formulation of clinical cases. In I. D. Turkat (Ed.), *Behavioral case formulation* (pp. 5–36). New York: Plenum.

Veenhoven, R. (1984). *Conditions of happiness*. Boston: D. Reidel.

Walen, S. R., DiGiuseppe, R., & Wessler, R. L. (1980). *A practitioner's guide to rational-emotive therapy*. New York: Oxford University.

Watson, D., Clark, L. A., & Carey, G. (1988). Positive and negative affectivity and their relation to anxiety and depressive disorders. *Journal of Abnormal Psychology, 97*, 346–353.

Wolf, M. M. (1978). *Social Validity: The case for subjective measurement. Journal of Applied Behavior Analysis, 11*, 203–214.

Young, J. E., & Beck, A. T. (1982). Cognitive therapy: Clinical applications. In A. J. Rush (Ed.), *Short-term psychotherapies for depression* (pp. 182–214). New York: Guilford.

SUGGESTED READINGS

Diener, E. (1984). Subjective well-being. *Psychological Bulletin, 95*, 542–575.

Frisch, M. B. (1989, June). *Quality of life therapy: An integrative model of etiology, assessment, and treatment of depression and related disorders*. Paper presented at the World Congress of Cognitive Therapy, Oxford, England.

Persons, J. B. (1989). *Cognitive therapy in practice: A case formulation approach*. New York: Norton.

Spilker, B. (1990). *Quality of life assessments in clinical trials*. New York: Raven.

4

Generalized Anxiety Disorder

Ellen Costello and Thomas D. Borkovec

Generalized anxiety disorder (GAD) involves excessive or unrealistic anxiety and worry over multiple life circumstances, with accompanying symptoms of autonomic hyperactivity, motor tension, and vigilance and scanning (DSM-III-R; American Psychiatric Association, 1987). From a cognitive-behavioral perspective, the disorder represents perhaps the most diffuse and complex cognitive/ affective state among the anxiety disorders (Barlow, 1988). To the person with GAD, the world and especially the future are seen as dangerous much of the time, and the individual feels that he or she does not have resources to cope. A vicious cycle of threat cue detection (Mathews, in press), a mixture of somatic activation and inhibition (Borkovec, Shadick, & Hopkins, in press), and worrisome thought activity (Borkovec & Inz, 1990) perpetuates habitual anxious responding.

Because of the absence of the circumscribed phobic avoidance characteristic of other anxiety disorders, cognitive-behavioral therapy for GAD has focused on interventions designed to provide the client with alternative cognitive and somatic coping responses to *internal* triggers (i.e., anxiogenic thoughts, images, and physiological sensations). This chapter presents a description of the treatment of a GAD case via such a package of techniques. The client participated in a controlled therapy outcome investigation; thus, the therapist was limited by the treatment protocol to the use of specific techniques and did not have freedom to employ additional interventions.

The therapy package was a multimodal treatment involving self-monitoring (with emphasis on learning to detect increasingly early anxiety cues), progressive and applied relaxation training, and self-control desensitization (Goldfried, 1971) with coping imagery and self-statements. Thus, in-depth cognitive therapy was not employed; rather, elements from cognitive therapy were primarily used to create self-statements for deployment in self-control desensitization rehearsal and in daily life. A worry program, in which the client postpones worrying to a 30-minute period later in the day, was an additional component of therapy—during the worry period, he or she engages in problem-solving and cognitive therapy exercises aimed at the content of the worrying. Twelve individual therapy sessions were provided on a twice-a-week basis with two fading sessions over the final month. The first five sessions were 90 minutes in length; all others were 60 minutes. The conceptual model underlying this package stresses the importance of rapidly terminating chains of anxious responding (especially worrisome thoughts) to prevent further strengthening of anxious associative network in memory and of rehearsing multiple

Ellen Costello • Butler Hospital, Providence, Rhode Island 02906. Thomas D. Borkovec • The Stress and Anxiety Disorders Institute, Department of Psychology, Pennsylvania State University, University Park, Pennsylvania 16802.

Comprehensive Casebook of Cognitive Therapy, edited by Arthur Freeman and Frank M. Dattilio. Plenum Press, New York, 1992.

coping responses to incipient anxiety cues in imagery and in daily living.

CLIENT BACKGROUND INFORMATION

Mike, a 34-year-old married male with one child, presented for treatment of chronic anxiety. At that time he was a doctoral candidate. There was no family history of anxiety, depression, or alcohol abuse. He was one of four children. At intake, Mike described himself as having worried "all my life" and as being "eager to please." He felt pressured by his family to achieve and was perfectionistic with high performance standards. His strengths included a good social support network and a history of career success.

ASSESSMENT AND DIAGNOSIS

The revised version of the Anxiety Disorder Interview Schedule (ADIS; DiNardo, O'Brien, Barlow, Waddell, & Blanchard, 1983) was used to determine diagnoses and was conducted separately by two independent assessors who both assigned a primary diagnosis of generalized anxiety disorder to Mike. The client also received secondary diagnoses of social phobia and simple phobia (air travel, animals, blood, and injury). At pretherapy, assessor severity ratings (0–8 point scale) were obtained for each diagnosis, and Mike completed several assessment questionnaires, including the STAI-Trait (Spielberger, Gorsuch, & Lushene, 1970), Zung Anxiety Rating Scale (Zung, 1975), the Penn State Worry Questionnaire (Meyer, Miller, Metzger, & Borkovec, in press), and the Beck Depression Inventory (Beck, Ward, Mendelson, Mock, & Erbaugh, 1961; see Table 4-1 for pretherapy, posttherapy, and 12-month follow-up scores). He also rated his level of anxiety three times a day on a daily diary form (1–100 point scale) throughout the duration of treatment and used this form for monitoring of thoughts.

From the interviews and questionnaires, several features of the client's disorder were revealed. Mike's current worries focused on finances, work and school performance, and marital and child-rearing responsibilities. Physiological symptoms included muscle tension in his neck and lower back, restlessness, easy fatigability when stressed, sleep disturbance, irritability, difficulties in concentration, shortness of breath, accelerated heart rate, and flushes. Cognitive beliefs centered around thoughts such as "I'm letting my family down," "I'll never get over my problem," "I'm inadequate," and "People will turn against me." Specific stressful situations contributing to

TABLE 4-1 Pretherapy, Posttherapy, and 12-Month Follow-Up Scores on Outcome Measures

	Pre	Post	12 Mo.
GAD-Assessor Severity (0–8 pt. scale)	4.8	1.0	0
Social Phobia-Assessor Severity	4.0	1.5	0
Simple Phobia-Assessor Severity	2.5	0	0
STAI-Trait	62	33	38
Beck Depression Inventory	14	4	5.5
Zung Anxiety Rating Scale	39	26	27
Penn State Worry Questionnaire	66	29	34
Client Daily Diary (0–100 pt. scale)	20	13	8

his generalized anxiety involved confronting authority figures, using computers, negotiating household and child-care responsibilities with his wife, public speaking, examinations, group projects, and meetings with his professors.

TREATMENT: OVERVIEW

Through frequent self-monitoring, Mike learned to detect increasingly early and mild anxiety cues and to let go of his worries through applied relaxation. He was taught to recognize maladaptive cognitions, challenge them, and substitute more helpful self-statements. These adaptive self-statements were practiced in imaginal self-control desensitization as he visualized himself relaxing while confronting stressors. Because he frequently engaged in catastrophizing, decatastrophizing skills were taught and practiced.

Homework was assigned regularly. Two daily 15-minute progressive relaxation sessions were suggested, with 5 minutes of self-control desensitization practice at the end of each relaxation session. In addition, he was instructed to check himself hourly, at any change in activity, or at any other time when he noticed incipient physiological or cognitive signs of anxiety and to practice letting go of these responses. By the eighth session, he began deliberately putting himself in stressful situations so that he could practice using his coping strategies. Elements of cognitive therapy began at the fourth session. As soon as he developed some skills in identifying and modifying self-statements, he used these techniques in daily life in response to incipient anxiety cues. He also set aside time daily for the worry program, either developing solutions and cognitive coping alternatives or relaxing away worries.

The therapist worked with Mike to identify the most effective interventions for him while encouraging him to use a broad and flexible array of coping techniques. A cooperative, open relationship was essential because of the need for the therapist to have access to information about compliance, signs of relaxation-induced anxiety (Heide & Borkovec, 1984), and cognitions.

More detailed description of intervention strategies and Mike's experience with them is provided below.

Applied Relaxation

Both progressive (Bernstein & Borkovec, 1973) and applied (Ost, 1987) relaxation techniques were used with Mike. Progressive relaxation began with training him in 16-muscle-group procedure and having him focus carefully on the difference between feelings of tension and relaxation in the muscle groups. Over the course of therapy, abbreviated relaxation was taught by combining muscle groups to seven and later to four major groups. Once he could relax easily, Mike was instructed to dispense with tensing and releasing his muscles, to pay attention to any feelings of tension in the various muscle groups, and to relax the tightness away. The final step involved counting from 1 to 10, letting go more and more on each count. Relaxation patter provided by the therapist during training emphasized being aware of the sensations of relaxation; letting go; slow, rhythmic breathing; and enjoying the pleasant resulting feelings. Diaphragmatic breathing techniques (slowed, 8–10 cpm stomach breathing) and positive imagery were also practiced and encouraged as means of rapid applied relaxation response.

Throughout therapy, relaxation application was emphasized. Self-monitoring helped the client identify increasingly early anxiety cues. Mike was instructed to check himself frequently for incipient cognitive or physiological signs of tension and then to spend a moment relaxing the tension away. For example, when he noticed tightness across his back and shoulders and shallow breathing as he was working on an assignment in the library, he immediately responded by taking four slow, rhythmic breaths and imagining his back muscles loosening up "like melted cheese." Mike discovered that early intervention was extremely effective in reducing his level of tension and, coincidental to greater relaxation, was surprised to discover the frequency of maladaptive cognitions, particularly his tendency to criticize himself for minor mistakes. He experienced much more difficulty in letting go of worrisome thoughts than in releasing muscle tension and found that a combination of redirecting his attention to his breathing pattern, focusing on enjoying the pleasant physical sensations of relaxation, and instructing

himself to "let go" were partially effective interventions prior to initiation of worry programs and cognitive therapy elements of therapy. His success in being able to eliminate intrusive thoughts was related to the amount of time spent practicing these skills both in therapy sessions and during daily activities.

While the most important practice of applied relaxation occurred outside of therapy, it was also rehearsed in the session: Whenever the therapist noticed observable signs of anxiety, she would instruct him to relax it away. Additionally, encouraging personal metaphors for relaxation was particularly useful. Mike once described the process by saying, "I look at it as an emptying thing: a bulldozer going through a vacant lot full of rubbish and cleaning it up quick."

Although circumscribed phobic situations are not always present in GAD, there are multiple situations that increase anxiety. As Mike was learning to apply relaxation skills in his daily life, he and the therapist worked together to identify situations in which he was frequently anxious. He then confronted these situations using his relaxation techniques before, during, and after these exposures. For example, he became tense whenever his routine was disrupted, so he deliberately created such situations and applied his new strategies. He would request meetings with professors who intimidated him, debate in class, or confront study group members who weren't pulling their weight so he could gain practice in applying his relaxation techniques to stressful events. As his relaxation skills improved, he repeatedly mentioned in therapy how amazed he was to discover how easy it was to let go of things like this, even when his anxiety was at severe levels. Mike reported that the combination of deliberately seeking these situations and responding differently to them with relaxation gave him an increased feeling of self-control.

Elements of Cognitive Therapy

Mike's relaxation applications to deliberately created stressful situations increased his opportunities to practice reacting adaptively in situations and also gave him a chance to collect new evidence to challenge underlying beliefs that were identified in the course of cognitive therapy. The following is an example.

I had done the whole routine, you know, the morning ritual, getting up, drinking coffee and all that sort of stuff, and everything was just hunky-dory and at 6:40 a.m. my wife said, "I have to go to town early today, so I'll drop you off on campus." Initially I thought, "Well, that's fine," and then I thought, "Wait a minute, that is not fine because I have, you know, we have to get everybody organized and out the door at the same time." In the morning my son has his little routine and I have my little routine, and I talk to the same professor every Monday, Wednesday, and Friday morning on the bus and I sort of enjoy him, it's a lot of fun. I realized that, boy, my routine is going to get wrecked up this morning. Well, it really wasn't. I got in here to campus and was at my carrel at the same time and everything and I had the same amount of time before class started and the whole business, but it seemed like for a while there that everyone, my whole world, had sort of been turned upside down and dumped on the floor and I had to sort through it to get it back together. Afterwards I felt like, "Get, it wouldn't have mattered 5 or 10 minutes one way or the other. I didn't have to be there at exactly the same time or earlier. I realized, before the bus was to arrive, I could have split, that I had a choice. I thought it was maybe better to deal with it than dash out the door and think about it. I thought it might be nice to see how well I could cope with it, and what I found interesting was that once I was out of the car and kissed everybody and said goodbye that it shut off and everything was OK.

In the above example, Mike remained in a stressful situation but was only mildly successful at containing his anxiety. However, he did get new information that helped him to begin to reevaluate the rules he imposed upon himself.

Although he was embarrassed to talk about it, Mike believed that his worrying actually kept disaster from striking. Somehow, if he focused on the worst possible outcome, it was less likely to occur and he would be prepared for it if it did occur. Related to this was a fear of losing control; consequently, he was afraid to let go and relax. To challenge these beliefs became an important task of therapy, because successful treatment depended on Mike's compliance in letting go of worry. As long as he believed it served an adaptive purpose, he would be conflicted about doing so. Other beliefs that were central to Mike's generalized anxiety disorder related to the benefits of self-criticism and perfectionism. A belief that he didn't have enough time to do all he had to do was also present. Some of Mike's worries had to do with his social phobia; Mike worried about the impression he made on others and feared their disapproval. This contributed to his anxiety about saying or doing the wrong thing. There were feelings of dread that "something bad will happen to my wife or son," although he couldn't articulate any specific concerns. As is typical of many clients with GAD, he believed prior to the therapy that he would never get over his problem; he had worried all his life ("It's just the way I am").

Cognitive therapy techniques to modify such maladaptive cognitions included self-monitoring of automatic thoughts, decatastrophization, logical analysis, and searching for alternative interpretations, the products of which were used in self-control desensitization. In addition to using the Socratic method within therapy sessions, the therapist had Mike gather evidence in support of alternative beliefs between sessions and practice substituting more adaptive cognitions in a range of situations in daily life. Within sessions, the therapist focused on possible alternative perspectives to the scenarios presented by Mike. Because anticipating future disasters is inherent in generalized anxiety disorder, decatastrophization is a particularly useful technique with this population. Mike was frequently asked what the worst possible outcome in a situation was, how likely it was to occur, how severe the damage would be if it did occur, and how he could cope in a worst-case scenario.

For example, one representative situation that distressed him was thinking about the comprehensive examination he needed to pass to obtain his doctorate. Within his department there was a high failure rate, and he had been through a recent experience of "freezing" in a test situation. Furthermore, his educational background differed from his classmates; he had earned his master's degree at another university. Prior to presenting this item in self-control desensitization, the therapist addressed certain elements of his logical errors in thinking;

THERAPIST: What would happen if you failed?
MIKE: Ah, well, I already checked that out. You have two options—one is you can take another one within four months or you can take an oral within two weeks.
THERAPIST: But you can't do both?
MIKE: You can't do both, no. If you fail the second written [exam], you can take an oral two weeks after that.
THERAPIST: What is the likelihood you would actually fail this thing twice? Three times, basically; to take it and fail and take it again within four months and fail it again, and take an oral and fail that?
MIKE: Pretty slim chance from what I have been able to judge so far. I don't think they are out to cream anybody. I don't see any maliciousness in the department committees or anything like that. My concern would be that I'd go in there and choke.
THERAPIST: Your mind would go blank?

MIKE: Yeah, which happened on an exam in the fall. A final and I sort of . . . it scared me.

THERAPIST: And what happened in that class?

MIKE: I got a B.

Through this exercise, Mike realized that even when the worst occurred—which in this case was "freezing" on an examination—the outcome was still acceptable to him. While his perfectionism pushed him to desire optimal performance, he was willing to accept an adequate performance that allowed him to advance on his career path. He had blown the incident out of proportion while failing to incorporate what actually had happened in the past into his view of the future. He experienced considerable relief in going through this exercise and had an immediate reduction in anxiety regarding his upcoming exam.

Through the use of the Socratic method, Mike's beliefs about the benefits of perfectionism, high performance standards, and negative self-evaluation shifted. He began to see these as having no evidential basis and as merely interfering with his functioning by creating anxiety. As a result he generated more adaptive self-statements, which he then substituted in his self-talk. He also practiced these new self-statements in his self-control desensitization sessions using images representative of situations that tended to elicit those previous maladaptive perspectives.

Worry Program

Mike was trained to recognize early signs of anxiety by checking himself often for anxious reactions and intervening immediately. To facilitate letting go of worrisome thoughts, he began using the worry program. He was told that upon recognizing a worry, he should let go of it through a combination of relaxation strategies and coping self-statements. If he wasn't successful in doing so or if the thought repeatedly returned, he was to postpone thinking about it until his worry period. Each day he was to set aside no more than one half hour for the worry program, preferably at the same time and place each day to facilitate discriminative control of worrisome activity. Mike became well rehearsed in verbalizing self-instructions that postponed worry and directed attention to the task at hand, as is demonstrated in the following session excerpt.

MIKE: I saw that the professor was correct and there was a feeling afterward, "Oh my God, if I can be that far off the mark on something that's relatively simple, I may be really in trouble in this course." But then that sort of passed and I kinda put it aside and hadn't really thought about it since.

THERAPIST: Do you have any idea of how or why it passed?

MIKE: Well, because I consciously said that I would put it aside. I said, "You don't have time this week to worry about this stuff. Get the homework done, get it out of the way, hand it in on Thursday morning and if you want to worry about it, worry about it some other time."

He was taught to divide his current worries into two groups during the worry period—those that could be helped through problem-solving techniques and those that could not. Part of the half-hour period was then used to develop realistic plans for dealing with those worries that might be eliminated through problem solving. The rest of the session was spent developing more adaptive self-statements to replace the remaining worries. This program was very effective in helping Mike terminate his daily worrying and providing structured time to apply cognitive therapy methods to his worrisome cognitions.

After three weeks of using the worry program, Mike came in apologetically, explaining he had curtailed his use of the worry program.

THERAPIST: How's the worry program going?

MIKE: (pauses) It seems I don't have a lot of—in fact, I skipped today and yesterday altogether because I just sorta sat down, looked out the window, and thought, "Well, what are you going to deal with today?" Didn't have anything. I mean if there were things I should worry about, I didn't know what they were.

The above dialogue presents a marked contrast to Mike's remark in his first therapy session that "When I don't have a lot to worry about, it's just one more thing to worry about."

Self-Control Desensitization

With Mike, self-control desensitization was used in sessions 4 through 11. By session 12 he reported that no imagery scenes were generating anxiety, so coping responses to three scenes that had previously elicited anxiety were practiced. In self-control desensitization, each scene is presented with the therapist attempting initially to elicit anxiety by elaborating anxiety cues. The anxiogenic scenes have three components: the situation, the physiological symptoms of anxiety most typically experienced in that situation, and negative cognitions characteristic in the situation. Once the client signals anxiety, relaxation patter begins while the client continues imagining the scene as if he or she were really in it. Remaining in the image, he or she imagines letting go of the anxiety through the use of relaxation and coping self-statements. Once anxiety is eliminated, he or she continues to imagine being in a relaxed state in the situation, continuing to use the coping responses. Throughout the use of self-control desensitization, the therapist draws external and internal cues flexibly from a hierarchy beginning with mild anxiety cues and continuing over sessions to higher items, so that the client has repeated exposure to and practice in responding differently to the full range of representative anxiety cues.

Mike's hierarchy from which items were constructed was divided into three clusters of low, medium, and high anxiety representing situational, somatic, and cognitive cues, examples of which are given below.

A self-control desensitization hierarchy is not a traditional hierarchy in the sense that one specific fear is broken into small steps and presented. Rather, a graduated range of representative situations and cues that elicit feelings of generalized anxiety are systematically employed. A typical scene presentation, taken from session 11, follows.

I want you [Mike] to imagine the following situation as vividly and realistically as possible, as if you were actually in the situation. Please signal by raising your finger at the first sign of anxiety and leave it raised until the anxiety has gone away. You are sitting in the examination room, looking at the exam. Your heart is beating rapidly and the muscles of your neck and shoulders are tense. As you read the questions, you realize you can't answer the first

---

Situations

Low	Medium	High
Seeing a snake	Course examinations	Being the focus of unexpected attention
Sharp knives	Financial transactions	Public speaking
	Saying no to anything work related	Being criticized by authority figures

Somatic Reactions

Low	Medium	High
Fatigued	Rapid heart beat	Irritable
Lower back muscle tension	Flushes	Muscle tension in neck
	Feeling on edge	Mind going blank
	Difficulty concentrating	Choking sensation

Cognitions

Low	Medium	High
"That was stupid."	"What if something happens, and we don't have enough money to cover it?"	"I can't function under the pressure of time constraints."
"You should have thought of that."	"I'm inadequate."	"I gave a poor performance."
	"I'm losing control."	"I'm letting my family down."
	"I'll never get over my problem."	"I don't express myself well."
	"I'm different from other people; I just don't fit in."	"Something horrible is going to happen to my family."
	"What if I fail?"	

---

two. Your heart races as you think, "I can't do this. I'm going to fail. My mind is going blank." (Client signals.) Now, continuing to stay in the situation . . . relax away the tension . . . slow, rhythmic breathing . . . slowing down your heart rate . . . melting your thoughts . . . muscles loosening up and unwinding as you focus on the pleasant feelings of muscle relaxation . . . just continue visualizing being in the exam situation as the muscles of your neck and shoulders continue to relax more and more deeply, more and more completely . . . as you just let go.

Such patter continued until Mike indicated he was relaxed by dropping his finger. He continued to image himself in the examination situation and relaxed himself in that situation for another 20 seconds. He was then instructed to turn off that scene, but to continue relaxing for 20 to 30 seconds. In the next scene presentation, further coping imagery was elaborated once anxiety was signaled, drawing from the products of earlier cognitive therapy.

You think to yourself, "I studied this. I feel confident I can do a reasonable job if I slow down, think it over, and take it one step at a time." You remain aroused, but relatively relaxed as you work on the exam.

Each scene is repeatedly presented until there is evidence of effective coping. Such evidence is seen in the increasing amount of time required for the imagery to elicit feelings of anxiety and in the decreasing amount of time necessary to eliminate the anxiety once elicited. The above exam scene was presented to Mike 10 times, and he then practiced it at home twice a day during his relaxation practice. By the end of therapy, this scene no longer elicited anxiety, nor in fact did any other scene from his hierarchy.

SUMMARY

This client responded well to treatment. At the end of therapy, he said, "I feel like a new person," and attributed his treatment success to relaxation, imaginal desensitization rehearsal, the worry program, and early intervention upon identification of anxious thoughts. His pretherapy, posttherapy, and 12-month follow-up scores are presented in Table 4-1. His compliance with the treatment regimen and homework assignments were major factors in his success. Other attributes that may have contributed to a positive outcome included high intelligence, excellent verbal skills, high motivation to change, and a strong

social support system. Treatment occurred in the context of a strong therapeutic alliance. By therapist observation, there was no evidence of a personality disorder or the occurrence of relaxation-induced anxiety, both of which are associated with poor outcome or premature termination in GAD. This client participated in a follow-up program of six months' duration. During that program, he completed a daily form on which he checked off which of eight coping skills he had used that day to manage anxiety and worry; these were mailed to the therapist once a month. The therapist would then have a brief telephone conversation with him reviewing successes and encouraging continued use of these strategies in daily life. The four techniques he used most frequently included structured relaxation practice, frequent checking for early signs of tension, applying breathing techniques to reduce tension, and postponing worry.

Potential challenges for the therapist in working with a GAD client include selecting the right balance among all the treatment components to individualize treatment successfully for the client; recognizing signs of relaxation-induced anxiety and dealing with them with flexible choices of types of relaxation strategies; insuring client compliance with a highly structured treatment approach and fairly extensive homework assignments; teaching the client to relax mentally as well as physically; and helping him or her to transfer these skills to real-life situations.

With regard to alternate treatments, there is some evidence that applied relaxation training alone, as well as cognitive therapy alone, may be successful in treating generalized anxiety disorder. However, research also shows that the comprehensive treatment package that integrates both approaches as described above yields consistently positive outcomes and has flexibility and sensitivity to client individual differences (Borkovec, Crnic & Costello, in press).

ACKNOWLEDGMENTS. Preparation of this chapter was supported in part by Grant MH 13759 from the National Institute of Mental Health to Thomas D. Borkovec.

REFERENCES

American Psychiatric Association. (1987). *Diagnostic and statistical manual of mental disorders* (rev. 3rd ed.). Washington, DC: Author.

Barlow, D. H. (1988). *Anxiety and its disorders*. New York: Guilford.

Beck, A. T., Ward, C. H., Mendelson, M., Mock, J., & Erbaugh, J. (1961). An inventory for measuring depression. *Archives of General Psychiatry, 4*, 561–571.

Bernstein, D. A., & Borkovec, T. D. (1973). *Progressive relaxation training*. Champaign, IL: Research Press.

Borkovec, T. D., Crnic, K., & Costello, E. (in press). Generalized anxiety disorder. In R. T. Ammerman & M. Hersen (Eds.), *Handbook of behavior therapy with children and adults: A longitudinal perspective*. Elmsford, NY: Pergamon.

Borkovec, T. D., & Inz, J. (1990). The nature of worry in generalized anxiety disorder: A predominance of thought activity. *Behaviour Research and Therapy*, *28*, 153–158.

Borkovec, T. D., Shadick, R., & Hopkins, M. (in press). The nature of normal and pathological worry. In R. Rapee & D. H. Barlow (Eds.), *Chronic anxiety and generalized anxiety disorder*. New York: Guilford.

DiNardo, P. A., O'Brien, G. T., Barlow, D. H., Waddell, M. T., & Blanchard, E. (1983). Reliability of DSM-III anxiety disorder categories using a new structured interview. *Archives of General Psychiatry*, *40*, 1070–1078.

Goldfried, M. (1971). Systematic desensitization as training in self control. *Journal of Consulting and Clinical Psychology*, *37*, 228–234.

Heide, F. J., & Borkovec, T. D. (1984). Relaxation-induced anxiety: Mechanisms and theoretical implications. *Behaviour Research and Therapy*, *22*, 1–12.

Mathews, A. (in press). Why worry? The cognitive function of anxiety. *Behaviour Research and Therapy*.

Meyer, T. J., Miller, M. L., Metzger, R. L., & Borkovec, T. D. (in press). Development and validation of the Penn State Worry Questionnaire. *Behaviour Research and Therapy*.

Ost, L. G. (1987). Applied relaxation: Description of a coping technique and review of controlled studies. *Behaviour Research and Therapy*, *25*, 397–410.

Spielberger, C. D., Gorsuch, R. L., & Lushene, R. F. (1970). *Manual for the State-Trait Anxiety Inventory*. Palo Alto, CA: Consulting Psychologists Press.

Zung, W. W. K. (1975). A rating instrument for anxiety disorders. *Psychosomatics*, *12*, 371–379.

SUGGESTED READINGS

Barlow, D. H. (1988). *Anxiety and its disorders*. New York: Guilford.

Beck, A. T., Emery, G., & Greenberg, R. (1985). *Anxiety disorders and phobias: A cognitive perspective*. New York: Basic Books.

Bernstein, D. A., & Borkovec, T. D. (1973). *Progressive relaxation training*. Champaign, IL: Research Press.

Ost, L. G. (1987). Applied relaxation: Description of a coping technique and review of controlled studies. *Behaviour Research and Therapy*, *25*, 397–409.

Smith, J. C. (1985). *Relaxation dynamics*. Champaign, IL: Research Press.

5

Performance Anxiety

Paul Salmon

INTRODUCTION

The use of cognitive-behavioral therapy (CBT) techniques in treating performing musicians for stage fright represents a useful application to a chronically underserved population. Highly skilled performers occupy a tenuous niche in contemporary society—valued for their artistic skills, but often forced to endure economic deprivation, stressful working conditions, and inadequate medical and psychological care. A popular misconception for years about artistic individuals has in fact been that creativity and deprivation go hand in hand, as if to imply that improving the psychological well-being of a performer might somehow diminish the quality of his or her art.

Fortunately, the situation show signs of rectification, as evidenced by the recent growth of arts-medicine organizations specializing in the treatment of artistic performance problems. A professional journal, *Medical Problems of Performing Artists*, enjoys widespread circulation among physicians, psychologists, and other specialists concerned with the health of performers, who are vulnerable to a wide range of physical, neurological, and psychological impairments (Brandfonbrener, 1986). Such vulnerability is especially evident in the psychological realm in fields where the achievement of professional stature normally comes only with years of formal training, single-minded preparation, intense competition, and a healthy dose of luck. Protracted solitude in the practice room punctuated by exposure to intense public scrutiny during concerts is the norm for many performers, whose efforts to cope with the resultant stresses often give rise to physical overuse injuries, drug and alcohol abuse, depression, and anxiety.

The vulnerability of this population has not yet been adequately recognized by psychotherapists. In contrast, the medical profession, spurred by the endorsement of several prominent performing artists who sought relief from physical injuries with appropriately trained specialists, has responded to the needs of this population by establishing treatment programs in several centers throughout the country. Systematic psychological intervention programs, though no less needed, are currently a comparative rarity, and there have been few large-scale studies in recent years focusing on treatment outcomes with this group. The focus of such studies as are available (see, e.g., Kendrick, Craig, Lawson, & Davidson, 1982; Sweeney & Horan, 1982) has been on musical performance anxiety (MPA), recently defined by Salmon (1990) as "the experience of persisting, distressful apprehension about and/or actual impairment of performance skills in a public context, to a degree unwarranted given the individual's musical aptitude, training, and level of preparation"

Paul Salmon • Arts in Medicine Program, Departments of Psychology and Psychiatry, University of Louisville, Louisville, Kentucky 40292.

Comprehensive Casebook of Cognitive Therapy, edited by Arthur Freeman and Frank M. Dattilio. Plenum Press, New York, 1992.

(p. 3). Despite a lack of therapy outcome studies, the topic of MPA is well represented in both the psychological and musical-pedagogical literature (see, for example, Aaron, 1986; Dunkel, 1989; Greene, 1986; Havas, 1976; Lehrer, 1987a, 1988; Reubart, 1985; Ristad, 1982; Triplett, 1983; Wilson, 1986). Available as well are helpful review articles on the pharmacological treatment of MPA (see, e.g., Lader, 1988; Lehrer, 1987b; Nies, 1986), though this topic is not considered in the present chapter.

Available evidence suggests that a broad spectrum of CBT (Beck, Emery, & Greenberg, 1985) and stress inoculation techniques (Meichenbaum, 1985), including self-monitoring, cognitive restructuring, and relaxation training, can be helpful in treating MPA. It is hoped that the present case example, in which several techniques are brought to bear on a problem of MPA, will provide a useful working model for clinicians interested in this approach.

PATIENT INFORMATION

Marty, age 47, is a highly skilled oboist with a large metropolitan orchestra in a midwestern city. After obtaining both undergraduate and graduate degrees at a music conservatory on the East Coast, she began a professional career as an orchestral musician in a position that she holds to this day. Married to a high school music teacher and the mother of three children, she has always felt partially responsible for the family's financial well-being and has thus treated music as something that is essential to her livelihood.

It gradually became apparent that a confluence of problems led Marty to seek professional assistance for performance anxiety, although she reported the precipitating cause to be anticipatory anxiety about a forthcoming concert. Among the general problems that contributed to her sense of psychological vulnerability were the following: First, the overall quality of the orchestra had improved in recent years with the addition of new, younger players who actively competed for prestigious "first chair" positions such as those held by Marty. Second, although Marty's practice time had actually increased recently, greater involvement in nonmusical orchestral activities created an uncomfortable burden for her. Third, she seemed somewhat troubled by a common prevailing attitude among some of her peers that professional orchestral musicians should be able to "get by" with less practice than may have previously been needed. Finally, health problems, including chronic respiratory distress related to smoking and a lack of regular exercise, had diminished

Marty's wind supply and breath control, resulting in greater difficulty producing the full, rounded tone for which the oboe is noted.

The precipitating event that brought Marty to therapy was her reaction to a forthcoming concert four months hence. A concerto was to be performed containing a passage for solo oboe that she dreaded playing. A famous soloist had been engaged for the performance, someone who was known both as an excellent musician and a perfectionistic critic. Marty had played the piece once before with the same soloist, who had been highly critical of the orchestra's supporting role. The music that she dreaded playing consisted not, as one might suspect, of a florid virtuoso passage but rather of several sustained notes in the slow (andante) movement of the concerto.

The mere thought of playing this passage evoked such intense anticipatory anxiety that Marty was actively considering finding a substitute oboist for the concert. Moreover, she reported fleeting thoughts of giving up music altogether because of her apparent inability to cope with what at one level she perceived as a "trivial" problem. It was obvious that Marty viewed this concert as a watershed event in her professional career and was putting enormous pressure on herself to pass the "test" that it posed for her.

Therapy was undertaken with two mutually agreed-upon goals. The first was for Marty to learn some basic anxiety management techniques, including self-assessment, cognitive restructuring, and relaxation training. The second was for Marty to reach a decision about whether or not to play for the performance, and to follow through on the consequences of her decision either way. By initially focusing on anxiety management skills and deferring somewhat the decision about performing, it was anticipated that Marty would gradually become more confident about her capacity to cope with the stresses she believed were inevitable.

Marty talked about her anxiety as a performer with a sense of both embarrassment and trepidation. Having no previous experience with psychotherapy, she, like many other musicians, harbored certain misconceptions that can impede therapeutic progress (Raimy, 1985). First, she tended to perceive the role of client as analogous to that of performer, trying to win the approval of the audience/therapist. Second, she feared being told she was "crazy" and overly obsessive for being concerned about playing a few notes that were hardly audible to anyone else. Third, she was concerned that talking about the problem would only make it worse, having previously preferred to deny being distressed both to herself and to others. She was careful to ensure that none of her colleagues knew of her predicament and believed that any sign of psychological weakness would undermine a performer's career.

To some degree, Marty's condition reflected a mixture of anxiety symptoms. Her anticipatory aversion to the forthcoming concert reflected elements of a phobic response, while her concerns about being negatively evaluated by others (either in terms of her performing skills per se or about being anxious) would suggest a pattern of social phobia. Marty's obsessive concerns about playing a brief (and, to an outside observer, perhaps insignificant) passage, as well as a somewhat more general style of ritualistic practice routines, made a consideration of either obsessive-compulsive disorder or a compulsive personality disorder not unreasonable. In reality, the pattern of psychological distress experienced by Marty as well as by many other performers is probably best described by the DSM-III-R diagnostic category of adjustment disorder with anxious mood. Many of the performers we treat manifest symptoms of anxiety in the context of an identifiable stressor—a major performance of some sort—and do not appear to be more globally impaired with respect either to the experience of anxiety or to undue distress at the prospect of performing. There is, however, a legitimate question as to whether the pattern should be considered a mental disorder or not, since in a consideration of social phobia, the DSM-III-R considers anxiety in the context of a stressful performance a normal occurrence.

Developing an accurate diagnostic impression of the anxious performer is the first step in cultivating effective therapeutic rapport. Many performers come from highly authoritarian, competitive training programs in which perfectionism, single-mindedness, egotism, and strong competitive instincts are all adaptive traits. Such characteristics may seem, however, maladaptive or even pathological to clinicians unaware of the context in which these individuals routinely function. Many performers are made unnecessarily anxious by the expectation that their behavior will be labeled as seriously disturbed, if not crazy, as a result of this. For this reason, it may be months or even years before psychologically troubled performers seek therapeutic assistance.

In addressing these problems, it is helpful to establish a collaborative working relationship in therapy such that the performer is encouraged to take a very active role in his or her own treatment. Performers are generally used to being told what to do by others, and although this may speed up the process of assimilating musical knowledge, it does little to promote the development of self-knowledge. Performers tend to rely on others for evaluative feedback, though they themselves are perfectly capable of realistic self-appraisal when given the chance. Encourag-

ing active collaboration at the outset of therapy helps give performers a clear message that they can deal with their anxiety in an active manner.

TREATMENT ILLUSTRATION

After a preliminary meeting and history-taking session with Marty, an entire session was spent discussing the basic tenets of CBT, and some preliminary baseline data were collected. Marty proved very receptive to this approach, and it was possible to move with her directly into an exploration of the relationship between thoughts and feelings, as the following exchange illustrates.

THERAPIST: I'd like to go into a couple of techniques having to do with thought monitoring, with keeping track of how you think about these things . . . and then I'd also like for you to do some playing, just to demonstrate what some of the circumstances are . . .

MARTY: See, just thinking about that (nervous laugh) makes me nervous . . . just thinking about showing you my problem . . .

THERAPIST: OK, all right, that's very instructive. Let's take a minute to consider something there. It's very good, and very important, for you to be aware of reactions like that, and you're convincing me of something I believe, that simply the thought, the idea . . .

MARTY: That's it!

THERAPIST: . . . of doing a lot of these things can almost automatically trigger this reaction. It's like a momentary freezing up . . .

MARTY: Right now I could feel my heart quickening . . . not, you know, overtly, but . . . just that little adrenalin push.

THERAPIST: In response to playing?

MARTY: In response to the idea that I could show you specifically the piece that I'm worried about, because . . . I don't have the music with me, but—it's so easy that I can remember it, it's only four notes—it's just how long they go on.

This brief exchange helped to confirm three hypotheses, suggested by Marty's responses to a series of assessment questionnaires.* First, much of Marty' anxiety was

*Basic pre- and postassessment measures that the Genesis Center routinely employs with performers seeking treatment for anxiety include the following: a clinical medical/psychiatric history questionnaire, the Symptom Checklist 90 (SCL-90; DeRogatis, 1983); Anxiety Sensitivity Index (Peterson & Heilbronner, 1987), and the Beck Anxiety Inventory (BAI; Beck, et al.,

anticipatory in nature, whether concerning playing in public or in sharing her problem with me. The suggestion that she actually demonstrate her difficulties by playing evoked nervous laughter, along with the insight that this indeed would be an anxiety-provoking task. Although Marty was intent on making a good impression, like many performers she instinctually anticipated criticism from others even where none was intended. This phenomenon carries over to perceptions of the therapist, toward whom many performers respond with varying combinations of anger, fear, and deference (Aaron, 1986).

Second, evident in this passage is Marty's capacity for introspection, a capability she shares with many other performers. Not only was she aware that the *thought* of playing made her feel anxious, but she could also identify the associated physical sensations, such as muscular tension, that she associated with the anticipatory anxiety. Third, this passage reveals a tendency to conceptualize her problem in terms of a highly encapsulated focus: that of playing a specific group of notes. She seemed a bit embarrassed about this, however, because she believed that people outside her field (including therapists) were not likely to understand the often subtle aspects of musical performance skills. Marty had in fact already contacted one therapist who suggested that her apparent anxiety about this musical segment was excessive and did not warrant psychotherapeutic intervention.

Indeed, it is tempting to consider this possibility. Why, for instance, should someone call into question their very professional identity over just a few notes? To accept a problem such as this as the focus of treatment might seem to play into—and even reinforce—the obsessive tendencies of many performers, who may practice untold hours to refine nuances of phrasing or expressiveness perceptible to only a very few others. On the other hand, in Marty's case, failure to take her complaint seriously would simply have reinforced her sense that psychological intervention had little to offer. Accepting her formulation at face value (a) reinforced her credibility and (b) provided a good starting point for a consideration of more broadly based issues.

We therefore undertook a detailed analysis of what was required to play the four notes in question. On the surface, they seemed simple enough, and not the sort of

thing that would tax a seasoned performer. But Marty quickly realized, upon reflection, that there was far more to playing this passage than was apparent on casual inspection. Among the factors which she enumerated as contributing to the problem were the following:

1. The notes were in a low range (register) and played at a slow tempo, which collectively required exceptional breath control.
2. The passage was "exposed," meaning that no other instruments save the soloist's piano were playing at the time.
3. The passage was not played in strict rhythm, but rather left to the discretion of the soloist to interpret. Thus Marty had to have ample breath to play the entire passage, but could not necessarily anticipate how long it would last.
4. This passage occurred at a point where she had not been playing for several minutes, and was therefore somewhat out of the "flow" of the piece. This also gave her more time to worry as that point in the piece approached.
5. She was aware that a less senior member of the oboe section had elsewhere disparaged her playing skills and was actively competing for her chair.
6. Although she had played the piece once before, she had never really studied it in detail and did not have a secure grasp of its overall structure. When questioned about this, she stated that at her stage of the game, a performer should not have to prepare so intensively, particularly for a piece where one's instrument served only in an accompanying role.

As she began to analyze the problem in detail, Marty began to realize that she harbored several erroneous underlying assumptions about performing, most notably that it should be easy to do, at least for a seasoned veteran such as herself. This is but one example of the many "shoulds" and "musts" that, in my experience, tend to dominate the thinking of performers such as Marty. "I *should* be able to play this perfectly," "I *have* to practice four hours a day," and "I *must* play this particular piece or people will think poorly of my abilities" are all examples of statements that exemplify the neurotic tendency Ellis (Ellis & Grieger, 1977) has characterized as "musturbation." Beginning at an early age (Marty had been eight when she began serious musical studies), musicians seem to internalize certain rules akin to "untested assumptions" about musical performance skills, many of which seem to have compulsive, even ritualistic, qualities. "Practice makes perfect" and "Play it 10 more times and you'll know it by

1988). Additional measures include a Performance History Questionnaire, in which performers reflect on their background, training, and performing experiences; and an analog-type measure of anxiety based on the BAI. Copies of the Performance History Questionnaire, the assessment photograph, and the modified BAI may be obtained by writing to the author in care of the Department of Psychology, University of Louisville, Louisville, KY 40292.

heart," they are told (among other things), never really stopping to determine if these timeworn rules are actually appropriate for them. What does it mean to play a piece of music "perfectly"? Why will 10 repetitions, and not 9 or 11, ensure that a piece is learned? What does it mean to *learn* a piece of music, to begin with?

Later on, during one's career, equally rigid and perfectionistic thinking is often evident in the self-talk of performers. The following passage, taken from the fourth session, illustrates the degree to which Marty's perfectionistic view of herself inhibited the assessment of her difficulties as a performer in realistic terms. The session took place shortly after she had played in a small concert, which took place after she had begun to work on some basic anxiety management techniques (including deep breathing and mental imagery) and had begun keeping notes of her rehearsal sessions.

MARTY: The next day [at rehearsal]—I've gotten a lot out of that one book on confronting fear [Agras, 1978]—I practiced learning how to manage the space before I played. And I could not . . . disassociate . . . and do beaches or anything like that. [I had suggested that she experiment with some relaxing imagery at some point prior, but not immediately so, before her entrance.]

THERAPIST: Uh-huh.

MARTY: But I really concentrated on my breathing, in rhythm with what was going on, and I concentrated on how I was going to pretend that I was tuning the note when I started the note, and in performance with the big audience . . . and I played it fine! But I had to really work hard to get that, and it was managing that time before the two measures . . . and I had to do it over and over, and I was thinking, "My God, I don't have time for this," and I was disappointed before, but I was very relieved afterward. So I wrote down my reactions afterward.

THERAPIST: It sounds as though this performance—this rehearsal and this first performance—was really the focus of the tension and depression this week.

MARTY: This week. (nods in agreement)

THERAPIST: Let's go back over this a bit; there are a couple of things you said that I want to pick up on. One is the reaction, the thought pattern that comes into play along the lines, "I *shouldn't* have to work so hard to manage one little section," and aside from whatever happens in the performance itself, I think we want to look at the mental reactions that we have afterwards, or beforehand, from the standpoint that they add certain pressures, and reflect certain beliefs and attitudes . . . that can promote depression or anxiety. I guess the idea is that one note seems so inconsequential . . . what are some aspects of your thinking on this?

MARTY: The first thing, I was surprised, and then throughout the piece I was thinking, "good God, I can't believe this." That was my first reaction. "Why can't I be relaxed enough to play it?" On the second day, I tried really hard to take deep breaths and just concentrate on body movements, rather than should, would, can, won't . . . that kind of stuff. And it really does bother me when I think I'm not perfect . . .

At this stage of treatment, Marty was becoming aware of how much her thoughts contributed to the way she felt about herself both as a person and as a performer. This particular session appears to have been important for Marty because it demonstrated to her how, despite her misgivings, she could cope with the stress of playing by actively focusing her concentration on the task at hand. Her inclination had been to believe that this was something that was more or less automatic, a capability to be taken for granted.

In this and other sessions, the focus was on helping Marty to adopt an active role in identifying, conceptualizing, and solving the problems she was having as a performer in a methodical manner. Used to letting others tell her what needed to be done, Marty was somewhat unsure of herself at first in this problem-solving role. But ultimately, she became quite adept both at evaluating problems and posing solutions. An important insight occurred as she became aware of the fears triggered by symptoms of anxiety, such as a rapid heartbeat or muscle tremors. Working in a collaborative fashion, we developed an "arousal analog" exercise in which she played the oboe immediately following a period of intense exercise, so as to become accustomed to playing in a physical state she considered less than ideal. So helpful did she find this that she eventually incorporated an exercise routine into her practice sessions, an action that had the added benefit of increasing her respiratory capacity! The success of this intervention was due, I believe, largely to Marty's capacity for accurate self-assessment—a capacity that is shared by many musicians, who may seem initially to adopt a rather passive stance toward their problems.

During the remaining five sessions, the focus of therapy shifted from being didactically oriented toward providing Marty with a forum to discuss and analyze the efforts she was making on her own behalf to deal with her anxiety. She soon discovered that she experienced manifestations of tension, apprehension, and anxiety under circumstances that were ostensibly far less pressure packed than the forthcoming performance.

An important issue that Marty had to settle early on

concerned the decision whether or not to play in the fall concert. Initially wondering what she "should" do, Marty at my recommendation delayed making a decision for several weeks until she had become proficient with some basic anxiety management CBT techniques and had a chance to review and practice the music in a detailed manner. When she abruptly announced during a subsequent session that she had decided to play the concert, her anxiety seemed to *increase* temporarily as she began to consider the implications of her decision. This is a common response of therapy clients as they begin to confront the source of their fears realistically and, as a result, engage in less denial and other forms of avoidant behavior. Performers, in particular, are especially prone to denial. In part a protective form of self-deception against the unpleasant experience of anxiety, and partly a concerned response to having one's anxiety discovered by others, denial is frequently a major obstacle to seeking help.

Marty had alluded to this in an earlier interview, in which she stated that she had waited years before seeking help, so convinced was she that therapists would either trivialize her condition *or* assert that she was seriously mentally ill. Having by this time incorporated some basic cognitive techniques, however, Marty was now able to begin to own up to her anxiety and to use it productively as a cue to engage in productive, preparatory coping activities. Prior to this time, thoughts about the upcoming performance tended to frighten her to the point where she tended to avoid practicing altogether—clearly a maladaptive response.

The anxiety management techniques that Marty eventually learned to practice and deploy consisted of both generic CBT procedures and more specific, musically oriented activities. Among the former were self-assessment activities (including thought listing, data collection, and problem conceptualization), cognitive restructuring procedures, and progressive relaxation training skills, which Marty practiced assiduously (being a musician, she appreciated the need for practice!). Exercises of the latter sort were developed in a collaborative fashion during actual playing sessions in which Marty experimented with different playing techniques and listened to tape recordings that we made. Among the procedures we developed together were the following:

- Marking her musical score with breath marks and other cues
- Playing along with different recordings of the music to accustom herself to differing stylistic variations
- Visualizing in great detail the music as she wanted it to sound, prior to playing it

- Playing when out of breath to simulate the experience of arousal under performance conditions
- Arranging "practice performances" in various settings, playing music making comparable demands on breath control
- Learning more about the soloist as a person, thereby helping reframe her perception of the performance as a collaborative, rather than adversarial, undertaking
- Allowing herself to make mistakes, then checking via live and taped feedback to determine just how perceptible such errors were

It is worth reiterating here that no particular one of these techniques is essential in dealing with MPA. Of greatest importance is encouraging the client to take an active role in developing strategies that address specific attributes of the problem. Marty's active involvement in this task-oriented, problem-solving phase of therapy appears to have been helpful in giving her a sense of coping effectively with the stresses that are inherent in the careers of professional performing artists.

DISCUSSION

The effectiveness of this treatment program might best be judged in practical terms, such as whether and how comfortably she subsequently played. But before addressing the specific issue of the concert in detail, let us consider the results of a series of more broadly based, pre- and posttreatment assessment measures. These measures not only helped to focus therapeutic interventions but provided an indication of changes that occurred in her psychological status. At the outset of therapy, Marty's description of the problem she was having (as she later came to realize) was so broadly based and vaguely described that she not unexpectedly lacked a clear sense of how to proceed and was on the verge of simply giving up playing altogether.

The desire for a thorough assessment of psychological functioning had to be balanced by the desirability, especially evident when working with performing musicians, to adopt a focused, problem-oriented approach. The following screening measures were therefore selected and administered both before and after treatment: Symptom Checklist 90 (SCL-90; DeRogatis, 1983), Anxiety Sensitivity Index (Peterson & Heilbronner, 1987), Beck Anxiety Index (Beck, Epstein, Brown, & Steer, 1988), and a self-assessment questionnaire requesting information concerning the performer's musical background (see note 1). Other measures that clinicians may want to consider but that were not employed here include the Performance Anxiety Self-Statement Scale (Kendrick et al., 1982) and the Report of Confidence as a Performer Scale (Craske & Craig, 1984).

To screen for general psychological distress, the SCL-90 was administered. It is helpful to examine the SCL both with respect to nonpatient and outpatient norms, since with performers a legitimate question can often be raised about the most appropriate comparison group. In a manner that appears to be generally consistent for this population, the three main index scores of the SCL-90—the General Severity Index (GSI), Positive Symptom Distress Index (PSDI), and Positive Symptom Total (PST)—were slightly in excess of the norm for a nonpatient comparison group, but considerably below that reported for an outpatient population (DeRogatis, 1983). Scores for the individual subscales that comprise the SCL-90 were likewise within a subclinical range, though a subscale that assesses interpersonal sensitivity was marginally elevated at pretreatment (a finding that is common with audience-oriented performers).

Overall, there were few changes in the major SCL-90 indices, and the individual scales that comprise the instrument likewise were relatively stable. The lack of apparent acute distress experienced by Marty is corroborated by fact that her overall scores on the SCL were only slightly higher than the average for a nonpatient sample, both pre- and posttreatment.

In comparison, pre- and posttreatment scores on measures more directly related to the experience of performance anxiety showed more pronounced change. A special administration of the Beck Anxiety Inventory (BAI) has been developed for use with performers, in which the client is shown a picture of the silhouette of a musician standing before a group of musical adjudicators, who appear to be listening intently and writing notes. The client is asked to visualize himself or herself performing for the group as if the circumstances involved an important audition. On the BAI, Marty's pre- to posttreatment raw score decreased from 23 to 6 (both essentially subclinical scores), suggesting that the prospect of playing before an imaginary evaluative audience had become significantly less threatening. The Anxiety Sensitivity Index (ASI) also suggested that a decrease in concern about the symptoms of anxiety had occurred; raw score values on the ASI decreased by more than 50% (from 27 to 13, the latter within normal limits).

The self-assessment inventory (see note 1) was notable chiefly in terms of some observations that Marty made concerning the history of her bouts with performance anxiety, which have much in common with those of other highly skilled performers:

I have been performing professionally for years and had normal ups and downs with nerves, but I had been able to manage it. After 1981, after a series of misfortunes with a colleague and coming from the front lines of orchestra political activities, my performance nerves got out of hand. I spent years [1983–1989] trying to deny the problem of putting it out of conscious mind until the actual experience.

In retrospect, she noted:

After exposing myself to a listener [the therapist], I see partners for the first time. I see my role as not so spotlighted but part of a very imperfect group. I'm working on listening to the good things I do and not dwelling on the imperfect. It is very hard, but I'm beginning to be more realistic about imperfection. I don't have to be a musician, but since I chose to do it, I might as well enjoy it.

As events turned out, Marty performed in the concert as planned, and during a follow-up session described her experiences in a pleased, though somewhat subdued manner. She had achieved an important insight with the recognition that whereas the symptoms of anxiety might well be present (or at least the associated indications of arousal), it was not obligatory that she either be frightened of the feelings or become self-critical of the way she felt. Her description of the concert the previous weekend therefore conveyed a sense of relief that it was over with, a recognition that she would be performing it in the near future, and a sense of confidence and a bit of resignation that a certain amount of distress seemed to come with the territory, no matter how expert a performer one is.

MARTY: When I arrived at the hall . . . the pianist was warming up, and I heard my section. I was overwhelmed with the fact that it was exceedingly slow . . . Then we did not have time to do a regular rehearsal without the soloist, and so we rehearsed with him. I had my score . . . and he took the cadenza entirely differently than the recordings I've listened to. He arpeggiated the notes to fast they almost sounded like chords . . . so I had to change the way I prepared a bit.

THERAPIST: All right.

MARTY: And when we played it, it was about the best performance I'd done, which surprised me a bit, because sometimes I have to work into it.

THERAPIST: Still the rehearsal?

MARTY: Right . . . it was the next day at the dress rehearsal that I discovered I had to breathe during my passage, and this went unnoticed, because he [the pianist] was trilling . . . so I thought to myself, "Aha! This is what I can do!" But then I was faced with the dilemma, that evening, of "Do I take the breath or do I not take the breath?" Well, we got to the performance and we were in that movement, and the first entrance I had was kind of shaky . . . and I didn't like the way it was coming out, and I got real nervous . . . and when we got to the cadenza I was concentrating on how I was going to do it, and there was never the feeling that "I can't do it" . . . I took a breath, then took another one, and that was noticed by some people . . . that was noticed. But I was able to recover . . . but it was much more controlled. I didn't feel my heart racing like crazy.

THERAPIST: Uh-huh . . . It really placed a premium on your ability to adapt, to kind of roll with the punches.

MARTY: We're all more relaxed . . .

THERAPIST: Almost like a kindling effect.

MARTY: Right . . . and now I have to look forward to doing this again at the end of the month.

SUMMARY

Altogether, Marty's treatment consisted of eight 90-minute sessions in the course of a two-month period, followed by booster and follow-up sessions at the time of the performance. Her assessment of therapy was that it had provided her with techniques useful in managing anxiety, which she had come to regard—at least for herself—as an inevitable part of performing. Like many performers, she was highly critical of herself for having the problem in the first place, but at the same time was cautious about psychotherapy because of concerns that it would not directly address her problems as a performer. Cognitive-behavior therapy, with its emphasis on client–therapist collaboration, self-assessment skills training, and a problem-oriented approach, proved to be an effective means of overcoming Marty's reservations about psychotherapy and ultimately helped her to surmount the fear of anxiety that had been blocking her musical expressiveness. By taking an active, problem-solving stance toward the issue of MPA, Marty was able to overcome her fears of being anxious, and also experience some relief in the overall intensity of her anxiety. The techniques that she employed blended elements of basic CBT and musical pedagogy, integrated within a framework that emphasized problem conceptualization, coping skills training, and application as described elsewhere by Meichenbaum (1985) and others.

REFERENCES

Aaron, S. (1986). *Stage fright.* Chicago: University of Chicago Press.

Agras, W. S. (1978). *Living with fear: Understanding and coping with anxiety.* New York: McGraw-Hill.

Beck, A. T., Emery, G., & Greenberg, R. (1985). *Anxiety disorders and phobias.* New York: Basic Books.

Beck, A. T., Epstein, N., Brown, G., and Steer, R. A. (1988). An inventory for measuring clinical anxiety: Psychometric properties. *Journal of Consulting and Clinical Psychology, 56*(6), 893–897.

Brandfonbrener, A. G. (1986). An overview of the medical problems of musicians. *Journal of American College Health, 34,* 165–169.

Craske, M. G., & Craig, K. (1984). Musical performance anxiety: The three-systems model and self-efficacy theory. *Behavior Research and Therapy, 22,* 267–280.

Derogatis, L. (1983). *SCL-90R: Administration, scoring, and procedures manual.* Towson, MD: Clinical Psychometric Research.

Dunkel, S. E. (1989). *The audition process: Anxiety management and coping strategies.* New York: Pendragon.

Ellis, A., & Grieger, R. (1977). *Handbook of rational-emotive therapy.* New York: Springer.

Greene, B. (1986). *The inner game of music.* New York: Anchor.

Havas, K. (1976). *Stage fright: Its causes and cures.* London: Bosworth.

Kendrick, M. J., Craig, K. D., Lawson, D. M., & Davidson, P. O. (1982). Cognitive and behavioral therapy for musical performance anxiety. *Journal of Consulting and Clinical Psychology, 50,* 353–362.

Lader, M. (1988). B-adrenoceptor antagonists in neuropsychiatry: An update. *Journal of Clinical Psychiatry, 49,* 213–223.

Lehrer, P. (1987a). A review of the approaches to the management of tension and stage fright in music performance. *Journal of Research in Music Education, 55,* 143–152.

Lehrer, P. (1987b). The use of beta blockers. *New Jersey Medicine, 84,* 27–33.

Lehrer, P. (1988). The causes and cures of performance anxiety: A review of the psychological literature. In F. L. Roehmann & F. R. Wilson (Eds.), *The biology of music making: Proceedings of the 1984 Denver Conference* (pp. 32–46). St. Louis: MMB Music.

Meichenbaum, D. (1985). *Stress inoculation training.* New York: Pergamon.

Nies, A. S. (1986). Clinical pharmacology of beta-adrenergic blockers. *Medical Problems of Performing Artists, 1,* 25–29.

Noyes, R. (1988). Beat-adrenergic blockers. In C. G. Last & M. Hersen (Eds.), *Handbook of anxiety disorders* (pp. 445–459). New York: Pergamon.

Peterson, R. A., & Heilbronner, R. L. (1987). The anxiety sensitivity index. *Journal of Anxiety Disorders, 1,* 117–121.

Raimy, V. (1985). Misconceptions and the cognitive therapies. In M. J. Mahoney & A. Freeman (Eds.), *Cognition and psychotherapy* (pp. 203–222). New York: Plenum.

Reubart, D. (1985). *Anxiety and musical performance.* New York: DaCapo.

Ristad, E. (1982). *Soprano on her head.* Moab, UT: Real People Press.

Salmon, P. G. (1990). A psychological perspective on musical performance anxiety: A review of the literature. *Medical Problems of Performing Artists, 5,* 2–11.

Sweeney, G. A., & Horan, J. J. (1982). Separate and combined effects of cue-controlled relaxation and cognitive restructuring in the treatment of musical performance anxiety. *Journal of Counseling Psychology, 29,* 486–497.

Triplett, R. (1983). *Stage fright: Letting it work for you.* Chicago: Nelson-Hall.

Wilson, F. R. (1986). *Tone deaf and all thumbs?* New York: Viking.

SUGGESTED READINGS

Barlow, D. H. (1985). *Anxiety and its disorders*. New York: Guilford.

Last, C. G., & Hersen, M. (Eds.). (1988). Handbook of anxiety disorders. New York: Pergamon.

Michelson, L., & Ascher, L. M. (Eds.). (1987). *Anxiety and stress disorders: Cognitive behavioral assessment and treatment*. New York: Guilford.

Woolfolk, R. L., & Lehrer, P. M. (1984). *Principles and practice of stress management*. New York: Guilford.

6

Social Phobia

Robert Becker

"I woke with dread in my stomach at 6:30 a.m. I knew I had to start my meeting at 9:00 a.m. My notes, where did I put my notes? Oh, God, I can't find my notes. Without my notes, I'll never be able to do it. The last thing I did with my notes was downstairs and they must still be down there. I'm sure I can't eat breakfast this morning, because I'll probably throw up on the front row of my audience. Wow, would that ever be embarrassing. Then they'll really think that I've lost it. How can I get them to listen to me after they have seen that I'm so weak and nervous? I won't be able to do my job. I can't take the risk of seeming so foolish in front of them. How can I face them the next day, the next week? I'm not ready to handle this, I don't think I can do it. So I call my colleague to ask him to do this morning's talk without me. While I'm dialing the phone this funny feeling comes over me. My vision seems to be leaving me. I can't see! How could I ever read my notes if this happened during my talk? Frank just has to do this talk for me. I'll be better for the next one."

Panic, avoidance, fear, negative thoughts, self-focus, autonomic nervous system arousal—are all hallmarks of an anxiety disorder. For social phobia, the crucial difference is in the evoking situations, which have to do with public humiliation and embarrassment. Social phobia and shyness, a closely related concept, appear to be very common. For example, Zimbardo (1977) and Pilkonis and

Zimbardo (1979) surveyed individuals across diverse cultures; from these samples, approximately 40% of respondents labeled themselves as shy, while 80% reported that they had been shy at some point in their lives. The same authors found that 41% of adults from their samples listed public speaking as their most serious fear, more than listed sickness and death.

> Hello, Dr. Becker, my doctor referred me to you. I've had this attack yesterday and I can't go to work today. It was really bad, almost horrible. I don't know what to do. Can I see you immediately? I'm so worried that this will happen again. Oh, by the way, my wife is very upset about this and I'm sure she'll be calling soon.

Many referrals for social phobia come in this fashion. By the time the call is made, most patients have tried several unsuccessful homegrown remedies and have reached a crisis point that is punctuated with desperation. The group I work with has found that a rapid evaluation and initiation of treatment is the best way to handle these types of referrals. A slower approach usually produces an avalanche of panic symptoms from the patient and phone calls from all of the concerned family members.

MY HASTILY REFERRED PATIENT

Mr. B. is a married gentlemen in his late 40s who has grown children, one of whom still resides with Mr. B and his wife. He is a deeply religious man, proud of his religious commitment. He has been married for over 25

Robert Becker • Private Practice, 501 Office Center Drive, Suite 290, Fort Washington, Pennsylvania 19034.

Comprehensive Casebook of Cognitive Therapy, edited by Arthur Freeman and Frank M. Dattilio. Plenum Press, New York, 1992.

years and is equally proud of his marriage. His work history has included continuous promotions with a very economically stable company. Now a senior-level manager, responsible for a large number of employees, he prides himself on being a good manager. He feels that he should listen to and understand his employees, that his approach to managing his people is informational and educational. Meetings organized by him are the main vehicle employed to carry out his management style.

PATIENT EVALUATION AND DIAGNOSIS

An initial diagnostic interview was carried out following the Anxiety Disorders Interview Schedule-R (ADIS; DiNardo et al., 1985). Further evaluation was carried out with the Fear of Negative Evaluation Scale (FNE), the Social Anxiety and Distress Scale (SADS: Watson & Friend, 1969), and the Personal Report of Confidence as a Speaker (PRCS; Paul, 1966). Results of these evaluations confirmed the diagnosis of social phobia (based on the ADIS), showing a normal score on the SADS and elevated scores on the FNE and PRCS. Further interview evaluation was carried out to determine a graded hierarchy of speaking situations and of negative thoughts. Physiological symptoms were investigated in detail and consisted of heart rate acceleration, narrowing of the visual field, blurring of vision, hyperventilation, chest discomfort, thought blocking, perspiration, and dry mouth. The physical symptoms appeared quite quickly, but could last for up to 60 minutes. An attack was always accompanied by an elevated SUDS (Subjective Units of Discomfort) report, along with an intense urge to avoid the situation or escape when in the situation. Avoidance spanned both situations and cognitions (i.e., not thinking about the embarrassing events). The following hierarchy was constructed:

1. Conversations with small groups at church (SUDS 10)
2. Conversations with small groups at work (SUDS 20)
3. In charge of formal meeting of very familiar employees (SUDS 40)
4. In meeting at work but not in charge (SUDS 50)
5. Presenter at large meeting at church (SUDS 80)
6. In charge of regular weekly work meeting (SUDS 80)
7. In charge of special work meetings (SUDS 100)
8. In a meeting as a participating speaker, but not in charge of the order of speakers (SUDS 100)

Next, a hierarchy of disturbing thoughts was created:

1. Someone in the audience could disagree with me. (SUDS 50)
2. I could make a mistake and someone would correct me. (SUDS 50)
3. I am going to start to shake. (SUDS 80)
4. My vision is going to change. (SUDS 70)
5. My heart is going to race. (SUDS 100)
6. My mind will go blank in front of everyone. (SUDS 100)
7. I am going to have to leave a meeting in the middle. (SUDS 100)
8. If my voice cracks, everyone will know I'm nervous, and they will not respect me. (SUDS 100)
9. Once they don't respect me, I won't be able to manage them any more. (SUDS 70)
10. No one will follow a leader who can't even control his own emotions. (SUDS 70)
11. If I can't lead, I can't do my job. I'm going to have to start a new career. (SUDS 80)
12. A new career means a salary cut, and I can't afford this. (SUDS 100)
13. If I leave my job, what will my wife think of me? (SUDS 80)
14. A panic attack in public will make me look foolish, and people will not respect me. (SUDS 100)
15. A panic attack in public will make me look weak, and no one will follow a weak leader. (SUDS 100)
16. Once some of my employees see a panic, they will pass the rumor around to everyone, and all will be laughing at me behind my back. (SUDS 100)

As a result of these evaluations, the following formulation of this man's disorder was hypothesized. Because of the normal score on the SADS and the elevated score on the FNE, the presumed potent stimuli for triggering a panic were primarily cognitive in nature and minimally affected by the actual reactions of the audience. These thoughts were hypothesized to begin with an impending public presentation situation and would be at their extreme under the following circumstances:

• With more alone time to focus on and rehearse these thoughts
• Under any set of circumstances that increased self-focus and triggered self-evaluation thoughts
• When a meeting was delayed and he could continue to be introspective in the presence of an audience

These hypotheses were tested in the office to see if they could support a functional relationship between these events and increasing anxiety. First, the patient was instructed in hyperventilation; he then hyperventilated while imagining a rather pleasant beach scene. This procedure produced the vision narrowing typical of his anxiety pattern as well as heart rate acceleration, but the psychological intensity of fear and dread did not appear. Next, he described an upcoming talk (without hyperventilating) and reported his SUDS every minute. The first description was deliberately constrained to describing the physical circumstances—the room, time of day, furniture arrangement, lighting, visual aids, and so forth. Minimal SUDS elevation occurred.

Next the scene was described again, but with an emphasis on self-focus (e.g., what he would feel, how his heart would race, how foolish he would look, how he would shake). SUDS was significantly elevated for this imagination. Lastly, the hyperventilation was combined with this last scene to illustrate how the psychology and physiology interacted to intensify further his attention to fear-evoking internal cues. A panic resulted. After calming him down, scenes were imagined, without hyperventilation, where people walked out of his talk, looked bored, asked hostile questions, looked at him in a hostile manner, and were generally unresponsive. None of these scenes produced much SUDS elevation.

These results were taken as confirmation of the original formulation, and an exposure treatment plan was created that included significant cognitive factors.

EXPOSURE-BASED TREATMENT

Part of the formulation for this treatment is drawn from Foa and Kozak's (1986) model, which describes the mechanisms through which exposure reduces fear. Both automatic (unaware) and controlled (aware) cognitive processes are involved; in order to maximize the effects of exposure, the fear structure must be aroused, and then information inconsistent with the propositions within the structure must be processed. To facilitate this processing, eliciting events are designated as CS+ and calming events are designated as CS−. A mix of CS+ and CS− events are used to create a manageable SUDS level so that the attentional narrowing of focus described by Barlow (1988) and the selective retrieval of memory described by Bower's (1981) model are of moderate proportion.

For example, the first exposure session was carried out at this man's church. The eliciting event factors of this meeting included a large audience (CS+), a comfortable setting (CS−), the presence of his wife (CS−), a group of speakers (CS−) control over the order of speakers (CS−), and a formal presentation with outline and notes (CS+). Most people in the audience were strangers, and he would not likely see them again (CS−); a small number of people were friends whom he would see again (CS+). The audience had printed copies of the materials to be presented, allowing a mistake to be easily detected (CS+). The client had to arrive early and wait for the audience to arrive and be seated (CS+). He continued to focus on how he would feel (CS+); he expected that he would have a panic (CS+). He saw this as a critical test of his ability (CS+). He was taught to control his speech rate and breathing to prevent hyperventilation (CS−), to shift his focus from himself to his audience (CS−), and was told that the anxiety would dissipate if he stayed long enough (CS−).

This combination of events produced intense anxiety, but not severe anxiety, so that the client was able to continue to process nonfear-relevant information and thereby benefit from the exposure. This exposure was carried out with the following instructions: He should arrive about 30 minutes ahead of the audience to set up his materials, making sure that all mechanical equipment worked (microphones, projectors, etc.) and that he knew how to control these items. He was to familiarize himself with the room seating and entrances and exits. (This was done to move these CS+'s toward CS−'s.) He was to be the first speaker, which reduced the amount of time for the CS+ cognitions to operate. Before and during his talk, he was to focus on his audience and not himself. He was to use thoughts like the following:

- They are here to learn this new information.
- My job is to pace the talk so that they can understand what I'm saying; going more slowly will allow them more time to understand the ideas better.
- The audience is here to learn from me not to evaluate me per se, but to evaluate the information I'm giving them.
- I should be looking directly at as many people in the audience as possible. Some people may not understand what I'm trying to say, and I'll be able to tell that from the expressions on their faces.
- I may have to slow down or go over a point to make it clear.

Also, he was told to expect the following pattern of autonomic nervous system arousal during his talk:

- A gradual, but consistent increase in arousal as the time for him to speak approached
- A peak in arousal just before he was to start his speaking

- A drop in arousal as he was able to speak
- An increase in arousal as soon as he moved his attention to self-focus (examples of self-focus include: "I'm doing pretty well so far. I haven't had a panic yet. I hope a panic doesn't happen now to spoil this. My hands are shaking, I hope no one notices.").

The results of this exposure were very much as predicted. The client experienced the anticipated arousal pattern. He found that he could make a panic happen by changing to a self-focus; he also found that he could continue his talk even if the panic happened because it subsided as he changed his focus. Toward the end of his talk, he moved to self-observation of how well he had done so far and caused an increase in anxiety.

The aftermath of this exposure changed several CS + 's. Many physiological cues were weakened, because the client could make them come and go. The audience size cues and the self-focus cues were among those weakened. The disruptive cognitions that took over during the anticipation of speaking were slightly weakened, but more needed to be done with them. The client felt a significant sense of accomplishment as a result of this exposure, and this feeling allowed movement to another more threatening CS+: his work setting. The work-setting plan included several of the meetings that he chaired as a part of his usual job responsibilities. Some of the dialogue from this session went as follows.

THERAPIST: We now need to expand the number of meetings that you can attend, and we eventually want you to go back to the administrative meetings where the worst panics happened. It will be more effective if we start with more comfortable meetings first. Would you look over your schedule for this upcoming week for meetings where we can start?

PATIENT: I've four meetings scheduled with week, and there are two meetings which I need to structure and start. These two meetings do not now exist, but I am going to need one to handle issues of employee safety and one to handle phase-in of this new equipment. I'm going to have to set the purpose and format of these meetings and decide who should attend. The memos have been sitting on my desk for over a month now. I can't see myself ever being able to make those meetings work, and if these don't work I'm not going to succeed as a manager.

THERAPIST: OK, that's fine. I am glad that we have plenty to choose from. Right now, let's not worry about the two meetings you have to start; let's choose from the ones that are ongoing. Can we look at those in more detail?

PATIENT: Two meetings involve routine reports from several of us. The setting is pretty informal. We go around the table and summarize progress on our various activities for the last week and highlight where any of us has a major problem. The other two involve people that I have worked with for a long time who know and respect me.

THERAPIST: Let's start with the last two meetings that you described. How likely do you think a panic is within these two contexts?

PATIENT: I feel very safe with these two groups. I can relax and really be myself, and I can even joke and enjoy the situation.

THERAPIST: OK. Can we start with these two meetings? What I'd like you to do is use the covert rehearsal technique that we learned before. Remember what this is?

PATIENT: I think so. That's where I first brainstorm about what I want to cover in the meeting. Then I organize these ideas into an outline and memorize the outline. The outline serves as my guide through the meeting to tell me where I want to go.

THERAPIST: That's right. You should rehearse that outline just before your meeting so that it is easily recalled, even if you get nervous. With these two meetings, I'd like you to announce your outline to your audience before you start. I would like you to stop talking—that is, pause—for a long time between each major part of your talk. During that pause, I want you to recall and rehearse your outline again, just so you keep your bearings.

PATIENT: That's just like what we did in our practices here, right? It was easy here, but if I pause for that long in front of these people, they'll think I am nervous, that I've lost my place and that I can't do this job. I think I can do the rehearsal all right, but I'm not so sure about the pauses.

THERAPIST: Well (long pause), that could happen and people might think those things about you. By the way did you notice that long pause when I started?

PATIENT: No, not really. I just thought you were thinking. I didn't pay much attention to it. But in front of an audience, this will be different.

THERAPIST: Let's have you try it here. Just a short pause and then go on. Can we use the presentation you did last week at church?

Once again, these various meetings contained a mixture of CS+ and CS− cues. A gradually increasing mixture of these was again employed to increase the SUDS level. Exposure to 10 meetings in the course of two weeks produced a strong and reliable habituation of anxiety within two minutes of the onset of a presentation. On one occasion the client deliberately tried to induce a panic, but this proved unsuccessful. Results of these exposures on cognitions included change in the expectations that a panic would go on forever and that he could not function when the anxiety struck. He now knew that the anxiety would stop after a short period of time, and he knew that he could continue to function with the anxiety.

More important, however, was what did not change. He was still very concerned about the appearance of being weak and foolish in front of his subordinates. Since this fear appeared to be a core belief in the fear structure and the one that was perceived by him as most damaging to his perception of himself and to his self-perceived ability to be a successful manager, any public presentation was still viewed as a necessary danger, but a danger nonetheless. Unless this perceived danger changed, he would be prone to anticipatory anxiety and to possible relapse.

THERAPIST: How did the last series of meetings go?

PATIENT: Pretty well, actually. Each one seems to build on the one before. As I do one and the anxiety melts away, my self-esteem goes up. The last few meetings were even fun. I found myself joking a little with people. But you know that when it really comes down to it, I really don't know what to say. I have to be careful that I say the right things, otherwise people will know that I don't have much to say. Especially around work, I could look like I am not knowledgeable, and people won't respect me.

THERAPIST: Let's see if I really understand this. Each idea has to be carefully weighed to make sure it's OK to say. So you have to think everything through before you say it, and then you discard most of it because you find that most of the ideas are foolish. Is that right?

PATIENT: Yes, that's what I do. That's why pauses are so uncomfortable. I just discarded something and now I'm left with nothing to say, so I look foolish. So if I say what I think I'll look foolish, and if I'm quiet I'll look foolish. That's when I panic.

THERAPIST: Each sentence must pass some pretty rigorous screening before you can say it, then. I'll bet that you often don't pay attention to what others are saying because you're so busy screening your thoughts. It seems too risky to you to just say what's on your mind.

PATIENT: Unless it's business or the other people learn something from me, what I think is not important.

THERAPIST: I guess that means that you could not say an idea that was only partially thought through. That would make you look too foolish.

PATIENT: Yes, and I couldn't do that in front of these groups.

The approach toward changing this core concept was twofold. First, he was told to observe other managers for signs of anxiety when they had to talk.

THERAPIST: So let me get this idea straight. If you show signs of nervousness or if say things that are not completely thought out, then people will lose respect for you. Is that right?

PATIENT: Yes.

THERAPIST: Is that true for other managers, too? Do they ever show signs of nervousness or say things that are not entirely thought out, and do they lose respect?

PATIENT: I've noticed several mangers who seem to be nervous when they talk, but I still think of them as effective. They still get the job done. But I wonder what other people there think of them.

THERAPIST: Well, you don't think badly of them. Is there some way we can find out about the reputations of these nervous managers?

PATIENT: When I talk to the crews, it is pretty easy to pick up this kind of information.

THERAPIST: Would you be willing to do this as part of your assignment for this week? I'd like you to watch the other managers carefully for nervous behavior, for pauses in their talks, and for saying things that are not entirely thought out. Then I'd like you to casually talk to your crews about these people to see what the crews think of them.

PATIENT: I can do that.

Such observation yielded a plethora of positive findings. Significant numbers of these other managers displayed quite observable signs of anxiety. Next, the client was to compare the reputations of these nervous managers to those who were not nervous. Stage one was accomplished by discussion with subordinates about these other managers' effectiveness. Results from stage two produced significant evidence that almost all of these mangers were considered to be quite capable and effective in spite of their displayed nervousness. The patient began to conclude that his reputation as a good manager did not appear to hang solely on his display of nervous behaviors.

Having accomplished stage one and stage two, in vivo exposure was next.

THERAPIST: It seems that other managers are nervous, and they still have respect. How do you understand that?

PATIENT: It might be like you said. Maybe other people don't pay as much attention to it as I do.

THERAPIST: I think we can move away from the amount of preparation that you feel you need to remain in control of the situation. I'd like to propose that we do several ad lib talks today in the office. I'm going to propose a topic that you know something about, but not a lot. Then I'd like you to use the brainstorming, organizing, and covert rehearsal techniques you've learned earlier to make up your outline. When we first start, I'd like you to put the outline on the board and then later to do the outline and keep it in your head. As you are going through the talk, I'll signal a pause to you, and I want you to stop until I signal a start. Are you ready?

PATIENT: I don't know a lot about other things. I don't know what I'll say.

THERAPIST: Yes, I know that it won't be expert and the very last word on the subject, but I'll bet that you do have something to contribute anyway.

PATIENT: OK. How long do I talk?

THERAPIST: The first one about three minutes, and then we'll get a little longer later. But let's not worry about talking to please the clock. Let's focus on getting across the desired information and let the clock take care of itself.

PATIENT: OK.

During this stage, the patient was told to carry out two of his presentations *without* the overprepared approach he has always used. He was encouraged to admit publicly that he did not know some parts of the operation and that he required assistance with a particular aspect. Furthermore, during his presentations, he was to pause *deliberately* in his talk in order to gather more thoughts for his next portion of the presentation. In-session treatment included a discussion and delineation of exactly how his reputation would be damaged by a display of "emotional weakness" in one of these public forums. The result of these discussions revealed that he felt that the only appropriate emotion for him to display in public was anger; such an emotion would not damage his self-perceived reputation in the eyes of his subordinates. An exploration of the concept of emotional display revealed that the concept transcended situations—there were virtually no situations in which he could display any emotion except anger. Yet, when asked if he thought his family would think less of him if he displayed other emotions, such as being frightened or sad, he unequivocally said no.

In another session, the main focus was on the possibility that display of emotion may not be seen by others as a weakness but as an asset. He, too, was human and had feelings, pain, and fear like everyone else. He could understand others feeling fear, pain, and sadness and not think of them as weak. If others saw these emotions in him, they would feel more like him and would like him better and respect him more, rather than less as he thought.

With this cognitive preparation accomplished and the previous, less fearful exposures accomplished with some SUDS elevation but no panic, the stage was set to move toward public situations that he perceived as quite dangerous. These situations involved his request for regular topical meetings with his subordinates. Such a situation was frightening because he would have made the request for a meeting and therefore could not back out; he would have to organize and run the meeting plus set the overall purpose of the group. Also, the content areas of the meetings were ones where he felt less mastery and could be shown not to know important information. These exposures were set up in a graduated fashion, moving from one requested meeting to another only after successful handling of the previous meeting. Results from these exposures were a significant drop in anticipatory anxiety and little anxiety during the performance part of the meeting. Even when the audience was aware that he was not a complete master of the topic, no panic happened.

After these last series of exposures, anxiety and panic remained very low. Further treatment was not needed, and a six-week follow-up visit was scheduled; if the gains made were retained, then a three-month follow-up would be next.

REFERENCES

Barlow, D. H. (1988). *Anxiety and its disorders: The nature and treatment of anxiety and panic*. New York: Guilford.

Bower, G. H. (1981). Mood and memory. *American Psychologist, 36*, 129–148.

DiNardo, P. A., Barlow, D. H., Cerny, J., Vermilyea, B. B., Vermilyea, J. A., Himadi, W., & Waddell, M. (1985). *Anxiety Disorders Interview Schedule-Revised* (ADIS-R). Albany: Phobia and Anxiety Disorders Clinic, State University of New York.

Foa, E. B., & Kozak, M. S. (1986). Emotional processing of fear: Exposure to corrective information. *Psychological Bulletin, 99*, 20–35.

Paul, G. L. (1966). *Insight vs. desensitization in psychotherapy*. Stanford, CA: Stanford University Press.

Pilkonis, P. A., & Zimbardo, P. G. (1979). The personal and social dynamics of shyness. In C. E. Izard (Ed.) *Emotions in personality and psychopathology*. New York: Plenum.

Watson, D., & Friend, R. (1969). Measurement of social-evaluative anxiety. *Journal of Consulting and Clinical Psychology, 33*, 448–457.

Zimbardo, P. G. (1977). *Shyness: What it is, what to do about it*. Reading, MA: Addison-Wesley.

SUGGESTED READINGS

Dodge, C. S., Hope, D. A., Heimberg, R. G., & Becker, R. E. (1988). Evaluation of the social interaction self-statement test with a social phobic population. *Cognitive Therapy and Research, 12*, 221–222.

Heimberg, R. G., & Becker, R. E. (1985). Cognitive-behavior group treatment for social phobia. *Behavioral Group Therapy*, *6*, 2–7.

Heimberg, R. G., Becker, R. E., Goldfinger, K., & Vermilyea, J. A. (1985). Treatment of social phobia by exposure, cognitive restructuring and homework assignments. *Journal of Nervous and Mental Disease*, *173*, 236–245.

Heimberg, R. G., Dodge, C., & Becker, R. E. (1987). Social phobia. In L. Michelson & M. Ascher (Eds.), *Cognitive-behavioral assessment and treatment of anxiety disorders* (pp. 280–309). New York: Plenum.

Heimberg, R. G., Hope, D. A., Dodge, C. S., & Becker, R. E. (1990). DSM-III-R subtypes of social phobia: Comparison of generalized social phobics and public speaking social phobics. *Journal of Nervous and Mental Disease*, *178*, 172–179.

7

Posttraumatic Stress Disorder

Constance V. Dancu and Edna B. Foa

INTRODUCTION

Rape is a traumatic event often followed by emotional reactions that can severely disrupt daily functioning. The responses following rape have been labeled *post-traumatic stress disorder* (PTSD), a relatively new diagnostic entity that was introduced in the DSM-III as an anxiety disorder (American Psychiatric Association, 1980). In the revised manual (DSM-III-R; American Psychiatric Association, 1987), the characteristic symptoms of the disorder were divided into three classes: (a) reexperiencing of the traumatic event (e.g., nightmares, flashbacks, intense emotional distress when exposed to reminders of the trauma); (b) avoidance and numbing (e.g., avoidance of thoughts and reminders of the trauma, psychogenic amnesia, detachment); and (c) increased arousal (e.g., sleep disturbance, trouble concentrating, hypervigilance, exaggerated startle response, physiologic reactivity upon exposure to events that resemble the traumatic event).

In a prospective study, 94% of rape victims met symptomatic criteria for PTSD shortly after their assault;

three months after the assault, 47% still manifested the disorder (Rothbaum, Foa, Murdock, Riggs, & Walsh, in press). In a study investigating lifetime prevalence of crime, 16.5% of rape victims had PTSD an average of 17 years after their assault (Kilpatrick, Saunders, Veronen, Best, & Von, 1987). It has been estimated that approximately 25% of American women will experience rape at some point in their lifetime (Koss, 1983). The high incidence of rape and high percentage of rape victims who develop chronic PTSD point to the urgent need for development of effective therapeutic procedures.

Two treatment programs, stress inoculation training (SIT) and exposure treatment, have been studied. The SIT program aims at teaching rape victims to manage fear and anxiety via a variety of coping skills. Several studies have found this program effective in alleviating target symptoms such as anxiety and PTSD (Foa, Rothbaum, Riggs, & Murdock, 1991; Resick, Jordan, Girelli, Hutter, & Marhoefer-Dvorak, 1988; Veronen & Kilpatrick, 1982). Exposure treatment, which includes reliving the traumatic experience and confronting reminders of the trauma, has also been found effective in reducing PTSD symptoms following combat (Fairbank & Keane, 1982; Johnson, Gilmore, & Shenoy, 1982; Keane, Fairbank, Caddell, & Zimering, 1989; Keane & Kaloupek, 1982), accidents (McCaffrey & Fairbank, 1985; Muse, 1986), and rape (Foa et al., 1991). Whereas SIT focuses on training in coping skills to manage anxiety, exposure procedures involve repeated prolonged confrontation with the fear stimuli in order to facilitate habituation of anxiety and modify cognitive appraisal of the feared situations.

Constance V. Dancu and Edna B. Foa • Department of Psychiatry, Center for the Treatment and Study of Anxiety, Medical College of Pennsylvania/EPPI, Philadelphia, Pennsylvania 19129.

Comprehensive Casebook of Cognitive Therapy, edited by Arthur Freeman and Frank M. Dattilio. Plenum Press, New York, 1992.

BACKGROUND INFORMATION

Martha was a 19-year-old, single Caucasian woman with a middle-class background. One year prior to her participation in a PTSD treatment study, she was raped and shot by a young black male. The assailant followed Martha to a parking lot, forced her into the car by holding a gun to her head, threatened to kill her if she struggled or made any noise, and ordered her to drive to a secluded area by a lake, where he raped her (both orally and vaginally) in the car. He then ordered Martha out of the car, shot her in the back, and threw her into the lake. Immediately after he left, Martha crawled out of the lake and was later found near the road. She was seriously wounded and remained hospitalized for two weeks. The assailant was arrested, found guilty, and was incarcerated.

After the assault, Martha experienced significant disruption in all aspects of her life. She withdrew her plans to attend college. She also started a job from which she resigned a month later due to her extreme difficulty in concentrating and her severe panic reactions. One week after she left the hospital, Martha started to drink heavily when with friends. She attributed this excessive intake of alcohol to the extreme discomfort she experienced around peers who knew about the rape. Within seven months after the rape, Martha was involved in two car accidents, one while driving under the influence of alcohol and the other as a passenger. These accidents intensified Martha's post-rape reactions, and she ceased to engage in any activity by herself, spending the days at home with her mother and the nights with her boyfriend. Because of Martha's increased dependency on her mother, their relationship became strained and was characterized by frequent arguments.

Martha was first diagnosed and evaluated to determine initial level of pathology using the assessment procedure outlined in the appendix at the end of this chapter. She then participated in a treatment study comparing stress inoculation training (SIT) and prolonged exposure (PE). Clients in this study were assigned randomly to a treatment condition; however, as part of the study protocol, those who received treatment and did not improve satisfactorily (or who relapsed) were offered the other treatment. This practice was based on the view that individuals differ with respect to how much they will gain from each treatment and that those who failed to improve with one treatment might gain from the other. Specifically, we think that women who suffer from intense arousal would benefit more from SIT, which focuses on teaching anxiety management techniques. On the other hand, women who have severe symptoms of reexperiencing and avoidance will benefit more from prolonged exposure. Martha was first treated with the SIT program and showed considerable improvement, but relapsed two months later and therefore was offered exposure treatment.

INITIAL PSYCHOPATHOLOGY

According to the Structured Clinical Interview for DSM-III-R (SCID I and II; Spitzer, Williams, Gibbon, & First, 1989), Martha met criteria for PTSD, panic disorder with agoraphobia, and alcohol dependency in remission. There was no evidence of psychopathology prior to the rape. Symptoms of PTSD included nightmares, flashbacks, fears of being alone, and intrusive thoughts about the assault. Martha reported attempts to avoid thinking about the assault and about situations that reminded her of it, difficulty getting motivated to engage in daily activities, and feelings of detachment from others. She also complained of sleep problems, difficulty concentrating, exaggerated startle response, and hyperalertness. Martha's scores on the self-report measures are reported in Table 7-1.

The pretreatment assessment indicated marked depression (BDI) and anxiety (STAI). The elevated scores on the State-Anger Scale suggested that Martha also experienced intense anger. Initial scores on the RAST indicated severe rape-related fears (e.g., parking lots, being alone in the car, people behind her, strangers) and elevated general psychopathology (e.g., low energy, trouble sleeping, feelings of worthlessness, spells of terror or panic). Finally, the SAS overall assessment score corroborated Martha's reports of significant disruption in all aspects of her daily functioning.

TREATMENT

Stress Inoculation Treatment (SIT)

This treatment program was adapted from Veronen and Kilpatrick (1983), with the exception that no instructions for in vivo exposure to feared situations were given. Treatment consisted of nine biweekly 90-minute sessions conducted by Constance V. Dancu. The first two sessions were devoted to gathering information about the rape and providing an explanation of treatment, including education about the nature of fear and anxiety. In the remaining seven sessions, Martha was taught anxiety management skills. These included muscle relaxation, breathing control, thought stopping, cognitive restructuring, guided self-dialogue, covert modeling, and role-playing. Each session began with a 10-minute review of homework assignments. A new coping skill was then taught, using a

TABLE 7-1 Psychopathology Measures

	Initial evaluation	Post-SIT	2 Mos. Post-SIT (Preexposure)	2 Mos. Post-PE
PTSD measures				
PTSD severity	33	4	33	3
Avoidance symptoms	13	0	10	0
Intrusion symptoms	8	2	5	1
Arousal symptoms	12	2	18	2
General Psychopathology Measures				
SAS overall	4	1	5	1
RAST	210	69	150	51
STAI-State	58	36	71	33
STAI-Trait	52	39	43	40
BDI	26	6	36	6
STAXI-State	27	11	34	10
STAXI-Trait	19	21	20	19

nonassault-related situation first, followed by an assault-related situation.*

Session 1

During the first session, Martha described the entire assault and the painful feelings connected with this memory but did not show overt distress. She related the sequence of the rape as if she was telling a story about another person:

> The whole time he was raping me I had the thought he was gonna shoot me up there . . . inside me . . . cause he's so sick. . . . After he raped and shot me he still came after me. . . . Luckily he didn't come in the water, but he was throwing rocks at my head. . . . Afterward when I was lying in the road . . . I could tell my body was dying.

Session 1 was terminated with breathing exercises aimed at decreasing anxiety that may have been elicited by questions during the interview.

Session 2

In the second session, the treatment method was described to Martha, a rationale for treatment was given, and a verbal and written explanation for the origin of fear and anxiety was presented. Fear and anxiety were described as normal, learned responses that can occur in three channels—behavioral, cognitive, and physical. To illustrate this point, Martha was asked to relate a recent situation in which she became anxious and to describe her responses. She related the following event:

*Treatment manuals can be obtained from the authors by a written request.

> Last night I heard a noise outside my window, and I thought somebody was standing out there with a gun getting ready to shoot me . . . my heart started pounding . . . I thought, someone is out there, and they are going to kill me . . . this time they are not going to miss . . . I couldn't move.

This example was used in the session to illustrate that fear responses occur in stages. Martha was told that she would learn in treatment to identify the early indications of fear and to utilize coping skills to control her anxiety before it became unmanageable.

Session 3

Martha was taught deep muscle relaxation and breathing control to aid her in managing fear and anxiety expressed through the physical channel. The Jacobson (1938) tension–relaxation contrast training was used to teach muscle relaxation. This training included all major muscle groups; verbatim instructions for relaxation training were drawn from Goldfried and Davidson (1976). Martha was instructed to practice relaxation twice daily between sessions, which she found to be very helpful in reducing her daily tension. She also utilized the breathing control exercises in several situations that reminded her of the rape.

Session 4

The relaxation training continued in the first part of the session. Thereafter, thought stopping (Wolpe, 1958) was introduced in order to teach Martha how to control her intrusive thoughts, which characterize PTSD sufferers. Martha was asked to close her eyes and generate the distressing thought and indicate when that thought was clear in her mind by raising her index finger. The therapist then shouted loudly, "Stop." Martha, like most clients, startled in response to the unexpected loud voice, and the distressing thought disappeared. It is important to point out to the patient that the "stop" exercises demonstrate the ability to control intrusive thoughts. Next, Martha was asked to shout "stop" after generating the intrusive thought, followed by producing the thought and then silently verbalizing the word *stop*. Finally, she was asked to imagine a pleasant scene after the silent verbalization of the word *stop*. Martha was instructed to practice this procedure 10 times each day and to use it each time she had a distressing thought. For example, when Martha was shopping in the mall with her mother, she reported being extremely upset by people walking behind her and by men glancing at her. Her ruminative thinking was as follows:

> That guy is looking at me . . . He is going to rape me . . . I'm a likely candidate for something to happen . . . Everyone wants to hurt someone, and I'd be the someone they'd pick . . . I'm going to die young and in some violent way.

Martha was instructed to use the thought-stopping techniques when such thoughts came to her consciousness.

Another example comes from Martha's attitude about attending a trade school. She reported apprehension about the prospect of interacting with other students and having troublesome thoughts about how she would perform academically (e.g., "I'm going to mess it all up"). Martha's homework assignment was to use thought stopping after generating the thought "I'm going to die young" and "I'm going to mess up."

Session 5

The treatment goal in session 5 was to teach Martha to identify and modify irrational trauma-related beliefs that caused intense anxiety. To this end, the ABC method (Beck, Rush, Shaw, & Emery, 1979; Ellis & Harper, 1961) was introduced. First, the therapist presents an example that demonstrates how an event (e.g., hearing a loud noise in the next room) can lead to totally different responses (intense fear and leaving the house versus mild annoyance and entering the room) depending on one's interpretation ("There's a burglar in my house; I'm in danger" versus "What did the cat get into now?").

The instructions for cognitive restructuring are:

1. Write down the antecedent (A) and consequences (C).
2. Generate the belief (B) in order to establish the automatic assumption.

3. Question the reality of the assumption under B: Weigh the evidence for and against the assumption as in a court of law.
4. If the evidence is found to be insufficient, dismiss the belief.
5. If sufficient evidence exists, respond rationally and adaptively.

The rationality of the client's beliefs are challenged using the Socratic method of questioning (e.g., "What is the evidence for or against this belief? Is your belief based on your feelings rather than factual information? What are the advantages or disadvantages of holding onto this belief? What is the probability that what you fear will actually happen? What is an alternative adaptive statement you could say to yourself?"). It is important to note when assessing the rationality of the client's beliefs that many rape victims may live or work in areas that are not safe. Therefore, it is important to consider this when assessing the rationality of the client's belief. If the belief is realistic, safety guidelines should be developed.

Martha's beliefs were "I'm not going to succeed in school"; "I'm going to have AIDS as a result of the rape"; "black men are out to get you"; and "I'm more liable to get victimized than other people". An example of applying the ABC technique is as follows:

> A (antecedent): seeing a black male
> C (consequences): feeling scared and anxious
> B (belief): "He is going to shoot me. I'm going to die."

After examining the evidence for and against the belief, Martha concluded:

> The man who shot me is in jail and I would know if he was out . . . The chance that another black man would happen to shoot me is very low . . . What are the chances that the black man would have just shot me in the presence of hundreds of people . . . This is ridiculous . . . The probability that I would be killed is very low.

Session 6

In the beginning of the session, Martha reported that she no longer had any problems in concentrating, anxiety attacks, or feelings of being intimidated. She had begun trade school and felt comfortable in the classroom. Also, Martha's relationship with her mother had improved considerably.

After the homework review, guided self-dialogue was introduced to help the client cope with realistic stress. This procedure involved teaching the client to focus on her self-statements. A typical irrational, negative, or faulty dialogue is identified by the therapist and the client and is replaced by a rational, coping self-statement. The framework for this technique was adapted from Meichenbaum (1974). The four categories for stress management are reviewed with the client:

1. Preparation for stress
2. Confrontation with stressful situations and how to manage them
3. Coping with feelings of being overwhelmed
4. Self-reinforcement

For each of the four categories, the client and therapist generate a series of questions or statements.

Martha was afraid that she had contracted AIDS during the rape, although blood tests of both her and the assailant one month after the assault were negative. Given the realistic concern that a blood test one month following the assault could be false-negative, it seemed appropriate to use the guided self-dialogue technique to prepare for the one-year blood test. The final self-statements that Martha generated were as follows:

> There's nothing I can do about it . . . I can't turn back now . . . there is a possibility, but there is nothing I can do about it at this point except move forward . . . I will pretend I'm feeling okay and can handle it . . . I think about the fact that he got tested, and it was negative . . . one step at a time . . . easy does it.

The morning after Session 6, Martha's mother reported that after the session, on the way to their car in the parking lot, she and her daughter were approached by a black male with a gun tucked into the front of his pants. Although they managed to get into the car and leave without being hurt, this incident was particularly distressing because the sequence of events was similar to that of the original assault.

Session 7

In the beginning of this session, Martha described the recent incident in the parking lot and her reactions.

> He was walking straight at me and my mom . . . and then for a minute I was thinking, what does he want . . . and then I saw the gun and I was just standing there . . . I had the door open but I was standing there staring at him, and then my mom said, "Get in the car; get in the car," and I finally woke up and jumped in . . . but I couldn't stop staring at him. I was starting the car and I looked over and as I was pulling out, I was still watching . . . I was surprised that I didn't pass out. That's what I always thought I would do if something like that happened again . . . I would say take me and kill me . . . I was thinking, I'm a likely candidate for this kind of thing . . . now I think everyone I see is going to rape, rob, or hurt me.

Martha was encouraged to fully discuss the incident and her responses. According to the treatment program, covert modeling was to be introduced in this session, but because of the incident in the parking lot, the therapist decided to implement coping skills that Martha had found helpful. Thus, the ABCs and guided self-dialogue were used to help Martha deal with her reactions to the parking lot event.

Session 8

Martha reported "feeling good". She was practicing relaxation twice daily and had used thought stopping a few times since the last session. She was not having flashbacks and was able to concentrate in school.

Role-playing and its imaginal analogue, covert modeling, were introduced. First, the therapist and the client identify an anxiety-provoking situation. The therapist then imagines that situation and verbalizes the images, introducing successful coping statements. Next, the client is asked to visualize the identical situation and imagine coping with it successfully.

Because the incident in the parking lot was very similar to the original rape, its image was used to teach Martha coping responses during an attack. In this image, the freezing response was replaced with a more active behavior. The following scenario was introduced:

> I'm leaving school late. I have my keys in my hand ready to use. I'm walking to my car, and I feel there's someone watching me. I walk down toward my car, and I see a man walking toward me. He starts to yell, "Excuse me, excuse me," and I just keep walking faster . . . keeping an eye on him, but not looking straight at him. And he keeps walking toward me, and I am ignoring him . . . He's asking me what time it is. I continue to ignore him. I hurry up and get into my car and lock the doors immediately . . . and he's still walking toward me. I hurry up and start the car, and turn the lights on, and get on my way.

When the covert modeling practice was completed, role-playing was introduced. It consists of acting out behaviors and rehearsing lines that can help manage potential stressful situations. In this way, the client learns new behaviors and statements to replace old, ineffective habits.

Since Martha felt vulnerable and anxious when walking alone, this situation was selected for role-playing. Martha learned to modify her slow, slightly bent-over walk with eyes downcast in a nonassertive fashion, and to replace it with an active and erect posture. Martha practiced this walk in several areas around the clinic.

Session 9

In the first part of this session, practice with covert modeling and role-playing continued. However, the primary purpose of this session was to review coping skills learned during treatment and to discuss its termination.

Assessment of Treatment Efficacy

Immediately after the session, a posttreatment assessment was conducted; the results are presented in Table 7-1. As is apparent from the table, Martha had benefitted from the treatment. She no longer met criteria for PTSD and had only minor residual symptoms. She evidenced better social adjustment and considerable reduction of rape-related fear. Her scores on generalized anxiety and depression reached normal levels.

Relapse

Two months after treatment, Martha reported a reoccurrence of her problems. She had dropped out of school and was again staying at home. Arrangements were made to evaluate Martha's psychological status; the results of this are also presented in Table 7-1.

Martha's symptoms reappeared after she read a newspaper article that described a woman who was murdered under circumstances similar to her own assault. She started to have nightmares in which she was murdered following the sequence of events described in the newspaper article. She also reported frequent flashbacks of her assault and intrusive thoughts about dying ("I'm not going to die of natural causes"; "I can't see myself growing old"). Martha was offered a trial by prolonged exposure.

Prolonged Exposure Treatment (PE)

Treatment consisted of seven twice-weekly, 90-minute exposure sessions. Imaginal exposure was conducted in the sessions and recorded on audiotapes to be reviewed daily for homework. In vivo exposure was assigned for homework. The clinic normally devoted the first two sessions of PE treatment to the gathering of background information; since such information was already available for Martha, prolonged exposure was introduced in the first session.

Session 1

During the first session, the rationale for exposure treatment was presented.

> It is not easy to digest painful experiences. If you think about the rape or are reminded of it, you may experience extreme fear and other negative feelings associated with the assault. It is unpleasant to feel this way, so most people tend to push away fearful, painful memories or

ignore them. We may tell ourselves things like "Don't think about it; time cures all." Other people may even advise you to use such tactics, believing that this is the best way to cope with traumas. Also, friends, relatives, or partners may feel uncomfortable hearing about the rape and may subtly influence you not to talk about it. Unfortunately, with highly traumatic events, ignoring your feelings and fears does not make them go away; therefore, these memories reoccur. Often the experience comes back to haunt you through nightmares, flashbacks, phobias, and other ways, because it is "unfinished business." What we are going to do is to help you overcome your tendency to avoid. We will help you to process the experience by having you remember what happened and stay with it long enough to get more used to it. The goal is to be able to have these thoughts, talk about the rape, or see cues associated with the rape without experiencing the intense anxiety that disrupts your life.

After the rationale for treatment was presented, a hierarchy of avoided situations was constructed to be used for in vivo exposure. The hierarchy for in vivo exposure included a list of the major situations that Martha avoided but were realistically safe. The following rationale and instructions for development of the hierarchy were presented.

> The treatment program involves having you confront situations and memories that generate anxiety and an urge to avoid. In order to prepare your treatment program, I need to obtain from you a list of specific situations that make you uncomfortable and how much discomfort each one generates in you. Let's talk about the degree of discomfort in numbers, with 100 indicating that you are extremely upset, the most you've ever felt. An example of this could be the rape. How much discomfort do you feel now using this scale? Have you ever experienced zero discomfort?

In vivo exposure begins with entering situations that evoke moderate levels of anxiety (e.g., subjective units of discomfort, or SUDS, = 50) and progress up the hierarchy to more feared situations (e.g., SUDS = 100). Clients are instructed to remain in the situation for 30 to 45 minutes or until anxiety decreases. Characteristics of the situations, such as time of day and others present, are adjusted to achieve the desired level of anxiety during exposure. For example, Martha reported that going to the mall with her mother evoked 60 SUDS and going alone was 85 SUDS. Examples of items in Martha's hierarchy were walking alone in a safe place, going to the store, being in a parking lot, going out with friends, and being in a car.

Sessions 2 to 7: Exposure to the Rape Scene

Imaginal exposure was introduced in the second treatment session and continued for the next six sessions. It consisted of having Martha imagine the rape and shooting as vividly as possible and describe it aloud in the present tense for 60 minutes. Because Martha reported nightmares as well as distressing thoughts about being murdered, she was asked to imagine that she was indeed murdered. Below are the instructions for the imaginal exposure.

> I'm going to ask you to recall the memories of the rape and shooting. It is best if you close your eyes so you won't be distracted. I will ask you to recall these painful memories as vividly as possible. I don't want you to tell a story in the third person; rather, describe it in the present tense—as if it was happening now, right here. You will close your eyes and tell me in detail what you see and feel as well as the thoughts you are having. We will work together on this. If you start to feel too uncomfortable and want to run away or avoid it by leaving the image, I will help you to stay with it. We will tape the entire scenario so you can take the tape home and listen to it. Every 10 minutes, I'll ask you to rate your anxiety level on a scale from 0 to 100. Please answer quickly and don't leave the image. Do you have any questions before we start?

During the first two imagery sessions, Martha was free to choose the level of detail she could tolerate. In the remaining sessions, she was encouraged to describe the assault in great detail, repeating it several times each session. The imaginal exposure scenes included external cues (e.g., walking to the car), internal cues (e.g., thoughts, images), physiological responses (e.g., heart pounding, hands sweating), and the feared consequences (e.g., death). Below is an excerpt from Martha's imagery.

> He is pushing my head down towards his penis to do oral sex. I feel the gun on my back. My heart is pounding and my hands are sweating; the smell is disgusting. If I don't do this, he is going to kill me . . . I'm feeling scared . . . my body is shaking all over.

Martha was able to recall and describe the rape and her responses without difficulty despite her high level of anxiety. Interestingly, she reported that "for the first time, I felt like it was real."

Martha complied with the treatment program despite the marked anxiety associated with reliving the assault and confronting difficult situations. As predicted, her anxiety (as measured) decreased both within and across sessions judging from her SUDS ratings. When treatment was terminated, the rape and murder scenarios did not elicit anxiety. Martha no longer avoided going into public places, cars, parking lots, or out with friends.

Follow-Up Assessment

A follow-up assessment was conducted two months after the completion of the exposure treatment; data are presented in Table 7-1. As is apparent from inspection of this table, Martha improved and returned to the symptom level she had following stress inoculation training. She no longer met criteria for PTSD and had only minor residual symptoms.

Interestingly, during the follow-up period two events that could provoke trauma-related symptoms occurred. First, a friend of Martha's was killed in a car accident. Second, she was going through the process of a civil suit associated with the assault. After the car accident, Martha reported "some thoughts about dying, but I kept on going using thought stopping and cognitive restructuring". In addition to a reduction of PTSD-related symptoms, Martha reported significant improvement in her social functioning. She instituted plans to attend college and completed the application process. She was working, dating a new boyfriend, visiting friends at college, and going to the beach with friends. Her family atmosphere was improved, as reflected in the many activities she shared with her parents, such as visiting friends, eating out, and going shopping. Martha's parents confirmed this report; her mother said, "We are back to where we were before it happened." A telephone call five months after treatment terminated revealed continued improvement. Martha is a full-time college student, dating and engaging in extensive social activities.

DIFFICULTIES IN TREATING RAPE VICTIMS

As implied by the DSM-III-R criteria, PTSD sufferers engage in extensive cognitive and behavioral avoidance. This may interfere with treatment for rape victims in several ways:

1. There may be a reluctance to attend treatment sessions that focus on confrontation with the painful images, thoughts, and situations. This difficulty can be partially overcome when the therapist conveys his or her understanding that the client's reluctance to attend treatment sessions is part of the disorder. The therapist allows more leeway in this matter than one would for clients with other types of problems.
2. Anxiety disorders usually include concerns that are largely unrealistic. Agoraphobic fears of having a heart attack in fear-evoking situations are indeed unrealistic, as is the obsessive-compulsive's concern of catching a venereal disease after using a public toilet. Assault victims were *actually* raped, and thus their fears are strongly rooted in reality. Therefore, it is important to consider carefully the degree of realistic danger when the treatment program for rape victims is designed.

3. Because of the close tie between post-traumatic stress disorder and reality, it is sometimes difficult to successfully use techniques such as cognitive restructuring that aim at changing the victim's perception of danger associated with specific events. While some situations that the clients avoid may be clearly safe and require altering perceptions, other avoided situations are more ambiguous. In these instances, rules for deciding what is safe and what is dangerous should be introduced.

4. Clients are often reluctant to engage fully in reliving the traumatic experience and in following homework assignments that include in vivo and imaginal confrontation with fearful material. This problem can be overcome by allowing the client to titrate her degree of emotional involvement during the first exposure session by selecting the level of detail in recounting the story.

5. During the imaginal exposure, clients who successfully overcome their tendency to avoid becoming emotional when discussing their trauma can become upset. It is important to provide enough time for the session to enable the client to gain control over her emotions before leaving.

RECOMMENDATIONS FOR TYPE OF TREATMENT

1. When the client's symptoms largely involve dissociative symptoms such as numbing or cognitive avoidance, treatment by exposure is indicated.

2. When the client's symptoms primarily involve chronic arousal (e.g., exaggerated startle response, hypervigilance), stress inoculation training is indicated.

3. When a client presents with the entire clinical picture of PTSD, a combination of exposure and stress inoculation seems to be an optimal program.

DISCUSSION

The case report presented in this chapter illustrates typical postrape responses and subsequent psychopathology as well as typical treatment issues with such clients. Martha's case is a clear example of a client who greatly improved after the implementation of the SIT program but showed considerable relapse triggered by the occurrence of a traumatic event that crystallized her belief that her life

was endangered. Prolonged exposure did, however, have lasting effects in the face of further stressful experiences. Similar results have been found in a controlled study that compared stress inoculation training, prolonged exposure, and supportive counseling (Foa, et al., 1991). Immediately after treatment, clients who received SIT showed the greatest improvement, although those who received prolonged exposure also improved significantly. Three months after treatment, some clients who received SIT showed varying degrees of relapse. However, those who received prolonged exposure continued to improve. It is possible that the optimal treatment for PTSD should include a combination of SIT and exposure. A study comparing the combination treatment with each component is being conducted by Foa and Dancu.

The importance of Martha's perception that her life was in danger, which contributed to the reoccurrence of PTSD, is consistent with repeated findings that perceived danger to one's life or to the life of a significant other leads to increased pathology following assault and predicts the occurrence of chronic PTSD (Ellis, Atkeson, & Calhoun, 1981; Kilpatrick et al., 1989; McCahill, Meyer, & Fishman, 1979; Norris & Feldman-Summers, 1981; Sales, Baum, & Shore, 1984). Riggs, Foa, Rothbaum, and Murdock (1990) found that severity of the assault, the use of a weapon, and injury during the assault were directly related to perception of life threat, which in turn was associated with severity of PTSD.

Riggs et al. (1990) also found two additional variables that predict PTSD: social adjustment and guilt related to the assault. Greater feelings of guilt were directly related to early PTSD severity. On the other hand, later severity of PTSD (3 months postassault) was influenced by two factors, early PTSD severity and subsequent social adjustment. Indeed, the important role of social support in mediating reaction to criminal assault has been documented in several studies (Burgess & Holmstrom, 1978; Ellis et al., 1981; McCahill et al., 1979; Norris & Feldman-Summers, 1981; Ruch & Chandler, 1983; Ruch & Leon, 1983; Sales et al., 1984).

The four major variables discussed above that contribute to the development of chronic PTSD are certainly amenable to change via psychotherapy. Accordingly, in a comprehensive PTSD program, PTSD symptoms should first be addressed. Additionally, therapy of victims who express feelings of guilt associated with the traumatic event should address this issue. Thirdly, treatment should include evaluation of the victims' perceptions regarding threat to their lives and address the realistic probability that a similar traumatic event may occur. Finally, support of family and friends should be elicited to facilitate victims' social adjustment. This may include educating significant others on the impact of rape and including them in the treatment program.

APPENDIX: DIAGNOSIS AND ASSESSMENT MEASURES

Pretreatment evaluation included the Structured Clinical Interview for DSM-III-R (SCID I and II; Spitzer, Williams, Gibbon, & First, 1989), a diagnostic interview to assess severity of PTSD, and self-report measures. The measures used to assess Martha are described below:

- The PTSD Symptom Scale (PSS) is a 17-item clinician-rated scale based on the DSM-III-R (American Psychiatric Association, 1987) diagnostic criteria for PTSD. Each item is rated for severity on a scale of 0 to 3 (total range 0–51). Interrater reliability was .90 for the diagnosis of PTSD (presence/absence), and $r = .97$ (Pearson product-moment correlations) for severity (Rothbaum, Dancu, Riggs, & Foa, 1990).
- The Beck Depression Inventory (BD) (Beck, Ward, Mendelsohn, Mock, & Erbaugh, 1961) is a 21-item inventory measuring depression. Beck et al. reported split reliability of .93 and correlations ranging from .62 to .66.
- The Rape Aftermath Symptom Test (RAST) (Kilpatrick, 1988) is a self-report inventory that includes 70 items differentiating rape victims from nonvictims. Items were derived from the SCL-90 (Derogatis, 1977) and the modified Fear Survey Schedule (Veronen & Kilpatrick, 1980) and consisted of psychological symptoms and feared stimuli rated on a 5-point Likert scale (total range 0–280). The authors reported internal consistency of .95 and test–retest reliability of .85 over a 2½ week interval for nonvictims.
- The State-Trait Anxiety Inventory (STAI) (Spielberger, Gorsuch, & Lushene, 1970) contains 20 items for state anxiety and 20 items for trait anxiety. The authors reported test–retest reliability for trait anxiety was .81; as expected, figures were lower for state anxiety (.40). Internal consistency ranged from .83 to .92.
- The State-Trait Anger Expression Inventory (STAXI) (Spielberger, 1988) includes 10 items for state anger and 10 items for trait anger that are rated on a 4-point scale. Internal consistency ranged from .95 to .99.
- The Social Adjustment Scale (SAS) (Weissman & Paykel, 1974) is a semistructured interview to assess functioning in eight specific areas (work, social and leisure activities, extended family, romantic partner, sexual activity, parental, family unit, and economic) as well as overall adjustment.

ACKNOWLEDGMENT. Preparation of this chapter was supported by NIMH Grant No. MH42178 awarded to Edna B. Foa.

REFERENCES

American Psychiatric Association (1980). *Diagnostic and statistical manual of mental disorders* (3rd ed.). Washington, DC: Author.

American Psychiatric Association (1987). *Diagnostic and statistical manual of mental disorders* (rev. 3rd ed.). Washington, DC: Author.

Beck, A. T., Rush, A. J., Shaw, B. F., & Emery, G. (1979). *Cognitive therapy of depression.* New York: Guilford.

Beck, A. T., Ward, C. H., Mendelsohn, M., Mock, J., & Erbaugh, J. (1961). An inventory for measuring depression. *Archives of General Psychiatry, 4,* 561–571.

Burgess, A. W., & Holmstrom, L. L. (1978). Recovery from rape and prior life stress. *Research in Nursing and Health, 1,* 165–174.

Derogatis, L. R. (1977). *SCL-90: Administration, scoring, and procedures manual, 1 (for the revised) Version.* Towson, MD: Clinical Psychometrics Research.

Ellis, E. M., Atkeson, B. M., & Calhoun, K. S. (1981). An assessment of long-term reaction to rape. *Journal of Abnormal Psychology, 90,* 263–266.

Ellis, A., & Harper, R. A. (1961). *A guide to rational living.* Hollywood, CA: Wilshire.

Fairbank, J. A., & Keane, T. M. (1982). Flooding for combat-related stress disorders: Assessment of anxiety reduction across traumatic memories. *Behavior Therapy, 13,* 499–510.

Foa, E. B., Rothbaum, B. O., Riggs, D., & Murdock, T. (1991). Treatment of PTSD in rape victims: . A comparison between cognitive-behavioral procedures and counseling. *Journal of Consulting and Clinical Psychology, 59,* 715–723.

Goldfried, M. R., & Davidson, G. C. (1976). *Clinical behavior therapy.* New York: Holt.

Jacobson, E. (1938). *Progressive relaxation.* Chicago: University of Chicago Press.

Johnson, C. H., Gilmore, J. D., & Shenoy, R. Z. (1982). Use of a feeding procedure in the treatment of a stress-related anxiety disorder. *Journal of Behavior Therapy and Experimental Psychiatry, 13,* 235–237.

Keane, T. M., Fairbank, J. A., Caddell, J. M., & Zimering, R. T. (1989). Implosive (flooding) therapy reduces symptoms of PTSD in Vietnam combat veterans. *Behavior Therapy, 20,* 245–260.

Keane, T. M., & Kaloupek, D. G. (1982). Imaginal flooding in the treatment of post-traumatic stress disorder. *Journal of Consulting and Clinical Psychology, 50,* 138–140.

Kilpatrick, D. G. (1988). Rape aftermath symptom test. In M. Hersen & A. S. Bellack (Eds.), *Dictionary of behavioral assessment techniques.* Oxford: Pergamon.

Kilpatrick, D. G., Saunders, B. E., Veronen, L. J., Best, C. L., & Von, J. M. (1987). Criminal victimization: Lifetime prevalence, reporting to police, and psychological impact. *Crime and Delinquency, 33*, 479–489.

Kilpatrick, D. G., Saunders, B., Amick-McMullan, A., Best, C., Veronen, L., & Resnick, H. (1989). Victim and crime factors associated with the development of post-traumatic stress disorder. *Behavior Therapy, 20*, 199–214.

Koss, M. P. (1983). The scope of rape: Implications for the clinical treatment of victims. *Clinical Psychologist, 38*, 88–91.

McCaffrey, R. J., & Fairbank, J. A. (1985). Post-traumatic stress disorder associated with transportation accidents: Two case studies. *Behavior Therapy, 16*, 406–416.

McCahill, T. W., Meyer, L. C., & Fishman, A. M. (1979). *The aftermath of rape*. Lexington, MA: D. C. Heath.

Meichenbaum, D. (1974). *Cognitive behavior modification*. Morristown, NJ: General Learning Press.

Muse, M. (1986). Stress-related, posttraumatic chronic pain syndrome: Behavioral treatment approach. *Pain, 25*, 389–394.

Norris, J., & Feldman-Summers, S. (1981). Factors related to the psychological impacts of rape on the victim. *Journal of Abnormal Psychology, 90*, 562–567.

Resick, P. A., Jordan, C. G., Girelli, S. A., Hutter, C. K., & Marhoefer-Dvorak, S. (1988). A comparative outcome study of behavioral group therapy for sexual assault victims. *Behavior Therapy, 19*, 385–401.

Riggs, D. S., Foa, E. B., Rothbaum, B. O., & Murdock, T. (1990). *Post-traumatic stress disorder following rape and non-sexual assault: A predictive model*. Unpublished manuscript.

Rothbaum, B. O., Dancu, C. V., Riggs, D., & Foa, E. B. (1990, September). *The PTSD symptom scale*. Presented at the European Association of Behaviour Therapy Congress on Behaviour Therapy, Paris.

Rothbaum, B. O., Foa, E. B., Murdock, T., Riggs, D., & Walsh, W. (in press). A prospective examination of post-traumatic stress disorder in rape victims. *Journal of Traumatic Stress*.

Ruch, L. O., & Chandler, S. M. (1983). Sexual assault trauma during the acute phase: An exploratory model and multivariate analysis. *Journal of Health and Social Behavior, 24*, 184–185.

Ruch, L. O., & Leon, J. J. (1983). Sexual assault trauma and trauma change. *Women and Health, 8*, 5–21.

Sales, E., Baum, M., & Shore, B. (1984). Victim readjustment following assault. *Journal of Social Issues, 40*, 17–36.

Spielberger, C. D. (1988). *Manual for the State-Trait Anger Expression Inventory*. Unpublished manuscript.

Spielberger, C. D., Gorsuch, R. L., & Lushene, R. E. (1970). *Manual for the State-Trait Anxiety Inventory (self-evaluation questionnaire)*. Palo Alto, CA: Consulting Psychologists Press.

Spitzer, R. L., Williams, J. B. W., Gibbon, M., & First, M. B. (1989). *Structured clinical interview for DSM-III-R*. New York: Biometrics Research Department, New York State Psychiatric Institute.

Veronen, L. J., & Kilpatrick, D. G. (1980). Reported fears of rape victims: A preliminary investigation. *Behavior Modification, 4*, 383–396.

Veronen, L. J., & Kilpatrick, D. G. (1982, November). *Stress inoculation training for victims of rape: Efficacy and differential findings*. Presented in a symposium entitled "Sexual Violence and Harassment" at the 16th annual convention of the Association for Advancement of Behavior Therapy, Los Angeles, CA.

Veronen, L. J., & Kilpatrick, D. G. (1983). Stress management for rape victims. In D. Meichenbaum & M. E. Jaremko (Eds.), *Stress reduction and prevention* (pp. 341–374). New York: Plenum.

Weissman, M. M., & Paykel, E. S. (1974). *The depressed woman: A study of social relationships*. Chicago: University of Chicago Press.

Wolpe, J. (1958). *Psychotherapy by reciprocal inhibition*. Stanford: Stanford University Press.

SUGGESTED READINGS

Foa, E. B., Steketee, G., & Rothbaum, B. O. (1989). Behavioral/cognitive conceptualization of post-traumatic stress disorder. *Behavior Therapy, 20*, 155–176.

Koss, M., & Harvey, M. (1987). *The rape victims: Clinical and community approaches to treatment*. Lexington, MA: Stephen Greene.

Resick, P. A., Jordan, C. G., Girelli, S. A., Hutter, C. K., & Marhoefer-Dvorak, S. (1988). A comparative outcome study of behavioral group therapy for sexual assault victims. *Behavior Therapy, 19*, 385–401.

Rothbaum, B. O., & Foa, E. B. (in press). Cognitive-behavioral treatment of post-traumatic stress disorder. In P. Saigh (Ed.), *Post-traumatic stress disorder: A behavioral approach to assessment and treatment*. New York: Pergamon.

Veronen, L. J., & Kilpatrick, D. G. (1983). Stress management for rape victims. In D. Meichenbaum & M. E. Jaremko (Eds.), *Stress reduction and prevention* (pp. 341–374). New York: Plenum.

8

Panic with Agoraphobia

Frank M. Dattilio and Robert J. Berchick

Carole had just turned 33 years old as she rounded off her 9th year of marriage to Ross. There had been an ongoing discussion between the two of them during the past year about whether or not to have a fourth child. This issue created some tension for Carole; she remained the undecided one. She put further discussion off with the excuse of waiting until after the Christmas holidays to make a decision. They had been in their new home for less than one year, and with all of the commotion, Carole had neglected to start her Christmas shopping—another burden on her mind. The combination of these events made for a very stressful period in her life, rendering her vulnerable to overload.

Carole decided one day to put all other pressures on hold and go into the city to do some of her Christmas shopping. Because she had overslept that morning, she had to rush to make breakfast for the children and to get them off to school. Consequently, she missed breakfast herself, quickly gulping several cups of coffee in lieu of her morning meal. Taking the subway into the city, Carole bustled from store to store doing her errands. She man-

aged to take care of everyone and everything on her shopping list, then reached the train station with 15 minutes to spare before the local line she wanted to take home was scheduled to depart.

In the 15 minutes remaining, Carole decided to make one last stop, at a nearby bakery. As she stood in front of the counter waiting for her order, she experienced some momentary dizziness. At first she brushed it off as a consequence of skipping breakfast and lunch, but as seconds passed, her dizziness began to worsen, with a rapid increase in her heart rate. This was accompanied by more dizziness, along with shakiness and sweating. Needless to say, this began to frighten her, particularly since it seemed to occur "out of the blue." By this point, Carole's heart was pounding as if she had just run a 100-yard dash, and she began to breathe more rapidly in response. The harder her heart pounded, the more she gulped for air. Her body was now hot all over, with a tightness in the chest and a dry mouth. Certain that she was going to die, she was ravaged by terror. She subsequently ran out of the store without her packages and anxiously awaited her train. She reported that the ride home for her "was hell."

What Carole experienced was a disorder common to over 4 million Americans (Clum, 1990; Dattilio, 1987, 1990; Solkol, Beck, Greenberg, Wright, & Berchick, 1989) that has been referred to in both the professional literature and the media as a *panic attack*. Carole's first panic attack was followed by similar episodes over the following months. As a result, she began to avoid certain public places and soon reached the point where she would not shop, attend church, or participate in any social situa-

Frank M. Dattilio and Robert J. Berchick • Center for Cognitive Therapy, Department of Psychiatry, University of Pennsylvania School of Medicine, Philadelphia, Pennsylvania 19104.

Comprehensive Casebook of Cognitive Therapy, edited by Arthur Freeman and Frank M. Dattilio. Plenum Press, New York, 1992.

tion without being accompanied by an adult (e.g., her mother or husband).

Carole eventually consulted with her family physician, who after conducting a full medical evaluation (including blood studies, electroencephalograms, and electrocardiograms) diagnosed her as having a "nervous condition." He prescribed a benzodiazepine (alprazolam) and continued to monitor her for approximately eight months, at which time she reported less frequent panic attacks. However, when the physician began to titrate her daily dose of alprazolam, Carole experienced an increase in both the frequency and intensity of her panic attacks. Consequently her agoraphobic avoidance became more severe and restrictive.

After learning about the nondrug treatment program at the Center for Cognitive Therapy in Philadelphia, Carole scheduled an intake evaluation.

PRESENTING SYMPTOMS

At the time of intake, Carole's reported symptoms fulfilled more than four of the criteria for a diagnosis of moderate panic disorder with agoraphobia (300.21 as outlined in the DSM-III-R) (American Psychiatric Association, 1987). Asked about the accompanying cognitions, she reported a decrease in her ability to concentrate as well as thoughts of losing control or fainting. Her mood and affect were characterized by vigilance and cautiousness. She reported avoidant behavior that included a reluctance to venture into public places alone and the need for escape to her home when experiencing the onset of any anxiety. In addition, she fulfilled the criteria for generalized anxiety disorder (300.02).

HISTORY

Carole was born in northern Pennsylvania. She lived with her grandmother for three months when she was 9 years of age because of her mother's inability to cope emotionally with seven children after the last child was born. Carole is the eldest child, with 11 years between her and the youngest child, whom Carole says she "helped rear." She described her father, who is now deceased, as a "real perfectionist." He experienced a period of depression in 1956 and was treated with electroconvulsive therapy (ECT); Carole had only vague information regarding his condition and treatment. She had a good relationship with him but was closer to her mother, who was "very supportive, outgoing, and helpful." Her mother had no formal history of mental illness.

Her parents got along well together but never socialized with others due to money problems and her father's depression. Carole generally related well with her brothers and sisters and served as a mother figure to the younger children. She enjoyed school and made many friends, but would become very worried about exams even though she performed well. Upon being graduated from high school, she was employed as a legal secretary. She had no sexual relationships prior to meeting her husband at age 19. They married five years later and Carole reported that it had been a good marriage, though recently it had been under some strain due to the conflict over having a fourth child and the difficulties created by Carole's agoraphobia.

INTAKE EVALUATION

During the initial intake examination, which lasted approximately 2½ hours, Carole was administered the Structured Clinical Interview for DSM-III-R (SCID), the Beck Depression Inventory (BDI), and the Beck Anxiety Inventory (BAI). The SCID yielded a DSM-III-R diagnosis of panic attacks with agoraphobia (moderate) and generalized anxiety disorder, with a global assessment of functioning (GAF) of 55. Results indicated that she did not meet full criteria for major depression or dysthymic disorder, although it was noted that some mild depression did coexist with her panic and she was possibly premorbid from late adolescence or early adulthood. An underlying depression was therefore ruled out along with any other psychopathology.

Subsequent to the intake evaluation, Carole was seen on a separate day for a full 1-hour psychiatric evaluation to rule out any possible biochemical disorder. As a part of the cognitive therapy approach (in addition to her request), Carole was gradually weaned from the alprazolam by the consulting psychiatrist. Her dose at that time was 0.5 mg, twice per day as needed.

SESSION 1

The goal of the initial psychotherapy session was to ascertain more specifically Carole's patterns of anxiety and also to orient her to the cognitive therapy model. The symptoms that she had related at intake were reviewed. Carole was asked to discuss the emotion and cognition accompanying each symptom.

THERAPIST: Carole, what I would like to do in this session is to try and understand more clearly how and when your panic attacks occur and under what circumstances. Also, I would like to try to see whether or not we can link up any of the thoughts and emotions that you have with the actual sensations themselves.

CAROLE: Okay, I'll try.

THERAPIST: Good, now can you recall the last several episodes in which you experienced a panic attack?

CAROLE: Yes, unfortunately.

THERAPIST: Do you remember where you were and what you were doing?

CAROLE: Yes. In fact, the last three attacks all occurred while I was taking the kids to school.

THERAPIST: Okay. Now, I would like you to close your eyes and see if you can recall distinctly what you were doing right before you experienced your initial symptoms.

CAROLE: Well, yes, but I am really not too keen on this.

THERAPIST: Why is that?

CAROLE: Because, well, this might sound silly, but every time I start recalling incidents like this, I start to have an attack again—so I just try not to think about it.

THERAPIST: Well, okay—actually, that is not so unusual. Later on, I will show you how to use that to your advantage. Right now I need you to persevere and just bear with me for the sake of the treatment. Do you think you can hang in there with me?

CAROLE: I'll try my best.

THERAPIST: All right. Now, go back again and try to recall these past three attacks. Can you remember exactly what you were doing?

CAROLE: Yes, it was about the same each time. The attacks began to occur while I was actually driving on the road with the kids in the car taking them to school.

THERAPIST: Okay, now can you recall what the initial symptom was each time you experienced the attack?

CAROLE: Oh, yes! That's easy—it always starts with my heart pounding rapidly and just goes out of control.

THERAPIST: And then what?

CAROLE: And then I freak out.

THERAPIST: Freak out? Can you explain to me more in detail?

CAROLE: I am not totally sure, but I just get worse—more nervous.

THERAPIST: Okay, but we really need to try and pin down exactly how the symptoms unfold so that we can trace the cause of the attack.

CAROLE: Well—I am trying to think . . . (pause) I'm drawing a blank.

THERAPIST: Okay. Let's try this—close your eyes again and try to imagine yourself back in the same situation. Try to imagine your heart pounding rapidly.

(Carole closes her eyes in an attempt to recreate this image.)

CAROLE: Oh—I think after the heart pounding, I begin to breathe a lot . . . yeah, that's it. I start breathing really heavily.

THERAPIST: Anything else?

CAROLE: Uh—I start to get a little hot and sometimes I notice that I sweat, too . . . Oh my! I'm starting to get a little anxious just talking about this.

THERAPIST: Okay, good. So we have an increased heart rate with increased respiration, heat flash and accompanying perspiration—anything else?

CAROLE: Well, yeah—if I'm somewhere where I am standing or waiting, I usually get dizzy or light-headed and either have a tightness in the chest or wobbly legs. Sometimes both.

THERAPIST: Okay. Let us go back and list these—and as we do this, I would like you to now state for me the thought and the emotion, if you have one, that comes into your head while you're experiencing these symptoms. For example: You say that the first thing that you experience is a rapid increase in your heart rate. Now, what is the first thought that comes into your mind immediately upon experiencing this sensation?

CAROLE: You mean when my heart starts pounding like that? Oh, probably something like: "Here it goes again!"

THERAPIST: Here what goes again?

CAROLE: The panic!

THERAPIST: Then what?

CAROLE: Well, that's when I begin to breathe really heavily.

THERAPIST: And the thought that accompanies that sensation?

CAROLE: Ah, let me think—I guess just that "I'm getting worse."

THERAPIST: Is there an emotion that you experience from this?

CAROLE: Yes! Fear and worry—you now, I get really sensitive to what is going on with my body.

THERAPIST: All right, so after the increase in your respiration, what do you experience next?

CAROLE: Well, then I usually get hot all over and start to sweat.

THERAPIST: And the thought that comes as a result of this sensation?

CAROLE: That's when I really start to think that I'm losing it. This is what seems to throw me into a tailspin, and I just get worse.

THERAPIST: What are your thoughts at this point?

CAROLE: Oh, I start saying things to myself like, "I am out of control," and start crying, thinking that I am going to faint for sure. All that I think about is fainting or sometimes even dying on the spot.

THERAPIST: OK, that's fine. Now, let us try to get this

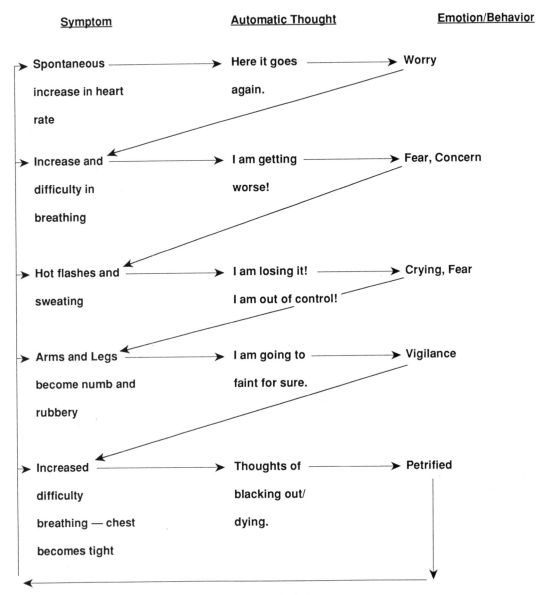

Figure 8-1. Carole's Panic Sequence.

down on paper and see if we can link up the sensations with any specific thoughts or emotions that might make a pattern.

Carole and I collaboratively constructed a diagram portraying the sequence of Carole's cognitions and how they directly affected her emotions and symptoms at the onset and during the course of her panic episodes (see Figure 8-1). By constructing the diagram, Carole and I established that each time Carole experienced an increase in heart rate, she passed through the sequence represented in Figure 8-1, except when she was in the company of others. While she did experience anxiety when with others, it would rarely escalate as it did when she was alone outside the home.

Once this diagram of her panic was constructed, Carole began to understand how she was escalating her symptoms by virtue of her catastrophic responses and emotional reactions to bodily sensations. It was explained to her in further detail that it was her misinterpretation of

Figure 8-2. Weekly Panic Log*

Name: Carole _____ Date: _____

Date, Time and Duration of the Panic Attack	Situation in which Panic Attack Occurred and Severity of the Panic Attack (1–10) units (u)	Description of the Panic Attack Symptoms and Sensations Experience	Your Response to Panic Attack. What Did You Do?
1. Sat. 2/21/88 5 min. 11:50 AM	At home sorting the wash 5-U	Heart Beating Fast, Tightness in Chest, Dry Mouth, Dizzy, Hands Sweating	Took Deep Breaths It worked!
2. Sun. 2/22/88 3 min. 7:00 PM	At home just after bathing girls 3-U	Dizzy, Heart Pounding, Legs Wobbly, Hot, Hands Sweating	Same as above
3. Mon. 2/23/88 Couple of minutes 10:00 AM	At home doing breakfast dishes 3-U	Heart Beating Fast, Tightness in Chest, Dizzy, Legs Wobbly, Dry Mouth	Same as above
4. Fri. 2/27/88 15 min. 8:55 AM	Driving daughter to school; waiting at a red light 9-U	Heart Beating Fast, Dizzy, Shaky, Sweating, Dry Mouth, Fear of Losing Control & Fainting in the Car.	Took Deep Breaths
5.			

Please indicate any additional Panic Attacks on the reverse side.
Circle the days you did not have a panic attack: M T W Th F S Sun   M T W Th F S Sun   u = units of anxiety

*Developed by the Center for Cognitive Therapy, University of Pennsylvania, 133 South 36th Street, Philadelphia, PA 19104.

bodily cues along with her catastrophic thought content that contributed to the exacerbation of her anxiety symptoms. In order to help her better understand this concept, Carole was asked to recall a recent incident in which she experienced panic and to trace the course of symptoms in that particular attack. Once again, her cognitions were aligned to each symptom and examined for their potential to escalate the subsequent symptom. Carole was also requested to keep a daily "panic log" (see Figure 8-2) for recording all attacks, so that we could examine together the cognitions and behaviors involved in the sequence of her attacks. As a homework assignment, she was instructed to keep this log and bring it into the next session.

SESSION 2

In session 2, Carole's panic log was reviewed in order to continue to examine the sequence of her symptoms and to identify her cognitions. Once again, specific focus was placed on catastrophic thought content as well as the pattern of escalation of her anxiety. It was also recognized that Carole would engage in overbreathing at times, which would occasionally cause an imbalance in her carbon dioxide level, resulting in dyspnea and the onset of hyperventilation. In order to aid her in correcting this, she was taught regulated breathing techniques (Clark, Salkovskis, & Chalkley, 1985) in addition to a traditional course of Jacobsonian progressive muscle relaxation (PMR; Jacobson, 1962). This involved having her breathe in through the nose and exhale slowly and continuously through the mouth. She was also provided with an audiotape that I recorded providing instructions in PMR. It was explained that the method was valuable both for controlling her breathing and for de-escalating her panic symptoms. As a homework assignment, Carole was asked to listen to this tape and to practice PMR twice per day for 15- to 20-minute periods. She was also to continue maintaining a daily panic log keeping track of her symptoms and the course of her panic attacks.

SESSION 3

In session 3, Carole's panic log for the week was reviewed, highlighting specific areas of escalation and anxiety, and linking these sensations to the automatic thoughts that underlay her catastrophic thought content. Her understanding of the escalation pattern of her symptoms was reinforced, and Carole was supported in the use of cognitive coping statements to thwart the onset of panic. In addition, an emphasis was placed on her practicing PMR with attention to specific difficulties she experienced in relaxing tense muscles. Once again, the controlled breathing technique was reviewed with her and she was taught to focus and concentrate on this state of relaxation. For the rest of the one-hour session, Carole and I worked together to construct a model of a hierarchy of situations she had come to avoid as a result of her anxiety and panic. A value was assigned to the units of anxiety and fear that she experienced in each situation. These are referred to as "SUDS" (subjective units of discomfort; Wolpe, 1973).

Carole's Hierarchy

SUDS

10	At home alone sorting laundry or doing breakfast dishes
20	Driving home alone after having dropped off her two children at school (four blocks from home)
30	Driving two traffic lights past the local drug store six blocks from home
40	Driving to the drug store alone and going in for one quick item
50	Going grocery shopping alone for a load of groceries
60	Taking the local train to the therapist's office alone and back (15 miles)
70	Driving to the shopping mall alone in the next town over to shop for several hours
80	Driving across the bridge alone into New Jersey
90	Driving to the New Jersey shore alone and back
100	Taking a bus trip alone to New York City

As a homework assignment, Carole was instructed to review the hierarchy that we constructed and make any changes or additions necessary for accuracy.* She was also advised to continue PMR exercises and to maintain the panic log on a daily basis.

SESSION 4

In session 4, Carole was taught to recognize very early signs of anxiety and the onset of panic. This was done by recapitulating a situation that occurred during the past week and reviewing the coping strategies used to control panic, namely, the cognitive self-statements and the breathing techniques. In this particular session, Carole cited two panic attacks that had occurred the previous week while taking her children to school. She said that in the morning just prior to leaving the house, she began to feel an overall uneasiness and shakiness. When she became alarmed by these sensations, she experienced an increase in heart rate and at that point began to engage in catastrophic thoughts (e.g., "I am starting to lose control again!"). During the session, the therapist had her imagine herself in that scene once again and try to reconstruct the circumstances as well as she could recall them.

While Carole was able to imagine this scene, she was unable to reproduce any of the symptoms by virtue of sheer imagery. Therefore, the use of panic induction was utilized in order to reproduce the identical symptoms that she experienced during the attack.

THERAPIST: Carole, I would like to try a short exercise with you that may aid in reproducing symptoms similar to those that occurred during your panic attacks.

CAROLE: On, no!

THERAPIST: Well, now, don't get upset. The idea is to help you learn how to control these symptoms in the way that we've talked about, through breathing retraining, progressive muscle relaxation, and the restructuring of your automatic thoughts. Okay?

CAROLE: I don't know—I mean, what if I begin to panic and I can't stop?

---

*Sometimes clients will unintentionally underestimate or overestimate a particular level of the hierarchy when constructing it in the office with the therapist only to realize its true impact when carrying it out in vivo. Therefore, therapists should always be prepared to make constant adjustments to the hierarchy in order to help the client overcome his or her fear.

THERAPIST: We'll address it should that occur—but again, I really need your cooperation with this exercise in order for me to help you overcome this problem.*

CAROLE: I'll do anything to try to overcome this problem—I just can't continue to live like this.

THERAPIST: Okay then, let's start. Now I would like you to begin to breathe by inhaling and exhaling through you mouth very quickly, almost as you would if you were really out of breath. (Therapist demonstrates technique.) Okay, now you do it along with me. (Carole mimics the same technique.)

THERAPIST: Good. Now, I'm going to say "go," and I want you to begin breathing along with me in this manner. However, I'm going to stop, but I would like you to continue on for about . . . oh, let's say 1½ to 2 minutes nonstop. Okay, are you ready?

CAROLE: I think so.

THERAPIST: Okay—let's start.

(Therapist and Carole begin the exercise together. Through the period of the exercise, the therapist supports Carole in her breathing and keeps track of the time.)

CAROLE: (as 1 minute and 10 seconds pass) Oh! (panting heavily) I don't know if I can breathe anymore!

THERAPIST: That's okay, keep going, we're almost through.

(Carole continues and finishes at the 2-minute mark.)

THERAPIST: Okay, stop. Good! Now stand up.

(Carole reluctantly stands.)

CAROLE: Oh, God, I feel like I'm going to pass out!

THERAPIST: What else do you feel?

CAROLE: I am having an attack right now—my mouth is dry.

THERAPIST: Okay. Now sit down and close your eyes and just begin to breathe slowly and continuously, inhaling through the nose and exhaling through the mouth—in the same way that I taught you in the PMR exercises. Just concentrate on your breathing and begin to slow everything back down to its normal resting state.

(Carole takes several minutes to do this.)

THERAPIST: Okay, how do you feel?

CAROLE: Much better.

THERAPIST: So, let's talk about what just occurred. This little exercise was designed to activate the autonomic nervous system and mimic some of the symptoms that you have during an attack. So what thoughts went through your mind during the exercise?

CAROLE: The exact same thoughts that I usually have during an attack, only I felt safer because you're here with me.

THERAPIST: What did you tell yourself about my presence?

CAROLE: Well—that if anything bad would happen, you would be here to help me through it . . . which you in fact just did.

THERAPIST: You mean by talking you down.

CAROLE: Yes.

THERAPIST: Do you think that this might be something that you could do by yourself?

CAROLE: Oh . . . I don't know.

THERAPIST: Why?

CAROLE: I don't know, I just always view it as such an overwhelming thing.

THERAPIST: Well, suppose we try a little experiment. Let's try having you expose yourself to a situation which is extremely low on the hierarchy that we constructed—let's say level 10, which is "at home alone sorting laundry or doing breakfast dishes." So, while you are doing your morning chore, try to identify the earliest onset of your symptom as it occurs. As soon as this happens, I would like you to begin focusing on your breathing to reduce your heart rate, de-escalating the symptoms from going any further. Do you think you can do this?

CAROLE: I'll try.

THERAPIST: Okay, and also we need to develop a cognitive self-statement for you to say to yourself during this time. Something to replace the catastrophic self-statements that you have made in the past. What might help you feel less threatened about your bodily sensations?

CAROLE: I don't know . . . I guess if I could convince myself that it will be all right and that I won't faint or die or anything like that—that might do it.

THERAPIST: Well, okay. Let's use this exercise that you just participated in. That's one example of how you controlled yourself. So, let's see if you can use the same thing on your own the next time you have symptoms. Just remember to reassure yourself that anxiety is limited and benign—it will always pass and not hurt you—and use this past experience as reinforcement.

CAROLE: All right—I'll give it a try.

This session introduced the technique of de-escalation and gave Carole direction for maintaining controlled breathing during her panics. Her homework and the panic log were reviewed and the de-escalation techniques reinforced. In addition, one of the lowest levels of the hierarchy was targeted as a homework assignment for begin-

---

*Prior to implementing this exercise, the therapist must have medical clearance from a physician to be certain that the client does not have any significant cardiovascular disorder, such as coronary artery disease, arrhythmia, or seizure disorder.

ning some self-exposure. The second lowest unit of anxiety on Carole's hierarchy, level 20, involved driving her children to school and returning home alone. Exposing herself to this situation was discussed, with the expectation that she would become anxious but would use the techniques she had learned for anxiety reduction. She was instructed to remain in the situation, regardless of her level of anxiety, until she experienced a significant decrease in anxiety level.

SESSION 5

In session 5 I continued to monitor Carole's exposure to the lower levels of the anxiety hierarchy. As her anxiety lessened, we moved to the next level and began to have her expose herself in the same fashion. As we progressed up the hierarchy in succeeding sessions, coping with her anxiety became increasingly difficult as the level of intensity grew. The same techniques for de-escalation and controlled breathing were utilized, along with cognitive coping statements about the effect that the anxiety had on her body. For example, one of her cognitive distortions was a belief that she might faint during heightened periods of anxiety. It was explained to Carole that there must be a significant decrease in blood pressure in order for one to faint—thus making fainting very unlikely during panic, which is associated with a rise in blood pressure resulting from the increase in heart rate. Carole was therefore instructed to remind herself of this fact each time she anticipated fainting and to repeat it out loud if necessary.

SESSIONS 6 THROUGH 15

During sessions 6 through 15, the focus remained on ascending the hierarchy. The range of 40 to 70 units of anxiety, which involved driving to the local drug store alone, going grocery shopping, taking a local train to the clinic for therapy, and driving to the shopping mall in the next town, was more challenging for her. Several of the situations required my assistance in actually accompanying her to the sites (in vivo). For example, at the point at which she was ready to begin taking the train alone, Carole's husband was asked to ride the subway train with her to the therapy center, but then leave her on her own. I then accompanied Carole to the subway station and rode one stop with her until she became comfortable. During this subway ride, I reinforced the techniques of controlled breathing and de-escalation in an in vivo setting. Carole then took the train alone to the next stop, where her husband was waiting to accompany her for the remainder of the trip

home. For the next visit, Carole came in again with her husband, but this time attempted to ride three stops alone, and so on until she was able to ride the train completely by herself. This was with her full agreement and involved a joint decision that she was ready for this step.

This practice of accompanying the client to some of the anxiety-provoking sites constitutes a graduated approach to helping the client approximate the goal and reinforce her coping strategies. It would be quite difficult, particularly with clients with panic disorders, to achieve results without using a behavioral follow-through on such coping strategies. The subsequent sessions involved similar exposure exercises; however, by this point Carole was assertive and motivated enough to attempt new situations on her own.

SESSIONS 15 THROUGH 28

Sessions 15 through 28 involved focusing on the levels of the hierarchy between 70 and 100 SUDS. Once Carole was able to take the train back and forth to our clinic for therapy sessions, she was then asked to generalize her ability to ride the train in different directions of the same length until she was able to take subway trains through the city during the daytime with relatively little or no anxiety. This again was a collaborative decision involving a joint agreement that she was ready.

The next level involved extending this ability to driving a car. This was a particular area of concern for Carole, since one of her catastrophic thoughts during anxiety was that she would lose control of herself. We proceeded with the same type of graded steps used to increase her exposure to taking the subway trains. She began by driving two blocks from her home, then gradually expanded to driving throughout the town and somewhat into the city. I later attempted to have her drive across the bridge from Philadelphia into New Jersey. This again was a very difficult undertaking, since she was afraid that she would lose control while on the bridge, which would be even more dangerous than having an attack in the city. The reinforcement of cognitive coping strategies and breathing techniques was a great aid in helping Carole keep her level of anxiety very low. Flash cards and coping cards containing positive self-statements were used to correct her maladaptive cognitions regarding her ability to function during attacks. I continued to progress through the hierarchy with Carole by having her make other driving trips as well as take the bus to different cities, such as New York and Atlantic City. These trips were all done on a solo basis using the techniques that Carole had been taught.

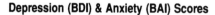

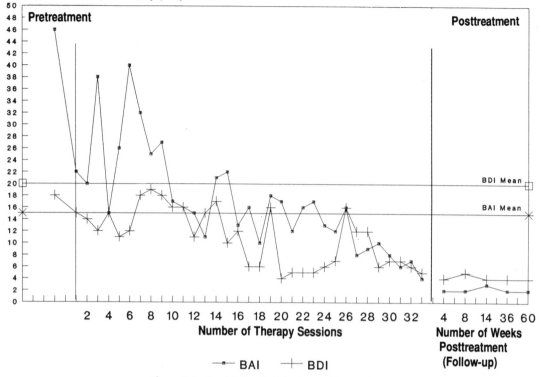

Figure 8-3. Carole's Level of Anxiety and Depression.

SESSIONS 29 THROUGH 33

Sessions 29 through 33 involved continuing to monitor Carole's anxiety and exposure treatment. In addition, we focused on handling daily stressors in her life. We discussed the strain and stress in her marriage and her difficulties with child rearing. The primary focus revolved around restructuring her underlying beliefs regarding child-rearing practices. Throughout the course of treatment, other issues would periodically be discussed as to whether or not they were possible underlying difficulties contributing to her panic.

A number of interesting points were uncovered that involved her self-esteem and self-concept. At times, dealing with her children reminded her of many periods of her upbringing in which she had to function as an adult role model. These occasions stirred up underlying anger and resentment that Carole had harbored since her childhood and that she had never felt free to express. Feelings of worthlessness caused her to develop conditional coping assumptions such as perfectionism and other rigid standards, which led to further low self-esteem. These feel-

ings were accompanied by a sense of guilt, which often appeared to serve as a trigger for her anxiety. All these issues were explored in greater depth once they were identified as precursors to Carole's panic and generalized anxiety disorder. In addition, we focused specifically on stress-reducing agents and ongoing techniques for maintaining a low level of anxiety.

The last three sessions (sessions 31 through 33) were reinforcement of the previous treatment strategies. The goal was not only to reduce or eliminate the level of panic and avoidance that she had been experiencing but also to reinforce and solidify techniques needed to prevent relapse.

Carole's therapy sessions ended with a recommendation that at some point in the future she again become involved in ongoing therapy in order to deal with some of the underlying issues regarding her upbringing. It was also suggested to her that some marital counseling might serve to enhance her relationship with her husband, particularly since the entire ordeal of her anxiety had taken a toll on the marriage. It was suggested that there may be some additional issues in the relationship that contributed to her anxiety.

FOLLOW-UP

Five follow-up visits were conducted following termination. The first follow-up session took place four weeks subsequent to session 33, with the second at eight weeks posttreatment. These two sessions showed no recurrence or increase of anxiety or depression and no report of relapse into avoidance. The subsequent follow-up sessions were conducted at 14 and 36 weeks posttreatment, with the last at 60 weeks (see Figure 8-3). Once again, all three follow-up sessions indicated a stable level of functioning. By that time, Carole had given birth to her fourth child (a boy)!

SUMMARY

This is the case of a 33-year-old, married woman who was treated for generalized anxiety and panic with agoraphobia. The case illustrates the successful implementation of cognitive-behavioral treatment with no relapse evident during a 14-month follow-up.

This is an interesting case that is in some ways atypical. For one, it is often found that the level of depression is highly correlated with the level of anxiety, particularly panic and agoraphobia. Several studies in the past have indicated that the overlap of symptomatology is quite high (Foa & Foa, 1982). In this particular case, it was somewhat unusual that Carole's level of depression remained relatively low as indicated on the BDI scores. In addition, Carole had also experienced little exacerbation of symptoms after being weaned from alprazolam, even though individuals experiencing panic commonly report an increase in frequency of panic and symptoms following benzodiazepine withdrawal (Wardel, 1990).

REFERENCES

Alford, B. A., Beck, A. T., Freeman, A., & Wright, F. (1990). Brief focused cognitive therapy of panic disorder. *Psychotherapy*, *27*, 230–234.

American Psychiatric Association (1987). *Diagnostic and statistical manual of mental disorders* (rev. 3rd ed.). Washington, DC: Author.

Beck, A. T., Emery, G., & Greenberg, P. L. (1985). *Anxiety disorders and phobias: A cognitive perspective*. New York: Basic Books.

Clark, D. M., Salkovskis, P. M., & Chalkley, A. J. (1985). Respiratory control as a treatment for panic attacks. *Journal of Behavior Therapy and Experimental Psychiatry*, *16*, 23–30.

Clum, G. A. (1990). *Coping with panic: A drug-free approach to dealing with anxiety attacks*. Belmont, CA: Wadsworth.

Dattilio, F. M. (1987). The use of paradoxical intention in the treatment of panic attacks. *Journal of Counseling and Development*, *66*, 66–67.

Dattilio, F. M. (1990). Symptom induction and de-escalation in the treatment of panic attacks. *Journal of Mental Health Counseling*, *12*, 515–519.

Foa, E. B., & Foa, U. G. (1982). Differentiating depression and anxiety: Is it possible? Is it useful? *Psychopharmacology Bulletin*, *18*, 62–68.

Jacobson, E. (1962). *You must relax*. New York, McGraw-Hill.

Solkol, L., Beck, A. T., Greenberg, R. L., Wright, F. D., & Berchick, R. J. (1989). Cognitive therapy of panic disorder: A non-pharmacological alternative. *Journal of Nervous & Mental Disease*, *177*, 711–716.

Wardel, J. (1990). Behavior therapy and benzodiazepines: allies or antagonists? *British Journal of Psychiatry*, *156*, 163–168.

Wolpe, J. (1973). *The practice of behavior therapy*. New York: Pergamon.

SUGGESTED READINGS

Beck, A. T., Emery, G., & Greenberg, P. L. (1985). *Anxiety disorders and phobias: A cognitive perspective*. New York: Basic Books.

Barlow, D. H. (1988). *Anxiety and its Disorders*. New York: Guilford.

Clum, G. A. (1990). *Coping with panic: A drug-free approach to dealing with anxiety attacks*. Belmont, CA: Wadsworth.

Goldstein, A. J., & Chabless, D. L. (1978). A reanalysis of agoraphobia. *Behavioral Therapy*, *9*, 47–59.

Tuma, A. H., & Maser, J. D. (Eds.). *Anxiety & the anxiety disorders*. Hillsdale, NJ: Lawrence Erlbaum.

9

Stress

Adrian Wells

Cognitive approaches to stress have focused on the role of individual differences in the appraisal of situations and coping responses in determining behavioral and emotional responses to stressful situations (e.g., Bandura, 1977; Beck, 1984; Lazarus & Folkman, 1984). Lazarus and Folkman (1984) define stress as "a particular relationship between the person and the environment that is appraised by the person as taxing or exceeding his or her resources and endangering his or her well-being" (p. 19). In their view, stress appraisals include harm or loss, threat, and challenge. Beck (1984) on the otherhand refers to three "stress syndromes" (hostility, fear, and depression) that represent emotional responses. In the hostility syndrome, individuals are hypersensitive to events that signal restraint or assault, whereas in the fear syndrome individuals are highly sensitive to danger. In the depression syndrome, the negative cognitive triad is activated. The basic tenet of this theory is that stress consists of the activation of cognitive schemas, with an idiosyncratic content specific for each syndrome.

Appraisals of the significance of an event (primary appraisal) and of the availability and effectiveness of coping responses (secondary appraisal) interact in determining the nature of stress reactions. Individuals may have to cope with external and internal demands in managing stress. Internal demands include the control of heightened emotion; expectations and situational appraisals concerning the intensity and controllability of emotion can shape anticipated outcomes. For example, since intense anxiety can interfere with effective coping, coping must also be emotion focused. Thus, in any situation, coping efforts can be directed toward managing threat imposed by external events and/or internal events (emotions).

These theoretical approaches to stress clearly suggest the need for multicomponent conceptualizations of stress-related problems. The relative contributions of cognitive processes and the nature of individuals' coping responses need to be considered in formulating a case. Stress results from appraisals that constitute an overestimation of threat and underestimation of the efficacy of coping resources. Appraisals of this type can interfere with the elicitation of coping responses even when responses are available. On the other hand, skill deficits can exist in which appropriate responses for managing situations are not available or have not been learned. In such circumstances, individuals may adopt specific strategies that may be functional in the short term but have negative long-term consequences because they maintain the stress cycle. For example, behavioral avoidance of stressful situations can produce immediate relief from anxiety, yet it deprives the individual of an opportunity to test the validity of catastrophic appraisals and to learn new coping

Adrian Wells • University of Oxford, Department of Psychiatry, Warneford Hospital, Oxford OX3 7JX, England

Comprehensive Casebook of Cognitive Therapy, edited by Arthur Freeman and Frank M. Dattilio. Plenum Press, New York, 1992.

responses. Since internal and external feedback concerning the effect of coping responses in situations shapes future appraisals, avoidance of situations means that preformed negative assumptions concerning self-efficacy remain unchanged.

The case presented in this chapter was selected because it illustrates a multimodal cognitive-behavioral intervention based on the cognitive model of stress.

CASE REPORT

Thomas was a 38-year-old engineer, married with an 11-year-old daughter. He was referred for treatment by his physician after he had sought help for anxiety associated with problems at work. His problems had culminated in him spending four months away from work; however, he had returned to work five weeks prior to the assessment session.

ASSESSMENT INFORMATION AND PRESENTING PROBLEM

During the two-hour assessment, a detailed description of Thomas' presenting problem (affective, behavioral, and cognitive aspects) was obtained. Specific situational antecedents for his symptomatic responses were identified, along with information pertaining to the development of the problem. A comprehensive personal history was also obtained.

Thomas's problem centered on recurrent feelings of anxiety that were accompanied by a number of psychosomatic symptoms, the most troublesome of which were abdominal discomfort, shoulder pain, and sleep-onset insomnia. A previous medical workup consisting of a barium enema had failed to show organic pathology. These symptoms were worse when Thomas was at work and were exacerbated by situations in which he was required to assert himself. More specifically, problematic situations consisted of giving directions to colleagues whom he supervised and offering critical feedback concerning their work. His anxiety in these situations centered around appraisals of potential conflict with supervisees. He felt that his "unassertiveness" was responsible for an apparent lack of respect that the supervisees showed for him, and this was also evidenced in the tardiness with which they acted on his suggestions.

Thomas was employed as a mechanical engineer and worked for a small engineering firm. His problem had developed over the preceding two-year period and was triggered by a promotion to a supervisory role, the first supervisory role he had ever occupied. With this new territory came greater responsibility for others and the task of ensuring that deadlines were met. Soon after assuming this new role, Thomas experienced difficulties dealing with one of the supervisees, who seemed to react negatively to being told what to do. A situation developed where the supervisee refused to take instructions from Thomas, and this resulted in recurrent verbal battles. Eventually, disciplinary action was brought against the supervisee, and he was required to leave the job. Nevertheless, Thomas's problems with anxiety did not remit after the supervisee left; instead, the symptoms appeared to worsen as they themselves became an additional focus for concern.

In order to elicit the cognitive concomitants of Thomas's anxiety, he was asked about the thoughts that he had in typical anxiety-provoking situations. His automatic thoughts were as follows:

- They don't respect me; they're trying to be difficult.
- What if they see I'm anxious?
- I don't have what it takes to do this.
- What if they argue? I can't tell them what to do.

These automatic thoughts suggested that Thomas was anticipating negative consequences of giving instructions to supervisees. Furthermore, he appraised their behavior as a sign that they didn't respect him and wanted to make his life difficult. These appraisals were doubly threatening because they were accompanied by negative appraisals of his ability to cope with the situation.

In addition to information concerning the presenting problem, background information was also obtained at assessment. Thomas stated that he had experienced a stable childhood. He had a slight speech impediment as a child (not strongly evident now), and this occasionally caused him embarrassment at school. However, he claimed not to have been socially inhibited by this problem, and his social history was unremarkable. His academic performance at school was average. Thomas left school at 15 years of age and took an engineering apprenticeship, but unfortunately, he failed the examinations. Following this, he held a number of jobs, but they were not what he was looking for. He had been married 16 years and had dated his wife for 2 years prior to their marriage. No problems in the marital relationship were evident.

SELF-REPORT ASSESSMENT

During the initial assessment, Thomas was presented with two self-report inventories that were to serve as treatment outcome measures. One of these was the state-anxiety subscale of the State-Trait Anxiety Inventory (STAI; Spielberger, Gorsuch, & Lushene, 1970), a 20-item self-report inventory consisting of statements relating to anxiety symptoms. It includes statements such as "I am tense" and "I am presently worrying over possible misfortunes"; responses are required on a 4-point scale ranging from "not at all" to "very much so." The Mulhall (1978) Personal Questionnaire (PQRST) was also administered in order to provide a more objective measurement of idiosyncratic symptoms, changes in which could be monitored on a session-by-session basis. The symptoms entered on the questionnaire were assertiveness at work and abdominal pain. The questionnaire requires choices between a series of randomized word pairs indicating symptom intensity; the word chosen in each case should be the one closest to how the patient feels. The state-anxiety subscale was administered at assessment and again at the end of treatment. The PQRST was administered at each session and at follow-up.

At the end of the assessment session, a brief overview of cognitive therapy and the cognitive model of anxiety was presented.

SESSION 2

The primary aim of this session was to develop collaboratively a comprehensive conceptualization of Thomas's problem, based on the information obtained in the assessment session. More information was required in order to determine the nature of his unassertiveness at work. Although he appeared socially skilled at assessment, this skilled behavior could have been absent in specific work situations. Aside from an exploration of his skills, his automatic thoughts were probed using socratic questioning (Beck et al., 1985) and the "downward arrow" technique (Burns, 1980, pp. 235–241) to elicit underlying assumptions and beliefs characteristic of his schemas. The following assumptions were elicited:

- If I tell them what to do, they will get angry at me.
- I'll go to pieces if they shout.
- If they don't like me, I won't be able to get the work done.

The data obtained in this session confirmed that Thomas's inability to assert himself at work stemmed from negative anticipated consequences of doing this. In addition, he had never before been in a position where he had to assert himself in this way.

Socializing Thomas in the cognitive model continued in this session, and the relationship among his under-lying assumptions, automatic thoughts, behavior, and anxiety was mapped out. He was introduced to the Dysfunctional Thoughts Record (DTR), and his most recent anxious encounter was recorded on the record as an illustrative exercise. Thomas was asked to fill out the first three columns of the record (situation, emotion, and automatic thoughts) for homework when he experienced anxiety or somatic symptoms. His goals for therapy were also delineated in this session: to reduce anxiety at work, to be more assertive at work, and to reduce the intensity of psychosomatic symptoms.

SESSION 3

On the basis of data obtained in the first two sessions, a more detailed conceptualization of Thomas's problem was formulated. It was evident that his problem was elicited and maintained by catastrophic appraisals of the effects of self-assertion, plus negative appraisals of his emotional control capabilities in potential conflict situations. In view of this conceptualization, cognitive restructuring and relaxation training were implemented in session 3 in order to facilitate modification of dysfunctional appraisals.

The session opened with a review of the previous homework assignment. Thomas had recorded several anxious episodes on the DTR. These episodes were accompanied by the types of automatic thoughts that had already been elicited in the earlier sessions. Although Thomas had successfully identified his automatic thoughts, he had also noted some secondary thoughts; thus, one task in this session was to facilitate him in differentiating between these cognitions, since automatic thoughts were to be targeted for restructuring. The rationale for challenging automatic thoughts was presented, and standard restructuring techniques were employed (e.g., Beck, Emery, & Greenberg, 1985). These consisted of questioning the evidence for specific thoughts listed on the thought record, evaluating the probability of feared outcomes, and generating alternative appraisals.

In addition to the introduction of verbal cognitive restructuring, relaxation training was initiated as a behavioral experiment to challenge his belief in his lack of emotional control capabilities. The relaxation method chosen was based on autogenic training (Schultz & Luthe, 1969). More specifically, it incorporated the autogenic themes of heaviness and warmth, which were presented in the form of therapist suggestions and then used in an auto-suggestion mode. The following is an excerpt from the exercise.

THERAPIST: Begin by relaxing the muscles in your neck and shoulders. Let the muscles relax and unwind, and as they do so notice that your shoulders begin to feel heavy. Concentrate on feelings of heaviness in your shoulders. Let the muscles relax more and more, and as they relax notice that your shoulders are becoming heavier and heavier. Concentrate on those feelings of heaviness; so very, very heavy and relaxed. Your shoulders are so heavy it feels as if they are made of lead, or as if someone has placed lead weights upon them, they are so heavy and so relaxed. Heavy and relaxed, heavy like lead, so very, very heavy. Repeat over to yourself five times the phrase: "My shoulders are heavy and relaxed, heavy like lead."

This formula was repeated for each arm in turn, and then each leg, for sensations of heaviness and then warmth. The sequence was presented in a slow and even-paced manner and lasted approximately 15 minutes. Thomas was instructed to practice the exercise at home for a period of 15 to 20 minutes each day. He was also instructed in basic techniques for questioning his automatic thoughts in problematic situations, and he was asked to record automatic thoughts on the DTR, along with rational responses.

SESSION 4

In the fourth session, the therapist reviewed the DTR with Thomas and introduced the concept of "cognitive distortions" as another variable that could be used to distance him from his automatic thoughts and to reinforce the efficacy of his cognitive disputations. Thomas had successfully completed the previous homework assignment and had found questioning automatic thoughts helpful in reducing the amount of time spent ruminating over work situations. However, he reported experiencing difficulty questioning thoughts and generating alternative responses while in the work situation itself. In view of this problem, a cognitive rehearsal exercise was also included on the agenda for this session. This consisted of re-imaging a specific episode from the previous week and restructuring cognitions within the image as the situation unfolded. The situation and automatic thoughts were first recalled as they had actually happened and Thomas was asked to rate his anxiety on a scale of 0% to 100% at key points in the scenario. Automatic thoughts and anxiety intensity ratings were recorded on a chalkboard by the therapist at specific points in the scenario. Thomas was instructed to recall the event in as much detail as possible

and as if it were happening in the "here and now." The following is an excerpt from this first stage of the procedure.

THERAPIST: I want you to cast your mind back to the stressful event of last Tuesday. Try and put yourself back in that situation, as if it were happening again right now for the first time. Describe to me where you are right now.

THOMAS: I'm standing in the workshop, and one of the men calls me over because he wants some advice.

THERAPIST: Describe what you can see as you stand in the workshop.

THOMAS: Well, I'm looking over towards the trainee who has asked my advice.

THERAPIST: OK, that's fine. What is the trainee wearing?

THOMAS: He's wearing a light blue smock, and I think he has blue trousers on.

THERAPIST: What are you wearing?

THOMAS: I have my overalls on; they're also blue.

THERAPIST: How do you feel right now? Do you feel anxious?

THOMAS: A little anxious, I suppose.

THERAPIST: You're looking over at the trainee, and you feel a little anxious. How anxious are you on a scale of 0 to 100 percent?

THOMAS: About 10 percent.

THERAPIST: So your anxiety level is about 10 percent; what thoughts are going through your mind?

THOMAS: Some of the men are looking at me an I'm worried that I may make a fool of myself.

THERAPIST: So the thought is, "What if I make a fool of myself?" Is that right?

THOMAS: Yes, that's it, and I'm worried that they may see that I'm nervous.

THERAPIST: OK, tell me what you are doing now.

THOMAS: I'm walking over to the lathe where the trainee is working.

THERAPIST: How is your anxiety level now on a scale of 0 to 100?

THOMAS: It's about 35 or 40 percent.

THERAPIST: What thoughts are going through your mind?

THOMAS: I'm thinking that if I have to tell him what to do, I will make a fool of myself.

This strategy was pursued until the entire scenario was complete. At specific stages, the therapist asked Thomas to rate his anxiety and to report his automatic thoughts. The process was repeated a second time, but at each specific stage Thomas was instructed to question his automatic thoughts and generate a rational response. His anxiety was rerated at each stage in this rational scenario. The following is a segment of this exercise.

THOMAS: I'm checking the work he has already completed with calipers. One of the pins he has turned is not the right diameter; it's too small.

THERAPIST: How anxious do you feel?

THOMAS: I feel anxious, about 80 percent.

THERAPIST: What are you thinking at this point?

THOMAS: I have to tell him it's wrong and he has to do it again.

THERAPIST: What' so bad about that?

THOMAS: I'm afraid that he won't like that, and he'll get annoyed and think I'm being picky.

THERAPIST: So, what's the automatic thought?

THOMAS: That he'll get annoyed and won't like me.

THERAPIST: Continue imagining the situation, and I want you to question that thought. Have you any evidence to support it?

THOMAS: Not really, I suppose, but it could happen.

THERAPIST: Does the trainee look annoyed right now?

THOMAS: No, I don't think so.

THERAPIST: Ask yourself what the probability is of that happening. Think of the worst thing that can happen, the best thing that can happen, and the most likely think that can happen. What's your rational response?

THOMAS: There's no evidence that he'll dislike me, and anyway, I'm only doing my job.

THERAPIST: OK, that's very good. How anxious do you feel now?

THOMAS: I feel less anxious, say about 40 percent.

By noting specific thoughts and anxiety intensity ratings, it was possible for the therapist to present feedback concerning the association between the threatening nature of the thoughts and anxiety intensity. This served as additional evidence of the relationship between thoughts and affect, and was presented as further support for the cognitive model.

A list of cognitive distortions was presented (adapted from Burns, 1980), and these were briefly reviewed with reference to the automatic thoughts recorded on Thomas's DTR and those elicited in the cognitive rehearsal task. There was insufficient time in this session to review these in detail, and so the identification of thinking errors was set as a homework assignment. The last part of the session was devoted to practicing the relaxation procedure. For homework, Thomas was instructed to work through his DTR and label his different thinking errors, to practice questioning his thoughts and generating rational re-sponses in real situations, and to continue with the relaxation exercises.

SESSION 5

The aim of this session was to review Thomas's homework and to focus on the identification of his thinking errors. In addition, a role play of a problematic work encounter was planned as an opportunity for Thomas to practice cognitive coping strategies and an opportunity for the therapist to explore Thomas's interpersonal skills.

The following thinking errors were identified:

- *Fortune telling*—In the absence of definite facts, the prediction that situations will turn out negatively; for example, supervisee's work is not up to the standard required, and Thomas predicts, "If I tell him it's wrong, he'll get angry and refuse to do the job"
- *Mind reading*—Assuming arbitrarily that someone feels negative toward you; for example, since Thomas's work colleagues seem reluctant to seek advice, he assumes, "They don't have any respect for me" (Note: Mind reading and fortune telling are both examples of arbitrary inference, that is, forming conclusions on the basis of insufficient evidence.)
- *Dichotomous thinking*—Appraising things in black-and-white terms; for example, given minor difficulties, Thomas assumes, "I just don't have what it takes to do this job"
- *Labeling*—Attaching a negative label to oneself if something falls short of personal standards or attaching a label to another person if they do something that leads you to have negative feelings; for example, Thomas's supervisees work slowly on certain tasks, and he thinks, "They're just being difficult."

Thomas's labeling thoughts were also an example of magnification. Many relatively benign situations in which individuals experienced hitches in their work or did not do the work the same way that Thomas would have done it were appraised as further evidence of their intentionally "difficult" behavior. These data were indicative of some rigid assumptions or "should statements" that were characteristic of Thomas's approach to work. Moreover, they seemed to suggest some inflexibility and perhaps obsessional personality components to his problem. This addition to the initial conceptualization was noted for possible later intervention.

The role play comprised a hypothetical scenario in which an angry work colleague (played by the therapist) had to be informed that a piece of work was not of the required standard and had to be done again. In the role play, it became evident that Thomas had difficulty dealing with the anger expressed by the work colleague. Moreover, his anxiety became evident in his increased hesitancy and lowered volume of speech. In response to these affect shifts, the therapist asked Thomas how he felt when they occurred and also elicited concomitant automatic thoughts. These thoughts were restructured in the standard way. An analysis of the role play suggested that some basic training in communication skills could increase Thomas's efficacy in conflict situations.

After discussion of this rationale, the therapist moved from a collaborative process to a didactic style of presentation in order to give new information aimed at developing specific interpersonal skills. A scheme for handling conflict was mapped out on a chalkboard. The scheme presented was a system of empathizing with others and complimenting them in combination with making specific requests. Similar techniques for enhancing interpersonal effectiveness have been presented in more detail elsewhere (e.g., Burns, 1989, chap. 21). After presentation of the system, the therapist briefly modeled the technique and then had Thomas practice the technique in the session. Thomas expressed some apprehension about giving compliments to work colleagues; his underlying assumption in this case was that they would think he was insincere. In view of this assumption, the therapist suggested a personal experiment in which Thomas had to compliment at least two work colleagues on some aspect of their work and note the nature of their responses.

Session 5 ended with a discussion of homework assignments for the following week. Assignments included a continuation of relaxation, rational responding with use of the DTR, complimenting at least two work colleagues on their efforts, and practice of new interpersonal techniques (if appropriate).

SESSION 6

The initial aim of this session, as in previous sessions, was to review the outcome of Thomas's homework assignments. The self-report measures were indicative of significant symptom relief, and therefore a review of treatment to date and the procedures that Thomas had found helpful was also undertaken so that treatment gains could be consolidated. Given the significant level of symptom relief and the provision of effective cognitive and behavioral coping strategies, the focus of intervention shifted to

a conceptualization of underlying schemas (beliefs and attitudes) and restructuring of these potential vulnerability factors.

In order to determine the content of schemas, the therapist looked for themes in Thomas's automatic thoughts and assumptions (which had been elicited in earlier sessions) and used the downward-arrow technique on specific automatic thoughts. This technique facilitated Thomas in articulating the core belief of "I'm inadequate." This belief seemed to be particularly relevant, as it was consistent with the content of automatic thoughts and also the nature of Thomas's behavioral responses. Aside from a cross-sectional derivation of this self-concept, the therapist asked about Thomas's earliest thoughts or feelings of inadequacy (i.e., a longitudinal assessment of the development of this schema was sought). Thomas reported first having the feeling after being teased at school about his speech impediment, and this feeling had been reinforced when he failed his engineering apprenticeship. Moreover, his rigid and perfectionistic approach to work (which had become apparent during therapy) could have been an adaptation to feelings of inadequacy, thus representing an attempt to conceal his inadequacy and prove himself to others.

Since this formulation was agreed to by patient and therapist, this latter attitude (perfectionism) was not specifically targeted for intervention, and treatment focused on the core inadequacy schema. Many patients do not find it easy to articulate core beliefs, and this can be compounded by personality factors such as those associated with avoidant personality. When patients experience this difficulty, the therapist can make inferences about beliefs based on the available data and then check the validity of these with the patient (in stating beliefs, it is important to use the patient's own words as much as possible).

SESSION 7 THROUGH 9

The remaining three sessions were devoted to restructuring beliefs and assumptions. This was accomplished by using specific cognitive restructuring strategies like those adopted in previous sessions; more emphasis was given to Thomas designing and implementing his own personal experiments. Part of session 8 and most of session 9 were devoted to relapse prevention issues. This consisted of reviewing the things that Thomas had learned in therapy and listing the techniques that he had found helpful. As a homework task at the end of session 8, Thomas was asked to compile a list of effective strategies learned in therapy and a description of each strategy. In session 9, the list was reviewed and appropriate elabora-

PQRST
score

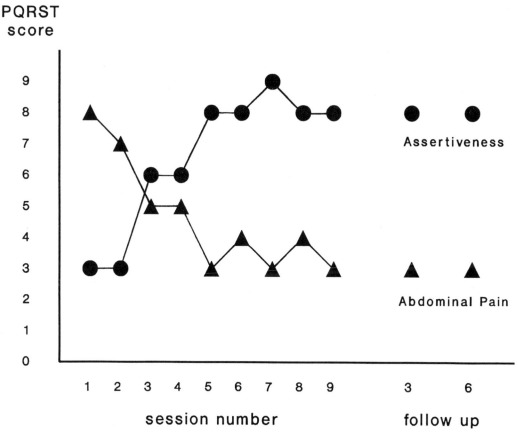

Figure 9-1. PQRST Intensity Ratings for Assertiveness at Work and Abdominal Pain (Across Treatment and at Follow-Up).

tions were made. The importance of designing and implementing personal exposure experiments in the future was delineated.

FOLLOW-UP

Follow-up and booster sessions were conducted at three and six months after termination of therapy. Thomas had maintained the treatment gains across this period. He reported that he was feeling more confident in work, and that he was handling encounters with work colleagues in a more relaxed manner. His self-report PQRST scores are displayed in Figure 9-1.

At pretreatment, Thomas's score on the Spielberger et al. (1970) state-anxiety subscale was 54, and at termination (session 9) his score had dropped to 26.

SUMMARY AND CONCLUSION

This case illustrates the use of a multimodal cognitive-behavioral intervention that was designed to explore and modify dysfunctional cognitive appraisal processes and increase cognitive-behavioral coping and interpersonal skills. The treatment strategies employed were based on a continuously evolving cognitive case conceptualization. The main elements of treatment may be summarized in terms of their primary focus as follows: (a) socialization and goal setting; (b) modification of affect and somatic symptoms via mini experiments (e.g., relaxation) and verbal cognitive restructuring; (c) improving interpersonal effectiveness; (d) schema work; and (e) relapse prevention. In designing this intervention, the relative contribution of disruptive cognitive processes (cognitive excesses) and the effect of cognitive-behavioral deficits was considered.

Abbreviated autogenic relaxation was used as a component of self-control training. Some individuals show an adverse reaction to self-focused relaxations that is marked by intensified anxiety. In such cases, relaxation techniques that do not require increased self-focus can prove less problematic (Wells, 1990). Alternatively, the anxiogenic effects can be utilized in an interoceptive exposure format aimed at reappraisal of the sensations released through relaxation. In the present case, the patient reported feeling self-conscious in certain situations; although this symptom was not specifically dealt with in treatment, distraction and task-focusing exercises could have been employed to reduce self-consciousness when problematic (see Wells, 1990, for a description of an external-focused relaxation technique designed to reduce self-awareness).

REFERENCES

Bandura, A. (1977). Self-efficacy: Toward a unifying theory of behavior change. *Psychological Review*, *84*, 191–215.

Beck, A. T. (1984). Cognitive approaches to stress. In R. Woolfolk & P. Lehrer (Eds.), *Principles and practice of stress management*. New York: Guilford.

Beck, A. T., Emery, G., & Greenberg, R. L. (1985). *Anxiety disorders and phobias: A cognitive perspective*. New York: Basic Books.

Burns, D. D. (1980). *Feeling good*. New York: Signet.

Burns, D. D. (1989). *The feeling good handbook*. New York: William Morrow.

Lazarus, R. S., & Folkman, S. (1984). *Stress, appraisal and coping*. New York: Springer.

Mulhall, D. J. (1978). *Manual for the Personal Questionnaire Rapid Scaling Technique*. Windsor, England: NFER/Nelson.

Schultz, J. H., & Luthe, W. (1969). *Autogenic therapy, volume 1: Autogenic methods*. New York: Grune and Stratton.

Spielberger, C. D., Gorsuch, R. L., & Lushene, R. E. (1970). *Manual for the State-Trait Anxiety Inventory*. Palo Alto, CA: Consulting Psychologists Press.

Wells, A. (1990). Panic disorder in association with relaxation induced anxiety: An attentional training approach to treatment. *Behavior Therapy*, *21*, 273–280.

SUGGESTED READINGS

Cox, T. (1978). *Stress*. London: Macmilan.

Meichenbaum, D. (1985). *Stress inoculation training*. New York: Pergamon.

Meichenbaum, D. (1986). Cognitive-behavior modification. In F. H. Kanfer & A. P. Goldstein (Eds.), *Helping people change: A textbook of methods* (3rd ed., pp. 346–380). New York: Pergamon.

Michelson, L., & Ascher, L. M. (Eds.). (1988). *Anxiety and stress disorders: Cognitive-behavioral assessment and treatment*. New York: Guilford.

10

An Adjustment Disorder

Mark Gilson

"We cannot think first and act afterwards. From the moment of birth we are immersed in action, and can only fitfully guide it by taking thought."

—ALFRED NORTH WHITEHEAD

INTRODUCTION

A 30-year history of cognitive therapy theory followed by a significant body of treatment research has given the practitioner credible and effective paths to conceptualize and remedy mood disorders (Beck, 1961, 1963, 1967; Beck, Rush, Shaw, & Emery, 1979; Ellis, 1962). This may be especially true for the client who is dealing with emotional problems associated with adjusting to demanding changes in life. The cognitive model promotes a collaboration with patients in defining problems in their own terms and using common sense to change thinking and to manage those problems (Beck, 1976; Beck et al., 1979). The therapist's role in this model of treatment is to work with clients' conscious ideas and to enhance or modify thought patterns and coping techniques to restore or improve functioning.

Cognitive therapy of depressive symptoms in adjust-

ment disorder goes beyond supportive contact that the therapist may give to a client suffering distress from major life changes. The sense of self-efficacy often diminishes when an individual has been subjected to difficult life transitions. The patterns in behavior and thinking in a previously highly functioning person can dramatically alter as a result of distress associated with stressors such as a change in livelihood, loss of a relationship, change in living circumstances, financial difficulties and so forth. Self-instruction may become maladaptive (Meichenbaum, 1977) in that a person's normal resourcefulness in problem solving and the ability to address oneself, the world, and the future in a confident and goal-directed manner may break down.

Cognitive therapy is directed, first of all, to the presenting situational and psychological problems. This is why cognitive therapy is considered a top-down approach that focuses on immediate problems and symptoms, rather than initially attempting to discover more deeply rooted areas of unconscious and preconscious processes (considered bottom-up techniques). The cognitive therapy premise is that one can achieve capability in dealing with more complex problems once initial problems in thinking and behavior are dealt with adaptively. This is especially true in adjustment disorder with depressed mood.

Mark Gilson • Atlanta Center for Cognitive Therapy, 1772 Century Boulevard, Atlanta, Georgia 30345.

Comprehensive Casebook of Cognitive Therapy, edited by Arthur Freeman and Frank M. Dattilio. Plenum Press, New York, 1992.

The cognitive approaches developed by Ellis (Ellis, 1962, 1970; Ellis & Dryden, 1987) and Beck (Beck, 1967, 1976; Beck et al., 1979) are similar in that they connect maladaptive thinking with distress and depression. Beck differed with traditional psychiatry in that he conceptualized negative thinking not just as a symptom of depression, but as a key factor in the maintenance of depressed mood. In treatment, the emphasis is placed on the patient expressing problems operationally in a here-and-now fashion while identifying specific goals for change. The patient in emotional distress is learning or recovering more flexible ways to think and act. These present the major challenges for therapist and client as they collaborate in the treatment process.

When dramatic changes occur in the course of a lifetime, a demand is made for the individual to revise his or her maps for living and, many times, to make revisions in the ways that he or she interprets experiences and lives life (Peck, 1978). This casebook focuses on the understanding and treatment of a broad range of emotional symptoms and disorders such as depression, suicide, anxiety, stress, avoidance, substance abuse, and family problems. Adjustment disorders often include symptoms of any or all of these. The emotional symptoms in adjustment can be just as intense and potentially dangerous to a client as other Axis I syndromes in DSM-III-R (American Psychological Association [APA], 1987), although the likelihood for improvement is usually greater, given the identifiable stressors that give rise to emotional distress and dysfunction and the short period of time between precipitating events and psychological symptoms. The key factors that distinguish adjustment disorder from other disorders are the identifiable life-disrupting events that occur within about a three-month period before the onset of symptoms and the partial syndrome of specific disorders (in the case-example here, depressed mood). Unlike other pathologies, the causes of the affective problems are quite evident and recent.

Although belief systems may play some role in this type of disorder, it is more likely that a patient's adaptive abilities are only temporarily malfunctioning due to the trauma of recent events. Key indicators in major depression are a minimum number of symptoms to complete a syndrome. In adjustment disorder with depressed mood, depressive symptoms are too few in number to meet the minimum criteria for major depression, although symptoms that are present can be severe. Adjustment is also not to be confused with uncomplicated bereavement, in that the symptoms go beyond the normal grieving process.

For those individuals who are especially susceptible, sometimes even a mild or moderate stressor will produce formidable symptoms. For example, Sara broke up with her boyfriend and had problems with her confidence about meeting another person. She had met her soon-to-be-ex-boyfriend the previous year and had not dated much prior to that time. She was feeling negative about her future, and thinking she would never again meet anyone who would love her, when she sought treatment. On the other hand, some individuals will have relatively benign symptoms in response to extreme and prolonged stressors. Bill is a good example; he lost his job last year and has been living on his savings. He reports he has liked the time off and believes that there will be work for him when he is ready to get back in the business world. He is confident of this abilities.

The intensity of the reaction to distressing circumstances cannot be predicted from the apparent severity of the situation. The degree of emotional strain a person might experience is relative to his or her interpretation of the events. This is consistent with the basic tenets of the cognitive model in that underlying cognitive structures appear to influence a person's affective state. There is a synthesis of a person's external stimuli (stressors) and internal processes (interpretation of stressors) that must be considered in understanding this disorder.

The methods and techniques used in the case chosen here exemplify the sensibility of the cognitive model and may serve as a review of its application to frequently experienced emotional problems.

BACKGROUND AND HISTORY

Captain Jerrold F. was a 50-year-old retired Navy flight commander who received an honorable discharge from the military under some pressure from his superiors. The years 1989–90 (before the Iraq crisis) produced a thaw in Soviet–American relations, and the subsequent changes in defense spending resulted in across-the-board shifts and cutbacks in all branches of the military. Early retirements were offered to "lifers" as an option to avoid less desirable assignments in ill-favored parts of the world or placements that involved boring desk work or isolation. The possibilities for advancement in the armed services were diminishing for all career military personnel. This was especially true if they experienced any personal problems. Jerrold had aspired to progress from captain to Navy air wing commander. He had a distinguished 20-year career in the military, having flown jets in battles during the Vietnam War and worked his way up the leadership ladder in subsequent years.

Some key events occurred in Jerrold F.s' life in 1989. His father had a serious bout with cancer that year, and although he was recovering well, it troubled Jerrold because this was the first time he ever thought he could actually lose his father, someone he took for granted would always be there. He started feeling doubtful of himself as well as of his control over his life, and this led him to seek psychiatric advice on the base.

At this time, Jerrold was a vice wing commander at a naval base where he was judged to be doing extremely well. Later that year, he was in contention for two different wing commander positions but was selected for neither. Given the stage of his career, Jerrold regarded this as possibly his last chance to achieve a career pinnacle for himself. Instead, he was now being considered for appointments that probably would not result in the position he had labored so long to achieve. Still, a reliable senior officer told him that if he accepted a transfer to another base and did well on the next assignment, he might still have a chance of commanding a wing. Although Jerrold was skeptical of this, he told his superiors that he would take a new assignment with the hope of fulfilling his career goals.

There was another type of personal distress involved in his decision to leave the base. He was also to bid farewell to his sons from a previous marriage, who were still living with their mother near the base. The older boy was in college and had for the most part achieved autonomy from the family; it was his 12-year-old son, Chet, who particularly worried Jerrold. Chet was having considerable communication problems with his mother and was also displaying behavior problems in school. Thus, Jerrold felt he was leaving his son in a bad situation, with the fear that things might get worse for Chet in his absence.

Jerrold F. believed he was withdrawing from a family predicament that troubled him and was headed toward a job that represented disappointment and lost hope. As a result, symptoms of depression began. These included a disrupted sleep pattern, loss of appetite and a subsequent 10-pound weight loss, diminished libido, and anhedonia. He again sought the assistance of medical services at the base, and spoke to another psychiatrist. He reported tearfulness when he thought about leaving his sons. He was given an antidepressant and a medical record that would ensure he would not become a flight wing commander.

Jerrold received two reviews by the military medical board. The first review found him to be fit for duty. The second review offered a retirement pension and 20% disability compensation, which meant a livable amount of monthly income and benefits. Jerrold looked at his options again and decided that he would take his pension and leave the military for civilian life. He moved with his current wife and family to the city where some of his family resided, but his mood was colored by his sense of disappointment and defeat.

Mood problems continued when Jerrold left the Navy and sought treatment after reading about cognitive therapy in a magazine article. He subsequently sought therapy at the Atlanta Center for Cognitive Therapy.

INITIAL EVALUATION

A structured extended clinical interview was administered at Jerrold's first visit. An effort was made to collect information about his symptoms, interpretation of emotional problems, and history. Objective measures such as the Beck Depression Inventory (BDI) and Beck Anxiety Inventory (BAI) were administered.

Jerrold's BDI score of 14 indicated a mild level of depression. His BAI score of 18 suggested mild symptoms of restlessness and agitation. Questions about symptoms endorsed on the inventory and in response to questions in the structured interview were categorized on several dimensions. *Emotions* included the descriptions he used for his distress to help establish a collaboration in understanding his vocabulary for difficulty. *Behavioral* descriptions of what he was doing served to provide a picture of how this man was conducting himself in his current situation, especially the behaviors associated with feeling better or worse emotionally. *Physical* symptoms that were possibly associated with distress were ascertained to rule out the necessity for seeking a physician and/or to establish a baseline for associated depression and anxiety symptoms that could be alleviated concurrently with the application of cognitive therapy. Cognitive appraisal during the assessment session targeted uncovering some of the thoughts that were experienced during low mood periods. Finally, visual *images* associated with depression were requested, given the potency of imagery in maintenance of depressed mood. Below is a summary of information collected during the initial evaluative interview:

- *Emotions*—Reported areas of distress included irritability, feeling overwhelmed, depression, anxiety, frustration, and intermittent hopelessness. Suicidal thoughts were denied.
- *Behavior*—Jerrold was currently involved in a job search. He had just returned from a vacation and felt rested. He was attempting to spend time in the library to explore employment possibilities. He also experienced difficulty falling asleep.
- *Physical*—Stomach problems such as indigestion and gas were described. There was a weight loss of 25 pounds in the past 10 months that was not due to diet. Physical condition and appearance were normal according to his physician.

- *Cognitive*—Am I capable? What's the use in trying? There's a plot to keep me from going where I want (although I know it's a ridiculous notion). I am too depressed to work. (Note: Neither the BDI nor direct questioning indicated that Jerrold had suicidal ideation, intent, or history.)
- *Images*: People looking at me as if I am strange. People turning me down for jobs.

DIAGNOSIS

It had been less than three months after leaving the military that Jerrold sought help for what he saw as an emotional problem. Unlike Axis II personality disorders where maladaptive traits are enduring and exhibited in a wide range of contexts, there was no formidable history of treatment or significant dysfunction before the previously described situation. Jerrold reported that he had gone through the stages of grief, including denial, anger, sadness, and resolution. He had given up his military career with a great deal of pain, but felt that his depressed symptoms were different than what he had experienced during and after his recent retirement. The relationship between psychosocial stressors and his emotional problems were evident. The criteria for adjustment disorder with depressed mood were met (APA, 1987, p. 330), along with symptoms of depression being a predominant manifestation of his symptomatology. Included in this was a negative view of self, situation, and future, sleep problems, and vegetative symptoms, as well as mild to moderate feelings of hopelessness and sadness.

TREATMENT

The therapeutic relationship begins at the very first contact, and treatment can start at the end of the evaluation session. I began immediately socializing the client to the collaborative relationship that is essential for good cognitive therapy. The process of therapy was explained to Jerrold as a two-way street in that both he and I would be exploring factor that precipitated emotional problems and looking for ways to solve problems. Near the end of the initial clinical interview, I told Jerrold that for the past couple of hours I had been examining aspects of his history, thoughts, feelings, character, and situation for the purpose of arriving at a diagnostic impression. At this point, I asked if there was anything he felt he wanted to know about me, emphasizing that his impression and confidence in me were extremely important for establishing the groundwork for a successful therapeutic relationship. Jerrold was able to establish rapport with me from the outset, which contributed to a good collaborative bond. Below is some dialogue that was extrapolated from the end of Jerrold's assessment session.

THERAPIST: It may seem like you have been given the third degree with all of these questions and I appreciate your patience and cooperation. Is there anything I said or did that bothered or concerned you?

JERROLD: Not really. You seem to know what you are doing. I hope this type of therapy can help me.

THERAPIST: I believe it can. The more you know about it, the more effectively we can work together. I could have all the skill and knowledge about treatment there is, but for us to accomplish goals in therapy, it is essential that we collaborate on ways to improve your situation and feelings. Before you leave, I will give you an article about this therapy and recommend a book you might read to help you before more familiar with cognitive therapy. Is there anything you would like to know about me?

JERROLD: You seem kind of young. What is your background?

THERAPIST: (after questions are answered specifically) I want to encourage you to ask questions of me and take an active role in your therapy. It's not just the process of you telling me how you feel or me lecturing about treatment. We can work together. No one knows more about your problems than you and I bring my knowledge and ability in applying cognitive methods of treatment in our efforts to solve some of your difficulties. The focus of treatment will be on your personal life and not mine. What do you think and how do you feel about what we've discussed so far?

JERROLD: It makes a lot of sense to me. I'm feeling hopeful that this is the right thing to help me get out of this slump that I've been in. I think I'm looking forward to getting things going.

Jerrold was asked to complete an activity schedule (Figure 10-1) in the five days prior to the initial therapy session in order to collect a baseline of his typical actions and level of emotional distress. He was instructed to rate his sense of both competence (mastery) and satisfaction (pleasure) for each activity on a scale of 1 to 10. Data was to be recorded at least once a day to make sure that his memory for events was fresh and accurate. The rationale was to allow both of us to see how he interpreted his experiences in a more concise manner than just relying on his recollection between sessions. Jerrold thought the assignment made sense and was motivated to follow through. At this point, collaborative empiricism had begun.

WEEKLY ACTIVITY SCHEDULE
NOTE: Grade activities *M* for Mastery and *P* for Pleasure

	M	T	W	Th	F	S	S
9-10		breakfast phone calls	breakfast coffee m-5 p-5	coffee m-8 p-6	brush teeth shower m-8 p-6	breakfast visit cousin	coffee. paper m-5 p-7
10-11	awake coffee,juice jog m-5,p-2	m-6 p-7 drive wife	drove to therapy	talk w/wife & father m-7 p-6	breakfast mow lawn	m-7 p-7	packed for trip
11-12	talk w/son re:future m-3 p-8	to work m-8 p-7		jogged m-7 p-7	m-6 p-6	jogged m-8 p-4	drove to base
12-1		library	wandered in shopping mall	drove dad to drugstore	look for job m-2 p-6		m-9 p-4
1-2	visit job opportunity m-8 p-7	m-9 p-7	m-5 p-5	m-9 p-5			
2-3	drive home			read pamphlet on job m- 8 p-7		rent canoe visit sister	
3-4	m-9 p-8		read info on CBT	library		m-5 p-7	
4-5	read paper m-8 p-8		Job search m-7 p-7	m-5 p-5			obtain room for night
5-6	eat	jog m-8 p-8	talked w/ wife	filled out applications	supper movie w/ wife	newspaper talk w/dad	m-9 p-5
6-7	m-6 p-7	eat go to support	m-5 p-6	m-8 p-6 dinner	m-8 p-7	m-5 p-5 shower, go	ate m-8 p-5 read, t.v.
7-8		group m-7 p-8	went to support group	groceries m-9 p-5	snack m-7 p-6	to baptism m-7 p-6	m-5 p-5 awoke early
8-12	chat w/wife sleep m-8 p-8	read job info m-8 p-6	m-3 p-7	t.v. m-5 p-6	t.v./problem sleeping m-2 p-3	dinner, t.v m-5 p-7 sleep prob.	m-2 p-4

Figure 10-1. Jerrold F's weekly activity schedule.

Upon review of the data collected at the initial evaluation, the diagnostic impression of adjustment disorder with depressed mood was made. Jerrold was a man who had recently experienced several stressors within a short period of time and was finding it difficult to maintain a balanced view of himself and his future. Events such as his father's illness, the stress from his efforts to attain a promotion, the move to another base, and the concern about his son had all taken a toll on his sense of well-being and confidence. He began to fear that nothing was going to go right for him and to have symptoms of depression. However, he did not sustain a syndrome of symptoms for any two-week period since the onset of his problems. He also did not experience a complete loss of interest in activity or of ability to experience pleasure. A diagnosis of major depression was therefore ruled out. Jerrold was reacting to circumstances that were difficult to cope with, but transient. There was no history of difficulties with depression or other psychopathology. His symptoms therefore warranted a diagnosis of adjustment disorder.

Prognosis for successful short-term cognitive therapy appeared good.

SESSION 1

Jerrold returned the next week with the two homework assignments. He had written goals for his treatment and completed an activity schedule for the previous week. The structure of sessions was clarified at the beginning of this meeting, and this was to set the format for therapy for the coming months. I explained the rationale behind setting an agenda. I first asked Jerrold if he thought it would be helpful if our sessions would consist of free association, where we could discuss whatever came to his mind at the time, and avoided any particular focus. Jerrold thought a moment and remarked that he would defer to my judgment, but that he believed it might not help him because sometimes he felt worse when there was no structure to the sessions. This was especially evident to him since he had recently left the regimentation of a miliary career, remarking that he sometimes missed the boundaries of a schedule and the sense of purpose he once felt when in the Navy. Since being home, he had noted that having free time and few obligations did not lead to his feeling at ease or having peace of mind.

Next, Jerrold was asked what problems he thought might occur if we did not structure the therapy meetings. He was able to identify potential difficulties such as avoiding dealing with important issues, wasting time that he was paying for, and potentially extending the period he would be in treatment. We then agreed that at the beginning of each therapy session we would outline some specific aims and objectives for our meetings, beginning with this session. Below is the agenda and homework for session 1:

1. Go over the homework (activity schedule and goals)
2. Therapist will explain some more about how cognitive therapy works
3. Consider other self-help tasks that would enhance goals

His goals for treatment were:

1. Become symptom free in 90 days and complete therapy in 6 months
2. Conduct a systematic job search that is less disorganized
3. Be able to deal with rejection during efforts to obtain a job
4. Be employed in a satisfactory position in 90 days
5. Be less critical of self and be more self-accepting

Jerrold and I both agreed that his goals appeared reasonable. Some questioning about the scope of the first goal was necessary. For clarification, I asked if he ever experienced himself as completely free of emotional distress. He smiled and first said that he might have felt that way when he was a child and then corrected himself, noting that even as a child, he sometimes felt distress. He recalled when he was 6 or 7 years old and his parents did not allow him to stay up late. When he was sent to bed, he would feel upset and cry. When his parents let him stay up a little later, he still would become upset, feeling frustrated that he could not stay up as long as he wished. He eventually learned that he wouldn't always get exactly what he wanted, but if he did not act whiny and demanding, his parents were more likely to allow him some flexibility to delay bedtime. This provided us with an entry point to discuss the cognitive biases, including dichotomous/all-or-nothing thinking characterized by the expectation that all symptoms would be eliminated with

treatment. We agreed that some relief from his symptoms was a reasonable and worthwhile modification of his goals, just as it was more successful for him as a child to adjust his expectations of his parents.

The activity schedule from the past week was then reviewed. This schedule provided Jerrold room to write in his activities on an hour-by-hour basis and rate his mastery (sense of competence) and pleasure (absence or presence of distress) associated with the activity he was involved with at each given day. His level of emotional discomfort appeared to be lowest when he was active, doing things such as looking for a job and reading about cognitive therapy; I noted to myself that I could come back to and use this subjective experience of activity lessening Jerrold's emotional discomfort. There were some evenings where he had problems getting to sleep because he ruminated about his situation and tossed and turned in bed.

I used the activity schedule as a means to explain basic principles of the cognitive model. I went to the eraserboard in my office and drew a diagram that represented a system of emotion (Figure 10-2). At the center of the chart was emotion, and surrounding emotion were the interrelated factors (situation, behavior, cognition, and biochemistry) that comprised its system. Jerrold's evening restlessness and fitful efforts to sleep were examined. It was found that he ruminated about his departure from the Navy, negatively interpreting his past and future relative to those events. The association between the situation (Jerrold's retirement and uncertain future), cognitions (I failed and will never solve my problems), behavior (inability to sleep), and biochemistry (stimulation when ruminating about past and future) were elicited by questioning him about each specific factor. We agreed to try an experiment to be attempted in the week prior to the next session.

I questioned the possibility of behavioral entry point designed to change the system of emotion with the hy-

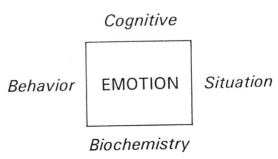

Figure 10-2. A system of emotion.

pothesis that if this part of the system of emotional distress was altered, discomfort might be lowered by producing better sleep and less rumination. Stimulus control was explained to Jerrold. He was to avoid any activity in bed except sleeping. If he started worrying (or to engage in any other activity, such as reading, watching TV, or eating) for more than 20 minutes, he would go to another location and perform those activities. His "worry couch" in another room was designated as the place he would go to ruminate until he felt sufficiently tired to go back to bed and sleep.

Homework also included an attempt to record thoughts and feelings associated with emotions such as depression and sadness. In the last few minutes of our meeting, Jerrold and I reviewed what happened in the session, and I checked to see if there were any questions or concerns.

SESSIONS 2 THROUGH 6

Jerrold's attempt at stimulus control for sleep was moderately successful, lessening the amount of time he spent worrying at night and increasing the amount and quality of his sleep. The socialization process during the previous session that involved a modification of expectations for treatment made the result of this experiment particularly rewarding. Although his symptoms were not totally eliminated, a satisfactory change was made toward improvement using a guided empirical approach. This was then used as evidence of his ability to take control of his life, thereby increasing his sense of self-efficacy.

Our focus in the next few sessions shifted from behavioral to cognitive techniques in an effort to reinstitute his previous high level of coping skills and to promote his adaptation to the current situation. Jerrold talked about his thoughts associated with the low points of the week. There were concerns about his sense of competence to solve problems and the possibilities for improvement in his situation. This information was put in the context of the Daily Record of Dysfunctional Thoughts (DRDT; Figure 10-3) during the session as a means of learning the technique. The thought record was collaboratively written on the eraserboard mounted on the wall in my office. The book *Woulda, Coulda, Shoulda* (Freeman & DeWolf, 1989) was assigned as bibliotherapy and as a reference for Jerrold as he attempted to identify and respond to automatic thoughts associated with his emotional distress.

Several rules of thumb for rational responding to distressing automatic thoughts in the DRDT were reviewed. These rules are described in the following paragraphs.

1. Address one automatic thought (AT) at a time in the rational response column; if several ATs are evident in a given situation, write them down and respond to the most potent one. For example, after Jerrold had a disagreement with his son, he was feeling discouraged. He identified several automatic thoughts associated with his feelings, including:

- He always wants to antagonize me. (A)
- I am a lousy father. (B)
- I wish something would go right in my life. (C)

Jerrold then sought to respond to B, bypassing A because it seemed to be a subset of B, and C because it seemed to be less specific to his distress from the current situation. He then identified reasons why he was not a lousy father, such as his consistent attention to his son's difficulties and the fact that he has supported and guided his son in such important areas as helping him to do better in school, listening to his feelings, and helping him work through difficulties with his mother and in finding a job. Jerrold also wrote that since his son was an adolescent, he was bound to disagree with his father sometimes. His son's school performance was generally improving, and for the most part, he was making an effort to get along with others better.

After making these responses to automatic thought B, Jerrold's level of discouragement decreased from 90% to 50%. Thoughts A and C no longer seemed valid to him, and he did not feel it necessary to go back and work on adaptive responses to them at this time. If the level of distress was significantly lowered, the other ATs could be circumvented. If emotional discomfort was still high, responding to the next AT would need to be done. The skill developed here was identifying the thought that was like the king, rather than the pawn.

2. Generate alternative interpretations in the response column, using specific examples and evidence. If the AT is a realistic problem, avoid trying to rationalize or to interpret the difficulties through rose-colored glasses. Be realistic and generate ways to solve the problem. Jerrold's other responses in the example above included trying to get his son to talk with him again about their disagreement, rather than just letting it slide. He actually called him and set a time for them to meet.

3. Consider being compassionate to yourself in a distressing situation. If your AT is self-punitive or blaming, try to find a more understanding response to the situation. Ask yourself what you would think if your therapist addressed you in a manner similar to your automatic thought when you were in a difficult situation and displaying distress (i.e., blaming, negative, and cruel versus sympathetic, patient, and hopeful). Continuing

<u>DAILY RECORD OF DYSFUNCTIONAL THOUGHTS</u>

DATE	SITUATION Describe: 1. Actual event leading to unpleasant emotion, or 2. Stream of thoughts, daydream, or recollection, leading to unpleasant emotion.	EMOTION(S) 1. Specify sad; anxious; angry, etc. 2. Rate degree of emotion, 1-100.	AUTOMATIC THOUGHT(S) 1. Write automatic thought(s) that preceded emotion(s). 2. Rate belief in automatic thought(s), 0-100%.	RATIONAL RESPONSE 1. Write rational response to automatic thought(s). 2. Rate belief in rational response, 0-100%.	OUTCOME 1. Re-rate belief in automatic thought(s), 0-100%. 2. Specify and rate subsequent emotions, 0-100.
6 Nov	In the evening watching T.V.	Sorrow 40% Despair 50%	I will never be able to find a job. I am deluding myself. 70%	–I have not really tried 70% –Job hunting is difficult work. It will require continued effort and there's bound to be discouragement until I find a job I want. 75% –I have a couple of good leads and I am going to go to a seminar that will help my effort. 80% –This thinking is all or nothing. Never is not the right word. It will be difficult. 80%	1. 25% 2. Sorrow 0% Despair 15% Optimistic 30%

EXPLANATION: When you experience an unpleasant emotion, note the situation that seemed to stimulate the emotion. (If the emotion occurred while you were thinking, daydreaming, etc., please note this.) Then note the automatic thought associated with the emotion. Record the degree to which you believe this thought: 0%=not at all; 100%=completely. In rating degree of emotion: 1=a trace; 100=the most intense possible.

Figure 10-3. Jerrold F's Daily Record of Dysfunctional Thoughts (DRDT).

with this example, Jerrold thought about kinder and more productive ways to interpret the situation. He came up with, "Give yourself a break. It's rare that parents get along with their teenage children. They are supposed to be rebellious, and that's bound to be aggravating."

4. Try to generate several responses to each AT. The AT is usually simplistic and vicious. It takes substance to combat the vindictive, emotional, and brutal accusations that are typical in automatic thoughts. As can be seen in the above example, there were several alternative interpretations to offset the conclusions drawn in the automatic thought, "I am a lousy father."

5. If you identify cognitive distortions and biases contained in your automatic thinking, be sure to follow with responses that are indicative of more flexible and adaptive thinking. The primary cognitive bias Jerrold identified above was overgeneralization. By being more specific about issues of fathering, he found that the evi-

dence did not support such an all-inclusive negative indictment of his abilities.

Jerrold continued to come to six weekly sessions. He produced dysfunctional thought records as homework for each meeting. Other self-help work included attending employment workshops at the university and participating in support groups that met in the metropolitan area (e.g., Emotions Anonymous).

RECOVERY

Within a few months after starting treatment, Jerrold F. found a job, and this may have been the single most important event associated with relief from the many symptoms he was experiencing. He attributed the success of his efforts in a variety of areas to his tenacity and to the therapy collaboration.

Although there did not appear to be problems generated from a dysfunctional personality structure, some underlying assumptions that were a result of his career in the military were identified. Civilian life and relationships outside of military structure required a change in his approach to other people. Two examples of assumptions needing change are listed below.

It's difficult to be myself and express my feelings around others. Jerrold was groomed to order people within a very clear chain of command. Expressing feelings and having conversations with others followed different rules in civilian life. I used role-playing as a method of modifying Jerrold's approach to casual conversation. Asking open-ended questions and developing active listening skills were points of focus to increase social effectiveness (Garner, 1981) in the civilian world. Jerrold practiced these methods in vivo at support groups he visited and was satisfied with the gains he made.

People feel uncomfortable around me. I don't fit in. This belief was closely connected to the previous one. Behavioral experiments were applied to allow Jerrold to develop some distance from the feelings associated with this belief and to test its validity. When he made an effort to apply his skills in real-life situations, he was able to have conversations and contact with people that produced experiences contradicting the meanings attached to the belief. He identified bias in the assumptions, including jumping to conclusions, emotional reasoning, mind reading, and fortune-telling.

Jerrold's recovery was progressive, but he did experience some setbacks. He persevered with his job search, but it took many months and included a series of dead-end interviews and some close calls that ended in disappointment. In behavioral terms, job hunting could be interpreted as a schedule of nonreinforcement that could lead to extinction of the behavior. Every attempt ends in a miss until employment is found. During his search, an effort was made to find elements of progress in each interview situation. Jerrold reframed the hunt for work as a process of elimination that allowed him to define and refine his goals and to concentrate on his strengths. When he received negative feedback in an interview, he made an effort to judge the credibility of the feedback instead of accepting it uncritically (Freeman & DeWolf, 1989). He attempted to use the constructive criticism he received to improve his self-presentation in subsequent interviews. If the commentary from prospective employers was irrelevant, unfounded, rude, or unnecessarily severe, he tried either to reject it or to put it in perspective with the positive feedback he obtained in most interviews. He and I collaborated on maintaining the focus on the challenges in his search rather than on the setbacks; some weeks were more difficult than others.

FOLLOW-UP SESSIONS

Jerrold F. continued treatment for six months. Sessions subsequent to the eighth week were scheduled every week; the last three sessions were three weeks apart. At the conclusion of therapy, Jerrold was able to understand the relationship among his life situations, feelings, thoughts, and beliefs and to use this understanding to his advantage. He moved from a depressed mood to behavioral activation and goal-directed behavior. Cognitive restructuring and acquisition and/or reactivation of adaptive skills led to recovery of function, mood elevation, and improved satisfaction with self-situation, and prospects for the future.

SUMMARY

The case of Jerrold F. illustrates how established methods of cognitive therapy furnish an efficient and effective means of providing short-term treatment for adjustment disorder. His transition from a military career to civilian life led to depressive symptoms including sadness, avoidance and diminished capacity. The lack of history of previous problems with depressed mood and the clear relationship between recent psychosocial stressors and adjustment problems led to Jerrold's diagnosis. Cognitive restructuring and therapeutic collaboration in treatment aided this man's effort to reach his goals, including gaining relief from symptoms, acquisition of social skills in a civilian milieu, and recovering a more positive self-concept. He was able to restore his previous level of functioning and to improve his mood through a short-term course of cognitive therapy.

REFERENCES

American Psychiatric Association. (1987). *Diagnostic and statistical manual of mental disorders (rev. 3rd ed.).* Washington, DC: Author.

Beck, A. T. (1961). A systematic investigation of depression. *Comprehensive Psychiatry, 2,* 162–170.

Beck, A. T. (1963). Thinking and depression. *Archives of General Psychiatry, 9,* 324–333.

Beck, A. T. (1967). *Depression: clinical, experimental, and theoretical aspects.* New York: Harper and Row.

Beck, A. T. (1976). *Cognitive therapy and the emotional disorders.* New York: New American Library.

Beck, A. T., Rush, A. J., Shaw, B. F., & Emery, G. (1979). *Cognitive therapy of depression.* New York: Guilford.

Ellis, A. (1962). *Reason and emotion in psychotherapy*. New York: Lyle Stuart.

Ellis, A. (1970). *The essence of rational psychotherapy: A comprehensive approach to treatment*. New York: Institute for Rational Living.

Ellis, A., & Dryden, W. (1987). *The practice of rational-emotive therapy*. New York: Springer.

Freeman, A., & DeWolf, R. (1989). *Woulda, coulda, shoulda*. New York: William Morrow.

Garner, A. (1981). *Conversationally speaking*. New York: McGraw-Hill.

Meichenbaum, D. H. (1977). *Cognitive-behavior modification: An integrative approach*. New York: Plenum.

Peck, M. S. (1978). *The road less traveled*. New York: Simon & Schuster.

SUGGESTED READINGS

Peck, M. S. (1978). *The road less traveled*. New York: Simon & Schuster.

Clance, P. R. (1985). *The imposter phenomenon*. Atlanta: Peachtree.

Beck, A. T., Rush, A. J., Shaw, B. F., & Emery, G. (1979). *Cognitive therapy of depression*. New York: Guilford.

Frankl, V. F. (1978). *The unheard cry for meaning*. New York: Simon & Schuster.

Freeman, A., Simon, K. M., Beutler, L. F., & Arkowitz, H. (Eds.). (1989). *Comprehensive handbook of cognitive therapy*. New York: Plenum.

11

Recurrent Major Depression

M. Jane Yates

INTRODUCTION

Cognitive therapy has been shown to be a powerfully effective approach for treating depression (Beck, Hollon, Young, Bedrosian, & Budeny, 1985; Blackburn, 1988; Elkin, Parloff, Hodley, & Autry, 1985). The model as developed by Beck and his colleagues (Beck, 1963, 1964, 1967, 1976, 1979, 1982, 1985; Beck et al., 1978; Bedrosian & Beck, 1980) is presently recognized by the professional community as a major force in psychotherapeutic practice. This is in large part due to its strong theoretical base and empirical support in clinical trials (Elkin et al., 1985; see Blackburn, 1988, for a review). Widespread recognition of the model has extended beyond the professional arena, through self-help books in the popular press, to the public at large (Beck, 1988; Burns, 1980, 1989; Freeman & DeWolf, 1989).

Clinical depression is so prevalent that it has been described as "the common cold of psychiatric disturbances." The Diagnostic and Statistical Manual of Mental Disorders (DSM-III-R; American Psychological Association [APA], 1987) reports that in Europe and the United States, 26% of adult females and 12% of adult males have experienced major depression. The competence of clinicians may be judged by the extent to which they can effectively help clients overcome depression and lead meaningful, functional lives.

The DSM-III-R defines several different types of depression under the broader category of mood disorders. The mood disorders are further divided into bipolar disorders and depressive disorders. The diagnostic criteria for bipolar disorders include (in addition to depression) a history of manic or hypomanic episodes. Bipolar disorder per se includes one or more manic episodes and one or more major depressive episodes; cyclothymia includes numerous hypomanic episodes and episodes of depressive symptoms. When major depressive and hypomanic episodes exist, the condition is sometimes known as bipolar II disorder but is included in the category of bipolar disorders, not otherwise specified (NOS).

Depressive disorders include major depression and dysthymia. Major depression is a condition in which five out of the nine diagnostic criteria have been met for a duration of not less than a continuous two-week period; the episode represents a change from previous higher functioning (APA, 1987). Major depression is further differentiated by type (melancholic or chronic) and episodes (single versus recurrent). Melancholic type is more severe, and includes early morning waking, failure to respond (even temporarily) to pleasurable stimuli, previous depressive episodes, and previous good response to specific somatic treatment or antidepressant medication or lithium. Chronic type lasts two years without a two-month alleviation of symptoms (APA, 1987).

M. Jane Yates • Atlanta Center for Cognitive Therapy, 1772 Century Boulevard, Atlanta, Georgia 30345.

Comprehensive Casebook of Cognitive Therapy, edited by Arthur Freeman and Frank M. Dattilio. Plenum Press, New York, 1992.

Dysthymia refers to chronic dysphoria (more days than not) over at least a two-year period in which, during the first year of the condition, diagnostic criteria for major depression were not met. A diagnosis of major depression may be superimposed on a diagnosis of dysthymia (APA, 1987).

Current episodes of major depression and bipolar disorders are further described as mild, moderate, or severe, and with or without psychotic features. For bipolar disorder, dipolar disorder NOS, recurrent major depression, and depressive disorder NOS a seasonal pattern may be noted, indicating a regular cyclic relationship between a specific 60-day period of the year and onset of the mood episodes (APA, 1987).

In treating the person who is suffering from a major depressive episode, it becomes evident that there are identifiable dysfunctional thought patterns involving a negative view of self, world and experience, and the future (Beck, 1963, 1964, 1967, 1976, 1979, 1982, 1985; Beck et al., 1978; Bedrosian & Beck, 1980). When using traditional cognitive-behavioral approaches to deal with these thoughts, the clinician quickly discovers underlying dysfunctional beliefs and maladaptive schemas. When a person's depression is recurrent, it becomes apparent that despite differences in the precipitating events, the same identifiable maladaptive belief patterns and schemas present themselves, full force, during each depressive episode.

Recurring depressive episodes often have the effect, over time, of further solidifying these maladaptive belief systems and schemas through a downward spiral, with each subsequent depression reinforcing the previously held negative beliefs. It is at this point that the inexperienced or narrowly focused cognitive therapist is tempted to question the efficacy of the model rather than to appreciate that these early learned, more complex and enduring problems are also amenable to cognitive interventions.

Specifically, women who were sexually abused as children are more likely to experience depression than are women who were not (Briere, 1984, 1985; Brown & Finkelhor, 1986; Gelinas, 1983; Sedney & Brooks, 1984). These survivors may experience depressive symptomatology intermittently or continually throughout their early life into adulthood. They often feel low self-esteem specifically related to self-blame for the abuse, shame, disgust, and a general perception of themselves as defective, bad, unloved, and undeserving of care from others (Courtois, 1988). When care is given, it is frequently not believed to be deserved. Feelings of emptiness are often reported and are believed to be associated with loss and grief (Courtois, 1988). Feelings of helplessness and pow-

erlessness initially experienced in the abusive situations continue and are generalized throughout the survivor's life experience; learned helplessness and its relationship to depression were described by Seligman (1975) and are specifically applicable with sexual abuse survivors. As a group, these women are more likely to consider or attempt suicide and to engage in self-harmful behavior (Briere & Runty, 1986).

In treating survivors of childhood sexual abuse whose depression and other psychological problems are related to that abuse, it is important to explore the meaning of present thought processes and behaviors in relationship to schemas (Peasicki & Hollon, 1987). Young (1987) has theoretically identified and categorized schemas and proposed that they continue by three functional processes: maintenance, avoidance, and compensation. These concepts are particularly valuable in working with sexual abuse survivors. As the above discussion would suggest, these women are likely to have schemas involving undesirability (defectiveness and shame), disconnection (emotional deprivation, abandonment, mistrust, and social alienation), and impaired limits (entitlement and insufficient self-control). They could be expected to (a) maintain these schemas by using cognitive distortions along related themes (assuming a victim role), (b) avoid manifestations of the schemas by dissociating feelings and thoughts and avoiding triggering situations, and (c) compensate for schemas by sexually acting out or by assuming the role of the abuser in an effort to regain control that was lost in the initial abusive situation.

The woman who is the focus of this chapter reported major depressive episodes dating back at least to her college days. At the time of initial treatment, she was diagnosed as having recurrent major depression. In addition, she displayed traits of borderline personality disorder; however, her positive response to treatment and the sustaining of her higher functional level over time argue against a primary diagnosis of a personality disorder.

BACKGROUND INFORMATION

Mary S. was a 39-year-old, twice-divorced woman with two sons (ages 8 and 10) and one stepson (age 20). She had completed college and two years of law school and was employed as a computer programmer. Mary was brought to the psychiatric hospital by a friend and coworker to whom she had been voicing suicidal intentions for several days. In the hour prior to admission, the coworker had taken a loaded gun away from Mary and then taken her to the hospital. Upon initial evaluation, the on-call psychiatrist signed an involuntary admission order that allowed a 48-hour psychiatric evaluation. Immediately upon admission, Mary agreed to a voluntary admission status.

While in the hospital, in order to prevent Mary from attempting suicide, she had to be restrained on one occasion and moved to a closed unit on another. These instances followed expressions of criticism and contempt on the part of other patients. Due to her lack of response to milieu therapy and medication, she was referred by her psychiatrist for cognitive therapy.

Mary described dysphoria, insomnia, hopelessness, self-contempt, low energy and motivation, crying spells, and a 30-pound weight gain due to overeating as symptoms. She also described increasing suicidal thinking and intent over the previous six to eight months, reaching crisis proportion two weeks prior to admission.

The first precipitating event leading to the present depressive episode was an automobile accident eight months previous in which her 10-year-old son sustained multiple fractures. The hospital bills had not been paid by the insurance company of the other person involved in the accident, reportedly due to the company's bankruptcy. Mary was in financial distress and planned for her own life insurance monies (from her death) to pay debts she owed. Within the previous year she also had been threatened with physical reprisal for her political activism on behalf of certain minority groups. In addition, her ex-husband had threatened to withhold child support. Most recently, she had terminated a wholly unsatisfying romantic relationship with a married man.

Mary is the second of three children, with a sister three years older and a brother two years younger. Her father, a dentist, was the son of a Russian Jewish immigrant. He also was verbally abusive to all the children. He had been sexually abusive to Mary since she was 3 years old, and possibly to her sister as well. He would punish Mary in unusually cruel ways, such as drilling her teeth without benefit of anesthetic and forcing her to walk around her neighborhood for hours in the hot summertime wearing a rubber rain suit. He had been admitted for several psychiatric hospitalizations during her childhood. Despite his abnormal behavior, Mary's father was a prominent member of their community and earned a very comfortable living. Her mother was a Roman Catholic of Italian origin; Mary described her as a "mouse" because she did not assert herself in the relationship with her husband or protect any of her children from his abuse.

Mary is presently estranged from her father. When she confronted him regarding his abuse of her, he denied it and essentially blamed her. Her relationship with her mother has been erratic. Her mother has always been critical of Mary and holds her responsible for the problems of the entire family.

Throughout her childhood, Mary was the scapegoat of the family, probably because she tended to act out her feelings and impulses—unlike her siblings, who were more compliant. As an adolescent, Mary was difficult to manage, defying the attempts of both parents to control her and running away from home numerous times. She was sexually promiscuous and engaged in numerous high-risk sexual activities during her absences from home.

Despite her tumultuous adolescent years, Mary's performance in school throughout her academic years was excellent. She went to college, achieved good grades, and was graduated with her class. She married shortly after college, but that marriage ended in divorce after two years.

Her second marriage was to a Greek man with two sons from a previous marriage. Both stepsons (ages 8 and 10 at that time) came to live with Mary and her husband after they were married. The younger son returned to Greece after a short period of time; the older son, Nick, continued to live with Mary and her husband. This second marriage lasted about six years and resulted in the birth of two more sons, who were 8 and 10 at the time of the evaluation.

Mary had been divorced from her second ex-husband (the father of her two children) for six years. The husband had been verbally abusive to both her and the children and was particularly critical of Nick, his son by his previous marriage. In response to this, Mary overidentified with her stepson Nick as the "victim" of an abusive father and became overprotective. Mary and Nick were interdependent, and their overinvolvement eventually evolved into a sexual relationship that Mary began with him when he was 14. This relationship ultimately became the basis of her self-contempt.

When Nick was 16, Child Protective Services (CPS) became involved in the situation following Mary's plea for help from Parents Anonymous. Mary was not allowed to see Nick for six months, and she received psychiatric help through a number of agencies. She attended a sexual abuse survivors group and received medication and infrequent supportive psychotherapy from a community mental health center. Later she received individual therapy from a counselor in her employee assistance program.

During this period, Mary attempted suicide twice by overdosing with prescription drugs. Following one of these attempts, she was admitted to a state hospital. While receiving active support and participating in frequent therapy sessions, Mary was able to abstain from having sexual contact with her stepson, but financial constraints and faltering motivation often interfered with her sustaining active involvement in the therapy to the extent necessary. Thus, the sexual relationship continued, with initiation by both Mary and her stepson, despite CPS involvements and her intermittent attempts to sever the relationship.

Mary and her stepson resumed their relationship in September 1988 after he was thrown out of his father's house and came to live with her. At this time he began to assume increasing responsibility in the household, and they began to be emotionally involved again. A continuing threat came from her second ex-husband to expose her previous sexual relationship with her stepson by telling her other two sons and her employers. In January 1989, after resuming their sexual relationship, Mary sought treatment and was referred to another therapist by her employee assistance program. This therapist told her she had an incurable personality disorder and that the best she could hope for was to learn to live with her depression. This further contributed to her hopelessness regarding her ability to control acting on her sexual feelings, and to her subsequent guilt and depression.

Four or five months before the evaluation, Mary once again terminated her sexual relationship with Nick. This time she substituted a romantic relationship with a married man, a relationship that had ended three days prior to her suicidal crisis and subsequent hospitalization. With this loss, she began to long for the comfort of her sexual relationship with her stepson, which in turn overwhelmed her with feelings of guilt and self-contempt. She felt hopelessly out of control regarding these feelings and determined that suicide was her only possible solution.

ASSESSMENT, DIAGNOSIS, AND CONCEPTUALIZATION (SESSIONS 1 THROUGH 3)

The initial evaluation consisted of a structured clinical interview. At that time, Mary was tearful, tangential in her presentation, and unfocused in her verbal presentation. She was feeling ostracized by other patients, and this seemed to confirm her feelings of self-contempt.

She was very articulate and somewhat dramatic in her presentation, focusing on the fact that her previous therapist told her the best she could hope for was to live with her problems. She used such words as "devastated" and "tragedy," and appeared to be overwhelmed by the numerous problems she faced.

Formal assessment measures included the Beck Depression Inventory (BDI), Hopelessness Scale, Minnesota Multiphasic Personality Inventory (MMPI), Wechsler Adult Intelligence Scale-Revised (WAIS-R), and Rorschach Inkblot Test.

On the BDI, Mary scored 37, indicating severe depression. Particularly significant were her endorsements of the following statements reflecting hopelessness and suicidal intent:

- I feel that the future is hopeless and that things cannot improve.
- I would kill myself if I had the chance.

Mary scored 18 out of a possible 20 points on the Hopelessness Scale, indicating extreme hopelessness. Both measures confirmed her extreme hopelessness and despair. Hopelessness has been shown to be more correlated with suicidal thinking than the severity of depression (Minkoff et al., 1973).

Despite a guarded response set, Mary's Rorschach responses resulted in 5 out of 12 indicators on the suicide constellation as scored by the Exner system. Her suicidal risk was considered extremely high, as reflected by all measures, especially the BDI and Hopelessness Scale. Her expressed intent, history of previous attempts, recent interrupted attempt, and behavior while in the hospital further confirmed the seriousness of her suicidal risk.

On the WAIS-R, her full-scale IQ of 134 placed her in the very superior range of intelligence, with somewhat higher verbal than nonverbal functioning. Her strong verbal skills would allow her to understand easily the concepts of cognitive therapy and to identify her own patterns of maladaptive thinking.

On the MMPI, Mary scored in the elevated range on scales 2 (Depression), 4 (Psychopathic Deviate), and 8 (Schizophrenia). With the highest score being on the Depression scale, her elevated scores on scales 4 and 8 were interpreted to reflect her social alienation and lack of ego mastery.

In addition to dichotomous thinking and overgeneralization noticeable in the clinical interviews, her capacity to distort cognitively was evident in the Rorschach protocol. This was especially true when strong affect was involved. Her responses, as interpreted by Exner's system, identified her as an "underincorporator," suggesting her capacity to distort the cognitive meaning of her experience by considering only partial information. This distortion tendency could alert the therapist to the possible use of arbitrary inference and selective abstraction. Certainly, catastrophizing was already evident. Behaviorally, she could be expected to act impulsively on her feelings (confirmed by history), subsequently perceiving herself as helplessly out of control. This was evident in her inappropriate relationship with her stepson, as well as her overeating. Mary was so overwhelmed by the multitude and magnitude of her problems that she was not able to view them separately.

The following dialogue from one of the evaluation sessions illustrates this, as well as Mary's negative view of herself, the world, and the future.

THERAPIST: Can you tell me how you see your problems right now?

MARY: Well, my life is just one big glob of misery. My whole life has been a tragedy.

THERAPIST: Can you tell me what you mean by your life being a "glob of misery" and a tragedy?

MARY: (begins to cry) Like when I saw that dog beaten on the side of the road. That just shows that the world is a horrible, despicable place, and I'm just the epitome of its despicableness.

THERAPIST: I can see this must be very painful for you. (pause) So you are seeing both the world and yourself in an altogether negative life.

MARY: Yeah.

THERAPIST: This is quite typical of people who are depressed. You sound pretty overwhelmed.

MARY: Well, things are not going to get better either. My other therapist said so. She said I would just have to learn to live with my depression, and I can't imagine how I can do that.

THERAPIST: You should like you feel pretty hopeless.

MARY: I *am* hopeless.

THERAPIST: The thought of having to live with the way you're feeling now, is that part of what your hopelessness is about?

MARY: Well, yes, this is what my whole life has come to, just a glob of misery.

THERAPIST: It does sound like you have a number of problems facing you. You also seem to be seeing them as a whole, a "glob," like you said. When you think of them that way, they must seem completely unmanageable.

MARY: Yeah.

THERAPIST: Sometimes when people can separate their problems and focus on them one by one, they find ways to deal with them more effectively.

MARY: I really don't think I do that. They all blend together.

THERAPIST: Well, one of the first things we can do in therapy is to look at your problems individually and collaborate on developing possible solutions to try. (pause) Would you be willing to give that approach a try?

MARY: Well, at this point there's really nothing to lose. I guess I could try.

Mary's lifelong beliefs and assumptions, of which she was convinced, were reflected by all the evaluation measures and were particularly apparent during the initial interviews. These beliefs and assumptions were discussed openly during the evaluation process. They are summarized as follows and identified according to Young's (1987) categories:

- I am a victim and powerless to change myself or my circumstances (insufficient self-control, incompetence).
- My emotions and impulses are beyond my control (insufficient self-control).
- I am a despicable person, permanently defective and not worthy of living (defectiveness, shame, unlovability, alienation, self-punishment).

Mary saw the world as "despicable" and herself as the "epitome of its despicableness." She hated herself and did not believe that she deserved anything better. She did not think of herself as capable of living without her stepson, and alternatively did not think she could live with the guilt of living with him. Thus, she considered herself worthy only of death.

Mary's symptomatology fit the DSM-III-R diagnostic criteria for recurrent major depression. Enduring, lifelong personality characteristics, as reflected in her history and evaluation, suggested a diagnosis of borderline personality disorder with histrionic and narcissistic traits. Her response to treatment and level of functioning following the alleviation of her depression serve to show, in this instance, that cognitive therapy is effective not only in the treatment of depression but with more deeply rooted character pathology as well.

TREATMENT (SESSIONS 4 THROUGH 13)

Mary's early treatment took place in the hospital, where she was seen daily. The therapeutic process began at the first contact.

Several very important foundation steps necessary for successful treatment outcome were laid down during the evaluation process. Rapport was established, collaboration and a problem-oriented focus were introduced into the treatment process, understanding was reflected by restatement and paraphrasing, and empathy was expressed by noticing and reflecting on feeling statements. During the initial sessions, these steps are particularly important because they foster the therapeutic alliance, actively engage the client in her own therapy (collaboration), and—perhaps most important in a very depressed person such as Mary—inspire hope.

It was rather difficult, at first, to set agendas for the sessions and stay focused on them. If not structured by the therapist, Mary tended to ramble in the sessions, and this inevitably led to her feeling of being overwhelmed and hopeless. This tendency was pointed out to her, and she was asked if she would feel less out of control in this one small area of her experience if she could agree on an agenda and focus on it throughout the session. She was able to see the benefit of the structure. Mary was better able to identify problems, set priorities, and sustain focus on the agenda when early in the session a specific amount of time was set aside for her to ventilate in an unrestricted way. This was most often limited to 5 to 10 minutes.

The stage was set for a problem-oriented approach to treatment. In the session when Mary's beliefs were discussed, the therapist gave her a pamphlet to read entitled "Coping with Depression" (Beck & Greenberg, 1984). Although her response was somewhat guarded, she seemed to be intrigued by the possibility that her negative view might be a product of distortion. When she thought of her present situation, she began catastrophizing and speaking of suicide. The therapist focused on her ambivalence, at first by suggesting to her that there must be a number of things keeping her alive, because she was in fact, living. She argued that not all of her wanted to die, but that she hated herself and did not believe herself worthy of living.

Later in treatment, Mary confided that two things had allowed her to give therapy a chance. One was that the therapist had not been judgmental and contemptuous of her for her sexual abuse of her stepson. Out of that experience, Mary was able to acknowledge her responsibility for her abusive behavior and at the same time explore the meaning, etiology, and function it served for her. The second was recognizing that there was an important issue of self-respect that related to her sexual relationship with her stepson, and that this issue could be faced and dealt with effectively. Until this point, Mary had been seeing herself as contemptible rather than seeing her *behavior* as unacceptable. When faced with criticism or shock from others regarding at her behavior, she loathed herself even more. There was an initial turning point in her treatment as a result of a Socratic method of questioning. When the therapist asked if she could imagine how she might feel if she did not act on her feelings for even a short period of time, Mary realized that a portion of her self-contempt had to do with her actions rather than her person. Her actions were, in fact, unacceptable to her. For the first time, she then could begin to distinguish her behavior from her self, and subsequently to view self-respect as something she could "earn" by changing her behavior.

The following dialogue took place during the session in which Mary's problem list was generated and she began to recognize the specific link between her relationship with her stepson and her suicidal feelings.

THERAPIST: You say your relationship with Nick is mostly what makes you feel suicidal, is that correct?

MARY: It's wrong, I know. It's just like what my dad did to me, but I just don't think I can stop myself. I *can't* live my life without him, and I can't bear destroying his whole life, too. I could never respect myself for that.

THERAPIST: So you lose your self-respect when you act on your feelings for Nick?

MARY: Yes.

THERAPIST: I hear that you don't think you can terminate your relationship with Nick right now, but does that necessarily mean you can't change it?

MARY: Well, I don't see any way to. He's moved back into the house and is taking care of the boys now. That's how it all started before, him moving back in.

THERAPIST: If you could keep from acting on your erotic feelings for him, for say a week, just a little while—would you feel any more self-respect than you do now?

MARY: Yes, I would, but that's not enough.

THERAPIST: Maybe not. Do you think it's a start in the right direction?

MARY: Yes.

THERAPIST: Perhaps it could make some difference in your hopelessness. Would you likely feel more, or less, or about the same?

MARY: Well, I guess I would feel more hopeful.

THERAPIST: It might let you know that you could make other changes, too.

MARY: (pause) I suppose it would. I've never really thought of it that way.

It was at this point that the discussion focused on Mary seeing her problems as unmanageable as a whole. She was urged to break them down into separate problems and to address them individually. She listed approximately seven problems and later organized and prioritized them as follows:

1. Relationship with Nick
2. Suicidal thinking
3. Finances
4. Few meaningful adult friendships
5. Not having enough time for her two sons
6. Being overweight
7. Antagonistic relationship with ex-husband

Because Mary's suicidal thinking and involvement with Nick were interrelated, both required priority focus. The Daily Record of Dysfunctional Thoughts (DRDT) was used to help Mary deal with both these problems. She responded well to the structure of the form and even took its use as an intellectual challenge.

When the assignment using the DRDT was given, two aspects of cognitive therapy were emphasized to Mary:

(a) the collaborative relationship between herself and the therapist, with active participation of her part, and (b) the experimental approach, involving increased awareness as she practiced graded task assignments. The "experimental" concept allowed Mary not to expect perfection or to judge herself harshly. She was asked to complete the first three columns as a first step, and rational responses were developed over the next two therapy sessions. Mary kept the record with her as a reminder. She was urged to refer to it frequently, especially when plagued with hopelessness. Figure 11-1 presents Mary's first DRDT after it had been the subject of two therapy sessions.

Since Mary's relationship with Nick was so closely related to her suicidal thinking, her discharge from the hospital required assurance of her ability to deal effectively with both. The one-week goal of not acting on her sexual feelings quickly became a short-term goal and a potential proving ground for Mary. Each session included preparing support plans for her to use when she left the hospital.

Mary and the therapist decided collaboratively that unless the relationship between her and Nick was confronted openly, Mary's one-sided attempts to reestablish limits and appropriate generational boundaries would probably fail. A joint session with Nick and Mary was planned, and Nick agreed to come in response to Mary's first invitation. At the session, Mary explained to Nick that she had entered the hospital feeling suicidal, primarily because she didn't feel she could limit her involvement with him. She confessed that she feared she had "ruined" his life. She apologized and expressed her desire that he enter therapy in order to deal with his own emotional issues related to her abuse of him. She attempted to frame the change in their relationship as her "need" (rather than a rejection of him) and urged him to enter therapy. She discussed what she referred to as their "secret language"—words, phrases, and behaviors encoded with special meaning to both of them.

Mary expressed appreciation to Nick for taking care of his brothers and for supporting her. She explained that he would have to move out of the house when she returned home from the hospital in order to help that assure they would no longer be sexually involved. He denied that there was any risk of sexual involvement and threatened to sever contact with her completely. General information about the expected effects of sexual abuse was given to Nick, along with the recommendation that he enter psychotherapy to deal with any such effects. Several names of therapists were provided. Nick denied that he needed to seek help or had any ill effects or problems resulting from their relationship.

Following this session, Mary seemed even more strengthened in her resolve to maintain limits for herself, as well as for Nick. She gave Nick a date to be out of the house and planned to change her locks. She was given several therapeutic leaves from the hospital to practice her self-control. To prepare for these leaves, sessions reviewed anticipated problems and involved role-playing specific situations.

In planning for discharge, Mary focused on things she could do to assure her necessary self-control. She decided to arrange some supportive contact every day, such as a therapy session, a codependency meeting, a phone call with a specific understanding person, or simply a "check-in" with her therapist or psychiatrist.

One of the most important issues addressed prior to her hospital discharge was how Mary would deal with suicidal impulses if they should occur. Following her face-to-face meeting with Nick, she became more confident in her ability to maintain the limits she had established, and thus became more hopeful and dramatically less suicidal. She and the therapist collaboratively developed a "crisis plan"; Mary vowed she would not make an attempt on her life, but instead would exhaust all 17 steps in her plan. Steps included referring to her dysfunctional thought record (to support her in challenging her automatic thoughts), telephoning friends, attending at least two therapy sessions and two support group sessions in which she would specifically discuss suicidal thinking, and finally—if needed—going to the hospital herself.

At the time she left the hospital, Mary's score on the BDI had decreased to 23 and her score on the Hopelessness Scale had decreased to 10, indicating alleviation of her depression to a moderate level and her hopelessness to a mild to moderate level.

SESSIONS 14 THROUGH 49

When Mary returned home, she faced many demands. Her young sons had missed her and naturally sought attention. Her home was in disarray, and the locks needed to be changed the first day back. Since Mary had been competent in her job, she looked forward to working again. Her return to her job was only difficult because many of her coworkers knew of her emergency hospital admission. Rather than being overwhelmed, she was able to apply the problem-solving approach learned in therapy to the demands of her daily life. Again, when she separated the specific problems and tasks, she found them quite manageable one by one.

A particularly useful technique in preparing for the challenge facing her was identifying and listing "enabling" versus "disabling" thoughts. Enabling thoughts were those that served to assist Mary in accomplishing her goals, and disabling thoughts were those that deterred or discouraged her from successfully reaching them. She already had a habit of writing notes to herself on the palm of her hand (phone numbers, reminders, etc.); the therapist suggested that she also could write several of her "enablers" across her palms in order to refer to them. These enablers were framed to her as supportive and nurturing rather than admonishing. Some examples of her enablers were "I don't have to be perfect" and "It's okay to learn from my mistakes." Regarding her first-week goal (following discharge) of not acting on her sexual feelings for Nick, she wrote "feelings/actions," "one week," "I deserve a life," and "Nick deserves a separate life."

Mary's first week out of the hospital was successful. Once she had demonstrated to herself that she was capable of maintaining her self-control and boundaries with Nick, she became increasingly motivated to make other changes as well.

Following the initial transition period, Mary's list of problems was reviewed. Although finances were a priority, therapy focused little on this. Mary instructed her attorney to mail letters to her creditors and developed a budget. Her weight was considered to be less of a priority for two reasons: (a) It would be emotionally stressful to diet at this vulnerable time, and (b) it was acknowledged that her obesity provided her some protection from her sexual impulses.

Establishing meaningful adult relationships was an immediate priority. When discussing this goal, Mary's underlying self-esteem and alienation issues had to be addressed. Mary saw herself as defective, unappealing to others, and deprived of emotional nourishment (love) and understanding. She viewed others as "regular," with "regular" lives and "regular" relationships. It was important that the therapist recognize the depth of these core issues while assisting her in the social skill-building necessary to form relationships.

The therapist emphasized that as a child, Mary had not had the guidance and opportunity to develop these skills, but in the present she could give herself these experiences with the support, protection, and guidance that previously had been lacking. By defining these as "parenting" functions, Mary was able to be more empathic toward herself and as a result develop more self-support. Often, her experience of parenting her two younger sons served as a prototype. Another concept that was especially useful in the imagery work was that of "ideal parents."*

*Credit is given to Albert Pesso (1969) for the specific use of the concept of "ideal parents." In psychomotor therapy, the messages of ideal parents are spoken and acted out by other people in role-playing exercises.

In working with the DRDT, the dysfunctional thoughts were identified (see Figure 11-1, e.g., "I am a miserable, despicable person"). The therapist assisted in generating more adaptive, rational thoughts by asking Mary to consider what kind of messages an "ideal" father might have given. After several messages had been generated, imagery was used to further reinforce them. Mary was instructed to close her eyes, relax, and focus on one representative time when her father told her how despicable she was. She was then asked to imagine what it would have been like to have another "ideal" father there, one who would have appreciated, understood, and respected her. The messages were slowly spoken by the therapist while she took them in as though being spoken by an "ideal" father. Using this technique, Mary gave herself guidance in making friends and experimenting with new behaviors.

Mary also began dating, which often brought up her fear of loss of control of her sexual impulses. Again, from the developmental perspective, the therapist suggested that she relate to herself as though she was dating for the first time at ages 14 to 16. In this way, she could develop confidence, learn interpersonal skills, and incorporate protection (appropriate caution) and limits into her life experience. She experimented with less demonstrative expressions of her sexuality and more thoughtful, conscious choices regarding demonstrations of affections and prospective partners.

Four months following her hospitalization, she was amazed to discover that some men found her attractive despite the fact that she was obese. Primarily in response to this realization, she decided that her obesity was not really a deterrent to her sexual expression and decided to engage in a medically supervised weight control program. She attended a support group with this program, and the therapist was primarily supportive rather than active in dealing with Mary's issues of overeating. Throughout the last four months of weekly therapy, she lost 42 pounds.

Nick did not sever contact with Mary in response to her limits on their relationship. Maintaining her boundaries with Nick was difficult for Mary and remained a standing agenda item throughout treatment. He included his girlfriend in family visits and kept a public facade. But privately, if allowed, he would express jealousy or sulk when Mary included her boyfriends in similar family gatherings. On two occasions, Mary and Nick came perilously close to resuming their sexual relationship. One of these occasions involved a lunch together following a quarrel Nick had with his girlfriend. Mary then phoned the therapist, and an appointment was immediately arranged. Mary was guided in reviewing the progress she had made, by reminding herself of her present capacity to enjoy life and how she previously felt suicidal when she

DAILY RECORD OF DYSFUNCTIONAL THOUGHTS

DATE / SITUATION Describe: 1. Actual event leading to unpleasant emotion, or 2. Stream of thoughts, daydream, or recollection, leading to unpleasant emotion.	EMOTION(S) 1. Specify sad, anxious, angry, etc. 2. Rate degree of emotion, 1-100.	AUTOMATIC THOUGHT(S) 1. Write automatic thought(s) that preceded emotion(s). 2. Rate belief in automatic thought(s), 0-100%.	RATIONAL RESPONSE 1. Write rational response to automatic thought(s). 2. Rate belief in rational response, 0-100%.	OUTCOME 1. Re-rate belief in automatic thought(s), 0-100%. 2. Specify and rate subsequent emotions, 0-100.
Hearing that Nick moved back into my house when I came into the hospital	Fear 65%	See now it's going to start all over again (95%)	1. It doesn't have to (60%) 2. I am getting help (95%) 3. I will stay in therapy as long as I need to	
		I won't be able to stop myself from having sex with him (95%) and The only way to stop myself is to kill myself	1. I can live with feelings (50%) 2. I am learning new ways to stop myself (70%) 3. I can stop myself for 1 week (70%)	
		There's no hope for me (90%)	1. If I can stop myself for 1 week there may be hope (80%) 2. I have more hope now than before (80%)	
		I am doing to him just what Dad did to me (90%)	1. No, I'm trying to change, he did not (80%) 2. No, I did not physically hurt Nick	
		I am a miserable, despicable person (95%)	1. My actions are not acceptable. That does not mean I'm bad (60%) 2. I am lerning to change my actions	

EXPLANATION: When you experience an unpleasant emotion, note the situation that seemed to stimulate the emotion. (If the emotion occurred while you were thinking, daydreaming, etc., please note this.) Then note the automatic thought associated with the emotion. Record the degree to which you believe this thought: 0%=not at all; 100%=completely. In rating degree of emotion: 1=a trace; 100=the most intense possible.

Figure 11-1. Mary's first daily record

(continued)

DATE	SITUATION Describe: 1. Actual event leading to unpleasant emotion, or 2. Stream of thoughts, daydream, or recollection, leading to unpleasant emotion.	EMOTION(S) 1. Specify sad/ anxious/angry, etc. 2. Rate degree of emotion, 1-100.	AUTOMATIC THOUGHT(S) 1. Write automatic thought(s) that preceded emotion(s). 2. Rate belief in automatic thought(s), 0-100%.	RATIONAL RESPONSE 1. Write rational response to automatic thought(s). 2. Rate belief in rational response, 0-100%.	OUTCOME 1. Re-rate belief in automatic thought(s), 0-100%. 2. Specify and rate subsequent emotions, 0-100.
			They would all be better off without me (85%)	3. I don't respect myself when I'm sexual with Nick (95%) 1. The boys need a mother (95%) 2. They would be damaged if I killed myself 3. Their father doesn't want them	

EXPLANATION: When you experience an unpleasant emotion, note the situation that seemed to stimulate the emotion. (If the emotion occurred while you were thinking, daydreaming, etc., please note this.) Then note the automatic thought associated with the emotion. Record the degree to which you believe this thought: 0%=not at all; 100%=completely. In rating degree of emotion: 1=a trace; 100=the most intense possible.

Figure 11-1. (continued)

did allow herself to act on her sexual feelings for Nick. She agreed that it was an appropriate time for her to implement her 17 steps. With the support of the therapist, she did so and regained her sense of control. She used the dysfunctional thought record and realized how in need of nurturing she felt and how responsible she felt for satisfying Nick's desires also. She again resolved to look to other relationships for her own nurturing.

For the most part, Mary was extremely proud of herself for what she termed "regular" life experiences, and that pride was self-reinforcing. Over time she came to accept that she and Nick would probably continue to have a special bond, and that from time to time she might have sexual feelings for him, but that she had the choice, capability, and support to not act on them.

As Mary began to structure her own life more effectively, she found that she had more time to spend with her two sons. Her depression steadily lifted as she became increasingly effective in dealing with her problems. There was a turning point regarding her commitment to living that related to an experience with her younger sons; they bought a box turtle, which became the entertainment and focus for the entire family. Mary described her pleasure and delight on one occasion of watching it "gobble up" food as she and the boys fed it. From that very simple experience, she realized her capacity for enjoying life and stated: "If I can find enjoyment in something so simple as feeding a turtle, then that in itself is enough to live for."

Mary's response to therapy was remarkable considering the nature of her abuse and the severity of her symptoms. At the conclusion of weekly therapy, her BDI score was 4, and her Hopelessness Scale score was 3. She was successful in maintaining an appropriate relationship with her stepson. She worked full time and supported herself and her two sons largely without financial support from her ex-husband. As she gained more confidence in her ability to deal with her problems, she independently began using her skills in other areas of her life.

Weekly therapy sessions ended after eight months, but check-in sessions continue on an infrequent basis, usually every six weeks. Mary has agreed to begin more frequent therapy sessions if stress increases or she has difficulty in maintaining appropriate control of her sexual impulses.

SUMMARY

Mary's therapy is an example of how cognitive therapy can be used effectively with someone suffering from recurrent major depression. Traditional techniques were useful in both inpatient and outpatient settings, especially in dealing with her suicidal thinking and impaired sexual impulse control. Mary's depression lifted as she was able to separate and deal with her problems specifically. Her childhood sexual abuse issues were dealt with by assisting her in establishing mastery and control in her life via a problem-solving approach. Underlying dysfunctional beliefs and schemas were addressed from a developmental perspective using imagery and concepts of symbolic reparenting.

The case study of Mary serves to show how cognitive-behavioral therapy can be used effectively with a person who has significant disruptive personality dynamics underlying their major depression. Mary's courage to transform herself from the role of a victim to that of a self-respecting human being and to see herself as an adult capable of learning life skills that she had not been fortunate enough to be taught as a child—is to be admired.

REFERENCES

American Psychiatric Association. (1987). *Diagnostic and statistical manual of mental disorders* (rev. 3rd ed.). Washington, DC: Author.
Beck, A. T. (1963). Thinking and depression I. Idiosyncratic content and cognitive distortions. *Archives of General Psychiatry, 9*, 324–333.
Beck, A. T. (1964). Thinking and depression II. Theory and therapy. *Archives of General Psychiatry, 10*, 261–571.
Beck, A. T. (1967). *Depression: Clinical, experimental and theoretical aspects*. New York: Hoeber. (Republished in 1972 as *Depression: Causes and treatment*. Philadelphia: University of Pennsylvania Press.)
Beck, A. T. (1982). Cognitive therapy of depression: New perspectives. In P. Clayton (Ed.), *Depression*. New York: Raven.
Beck, A. T. (1976). *Cognitive therapy and the emotional disorders*. New York: International Universities Press.
Beck, A. T. (1985). Cognitive therapy, behavior therapy, psychoanalysis and pharmacotherapy: A cognitive continuum. In M. J. Mahoney & A. Freeman (Eds.), *Cognition and psychotherapy*. New York: Plenum.
Beck, A. T. (1988). *Love is never enough*. New York: Harper and Row.
Beck, A. T., Freeman, A., & Associates. (1990). *Cognitive therapy of personality disorders*. New York: Guilford.
Beck, A. T., Hollon, S. D., Young, J., Bedrosian, R. C., & Budeny. (1985). Treatment of depression with cognitive therapy and amitriptyline. *Archives of General Psychiatry, 42*, 142–148.
Beck, A. T., Rush, A. J., Shaw, B. F., & Emery, G. (1979). *Cognitive therapy of depression*. New York: Guilford.
Bedrosian, R. C., & Beck, A. T. (1980). Principles of cognitive therapy. In M. Mahoney (Ed.), *Psychotherapy process (pp. 127–152)*. New York: Plenum.
Briere, J. (1984, April). *The effects of childhood sexual abuse on later psychological functioning: Defining a post-sexual abuse syndrome*. Paper presented at the Third National Conference

on the Sexual Victimization of Children, Childrens' Hospital, National Medical Center, Washington, DC.

Briere, J. (1985). *Symptomatology associated with prior sexual abuse in a non-clinical sample*. Paper presented at the annual meeting of the American Psychological Association, Los Angeles, CA.

Briere, J., & Ruty, M. (1986). Suicidal thoughts and behaviors in former sexual abuse victims. *Canadian Journal of Behavior Science, 18*, 413–423.

Brown, A., & Finkelhor, D. (1986). Impact of child abuse: A review of the literature. *Psychological Bulletin, 99*, 66–77.

Courtois, C. A. (1988). *Healing the incest wound*. New York: Norton.

Burns, D. D. (1980). *Feeling good: The new mood therapy*. New York: William Morrow.

Burns, D. D. (1989). *The feeing good handbook: Using the new mood therapy in everyday life*. New York: William Morrow.

Elkin, I., Parloff, M. B., Hodley, S. W., & Autry, J. H. (1985). NIMH Treatment of Depression Collaborative Research Program. *Archives of General Psychiatry, 42*, 305–316.

Freeman, A., & DeWolf, R. (1989). *Woulda, coulda, shoulda: Overcoming regrets, mistakes and missed opportunities*. New York: William Morrow.

Gelinas, D. J. (1983). The persisting negative effects of incest. *Psychiatry, 46*, 313–332.

Peasecki, J., & Hollon, S. D. (1987). Cognitive therapy for depression: Unexplicated schemata and scripts. In N. S. Jacobson (Ed.), *Psychotherapists in clinical practice*. New York: Guilford.

Pesso, A. (1969). *Movement in psychotherapy*. New York: New York University Press.

Seligman, M. E. P. (1975). *Helplessness*. San Francisco: Freeman.

Young, J. (1990). *Cognitive therapy for personality disorders: A schema-focused approach*. Sarasota, FL: Professional Resource Exchange, Inc.

SUGGESTED READINGS

Beck, A. T. (1982). Cognitive therapy of depression: New Perspectives. In P. Clayton (Ed.), *Depression*. New York: Raven.

Burns, D. D. (1980). *Feeling good*. New York: William Morrow.

Burns, D. D. (1989). *The feeling good handbook: Using the new mood therapy in every day life*. New York: William Morrow.

Hollon, S. D., & Evans, M. D. (1983). Cognitive therapy for depression in a group format. In A. Freeman (Ed.), *Cognitive therapy with couples and groups*. New York: Plenum.

Wright, J. H. (1987). Cognitive therapy and medication as combined treatment. In A. Freeman & V. Greenwood (Eds.), *Cognitive therapy: Applications in psychiatric and medical settings*. New York: Human Sciences Press.

12

Dysthymia

Arthur Freeman

When Aaron T. Beck first began to conceptualize his new therapy, he applied it to that most common of human conditions and clinical treatment problems, depression (Beck, 1966). As his ideas crystallized over the next decade, he refined the theory and therapy as it applied to the broad range of clinical problems (Beck, 1976). As a result of his weekly clinical meetings with the staff of the Center for Cognitive Therapy, a treatment manual for the treatment of depression grew organically. Starting as a mimeographed booklet of several pages, it eventually became the "treatment manual" that evolved into the now-classic *Cognitive Therapy of Depression* (Beck, Rush, Shaw, & Emery, 1979). Over the past decade, Beck and his colleagues have addressed the cognitive therapy treatment of other clinical problems, such as anxiety (Beck, Emery, & Greenberg, 1985) and personality disorders (Beck, Freeman, & Associates, 1990). Depression has, however, been the clinical problem that has been most studied in terms of treatment efficacy (Rush, Beck, Kovacs, & Hollon, 1977; Blackburn, Bishop, Glen, Whalley, & Christie, 1981; Murphy, Simons, Wetzel, & Lustman, 1984). While best known for the outpatient treatment of depression, cognitive therapy may be the psychotherapeutic treatment

Arthur Freeman • Department of Psychiatry, Cooper Hospital/ University Medical Center and Robert Wood Johnson Medical School at Camden, Camden, New Jersey 08103.

Comprehensive Casebook of Cognitive Therapy, edited by Arthur Freeman and Frank M. Dattilio. Plenum Press, New York, 1992.

of choice—along with appropriate pharmacotherapy—for depressed patients needing inpatient or day hospital treatment (Bowers, 1989; Coche, 1987; Freeman & Greenwood, 1987; Greenwood, 1983; Grossman & Freet, 1987; Perris, et al., 1987; Schrodt & Wright, 1987; Wright & Schrodt, 1989).

Given the active, directive, structured, and problem-focused nature of cognitive therapy, the therapist can start to focus and structure therapy from the onset of treatment by paying special attention to the depressive triad. The personal issues relating to self, world and/or experience, and future differ for each patient. By examining each component, the therapist can begin to develop a picture of the depressive problem. Since each constituent of the triad does not necessarily contribute equally to the depression, the therapist can begin to develop a visual conceptualization of the patient's problem(s). Virtually all patient problems can be subsumed under one or a combination of these areas. The summation of the content in each of these three areas is evident in the patient's overt and covert cognitions, including verbal and visual representations. Affect and behavior will typically correspond with the negative content of these views. For example, if a male patient views himself as physically unattractive, he may feel sad or disappointed in his looks, and may then avoid situations where physical attractiveness might be seen as a prerequisite for success (e.g., dating).

When the patient first comes to therapy, he or she is often unaware of the negative self-statements that fill his or her speech and thinking. For example, a male patient just beginning therapy was asked how many negative thoughts a day he had. The patient thought carefully and responded, "Three or four, no more than that." Inasmuch as the patient had a BDI of 32, this was seen by the therapist as unlikely. The patient was asked to obtain a small pad and record his negative thoughts over the next week. The therapist suggested to the patient that he (the patient) probably had more negative thoughts than he was aware of. The therapist then asked the patient to try to record at least 50 thoughts over the week. The patient responded, "Oh, that would be impossible; I couldn't do it. I'll probably fail as I have before." The therapist responded by telling the patient that the patient had just come up with at least 3 negative thoughts for his list and needed only 47 more.

Cognitive distortions (automatic thoughts) become the initial focus of the therapy. They occur in many combinations and permutations. The therapist works with the patient to make the distortions manifest by tracking the spontaneous thoughts associated with certain moods or situations. These spontaneously generated thoughts are then evaluated for their content, degree of patient belief, style, and impact on the patient's life. The distortions become the thematic directional signs that point to the underlying schemas. The main purpose of labeling the style or content of the distortion is to provide a conceptual tool to help the patient understand his or her thoughts and begin to alter those thoughts that are dysfunctional. Reinforcing the patient for questioning the possibility of a distortion and testing alternatives is far more important than the rightness of the label.

The focus of this chapter is to illustrate several strategies and techniques developed for the cognitive therapy treatment of depression. Of specific interest is the use of homework as an important part of the therapy.

CASE STUDY

Marie is a white, Catholic, 33-year-old married female who was referred by her family physician. She described herself as depressed—so depressed, in fact, that for the past year she reported that she had been "paralyzed." She described the depression as affecting her work life, her marital and sex life, and her social life. While not presently as depressed as she had been several months earlier, she did not feel that she was as functional as she had been at the peak of her productivity. She described her marital difficulty as being in part due to conflict with her career needs and her husband's life-style. Marie was fearful of making any changes in either her career or her marital status, as she was afraid of losing her

husband and then feeling that she was unlovable and would never be able to live with anyone.

She lived with her husband in a northern suburb of a large city and worked in a far southwestern suburb of that city; this amounted to a 2-hour daily commute in either direction. Her husband worked near their home. To ease the commuting problem, she maintained a small apartment near to her work. They had lived apart for two years, with Marie seeing her husband only on weekends to avoid the 140-mile round-trip commute. She was employed as an equal opportunity officer and assistant to the president of a large corporation. She thought that her work had been unsatisfactory and that she was in danger of being fired, although she had no evidence that the president of the corporation was thinking of firing her. The other major conflict regarded her marriage and her wanting to stay married. She had been married for seven years, but there had been no sexual intercourse in the marriage (or outside of it) for the last three years. Intercourse was painful for Marie, and therefore avoided.

Marie is the second youngest of four children, having two brothers (ages 36 and 35), and a sister (age 28). Her mother is a teacher, and her father a retired chemist; both are still physically active. Marie described her childhood as relatively unhappy, with episodes of depression from about age 12 on. She was the butt of insults and teasing from her second oldest brother, who would constantly call her "elephantiasis," a reference to her being overweight and later having acne.

Marie described herself as an unpopular child with very poor social skills. She was seen as "brainy" and uninvolved in the social activities of her childhood and adolescent peers. She had no dates throughout her adolescence and first started dating in college. She met her husband when she was 24 years old; they dated for two years and married. She reported having few friends, except friends at work with whom she did not socialize.

Marie always did well in school. She graduated from high school with high honors and attended a small, prestigious private college, where she received high honors and was a member of Phi Beta Kappa, graduating summa cum laude. She continued her graduate work at a large university, getting her M.A. and Ph.D. in history. For the past three years, she had been responsible for the implementation of equal opportunity and affirmative-action programs at her company.

A recent medical evaluation showed that Marie was in good health, 15 to 20 pounds overweight, with no other medical findings. Previous therapy included seeing a social worker once or twice a week for four years while she was a graduate student; Marie described the therapy as "helpful" but was unable to verbalize what she learned.

She felt that the therapist was supportive and offered a critical, listening ear. More recently, Marie had been involved in reevaluation (peer) counseling. For the past two years, she and her husband had been in sex therapy to deal with the lack of sexual activity, but the result of the sex therapy was that they terminated therapy without initiating sex.

At intake, Marie appeared well-groomed and neat. She was cooperative throughout the interview. Her mood was depressed, and she appeared sad and cried several times during the session. She was, however, able to smile and laugh appropriately, and her speech and thought were clear and appropriate. There were no hallucinations or delusions, but some minimal depersonalization. She was oriented in all spheres.

Major problem areas. The major areas of difficulty identified were: (a) her depression, (b) low self esteem, (c) marital difficulty, (d) sexual problems, (e) vocational difficulty. Marie's intake diagnosis was: Axis I—dysthymic disorder; Axis II—R/O obsessive-compulsive disorder; Axis III—none, Axis IV—marital difficulty, job difficulty (moderate); and Axis V—excellent functioning.

Results of testing. On intake, Marie's Beck Depression Inventory score was 42, placing her in the severely depressed range. She endorsed 10 of the 21 items at the highest level.

An assessment of her suicidal thoughts on the Scale of Suicidal Ideation (Beck, Kovacs, & Weissman, 1979) indicated a score of 6, endorsing a weak wish to die, with her reasons for living and dying about equal. Her general attitude toward suicide was ambivalent, with her reasons for contemplating a suicide attempt being to escape and to solve her problems through a surcease of the depression and difficulty she was presently experiencing. The major deterrents to her attempting suicide were her husband and the thought that "it is going to get better."

Marie was seen for a total of 28 sessions from the initial interview to the termination interview, over a period of eight months. She was seen twice weekly for the first two weeks of therapy and then approximately once weekly thereafter.

Formulation of the problem. The patient presented several discrete problems: (a) an overriding sense of hopelessness with a consequent suicidal ideation; (b) marital difficulty (i.e., relating to her husband and maintaining the marital relationship); (c) sexual difficulty involving abstinence from intercourse because of physical pain and discomfort; (d) career difficulty—specifically, a sense of dissatisfaction with her present position in terms of whether or not she could effectively do the kind of job that she felt she needed to do; and (e) lack of a social support network.

Conceptually, the patient was a perfectionist who utilized an all-or-nothing approach to problem solving. A major goal of treatment was to have her alter this dichotomous thinking to allow herself to experience and accept being successful. Because of the suicidal ideation, a rather immediate set of interventions focused on Marie's sense of hopelessness to relieve the suicidality and make it less likely for it to pose a danger to her. A second part of treatment protocol was an exploration of the marital/sexual difficulties with a part of the treatment discussion focused on the sexual problems.

After termination of therapy and in 2½ years of follow-up, the patient has (a) changed her job so that she now works at a job for higher pay and equal prestige only four miles from her home; (b) eliminated the issue of hopelessness and suicidality; (c) become more conscious of her health and physical appearance, lost weight, and maintained the weight loss; and (d) described her marital relationship as excellent, with she and her husband maintaining an active and gratifying sexual relationship.

By directly addressing her cognitive distortions and the often-irrational underlying belief systems, Marie was helped to think more clearly, behave more functionally, and cope more rationally. This initial session excerpt is from the sixth session.

THERAPIST: Okay, where do you want to pick up? What do you have on tap for the agenda today?

MARIE: Well, first item would be the purpose of the taping. I want to talk about that.

THERAPIST: Sure.

MARIE: What it will be used for and so forth. And then the topic that I wanted to discuss is body image, appearance, all related to self-esteem, being fat, feeling that I am fat and ugly. Clothes, buying clothes. When I categorized my problems, those came out as part of self-image.

THERAPIST: So, it relates to some of the homework you were working on?

MARIE: Right, and that's it for what I have.

THERAPIST: Okay, so we want to look at the homework and to review how things have been going since the last session.

MARIE: Okay.

THERAPIST: Okay, what do we have? We have three things. The purpose of the taping, the whole thing of body image and how that relates to your homework, and there is some other homework, too. And just how things have been going since the last session.

MARIE: Why don't we do that one second, since it is going to bring you up to date.

THERAPIST: Okay, and the taping first. What do I do—I

guess the body image is part of the homework, or the homework . . .

MARIE: Why don't we do the homework third, and then get into the body image from there?

THERAPIST: And let's save the majority of the session for that.

MARIE: Okay.

These interactions involved setting the basic agenda and then setting the priorities for the session. Note that both patient and therapist collaboratively established the session goals.

THERAPIST: Okay, fine. The purpose of the taping—any notions of it, any thoughts that you are having?

MARIE: I just don't know. It would be interesting for me to hear it.

THERAPIST: Sure, that's always available.

MARIE: Yeah, it will be interesting evidence for me. I'm always scared about seeing it because just that [sic] I hate hearing myself on audiotape. I also hate seeing myself on videotape.

THERAPIST: (Marie suddenly looks quite sad)What is going on? What are you thinking?

MARIE: I'm ugly. I'm awkward.

THERAPIST: She says with a quiver in her voice.

MARIE: This really is no good. (starts crying) The tissues are too far away.

THERAPIST: We can remedy that. That's easy to remedy. Here you go (hands her the tissues)

MARIE: My mannerisms are peculiar, annoying, and embarrassing. If I met me I would think I was pretty unattractive, both physically and in behavior.

THERAPIST: So there is a thought that goes, "I'm ugly, awkward, and if I met me, I would be pretty upset."

MARIE: Well, not just me, others would be unimpressed.

THERAPIST: Would *I* be unimpressed?

MARIE: Yeah.

THERAPIST: What might I say to myself?

MARIE: She's a loser. She's weird. I don't want to associate with her.

THERAPIST: She's weird, a loser, don't want to associate. So you have all of these—a whole stream of automatic thoughts that just kind of—not just a stream; sounds more like a cascade.

MARIE: Right, a waterfall. (Marie starts crying again)

THERAPIST: A waterfall and it really does begin to fall, doesn't it?

MARIE: Yes, right.

THERAPIST: That is probably an apt image, because as you start thinking those things, you're feeling what?

MARIE: Umh, sort of sorry for myself. Poor me, I'm so horrible.

THERAPIST: That is certainly sad.

MARIE: Yes, very sad, yes.

THERAPIST: Because even as I just ask you this, your voice begins to quiver again. And what evidence do you have that all this is true? That you are ugly, awkward? Or that it is not true? What data do you have?

In this way, the therapist helps Marie to look at the "hot cognitions," those that occur immediately in the session. Rather than the two of them talking about her sadness of last night or last week, the sadness sits on the desk between patient and therapist and can be used to explore the thoughts that generate fresh sadness within the session. This is followed by examining the data that Marie uses to maintain her dysfunctional ideas.

MARIE: (answering the last question above) Comparing myself to people that I consider extremely attractive and finding myself lacking.

THERAPIST: So if you look at this or that beautiful person, you're less?

MARIE: Yes.

THERAPIST: Or if I look at that *perfect* person, I'm less? Is that what you are saying?

MARIE: Yes.

The therapist introduces a schematic focus with this question. Marie's perfectionistic thinking has been discussed in previous sessions, and the present statements can move beyond the present case to reflect the more dynamic issues.

THERAPIST: (continuing) That they are somehow perfect and you are . . .

MARIE: Yeah. I always pick out, of course, the most attractive person and probably a person who spends 3 hours a day on grooming and appearance, clothes shopping, and I only compare myself to them. I don't compare myself to the run-of-the-mill . . . I have begun to try to contradict all this stuff, and that's why I know that.

THERAPIST: I would like to hear some of that.

MARIE: Okay, well, we are getting the body image stuff. Well, I have done very well this whole week. I'm a lot less depressed. I have done a couple of really tough dysfunctional thought analyses which I feel I have made very good progress on, and I find myself thinking in those terms so that the thoughts come up again and I find myself contradicting the negative thoughts, the automatic thoughts, almost automatically—especially the ones I have written out. I have enjoyed what I have been doing this week. I didn't commute much this week, so that helped. But I don't think that was just that. It seems that it was more than that because there have been days when I haven't commuted, when I have stayed and I have been depressed, too. I've been in bed all day.

THERAPIST: So, overall, you are saying that you had greater touch with the pleasure experiences.

MARIE: Yes.

THERAPIST: You felt more competent?

MARIE: Yes.

THERAPIST: Handled things much better?

MARIE: Yes.

THERAPIST: And less depressed?

MARIE: Yes, all of those.

THERAPIST: Phew!

MARIE: Yes, it's a lot.

THERAPIST: Quite a lot, isn't it?

MARIE: And it does seem to be related to some of the dysfunctional thought analyses I did.

THERAPIST: Can you just briefly capsule one for me?

MARIE: Well, actually there are two that I gave you last time which I keep sort of coming back to.

THERAPIST: Which two are those?

MARIE: 15 and 16, number 15 and number 16. I don't exactly remember what they were on, but I know they are very important. Ahh, [number] 15 was when I cancelled our therapy appointment right after the surgery because I felt a lot of pain and I didn't feel motivated to do the homework. I felt really lousy about myself because of that. And [number] 16 was when we decided I should work on more specific problems and I started out with low self-esteem, and that was the morning I spent ruminating in bed and had 250 automatic thoughts in three hours. And then spent the whole afternoon doing the homework and contradicting that.

THERAPIST: And the result was what?

MARIE: The result was that although I didn't immediately stop being depressed, gradually that evening I felt less depressed, and then that weekend I felt even less depressed and by Monday I felt pretty good, and then this whole next week from Monday to Monday.

THERAPIST: You are getting a sense of mastery.

MARIE: Yes.

In the next part of the session, the purpose of the audiotaping was discussed. The tape was available for Marie to take home for listening. The next portion of the interview focused on buying clothes and dressing properly.

THERAPIST: It has to be the exact size, color, fit?

MARIE: Right, and if it isn't, then that means there is

TABLE 12-1 Problems About Which I Have a Lot of Dysfunctional Thoughts (Marie)

Priority	Problem
8	Relationship with Alan
1	Feelings of low self-esteem
5	Resistance to doing "work" work
5	Resistance to doing *any* work (correspondence, washing clothes, etc.)
12	Sex with Alan
9	Food, especially chocolate
6	Career—goals in general, and should I change jobs now in particular
2	Meaninglessness of life
11	Body image, exercise
10	Appearance, grooming, clothes shopping
14	House maintenance
13	Money—feelings about spending it, earning it
7	Wasting time—frittering my life away, not accomplishing anything important
21	Aging
20	Children—OK not to have any?
18	Relationships with men in general
19	Relationships with women in general
15	Relationships with secretaries at work
16	Relationships with president's staff at work
17	Friendships—role of, place in my life, "usefulness of feelings about"
3	Work (career) generally—role and place in my life
23	Mechanical abilities
24	Athletic abilities
22	Aesthetic sense and interior decorating
4	Regrets over fast decisions

something wrong with me. It doesn't mean that that store doesn't have enough sizes, colors . . .

THERAPIST: Maybe that is something you can work on.

MARIE: It is a good candidate for dysfunctional thought analysis.

Again, the issue of perfectionism is addressed. The idea that "if the store does not have what I want, it is my fault" is raised by Marie. The next portion of the session develops the homework assignment. The goal of the homework assignment was to collect evidence that she could use to test her thoughts and to begin to dispute some of her active dysfunctional thoughts.

THERAPIST: I think I agree, it would be good to really look at yourself. With a mirror.

MARIE: Uh-huh. That's a good idea.

THERAPIST: To really sit down in front of mirror and just look at yourself and write down what you see and then deal with that, and I think it might be helpful to . . . hmm, do you have a full length mirror?

MARIE: Yes.

THERAPIST: . . . to do it in the nude. Do it dressed and do it in the nude, and write down what you are feeling about your body and the thoughts that you have. And then sit down and knock the hell out of it. Not your body but your negative thoughts.

MARIE: Okay.

THERAPIST: Then challenge that. That it is there and to really, almost, to desensitize yourself to look in the mirror until you don't have to have that feeling anymore, because the feeling clearly stems from the thoughts. So that you then can remove that one more piece of anxiety about going clothes shopping. You can look in the mirror and . . .

MARIE: That's a good idea.

THERAPIST: So that is something you can work on. And then, I think, deal with some of these issues of the "ugly, awkward" speech. I guess it is always, too, a matter of a perspective. As you look towards the reserved, chiseled profile you have envied, I wonder how many reserved, chiseled types are looking for your curly hair.

MARIE: Nowadays, a lot. They are all going and getting permanents.

THERAPIST: I guess it's the perspective that they look and say, "Gee, I wish I had naturally curly hair."

MARIE: Yeah, it is hilarious. We all want to be different than what we are. Society tells us we're not good enough the way we are, we've got to be different. Hairdressers—every hairdresser that a women goes to tells her that she ought to do this, that, and the other to her hair, no matter what kind of hair she has. Just resisting that takes a lot of self-confidence.

THERAPIST: But, given what society says, it's what we say.

MARIE: Yeah, we internalize that and say it to ourselves, yeah.

THERAPIST: Okay, let's see where we have been. We've talked about the taping, we've gotten through the homework, and you've brought me up to date since last session. We've spent a good part of the session on this issue of body image and talking about how you think about yourself, especially covering yourself with either makeup or clothing. Then you have to deal with it in terms of "Am I doing it for society or for me?" But to change how you look on the exterior because on the inside maybe you are not so bad. That might go along with changing that negative self-image. One piece of specific homework you'll be working on is doing some dysfunctional thoughts, specifically about your body image and your body. That will deal with several of the

issues here of appearance, grooming, body image. We've talked about some of the issues about money and spending it. If you buy clothes, it is going to cost you a bundle. No way around that.

(This final part of the session is a review and summary of the session content.)

MARIE: Yes.

THERAPIST: It means, I think, I'm going to spend money. That's what it is all about. And it depends whether you then want to choose to try to go and buy as much as you can as cheaply as you can or buy what you are really talking about, which may cost more. To get those fine, tailored pieces, like a camel's-hair coat, you can get a Dacron and tissue-paper version or the real one, which won't go out of style. So, OK, we're running close to the end of our time. Any thoughts on the session, thoughts you have had? Anything about me today?

MARIE: Ummm. I don't think so.

THERAPIST: Anything I have said today that has upset you, annoyed you? (Marie shakes her head) OK. Any closing comments? OK, I will see you on Thursday.

MARIE: OK. I'm having my six week evaluation just before the session.

THERAPIST: OK.

The next session excerpt is from the session immediately following the one described above. Marie came into the session very upset.

THERAPIST: Well, where do you want to pick up today?

MARIE: The week has been OK. But this thing that I did with, you know, the mirror has really upset me.

THERAPIST: Upset you in what way?

MARIE: Well, it just confirmed all of my negative views of myself. It didn't help me. I don't know why you made me do it.

THERAPIST: Before we go into that, do you want to spend the majority of the session on that? Is that why your Hopelessness Scale is so high today?

MARIE: As upset as I am, I think so!

THERAPIST: Let's get right to it. What is so upsetting?

MARIE: (starts crying) Ever since I did it last Thursday after our session, I've been upset. I did what we agreed, I stood in front of the mirror nude. I had a pad and pen with me, and I made a list of all of the parts of my body that I didn't like. Here, here's the list. (hands therapist the list).

THERAPIST: (looking at it) Its quite a list.

MARIE: It sure is. That's why I feel so hopeless. I didn't think about what the impact of the homework would be. As I wrote, I got more and more upset. Everything is wrong with me. It's just as I have always feared. I really hate the way that I look, and now I not only have the evidence, but hate myself with greater specificity.

THERAPIST: It's a long list. (counting items) 27 different things that you hate [see Table 12-2].

MARIE: Yes. From the top of my head to the tips of my toes.

THERAPIST: What do you think of . . . let me back up. What did you think of as you were doing it?

MARIE: I'm ugly, I've always been ugly, it will always be the same.

THERAPIST: As you look at the list right now, what do you think?

MARIE: I feel lousy.

THERAPIST: What thoughts go through your mind?

MARIE: That's it. I feel lousy.

THERAPIST: You're saying what to yourself?

MARIE: I'm what I've always been and will always be. I have been cheated. Others have good looks, and look at my list.

THERAPIST: Hmm. So the list is really bugging you. You've been cheated, and there's nothing, absolutely nothing you might do?

TABLE 12-2 Things I Hate About Myself (Marie)

My hair is cut poorly
My hair is a mousy color
I have gray hairs, which make me look old
My hair is too curly
My hair is thinning
My forehead is too high
My glasses make my eyes look beady
My poor eyesight makes me wear thick glasses
I have squint wrinkles near my eyes
My nose is too wide
My lips are too full
My face is too broad
My shoulders are too wide
My breasts are too small
My stomach sticks out
My hips are too wide
My thighs are heavy
My ass is huge
My knees are bony
My calves are too heavy
I have ugly ankles
My toes are too long and ugly
My skin is a sallow color
My skin is too grainy
I'm too short
I have a thick waist
I have saddlebags on my hips

MARIE: Sure, I can always kill myself.

THERAPIST: Anything else?

MARIE: Not that I can think of.

THERAPIST: I wonder . . . I wonder what would happen if we looked at this list in some different ways.

MARIE: Such as?

THERAPIST: Well, what if we divided this list into three lists? List one would be things that you might easily change. List two would be things that you could change with difficulty, and finally list three would be those things that you could not change.

MARIE: What would that do? This list would be as long.

THERAPIST: The overall list would be as long, but we might have some things you could work on. Would you be agreeable to trying it?

MARIE: Sure.

THERAPIST: How about if I read the list, and you assign it to one of the three categories? Let's try it.

MARIE: OK. My hair is cut poorly. I could always have it recut. But it's so short now, what are they going to cut? It will just look worse. I'm getting bald as it is . . .

THERAPIST: Whoa! You're going too fast for me. Let's separate things. Can you get your hair recut?

MARIE: I guess so.

THERAPIST: Will having your hair recut be something easy, some difficulty, or impossible?

MARIE: Easy. But . . .

THERAPIST: Hold the "but" for a moment until I write down the first hair issue in the easy column. (writes it down) Now, what thoughts did you have?

MARIE: This won't work, it won't make any difference. My hair is awful, and this won't make it any better.

THERAPIST: Lots of thoughts! Can we do two different things here? First, can we do the columns, and then can we deal with the thoughts? I've written them down so that we won't lose them.

MARIE: OK. It's just that this seems like a waste of time.

THERAPIST: I've written that down as another negative thought.

MARIE: Well, the hair can be dealt with rather easily. I could always go to another barber.

THERAPIST: A barber?

MARIE: Yes. The closest shop to my apartment, and also the one that's open late, is a barber shop. I have always avoided women's beauty shops as places to advance one's narcissism. All of that primping and women's stuff is awful.

THERAPIST: Between a men's barber shop and a women's beauty parlor, there must be other choices. Possibly ones that are more inconvenient, but will better meet your needs in this regard.

MARIE: I suppose there must be.

Marie's all-or-nothing thinking once again governs her choices. She must either go to a barber who cuts her hair poorly or to a beauty parlor that represents an image she hates. The assignment of each of the various body part concerns to one of the three columns proceeded throughout the session. The following excerpt picks up the session at the end.

THERAPIST: We're almost out of time, and we have several more of these to go. How do you want to handle that?

MARIE: I could do it for homework. I feel much better. I see where you were going with this. Its obvious that the longest list is composed of things that I can do rather easily. There are far fewer on the next list [with difficulty]. I'm not going to have my nose done!

THERAPIST: How about the last list?

MARIE: I know, it's the shortest. I get the idea. But I'm still overwhelmed by the number.

THERAPIST: Do you have to do everything at once? Is it all or nothing?

MARIE: (laughs) No. You've made that all-or-nothing point enough. I can do something.

THERAPIST: When you came in, you were not feeling good about the homework, and about me. How are you feeling now as we end?

MARIE: Better. I believe that I can do something. I'm not sure what, and when it will all get done . . .

THERAPIST: All?

MARIE: OK, OK.

THERAPIST: Good luck with this. I'll see you next week.

The sexual issue was addressed in sessions 14 through 19. Marie's husband refused to come in for any therapy sessions. His position was that therapy did not help their sex life, so he saw no reason to start therapy again. Marie wanted to change the sexual situation, so the sexual issue became a focus in her individual therapy. An assessment of Marie's sexual history included a detailed discussion of the present sexual problems in addition to her early sexual learnings and experience.

What emerged was that Marie had often experienced painful intercourse. The issue was that she did not generate vaginal lubrication; when penile penetration was attempted, the result was painful. Oral stimulation was enjoyable but not her preferred sexual activity. When questioned as to why she did not enjoy the oral sex, inasmuch as she enjoyed it and was gratified by it, Marie said, "It's not the right way." Once again, her schema become manifest in her sexual activities. The schematic issue was tested when she was questioned about the possibility of using a vaginal lubricant prior to intercourse

(e.g., K-Y Jelly). Marie responded, "I want to do it the right way. These jellies are not natural. I should be able to do it the way that everyone does it."

When Marie was asked about her sexual fantasies, she responded that she did not have any. Given that sexual arousal is largely a cognitive event, it would seem antisexual to not have (or be able to generate) sexual fantasies. When she was asked to generate sexual fantasies in the office, she seemed flustered. She finally said, "I'm having sex with a man." Given her intelligence, this seemed a rather sparse response. When asked to elaborate on the fantasy, Marie responded, "I'm having sex with two men."

The sexual focus involved Marie agreeing to a six-session program. In her first homework assignment, she was asked to read *My Secret Garden*, a volume of women's sexual fantasies, by Nancy Friday. The next series of excerpts are from the sexual-focus sessions.

MARIE: (commenting on the homework) I never have fantasies like that. I have always written off these kinds of stories or fantasies as pornography. But I must say that I found them to be rather exciting. It made it easier when you assigned this book, but I noticed a certain, um, tickle.

THERAPIST: A tickle?

MARIE: Must I say it?

THERAPIST: Yes.

MARIE: I felt excited. It was fun.

THERAPIST: Were there any particular stories that tickled you more than others?

MARIE: I haven't finished the book yet, but there are several that I found especially exciting. Some didn't appeal to me at all.

THERAPIST: Did you share the book with Alan?

MARIE: No. I read it during the week at my apartment.

THERAPIST: Were there any special images that you enjoyed?

MARIE: Yes. There was one about a women . . . do you want me to tell you the one that I found sexy?

THERAPIST: Would you be comfortable in doing that?

MARIE: No.

THERAPIST: Then it's not necessary. Let's deal with it without your having to tell me the details. What could you do to make the fantasy more "you"?

MARIE: What do you mean?

THERAPIST: Well, what you read was somebody else's fantasy. What could you do to place yourself into the fantasy? You know, make it more Marie.

At this point, Marie described the fantasy and tried to rework the images to place herself into the picture. The next parts of the treatment strategy would include having

Marie image the arousal scene and then masturbate in response to the scene. In the second session, the arousal practice was altered to include practice imaging the arousal scene and then using a nonsexual image to decrease arousal. This homework came from the session material where Marie discussed the problem of trying to maintain her arousal. She described her sexual arousal state as so tenuous that any interruption would cause her to lose her arousal. Once the arousal was gone, it could not be recaptured. Marie then practiced arousal, masturbation, interruption of the image, and then trying to regain the arousal. She reported in the third session that she had been successful at regaining arousal after losing the image.

Her homework for the fourth session was a result of the third session material. Marie reported that if she became aroused, she could achieve an orgasm, but only once each time that she was aroused. Her homework involved trying to stimulate herself mentally and then to masturbate to orgasm. After a brief period of time, she was to try to become aroused again and to reach a second orgasm. During the fifth session, she reported having multiple orgasms. She seemed surprised that it was so simple.

MARIE: I have an orgasm, and then another . . . and another.

THERAPIST: You seem surprised.

MARIE: I am. I've never had several orgasms in a row. I've read about it, but, well . . .

THERAPIST: So the equipment works. What do you make of that?

MARIE: I can't believe all of the orgasms that I've missed over the years.

THERAPIST: What are you doing right now?

MARIE: I'm not sure.

THERAPIST: Let's look at it. You start by being surprised and happy about the orgasms, but then do something to yourself.

MARIE: I focused on what I didn't have. The many years of missed orgasms.

THERAPIST: Exactly.

In this exchange, the schematic issue of all-or-nothing is once again a focus. In the sixth session, Marie discussed the antisexual images and thoughts she had; when she could focus on the sexual images, she was easily aroused. A final test was the weekend when she went home. She left *My Secret Garden* on the kitchen counter. Her husband found the book and was quite interested. They decided to take the book to the bedroom and to read the fantasies to each other. The result was sexual intercourse without difficulty.

CONCLUSION

In the course of the therapy with Marie, several issues were dealt with. The goal of the therapy was not to achieve a cure of her long-term depression. In the short-term treatment model of cognitive therapy, Marie was taught several basic skills. By looking at her negative thoughts, identifying the nature of her distortions, and then testing the thoughts using the format of the Daily Record of Dysfunctional Thoughts (DRDT), Marie learned that she could take control of her life by controlling her depression. The schematic focus of pointing out several of her prominent life rules was helpful in helping her to generalize her gains in one area to other life areas. Marie's self-esteem was enhanced by her taking control. Her depression lifted and, at follow-up, remained under control. The focus on her sexual behavior allowed greater success and for Marie to increase her sexual behavior with her husband.

As Marie felt better, she began exploring the possibilities of jobs closer to home. She eventually accepted a position commensurate with her education, experience, and salary requirements. Homework was emphasized with Marie; as a lifelong academic, she understood its importance. The therapist stressed that the therapy in the session was akin to the lecture part of a course, while the homework was the laboratory part of the course. Without the opportunity to try out the various ideas and behaviors in real life, the material from the sessions would have remained an abstraction for Marie.

REFERENCES

Beck, A. T. (1966). *Depression: Causes and treatment.* Philadelphia: University of Pennsylvania Press.

Beck, A. T. (1976). *Cognitive therapy and the emotional disorders.* New York: International Universities Press.

Beck, A. T., Emery, G., & Greenberg, R. L. (1985). *Anxiety and phobia: A cognitive perspective.* New York: Basic Books.

Beck, A. T., Freeman, A., & Associates. (1990). *Cognitive therapy of personality disorders.* New York: Guilford.

Beck, A. T., Kovacs, M., & Weissman, A. (1979). Assessment of suicidal ideation: The Scale of Suicidal Ideation. *Journal of Consulting and Clinical Psychology, 47,* 343–352.

Beck, A. T., Rush, A. J., Shaw, B. F., & Emery, G. (1979). *Cognitive therapy of depression.* New York: Guilford.

Blackburn, I. M., Bishop, S., Glen, A. I. M., Whalley, L. J., & Christie, J. E. (1981). The efficacy of cognitive therapy in depression: A treatment using cognitive therapy and pharmacotherapy, each alone and in combination. *British Journal of Psychiatry, 139,* 181–189.

Bowers, W. (1989). Cognitive therapy with inpatients. In A.

Freeman, K. M. Simon, L. E. Beutler, & H. Arkowitz, *Comprehensive handbook of cognitive therapy* (pp. 583–596). New York: Plenum.

Coche, E. (1987). Problem-solving training: A cognitive group therapy modality. In A. Freeman & V. Greenwood (Eds.), *Cognitive therapy: Applications in psychiatric and medical settings* (pp. 83–102). New York: Human Sciences Press.

Freeman, A., & Greenwood, V. (Eds.). (1987). *Cognitive therapy: Applications in psychiatric and medical settings*. New York: Human Sciences Press.

Greenwood, V. (1983). Cognitive therapy with the young adult chronic patient. In A. Freeman (Ed.), *Cognitive therapy with couples and groups* (pp. 183–198). New York: Plenum.

Grossman, R. W., & Freet, B. (1987). A cognitive approach to group therapy with hospitalized adolescents. In A. Freeman & V. Greenwood (Eds.), *Cognitive therapy: Applications in psychiatric and medical settings* (pp. 132–154). New York: Human Sciences Press.

Murphy, G. E., Simons, A. D., Wetzel, R. D., & Lustman, P. J. (1984). Cognitive therapy versus tricyclic medication in the treatment of major depression. *Archives of General Psychiatry, 41*, 33–41.

Perris, C., Rodhe, K., Palm, A., Abelson, M., Hellgren, S., Lilja, C. & Soderman, H. (1987). Fully integrated in- and outpatient services in a psychiatric sector: Implementation of a new model for the care of psychiatric patients favoring continuity of care. In A. Freeman & V. Greenwood (Eds.), *Cognitive therapy: Applications in psychiatric and medical settings* (pp. 117–131). New York: Human Sciences Press.

Rush, A. J., Beck, A. T., Kovacs, M., & Hollon, S. (1977). Comparative efficacy of cognitive therapy and imipramine in the treatment of depressed outpatients. *Cognitive Therapy and Research, 1*, 17–37.

Schrodt, G. R., & Wright, J. H. (1987). In A. Freeman & V. Greenwood (Eds.), *Cognitive therapy: Applications in psychiatric and medical settings* (pp. 69–82). New York: Human Sciences Press.

Wright, J. H., & Schrodt, G. R. (1989). Combined cognitive therapy and pharmacotherapy. In A. Freeman, K. M. Simon, L. E. Beutler, & H. Arkowitz (Eds.), *Comprehensive handbook of cognitive therapy* (pp. 267–282). New York: Plenum.

SUGGESTED READINGS

Freeman, A., Epstein, N., & Simon, K. M. (Eds.). (1986). *Depression in the family*. New York: Haworth.

Freeman, A., Pretzer, J., Fleming, B., & Simon, K. M. (1990). *Clinical applications of cognitive therapy*. New York: Plenum.

13

The Suicidal Patient

Dennis Greenberger

Cognitive therapy has consistently been demonstrated to be effective in treating depressed patients. The cognitive therapy approach to treating suicidal patients is to focus on the thoughts, assumptions, and beliefs that accompany the suicidal intent. Understanding the cognitive component of the suicidal patient can be instrumental in treatment planning and eventual therapeutic success.

Research and clinical experience have indicated that depressed and hopeless patients are at high risk for killing themselves or making suicide attempts. Research has also demonstrated that the cognitive characteristic of hopelessness is the single best predictor of eventual suicide (Beck, Steer, Kovacs, & Garrison, 1985). Perhaps hopelessness is such an important variable in suicide because when one is in psychological pain, death may be seen as an alleviation of that pain—as a way out of what is perceived to be an unlivable situation. Hopelessness is expressed in such thoughts as:

- Things will never get better for me.
- I have nothing to look forward to.
- I'll never amount to anything.
- No one will ever want me.
- I'll never be happy.

In explaining the role of hopelessness as a predictor of suicide, Beck, Brown, Berchick, Stewart, and Steer (1990) suggest that a depressed patient "systematically misconstrues his or her experience in a negative way and anticipates dire outcomes to his or her problems" (p. 2). Suicide may appear to be the only solution to a seemingly unsolvable/unlivable situation.

Shneidman (1985) has also identified constriction and ambivalence as two other cognitive characteristics of the suicidal patient, noting that "the common internal attitude towards suicide is ambivalence." (p. 135). He also notes that most suicidal people want to live and simultaneously want to die: "The prototypical suicidal state is one in which an individual cuts his throat and cries for help at the same time, and is genuine in both of these acts (p. 135).

Shneidman notes further that "the common cognitive state in suicide is constriction" (p. 138). He goes on to write that "synonyms for constriction are tunnelling or focusing or narrowing of the range of consciousness when the mind is not panicked into dichotomous thinking. . . . The range of choices is narrowed to two—not very much of a range" (p. 138). There is a tendency for suicidal patients to think dichotomously. Examples of dichotomous thinking include "if my wife doesn't take me back, I'm going to kill myself" or "I would rather die than have to experience one more flashback."

When working with suicidal patients, one hopes that hopefulness is restored, ambivalence is replaced with a desire to live, and cognitive constriction is replaced with the ability to see different options, to think along a continuum or in shades of gray.

Dennis Greenberger • Private Practice, 1851 East First Street, Santa Ana, California 92705.

Comprehensive Casebook of Cognitive Therapy, edited by Arthur Freeman and Frank M. Dattilio. Plenum Press, New York, 1992.

The purpose of this chapter is to illustrate how cognitive therapy can be utilized with a suicidal patient. A case example is used to demonstrate how cognitive therapy is done (from intake, assessment, conceptualization, and diagnosis to treatment, termination, and follow-up) as well as to illustrate the cognitive characteristics described above.

CASE BACKGROUND

Lisa, a 36-year-old female, was referred by a psychiatric hospital that had admitted her following a suicide attempt. A clinical interview assessed Lisa's current problems, family history, marital history, occupational history, and mental health history, with a specific emphasis on her previous suicide attempts. The interview revealed Lisa as an overweight female who identified her primary difficulties as depression, suicidal ideas, two abusive marriages, abusive parents, and being "unable to deal with life." Lisa's suicide attempt on the night of admission into the hospital followed two previous suicide attempts. One occurred two years prior to this hospitalization, and one occurred when she was 15 years old. On the night of admission into the hospital, she had cut her wrists with a razor blade. Lisa indicated that she had thought she would die as a result of cutting her wrists, and she had made the suicide attempt in order to "stop hurting." She had planned out this suicide attempt for approximately 48 hours in advance, and for a time when it was probable that no one would be phoning her or coming to her home. Lisa had been psychiatrically hospitalized subsequent to her other two suicide attempts.

Further history revealed that she had been sexually molested by her father as a child and as an adolescent. Her mother had committed suicide when Lisa was 12 years old. Lisa had been married and divorced twice; both of her husbands were physically abusive. She had two sons, ages 19 and 16. Lisa was religious and considered her religion important in her life. She worked as a legal secretary and had maintained her present job for approximately five years.

Lisa described being depressed for approximately eight months. She indicated that she had, on at least three other occasions, gone through yearlong episodes of being depressed. She went on to say that in the previous eight months, she had gained 30 pounds, had early-morning sleep awakenings more than 50% of the time, felt fatigued almost every day, had been self-critical, could not concentrate as well as she used to be able to, and had experienced increasingly frequent thoughts about suicide. She also described having no close friends, wanting to be close to other people but being afraid of being rejected, and being very sensitive to criticism or feedback from others.

Lisa had been in psychotherapy on three previous occasions. She described two of the therapies as not useful, and the third therapist as being "understanding and caring" and moderately helpful.

In addition to a clinical interview, Lisa's intake evaluation included a Beck Depression Inventory (BDI), Hopelessness Scale, and a Beck Anxiety Inventory (BAI). Her BDI score was 39, her Hopelessness Scale score was 17, and her BAI score was 27. The purpose of administering these inventories is to ascertain initial levels of depression, anxiety, and hopelessness, and to have data by which to measure progress, lack of progress, and specific areas that may be changing or not changing. Additionally, the hopelessness scale is administered in order to help gauge suicidal risk; as indicated above, Beck et al. (1985) have reported that hopelessness is the single best indicator of eventual suicide in a prospective patient. The BDI and the BAI were also administered to detail the specific symptoms that Lisa was experiencing.

An assessment of her current suicidal ideation revealed that she continued to have suicidal thoughts and intent. She continued to be hopeless, as evidenced in her statements and by the score on the Hopelessness Scale. She had no immediate plans subsequent to her failed attempt the night before, or time frame in which to kill herself. A review of her three suicide attempts indicated that all three had been planned out and thought about for at least several weeks in advance, and that none of them had been impulsive attempts.

On initial assessment, Lisa was asked to describe her suicide attempt, with particular attention paid to the cognitions that were present when she decided to kill herself, and the cognitions that were present as she was overdosing on the medications.

THERAPIST: Can you tell me what you were thinking right before you cut your wrists?

LISA: I just wanted to die.

THERAPIST: What was going through your mind at the moment that you decided to kill yourself?

LISA: I just thought that I would be better off dead.

THERAPIST: What else were you thinking?

LISA: I had images of my father crawling into bed with me. I thought that the only way to stop the pain that I was in was to die. Life is not worth living.

THERAPIST: What does it mean about you that you were molested?

LISA: God has forgotten me, abandoned me. I've failed in some way.

Lisa described a recent recognition that she had been sexually abused as an adolescent by her father. Although she had known before this that she had been sexually molested by a neighbor, the memory of her father's abuse was new. She described thinking on the night of her most recent suicide attempt about her father molesting her, and feeling depressed. She described the following thoughts:

- Life is not worth living.
- I'm such a failure.
- The pain is so great I have to kill myself.
- Nothing will help me.
- I'm so empty inside.
- I just have to die.
- I want to go numb so I don't have to feel anymore.
- The only way to stop the pain is to die.
- I will never get better, and this pain will go on forever.

Her hopelessness is reflected in the thoughts "Nothing will help me," "The only way to stop the pain is to die," and "I will never get better, and this pain will go on forever." Additionally, Lisa described thoughts related to her abusive history that included:

- People who are abused are unimportant, invalid, and dispensable.
- I'm unimportant.
- I'm worthless.
- I'm incompetent.
- I'm helpless.

These thoughts and attitudes, which grew out of her family background and abusive history, seemed to have generalized into many dimensions of her functioning as an adult.

Lisa was given an Axis I diagnosis of major depression, recurrent, and an Axis II diagnosis of personality disorder, not otherwise specified, mixed personality disorder with features of borderline and avoidant personalities.

CONCEPTUALIZATION

Lisa's abusive background, critical parents, and family life left her with core beliefs about herself (self-schemas) that included:

- I'm worthless.
- I'm powerless.
- I'm helpless.
- I'm out of control.
- I'm no good.
- I'm inadequate.

Additionally, she was left with the core beliefs that:

- People are dangerous.
- Others will hurt or take advantage of you.
- There is no safe place.

Out of these schema grew the assumptions:

- If I get close to people, they will hurt me.
- If I try something, then I will fail.
- If others get to know me, they will reject me.

One can see how the core beliefs "I'm helpless" and "I'm out of control" would develop in the abusive background that Lisa was raised in. The sense of inadequacy and worthlessness seemed to have resulted from the constant belittlement and criticisms that she endured from her parents and spouses. Lisa used a number of different cognitive distortions; however, the predominant ones appeared to be all-or-nothing thinking, selective abstraction, and mind reading.

TREATMENT

Cognitive therapy occurs in the context of an interpersonal relationship, and it is critical that this relationship be a therapeutic one. Beck (Beck, Rush, Shaw, & Emery, 1979) notes that the cognitive therapist who is warm, genuine, and possesses accurate empathy will facilitate treatment. Trust, rapport, and collaboration are the hallmarks of the interaction between the cognitive therapist and the client. One differentiation between cognitive therapy and other forms of psychotherapy is the collaborative nature of the therapeutic interaction. In Lisa's case, the collaboration was formed as she and I worked together in order to understand the suicidality, and in order to uncover the thoughts and beliefs that contributed to her suicidal impulses. The collaborative relationship can be thought of as two people providing different areas of expertise in pursuit of a common goal (Beck et al., 1979). Lisa provided the information about what she was thinking and feeling in specific situations, while I provided information about what to look for and how to recognize the thoughts, beliefs, feelings, and behaviors that would become part of the therapy.

The issues of trust and a collaborative therapeutic relationship were more difficult with Lisa than with many patients. Her beliefs that "if others get close to me, they will hurt me" and that "if others get to know me, they will reject me" were addressed in the beginning of treatment and periodically as therapy progressed. Lisa was asked to rate her degree of belief in these thoughts and to think of these statements as hypotheses and predictions rather than as facts. In this way, we would be able to set up behavioral experiments to ascertain whether or not her predictions came true. Lisa was also asked to verbalize any thoughts she had about me as the therapist regarding trust, closeness, acceptance, or rejection. These thoughts were periodically ascertained as therapy continued.

After two sessions of assessment, treatment began during our third session. Lisa and I collaboratively decided that the primary treatment goal was to minimize or eliminate her suicidality. Secondarily, we wanted to focus on reducing her sense of worthlessness (low self-esteem), sense of helplessness, and chronic depression. To lessen her suicidality, we decided that it would be important to increase her sense of hopefulness.

As Lisa was psychiatrically hospitalized, she had individual psychotherapy sessions five times a week, in addition to the hospital milieu's three cognitive therapy groups per day, assertion training groups, relaxation training groups, recreational therapy, and numerous group activities that were offered through the social services department.

Part of the agenda of the initial treatment session was to explain the cognitive model and to demonstrate how it applied in Lisa's life. We talked about the importance of differentiating between thoughts, emotions, and behaviors, and thought records were introduced as a means of analyzing specific thoughts and emotions and determining whether or not they were connected. Lisa's initial homework assignment was to do one or two thought records per day. It was suggested that she may want to do thought records when she was thinking about killing herself, or in those situations when she was extremely depressed, anxious, or angry. It was also decided that it would be worthwhile to do thought records in situations relating to her therapy goals, which included suicidality, low self-esteem, and hopelessness. In order to simplify the thought records, Lisa was told that in the "situation" column, she should answer the questions:

- Who are you with?
- What are you doing?
- Where are you at?
- When is it?

Emotions can often be identified in one word. In Lisa's case, we were primarily focusing on depression, guilt, anger, and anxiety. Thoughts were explained to Lisa as being either verbal or visual; the visual images or the verbal messages that accompanied her feelings were to be listed on the thought records. Initially, Lisa was asked to complete only the first three columns of the thought records. The reasons for this were her short concentration span and the necessity of completing this part accurately as a foundation for completing the rest of the thought record. Lisa initially had difficulty focusing on specific situations, so we decided to try to delineate a time period that would not exceed 30 minutes, in order to be able to identify specific situations, thoughts, and feelings.

The following two sessions were spent fine-tuning Lisa's ability to fill out the first three columns of the thought record. In order to immediately address the immediacy of her suicidality, we jointly devised a list of alternatives to suicidal behavior, in case she became suicidal again before she had developed cognitive coping strategies. This list included (a) calling her therapist, (b) calling a family member, (c) talking to a hospital staff member, and (d) doing something that was likely to make her feel better (reading, exercising, etc.). Eventually, this list included doing thought records in order to assess any distortions that might be present.

Part of our initial therapy sessions involved reviewing the thought records that she had done for homework, or writing a thought record about a new situation that she would experience. Early in Lisa's therapy, she continued to have suicidal thoughts. Her suicidal thoughts were especially pronounced subsequent to phoning her brother to inform him that she had made a suicide attempt and was now in the psychiatric hospital. Table 13–1 shows the first three sections of a thought record that Lisa did regarding this situation.

As Lisa became proficient at completing the first three columns of a thought record, the idea of cognitive distortions was presented. Cognitive distortions were presented as "thinking errors" that prevent people from accurately perceiving themselves or the world. Although we did not know for sure that Lisa had cognitive distortions, what the remainder of the thought record would enable us to do would be to assess the accuracy of her thinking. In other words, we would put her thoughts out on the table between us and practice a method that would enable her to examine the validity or accuracy of these thoughts. At this point, Lisa learned to ask herself, "Where is the evidence?" This question, in response to the automatic thoughts that contribute to her depression and suicidality, was designed to look at the basis or data that her thinking was based on.

The last three columns of the thought record form that was utilized with Lisa had her examine the evidence supporting her thoughts, examine the evidence that would suggest that her thoughts were not 100% true, and develop a thought that was more reflective of the data if so indicated. In other words, Lisa was being taught to look at the validity of her thinking and perceptions, and to correct or replace any thinking that was determined to be inaccurate. The thought records that she was using prompted her to ask herself where the evidence was to support her thoughts or perceptions, and where the evidence was that suggested that this thought or perception was not entirely true.

Evidence was further defined as "data" or "facts," that would be as objective as possible. For example, if Lisa were examining evidence to support the cognition "I

TABLE 13-1 Thought Record #1

Date	Situation	Feeling(s)	Automatic thought	Facts that show it's true	Facts that show it's not 100% true	Rational response	Rerate feelings now (0–100)
	What were you doing or thinking about?	*(Specify: rate 0–100)*	*What was going through your mind just before you started to feel bad? Any other thoughts?*				
7/22	Thursday night, 8:00 p.m. After phone call to brother. Alone in room.	Depressed—99 Empty—99 Afraid—90	I can't handle this anymore. I've disappointed my family. I'm never going to get better. There is no use in trying anymore. Killing myself is the only way to end this pain.				

can't go on any more," "I always fail" would not constitute evidence, data, or facts. "I always fail" would be another cognition that could be scrutinized as well.

Lisa's hopelessness, suicidality, and growing ability to look for the evidence underlying her thoughts were highlighted in the following interchange:

THERAPIST: How was your day?

LISA: Don't ask.

THERAPIST: What happened?

LISA: It was an awful day. It started out in group therapy where I was afraid of talking in front of the other patients.

THERAPIST: What was it that you were afraid of?

LISA: I was afraid that they would ignore me or not like me after I opened up. So I didn't say anything, and I began to feel depressed.

THERAPIST: At what point were you feeling most depressed?

LISA: As soon as the group therapist announced the end of the group.

THERAPIST: At that point, what were you thinking?

LISA: That I'm never going to get better, and I might as well die. If I can't even talk in group therapy, there is no use in even trying any more. I'm never going to get better.

This interaction, in addition to highlighting Lisa's hopelessness and suicidality, demonstrates focusing attention on thoughts through questions, such as "What was it that you were afraid of?" and "At that point, what were you thinking?" Her hopelessness and suicidality are reflected in the thoughts "I'm never going to get better," "I might as well die," and "There is no use in even trying any more."

The remainder of this therapy session focused on times in the past when Lisa had felt this hopeless, and what she had done in order to change that. We also looked at evidence suggesting that perhaps there was some chance she would improve and feel better, and that she was in fact already changing in some small but important ways. An interchange later in the same session demonstrated some of the cognitive/affective shift that had taken place.

THERAPIST: Is there any evidence to suggest that perhaps you will get better?

LISA: Well, I am learning some new skills that may help in the future.

THERAPIST: What else?

LISA: Some days are better than others. Also, I have accomplished some things that other people would call success.

THERAPIST: Anything else?

LISA: My pain may mean that I am getting better.

THERAPIST: In what way?

LISA: Maybe I need to feel this bad before I can feel better.

Toward the end of this session, Lisa was asked to give an encapsulated summary of the session.

THERAPIST: How would you summarize what we have been talking about?

LISA: I guess it would be fair to say that even though I am in pain, and that sometimes I feel like giving up, there are other times that I realize that I am making progress in small steps.

The subsequent sessions in Lisa's therapy focused on improving her ability to identify and analyze the accuracy or validity of the thoughts and attitudes that were correlated with her suicidality and depression. Additionally, Lisa began to talk more about the abuse perpetrated by her father and her reaction to the memories of the abuse. These reactions became available for scrutiny in the same way that Lisa was beginning to question the functionality and accuracy of her other thoughts. The following interaction highlights both the issue of abuse and Lisa's growing ability to challenge the basis of her thinking.

THERAPIST: You mentioned that you had been thinking about your father?

LISA: I was remembering the times that he crawled into my bed at night. It makes me sick when I think about it. Most people treat their animals better than my father treated me.

THERAPIST: Does the fact that you were abused mean anything about you?

LISA: It means that I am unimportant, dirty, and worthless. Also, I believe that in some way it was my fault. If I had been a better child or if I hadn't misbehaved, maybe he wouldn't have done what he did.

THERAPIST: So you believe that because you were abused, you are unimportant, dirty, and worthless?

LISA: Yes.

THERAPIST: On a scale of 1 to 100, with 1 being slightly worthless and 100 being totally worthless, how worthless do you believe you are?

LISA: Right now . . . 95.

THERAPIST: What is the evidence that would indicate you are worthless because you have been abused?

LISA: I feel worthless. Does that count?

THERAPIST: Evidence usually consists of data, facts, or material that different people would agree on. I don't know that everyone would agree that you are worthless. Is there any other evidence that would indicate you are worthless because you have been abused?

LISA: If I had any worth, God would not have allowed this to happen to me. My father told me that I was there for his convenience. My needs, wants, and desires were a joke to him. That's all.

THERAPIST: Is there any evidence that would show the thought "I'm worthless because I've been abused" may not be 100% true?

LISA: I guess I have some value to some people. My sons tell me that I'm a good mother, and some people in the hospital seem to like me just for who I am.

THERAPIST: What else would suggest that the thought "I'm worthless because I have been abused" is not 100% true?

LISA: I do some things at work well, and I guess this gives me some worth. Part of me wants to keep trying, and I imagine that if I were completely worthless, I wouldn't be putting all this effort into getting better.

THERAPIST: Based on the evidence that you just came up with, what would be another way of thinking about how the abuse affects your worth?

LISA: It might be more accurate to say that the abuse has taken away my innocence and childhood, but not my worth. I don't know if I believe that yet, though. I'm going to have to think about it. Also, even though I was abused, I have been able to contribute some things of worth to the world, such as my sons and my work. It is not so much that I'm worthless, but I could have been and done so much more.

THERAPIST: Now, on a scale of 1 to 100, how worthless do you believe you are?

LISA: 15 to 20.

Paralleling these therapy sessions, Lisa was doing homework assignments that were intended to establish further her ability and skills in examining the validity of her thoughts and beliefs.

Approximately nine days into therapy, Lisa attended a group therapy session where several other patients were talking about their own suicidality. This seemed to trigger her own suicidal thoughts, which she talked about in individual therapy. As a homework assignment, she was asked to focus on her suicidal thoughts and complete a thought record. Table 13–2 shows the result.

SUBSEQUENT SESSIONS

Lisa's subsequent therapy sessions continued to focus on development of cognitive skills that would enable her to defuse the severity and frequency of her depression and suicidality. After 17 days in the hospital, it was mutually agreed that Lisa had developed the ability to defuse her suicidal thoughts when they occurred. At this point, she was transferred out of the full hospitalization program and admitted to the partial hospitalization program, where she attended all hospital activities between 8:30 a.m. and 4:00 p.m. five days a week. This enabled her to go home at night and on weekends while still receiving the level of care and intensity of treatment that she needed. Lisa's

TABLE 13-2 Thought Record #2

Date	Situation	Feeling(s)	Automatic thought	Facts that show it's true	Facts that show it's not 100% true	Rational response	Rerate feelings now (0–100)
	What were you doing or think-ing about?	(Specify: rate 0–100)	What was going through your mind just before you started to feel bad? Any other thoughts?				
7/30	Immediately following group therapy on July 30. Everyone was talking about their sui-cide attempts.	Depressed—99 Disappointed—90	Everyone would be bet-ter off without me. I'm worthless. I'm a failure. I'm inadequate. If I'm dead my children will no longer have to worry about how I am doing. I was relieved when my mother died. My kids will understand if I kill myself.	I'm better off without my mother. I believe they would be better off without me.	My sons tell me they don't want me to kill myself. I mean some-thing to other patients in the hospital. I felt im-portant to my kids when they were young, and I guess that I am still im-portant to them in some way. The pain in my family would never go away if I killed myself.	There are still many things that I can do for my family. There are still some ways that I am important to my sons. Suicide is an act of pain and frustration for everyone.	Depression—65 Disappointed—90

attendance in the hospital's program was gradually tapered down until it was decided that she could continue treatment on an outpatient basis.

Outpatient therapy sessions focused on addressing Lisa's core beliefs. The sense of herself as worthless, powerless, and inadequate was addressed in her outpatient treatment. Her sense of others as dangerous and hurtful was also addressed.

Eighteen months subsequent to her hospitalization, Lisa had not made another suicide attempt. Her BDI scores were consistently below 12, and her Hopelessness Scale scores were 5 or below. She continued in treatment to change her core beliefs and the personality disorder characteristics described earlier.

Several years after being hospitalized, Lisa, now moved from the area, wrote a letter, which is excerpted below.

Dear Dr. Greenberger:

The main reason that I am writing you is to let you know I'm feeling good. I feel the best I ever have in my life. My depression has really lifted. With thanks to you and other therapists, I have been able to put my life back together. It took awhile—a long time, actually. I can think clearly now—think things through, not only see black, but pros and cons. I feel human again. I don't distort things—and if I do, I'm able to see what I'm doing and to challenge my thinking. I make an agenda and a journal, and do thought records every day. I see a future for myself, and a good one at that. I want to thank you for your help. There *is* life after depression.

Thank you, again.

Lisa.

REFERENCES

Beck, A., Brown, G., Berchick, R., Stewart, B., & Steer, B. (1990). Relationship between hopelessness and ultimate suicide: A replication with psychiatric outpatients. *American Journal of Psychiatry, 147,* 2.

Beck, A. T., Rush, A. J., Shaw, B. F., & Emery, G. (1979). *Cognitive therapy of depression.* New York: Guilford.

Beck, A. T., Steer, R., Kovacs, M., & Garrison, B. (1985). Hopelessness and eventual suicide: A 10-year prospective study of patients hospitalized with suicidal ideation. *American Journal of Psychiatry, 142(5),* 559–562.

Shneidman, E. (1985). *Definition of suicide.* New York: John Wiley.

SUGGESTED READINGS

Beck, A. T., Resnik, H. L., & Lettieri, D. J. (1974). *The prediction of suicide.* Philadelphia: Charles Press.

Hawton, K., & Catalan, J. (1982). *Attempted suicide: A practical guide to its nature and management.* Oxford: Oxford Medical Publications.

Shneidman, E. (1985). *Definition of suicide.* New York: John Wiley.

Beck, A. T., Rush, A. J., Shaw, B. F., & Emery, G. (1979). *Cognitive therapy of depression.* New York: Guilford.

14

Childhood Depression

Mark A. Reinecke

INTRODUCTION

Cognitive therapy has developed rapidly since the early 1970s and has become a respected and established model for conceptualizing and treating a range of emotional and behavioral problems. As the chapters of this volume attest, the theory has yielded a family of important therapeutic techniques that have proven useful in treating a number of adult disorders, including depression, generalized anxiety, panic disorder, marital problems, alcohol and substance abuse, and personality disorders.

Cognitive therapy with children, however, has received less attention. Until recently, psychodynamic and behavioral models prevailed as the most popular approaches for conceptualizing and treating childhood psychopathology. Although cognitive therapy has provided us with intuitively appealing alternatives for understanding childhood depression, anxiety disorders, and attentional problems—and important advances in both the theory and application of cognitive therapy with children have been provided by Kendall, Meichenbaum, Hammen, DiGiuseppe, and others—we have not seen, as yet, the development of an established body of outcome research

Mark A. Reinecke • Center for Cognitive Therapy, Department of Psychiatry, University of Chicago, Chicago, Illinois 60637.

Comprehensive Casebook of Cognitive Therapy, edited by Arthur Freeman and Frank M. Dattilio. Plenum Press, New York, 1992.

or a fully articulated model of childhood behavioral problems. As DiGiuseppe wrote in 1981, "In the field of child psychotherapy, cognitive-behavior therapy is the new kid on the block. Nobody knows much about him and his skills are unproven." Although approximately 10 years have passed since those comments, his sentiments remain essentially true today.

As with adults, cognitive therapy with children is based upon the assumption that there is a fundamental interaction between how individuals think and how they subsequently feel and behave. A person's assumptions, memories, attentional biases, plans or goals, expectations, inferences, and attributions all influence his or her feelings and behavior. Behavioral and emotional problems in both children and adults are seen as stemming from distorted mental representations and maladaptive thought processes that had been learned at an earlier point in time.

COGNITIVE THERAPY OF DEPRESSION

Cognitive models of depression such as those proposed by Abramson, Seligman, and Teasdale (1978), Beck (1967), Rehm (1977), Rehm and O'Hara (1980), Cole and Kaslow (1988), and Ingram (1984) posit that depressive disorders stem from negativistic expectancies, attributions, and causal inferences. An individual's beliefs and ideations serve both to maintain and to exacerbate depressive emotions. Cognitive theory recognizes that intrapsychic as well as biological, social, and environmental factors play a role in the regulation of affect.

Depressed individuals tend, as a group, to believe that they should meet high standards, yet evaluate themselves critically and believe that they are unable to meet these self-imposed expectations or goals. They attribute these failures to global and stable characteristics of themselves. In essence, they view themselves as fundamentally flawed in important ways. As Beck (1976) stated, the depressed individual "regards himself as lacking some element or attribute that he considers essential for happiness."

Depressed individuals do not, as a consequence, view themselves as able to influence important outcomes, and as a result feel "personally helpless" (Abramson et al., 1978). As Rehm (1977) has observed, depressed individuals manifest deficits in self-monitoring, self-evaluation, and self-reinforcement. They show a generalized negative expectancy about life events, which in turn contributes to highly critical self-evaluations, excessive self-punishment, low rates of self-reinforcement, and selective attention to negative events. Moreover, depressed individuals often manifest poor social skills and behave in ways that elicit both rejection and overinvolvement from others.

DEVELOPMENTAL CONSIDERATIONS

Although the majority of research on cognitive contributions to depressive disorders has used adult subjects, we have no reason to believe that such factors should not also play a role in depression experienced by children and adolescents. A growing body of research suggests, in fact, that the cognitive patterns of depressed children are in many respects quite similar to those of clinically depressed adults (Asarnow, Carlson, & Guthrie, 1987; Blechman, McEnroe, Carella, & Audette, 1986; Blumberg & Izard, 1985; Haley, Fine, Marriage, Moretti, & Freeman, 1985; Hammen & Zupan, 1984; Kazdin, French, Unis, Esveldt-Dawson, & Sherick, 1983; Kaslow, Rehm, & Siegel, 1984; Kaslow, Tanenbaum, Abramson, Peterson, & Seligman, 1983; Leitenberg, Yost, & Carroll-Wilson, 1986; Mullins, Siegel, & Hodges, 1985; Nolen-Hoeksema, Girgus, & Seligman, 1986; Schwartz, Friedman, Lindsay, & Narrol, 1982). Like adults, depressed children demonstrate decreased self-esteem, feelings of hopelessness, cognitive distortions, a depressive attributional style, deficits in self-monitoring, poor social problem solving, and an impaired sense of personal efficacy or competence.

Although these studies suggest that important similarities may exist between depression experienced by adults and children, they do not imply that models derived from work with adults can be applied without modification to children. Changes in cognitive, emotional, and social

functioning during childhood and adolescence require that we adopt a developmental approach and that we modify cognitive models of depression accordingly (Cicchetti & Schneider-Rosen, 1986; Reinecke, Beck, & Stewart, 1990).

Cognitive therapy with adults has emphasized cognitive *contents* and has focused on assisting patients to change maladaptive or distorted perceptions and beliefs. Cognitive and behavioral techniques are employed to teach patients to become more aware of their perceptions of specific events and to aid them in monitoring and reevaluating recurrent maladaptive patterns of thinking. The ultimate goal of this is the development of alternative ways of looking at day-to-day events and of coping with potentially depressing problems that arise.

Cognitive therapy with children, in contrast, has largely focused upon impaired cognitive *processes*. Its literature has been derived from the work of Vygotsky (1962) and his student, Luria (1959, 1961), who emphasized training of reflective thought processes and the rehearsal of adaptive self-statements as a means of alleviating children's behavioral problems. Self-control training (Kanfer & Hagerman, 1981; Rehm, 1977) has been based upon these theories; it employs a range of procedures, including the modeling, rehearsal, and reinforcement of adaptive behavior, "sub-vocalization" of coping strategies, and role-playing of alternative responses for problematic situations. In addition to self-instructional techniques, social problem solving, perspective taking, relaxation training, and assertiveness skills training have been employed. The emphasis is upon compensating for poorly developed thought processes or behavioral skills and is directed toward developing children's reflective competence—in essence, training them how to think and behave (Abikoff, 1985; Braswell & Kendall, 1988; Craighead, Meyers, & Craighead, 1985; Kendall, 1977, 1982, 1985; Kendall & Braswell, 1985; Kendall, Reber, McLeer, Epps, & Ronan, 1990; Kazdin, Esveldt-Dawson, French, & Unis, 1987; Lochman, Burch, Curry, & Lampron, 1984; Mahoney & Nezworski, 1985; Swanson, 1985; Urbain & Kendall, 1980). These approaches have been effective in improving attention and reducing impulsivity among both subclinical populations and clinically referred children. Their effectiveness in treating childhood depression, however, has received little study, which is surprising given the quantity and quality of research into the treatment of depressed adults.

Cognitively oriented case studies of depressed children also have tended to emphasize the use of social skills training and social problem solving (Frame, Matson, Sonis, Fialkov, & Kazdin, 1982; Matson, et al., 1980; Petti, Bornstein, Delamater, & Conners, 1980). Only two controlled outcome studies examining the effectiveness of cognitive interventions for treating childhood depression have been completed (Butler, Miezitis, Friedman, & Cole, 1980; Stark, Kaslow, & Reynolds, 1987). Both found that active cognitive interventions (role-playing of social problem solving; cognitive restructuring; and self-control training) were effective in improving mood and differed from attention and wait-list controls.

One possible reason that childhood depression has received little attention from cognitive therapists is that the treatment of depression experienced by adults emphasizes conscious causal reasoning, a form of cognitive activity that is not fully consolidated until middle childhood. A goal of this chapter will be to show how cognitive therapy techniques such as those developed for the assessment and reframing of maladaptive beliefs in depressed adults can be adapted for use in treating prepubertal children. An attempt is made to use Beck, Rush, Shaw, and Emery's (1979) approach to conceptualizing and treating depression as foundation for work with children.

ADAPTATIONS OF COGNITIVE THEORY AND TECHNIQUE

For individuals to benefit from short-term psychotherapy, they must possess a number of capacities. These include the ability to form a trusting and collaborative relationship with a therapist, the capacity to identify a specific problem or therapeutic goal, the ability to identify and label how they are feeling in specific situations, the capacity to identify what they are thinking, an ability to see relationships between affect and behavior on the one hand and how they were thinking on the other, and an ability to develop and evaluate alternative points of view. Children, unfortunately, do not possess many of these requisite capacities. As a result, they might be seen as poor candidates for traditional forms of cognitive therapy. With this in mind, there are several alternatives. First, one might abandon the cognitive model, realizing that in its current form it is not applicable to childhood behavioral and emotional problems. Second, one might reframe cognitive theory from a developmental perspective, taking these concerns into consideration. Third, one might adapt cognitive therapy techniques as a means of circumventing these difficulties. Finally, one might address these shortcomings directly, identifying which of these requisite abilities an individual child lacks and training him or her in those specific skills.

Cognitive therapy with children has a number of conceptual and technical similarities to work with adults. As in cognitive therapy with adults, treatment of children focuses on specific beliefs, attributions, and cognitive distortions that contribute to depression. Verbal and behavioral interventions are employed in teaching the child to become more aware of his or her views and beliefs. In addition, however, drawings, stories and other metaphorical or "projective" techniques are employed as a means of gaining access to the child's beliefs and assumptions. As with adults, children learn to identify and label their emotions, as well as recurrent patterns of thinking. Although less emphasis is placed upon Socratic questioning as a means of evaluating the validity of automatic thoughts (the preoperational child does not as yet have the cognitive means for logically evaluating such alternatives), attempts are made to demonstrate that alternative points of view may be more helpful. Although such focused procedures as the Depressive Thought Record (DTR) or three-column technique can be used with adolescents, younger children often find this exercise confusing or difficult to complete. Younger children often lack sufficiently developed vocabularies or verbal abstraction capacities to write down specific feelings experienced, the thoughts that occurred at that time, and a rational disputation of those beliefs. With modifications, however, these approaches can be used by children. Asking the child to "draw a picture of how I was feeling," then using this as a point of entry for a discussion of "what was I thinking" and "how could it be different" can be quite useful in this regard.

A point of difference between cognitive therapy with depressed adults and that practiced with children centers on the role of underlying schemas and assumptions in maintaining emotional disorders and the importance of changing them as a means of reducing the potential for relapse. Arguments can be made on empirical grounds that depressive episodes experienced by children are phenomenologically different than those experienced by adults, and that depressive affect is more responsive to environmental change during childhood. The theoretical point can be made that school-aged children do not possess a fully consolidated sense of self; a fully articulated set of beliefs about their world; or a stable and broad-based set of expectations about the future. As a result, cognitive therapy with prepubertal children places less emphasis on the identification of core beliefs and dysfunctional assumptions.

Cognitive therapy with depressed children places a relatively greater emphasis, however, on work with parents and other important persons in the child's life. Active attempts are made to examine how parents may inadvertently be contributing to their child's behavioral or emotional problems, and toward identifying specific maladaptive beliefs they may be conveying to their child. Behavioral interventions, such as activity scheduling and operant reinforcement of appropriate behavior play an important role in treating depressed children, as does the development of social skills and social problem-solving abilities.

CASE REPORT

Bill C., a 10-year-old fifth grader, was referred for treatment by his parents due to feelings of sadness, anxiety, social isolation, and fighting with peers at school. Bill's parents were interviewed together for two hours as part of the initial assessment. Complete developmental, social, and medical histories were obtained, as was a history of their son's problems. Information was gathered as to when Bill's behavioral problems were most severe, what his parents had done to resolve them, and what they saw as the cause of these problems.

Initial Assessment

Bill's parents described his behavioral problems at school as "severe" and stated that they had become progressively worse over the past two to three years. Although Bill's feelings of dysphoria were of recent origin, his parents reported that he had "alienated other kids" for several years and stated that he now was involved in fights on an almost daily basis. His parents described few behavioral problems at home, however, and reported that he got along well with his older brother and younger sister.

Next, Bill was interviewed alone and was encouraged to share his views on the problems he had been experiencing. Although he acknowledged feeling depressed and lonely, Bill minimized the severity of his problems. As he stated, "No matter what school you go to, the kids are always mean . . . I just wish they'd leave me alone." Bill perceived his classmates as malicious and "immature," and stated that he felt his only course of action was to "fight or ignore them." Bill's responses on self-report mood rating scales and a sentence-completion test suggested that he was experiencing moderately severe feelings of depression, anxiety, and hopelessness, and that he viewed himself as "repellent" to other children.

Bill became tearful while describing his suicidal thoughts. He stated that he had experienced thoughts that he "deserved to die" and that the other children at school "would really be sorry" after he was dead for several months. Bill's suicidal ideations appeared to be exacerbated by frustrations at school, and were most common after he had "been humiliated" by losing a fight. Bill's referral for treatment was precipitated by his having engaged in suicidal "gestures," such as eating berries from local trees that he believed were poisonous.

Bill's teacher was asked to complete a number of behavioral rating scales and was interviewed by phone to gain her impressions. She characterized him as an "unhappy, depressed child" and reported that he had "stopped smiling or laughing or talking to his classmates . . . he only talks to adults." Bill's teacher also described him as "academically talented" and characterized him as "hardworking and very attentive" in class. She observed, however, that he was "very hard on his peers . . . he sees no shades of gray and makes no compromises." This tendency to dichotomize was similar to that seen among depressed adults, and became an important focus of treatment.

We asked Bill's mother to complete the Personality Inventory for Children-Revised (PIC-R) to gain a clearer understanding of his behavioral problems. As can be seen in Figure 14-1, clinically significant elevations were apparent on Factors II (social incompetence) and III (internalization, somatic complaints), as well as the adjustment (Adj-S), depression (D-S), anxiety (Anx-S), psychosis (Psy-S), and social skills (SSK-S) subscales of this measure. Although the psychosis subscale was highly elevated, this did not appear to stem from the presence of delusional beliefs or hallucinations. Rather, this was due to Bill's social isolation and the overlap between the content of the psychosis and social skills subscales.

Diagnosis and Cognitive Conceptualization

Diagnostically, Bill appeared to meet DSM III-R criteria for major depression and separation anxiety disorder. These problems were superimposed upon a self-critical and highly perfectionistic personality style. Bill maintained high standards for his own performance (believing, for example, that his parents "shouldn't give me any Christmas presents; I haven't earned them") as well as for the behavior of his peers. He was highly critical of mistakes made by his classmates and would flaunt his own knowledge by bragging in the class. Bill's feelings of dysphoria were accompanied by crying, social withdrawal, a loss of interest in his usual activities, and feelings of self-reproach. Given the information available to this point, one might conceptualize Bill's difficulties as follows:

Behavioral Coping Strategies
- Fighting
- Avoidance of peers
- Seeking support from adults

Cognitive Distortions
- Dichotomizing
- Catastrophizing

Personality Inventory for Children (PIC)
REVISED FORMAT PROFILE FORM: PARTS I AND II

R.D. Wirt, Ph.D., D. Lachar, Ph.D., J.K. Klinedinst, Ph.D., and P.D. Seat, Ph.D.

Published by

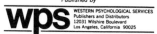

WESTERN PSYCHOLOGICAL SERVICES
Publishers and Distributors
12031 Wilshire Boulevard
Los Angeles, California 90025

MALE
Ages 6-16

Child's Name: _____ Birthdate: _____ Age: _____
Sex: M F   Race: _____ Grade: _____ Date Tested: _____
Informant: _____ Relationship to Child: _____
Reason for Assessment: _____

RAW SCORES: 8 18 10 | 1 | 4 | 5 11 27 8 | 8 | 3 3 21 4 12 2 11 12 15 21

*This scale is not a substitute for an individual assessment administered to the child.
NOTE: If Part III and/or IV was completed and the full scales scored, the original Profile Form (W-152C) must be used.

Figure 14-1. Bill's Personality Inventory for Children—Revised.

- Magnification/Minimization

Automatic Thoughts
- "I have to fight or leave."
- "People are either good or bad . . . nice or mean."
- "I don't deserve anything good unless I've earned it."
- "Kids just want to hurt me."

Assumptions
- "If only people would leave me alone, then I'd be happy."
- "If I'm successful, then people will approve of me."
- "If I know what you want from me, then I can avoid rejection."

Schemas
- "Kids are rejecting and malicious."
- "I'm smarter than everyone else."
- "The world is a dangerous, unpredictable place."
- "I'm no good."

Bill's feelings of depression and anger appeared to be exacerbated by his desire to withdraw from others, his decreased motivation to participate in enjoyable activities, and his social skills deficits. Bill's behavior toward his peers had been described as "obnoxious" and tended to contribute to rejection by them; his view of himself as "repelling" to others was in many respects accurate. His descriptions of interactions with his classmates suggested that he felt little empathy for them and that he was intolerant of their mistakes and shortcomings. He tended to be demanding toward his peers and insisted that they follow his rules while playing games.

Course of Treatment

As in therapy with adults, the first goal in cognitive therapy with children is to develop a therapeutic rapport. Like many children who are referred for treatment by others, Bill was anxious about attending sessions and felt that he wasn't "the person with the problem." Although he acknowledged feeling upset about what had been happening at school, he did not believe these problems could be solved and remarked tersely that he "didn't want to talk about it." With this in mind, a nondirective stance was adopted, and Bill was asked if there was anything he would like to talk about or do during the session. As might be expected, Bill responded, "No." A suggestion was then made that there were many toys and objects in the room, and Bill was asked if he would like to draw something, which he did. Bill's initial drawings were of his house and family (see Figure 14-2); as can be seen, Bill left himself out of the drawing—a notable omission. Also

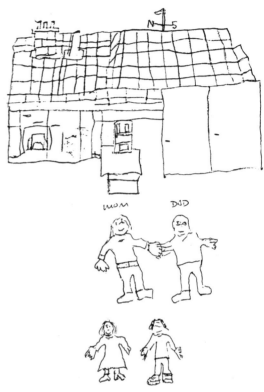

Figure 14-2. House and family.

notable was the amount of detail he provided in the drawing. Bill took more than 20 minutes to complete the drawing, frequently erasing and commenting that he "couldn't draw very well" and that he "didn't want to insult his family by making them ugly."

When asked to draw a person, Bill drew a small, monsterlike figure (see Figure 14-3). Traditional interpretations of the draw-a-person task as a reflection of one's self-image (in this case, small, angry, and repulsive) are quite consistent with Bill's automatic thoughts.

Bill's next drawings were particularly disturbing, and appeared to capture his view of his world and his relationships with others. His drawings of a crowd shouting "We hate you!" and of an isolated figure being bombarded by an entrenched army were consistent both with his parents' and teacher's reports of his social situation and with his view of himself as an isolated, rejected child (see Figures 14-4 and 14-5). Bill rarely spoke while drawing and appeared to be quite concerned as to whether the therapist would approve of his work. He frequently apologized for perceived "mistakes" and carefully selected his words when responding to the therapist's queries. He

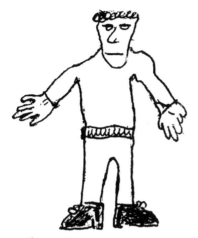

Figure 14-3. Draw-a-Person Task.

rarely smiled. In attempt to engage him in a more collab-orative activity, the therapist next drew a short "squiggle" (Winnicott, 1958) on a sheet of paper and asked Bill if he could make something out of it. Bill's drawing, presented in Figure 14-6, provides an interesting example of how techniques borrowed from other approaches to child psy-chotherapy can be employed in cognitive therapy with children.

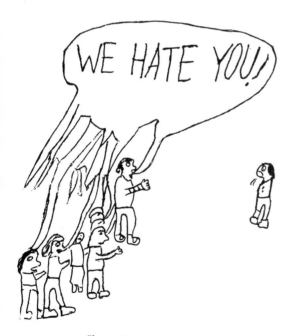

Figure 14-4. "We Hate You!"

Bill labeled his drawing "the invisible man" and remarked that "he's going nowhere." This might be inter-preted in several ways, depending on one's theoretical predilections. His drawing might, for example, express his feelings about himself at school in that he is misun-derstood or "invisible" to his peers. Alternatively, it might reflect his feelings about therapy (that he was invisi-ble to the therapist, and that treatment was going no-where), his relationship with his parents, or his feelings toward himself. Inasmuch as cognitive therapy empha-sizes the phenomenological meaning of each event to the individual, the best way of knowing which interpretation is correct was simply to ask him.

BILL: He's invisible, all right . . . he's going to work in the snow, he's 30 minutes late, and he's afraid of being punished by the boss because his subordinates are lazy and won't work for him like he tells them to . . . they'll just throw snowballs at him and they won't do what he says.

THERAPIST: What's going to happen?

BILL: He'll just hope that things will be better.

THERAPIST: No, I'm not sure. The workers seem to be really lazy. He'll have to do more than just hope that they'll change . . . what do you think he could do?

Bill's story bears a remarkable resemblance to his experiences at school, and his comment that the invisible man will "just hope things will be better" reflects his feelings of hopelessness, passivity, and limited problem-solving abilities. The therapist's response was a direct attempt to encourage Bill to consider alternative courses of action and new ways of thinking about his "subordi-nates." Bill was able to generate several alternative sce-narios, and came to feel that "maybe they can work together . . . just because they don't do it his way doesn't mean they don't like him." He recognized the possibility that "his boss might be understanding . . . it's OK for him to be late sometimes" and that the invisible man "didn't really think about how the workers felt." At the conclu-sion of the session, Bill commented that he "wanted to think about this for next time" and that he "really liked today's session . . . I was afraid I wouldn't, but I did." His story, then, may have reflected his sentiments about ther-apy as much as his feelings about school.

During subsequent sessions, attempts were made to apply the insights he had gained from the story more directly toward his problems at school. During the fourth session, for example, he reported having felt "bad" after his classmates got angry at him for making an error during a volleyball game. He remarked that he felt "angry and hurt that they wouldn't forget it . . . they wouldn't see that it was just a mistake and not the end of the world." An

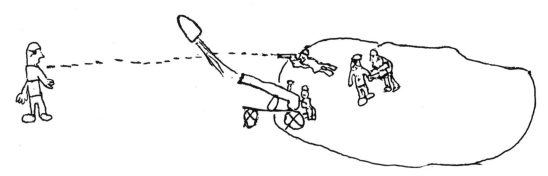

Figure 14-5. Bombarded by Army.

interesting shift occurred at that time, however, in that he continued by describing how a girl on the team, Sheila, had "missed *all* her shots."

BILL: I wanted to kill her she was so stupid . . . I wanted to yell at her because they were easy shots.
THERAPIST: It sounds like it really bugged you that she made those mistakes.
BILL: Yeah . . . I wanted to punch her to the moon.
THERAPIST: All the way to the moon? It must have been pretty bad, all those mistakes. You really wished that they'd cut you some slack for catching the ball. Do you think Sheila might feel hurt, too; that she'd like it if you cut her some slack?
BILL: She got mad, too . . . she didn't want to play any more because . . . they were all yelling at her. This is stupid; can we play some checkers?
THERAPIST: No, not just now. It's sounding like it's hard to talk about getting angry, hard to deal with it.
BILL: Yeah, I guess I don't [like talking about it] . . . I need to let off some steam . . I don't think it bothered her.
THERAPIST: You don't think it bothered her that you were so mad at her?
BILL: Nah . . . I wish they'd cut me some slack.

Although Bill wished that his classmates would be tolerant of his mistakes, it was quite difficult for him to recognize that others might appreciate the same patience. Although he attempted to shift our conversation away from this topic by asking to play checkers and to go for a drink of water, a problem focus was maintained. Bill, in fact, became quite angry at the therapist for directing the discussion back to the volleyball game. As he stated, "Slack? I'd like enough rope to go around this hospital and wrap it around the world . . . It's nothing against your profession, but I'd rather have seen a psychiatrist because they don't make you think so much." (Indeed.) As the

conversation continued, Socratic questioning was employed as a means of developing his tolerance for Sheila's mistakes as well as his own shortcomings. As he concluded, "It's not a big deal if I make mistakes . . . I'd like it if people would cut me some slack. But you know, I get mad at myself a lot . . . I should cut myself some slack, too."

A combination of direct discussion of problematic situations and metaphorical interventions (such as story telling, drawing, and playing with toy figures) were employed during subsequent sessions as a means of developing Bill's ability to empathize with others and tolerance for his own mistakes. Socratic questioning and rational responding were employed as a means of reducing his tendency to dichotomize people as "good or bad" and "friends or enemies" and to develop his ability to recognize that it was possible to experience two emotions simultaneously. The goal of the latter intervention was assisting him to see that people can disapprove of his behavior, yet still care for him. Bill came to see that other children might not intentionally wish to harm him but that his critical and demanding demeanor did little to engender friendship. Specific behavioral skills, such as negotiating with classmates about rules for games and "not quitting when they don't do it my way," were rehearsed.

Meetings were held with Bill's parents on a regular basis during his treatment. Their feelings about his depression were explored, as were possible origins of his underlying beliefs. Bill's father, it was learned, felt frustrated in his work as a lab assistant as his applications to medical school had repeatedly been rejected. He believed that "nothing less than the best work" was good enough and placed a high premium on academic accomplishment. Bill's mother was frustrated by her husband's frequent complaining, but felt powerless to help him. As she whispered at the conclusion of a parent guidance session, "Sometimes I think he's the one who needs help, but I

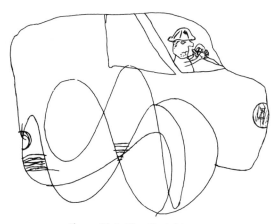

Figure 14-6. The "Invisible Man."

can't tell him so." Bill's parents encouraged their son's participation in enjoyable social activities, including Little League and a hockey team. Supervised social activities were selected because they were enjoyable for Bill and served to develop his social skills.

Therapy was terminated with Bill and his family after 22 sessions. His parents reported that "all was well" both at home and at school. Bill's mood had improved, and he had not been involved in a fight for approximately six weeks. Bill had not experienced suicidal ideations since the third week of treatment, and he appeared to be far less perfectionistic than at the outset. As he stated, "I know I'm not perfect . . . and sometimes I wonder where I got the idea that I had to be." Although Bill continued to criticize his peers, this occurred less often and was rarely accompanied by withdrawal or an angry outburst.

SUMMARY

This case example illustrates how cognitive, social, and familial factors interact in contributing to behavioral and emotional problems experienced by children. Focused cognitive and behavioral interventions were found to be highly effective in alleviating this child's depressive disorder and in improving his social adjustment. As in many depressed children, this patient's social perspective-taking ability and problem-solving skills were poorly developed. Moreover, he demonstrated many of the cognitive concomitants of depression found among depressed adults. He tended, for example, to attribute negative events to external factors and did not recognize how his behavior might inadvertently be contributing to his predicament. Negative views of himself, his world, and his

future were readily apparent, as was a negativistic attributional style and a lack of perceived self-efficacy (i.e., he did not feel that he had the ability to bring about meaningful changes in his life). This lack of perceived competence, in conjunction with his external locus of control, contributed to his feelings of pessimism. Bill's sensitivity to the feelings of others and his social problem-solving skills—specifically, his ability to develop, evaluate, and implement alternative approaches to resolving conflicts with his peers—were poorly developed. Bill's consequent feelings of hopelessness, combined with a desire to seek revenge by "making them feel sorry," appeared to underlie his suicidal ideations.

Given his level of cognitive and emotional development, however, it was not possible to apply traditional cognitive therapy techniques. Children's ability to differentiate emotions, identify thoughts and beliefs, generate hypotheses, and understand causal relationships are not fully developed. Modifications in technique were necessary, as a result, to compensate for these difficulties.

The treatment of this child was multifaceted. It included developing his social perspective-taking and problem-solving skills, modeling and practicing of more adaptive social behavior, and role-playing of alternative approaches to handling difficult situations at school. Cognitive interventions included attributional retraining (Braswell & Kendall, 1988)—a careful examination and reframing of his beliefs, expectancies, and attributions about the behavior of his classmates, and a demonstration of links between his attributions and behaviors—rational responding to his cognitive distortions, and affect monitoring (Beck et al., 1979). Beliefs about personal efficacy (that desired changes are possible, and that one has the ability to bring them about) are an important predictor of therapeutic improvement in children (Weisz, 1986). Bill initially showed little confidence in his abilities and was pessimistic about the possibility of change. With this in mind, it was important to encourage Bill's active attempts to develop friendships, and to assess how confident he was that he could accomplish his goals and what he felt might interfere.

The active participation of Bill's parents in the treatment process was essential as a means of encouraging his participation in enjoyable activities, developing his social skills, and addressing familial interactions that appeared to support the development of maladaptive schemas and assumptions.

Behavioral management techniques, such as operant reinforcement of appropriate social behavior, were not necessary given the dramatic decline in the frequency of Bill's fighting as thoughts underlying his feelings of anger were examined. A contingency management system could readily have been developed if his fighting had persisted.

DISCUSSION

Cognitive therapy with children, as with adults, is based on the premise that there is an essential interaction between how individuals think and how they consequently feel and behave. Although an emphasis is placed upon learning processes, including the modeling and reinforcement of behavior, these processes are seen as mediated by individuals' active attempts to understand and derive a sense of meaning from their experiences. Depression, anxiety, and anger are mediated by distorted cognitive processes and dysfunctional belief systems in both children and adults.

Although projective assessment techniques and the interpretation of fantasy are rarely employed as part of cognitive therapy with depressed adults, this case example illustrates how they can be useful in work with children. The projective hypothesis, that unconscious motivations, desires, and impulses will be reflected in one's response to ambiguous stimuli, is not entirely inconsistent with cognitive theory (Sobel, 1981). Although cognitive metatheory explicitly rejects hydraulic models of unconscious motivation and defense, it acknowledges that nonconscious belief systems and tacit knowledge structures guide one's perceptions and memories (Guidano & Liotti, 1983; Mahoney, 1985). As a consequence, one might predict that negativistic beliefs would be found in the dreams of depressed individuals (Beck & Hurvich, 1959; Beck & Ward, 1961) as well as in their responses on projective measures and in fantasy.

This case example illustrates how children's drawings and stories can be used as a tool for suggesting possible beliefs, assumptions, and attributions that can be explored in therapy. This is *not* to suggest that unconscious processes are at play in childhood depression. Rather, as children experience difficulty identifying and rationally evaluating the validity of automatic thoughts, we must creatively develop alternative means of assessing and reframing their beliefs. The reliability and validity of these approaches to cognitive assessment, of course, are yet to be demonstrated. Alternative approaches for assessing children's cognitions (e.g., think-aloud techniques, guided imagery, rating scales, thought records, tape recordings, and descriptive questionnaires) are worthy of examination.

Depression and suicidality are highly distressing for both child and family. This case study illustrates how cognitive and behavioral interventions developed for the treatment of depressed adults can be successfully adapted for treating children. The treatment of depressed children challenges us to test the limits of adult models of cognition and depression and to reexamine these models from a developmental point of view. Treatment of children further requires that we develop reliable and valid cognitive assessment techniques and that we modify our therapeutic approaches with the developmental limits of children in mind.

The usefulness of cognitive therapy for treating depression and suicidality among adults has been well documented; the techniques are powerful, and the model is compelling. The potential value of cognitive therapy for treating children, while not yet realized, is equally great.

REFERENCES

Abikoff, H. (1985). Efficacy of cognitive training interventions in hyperactive children: A critical review. *Clinical Psychology, 5*, 479–512.

Abramson, L., Seligman, M., & Teasdale, J. (1978). Learned helplessness in humans: Critique and reformulation. *Journal of Abnormal Psychology, 87*, 49–74.

Asarnow, J., Carlson, G., & Guthrie, D. (1987). Coping strategies, self-perceptions, hopelessness, and perceived family environments in depressed and suicidal children. *Journal of Consulting and Clinical Psychology, 55*, 361–366.

Beck, A. (1967). *Depression: Clinical, experimental, and theoretical aspects.* New York: Hoeber.

Beck, A. (1976). *Cognitive therapy and the emotional disorders.* New York: International Universities Press.

Beck, A., & Hurvich, M. (1959). Psychological correlates of depression. 1. Frequency of masochistic dream content in a private practice sample. *Psychosomatic Medicine, 21*, 50–55.

Beck, A., & Ward, C. (1961). Dreams of depressed patients: Characteristic themes in manifest content. *Arch. Gen. Psychiat., 5*, 462–467.

Beck, A., Rush, A., Shaw, B., & Emery, G. (1979). *Cognitive therapy of depression.* New York: Guilford.

Blechman, E., McEnroe, M., Carella, E., & Audette, D. (1986). Childhood competence and depression. *Journal of Abnormal Psychology, 95*, 223–227.

Blumberg, S., & Izard, C. (1985). Affective and cognitive characteristics of depression in 10- and 11-year-old children. *Journal of Personality and Social Psychology, 49*, 194–202.

Braswell, L., & Kendall, P. (1988). Cognitive-behavioral methods with children. In K. Dobson (Ed.), *Handbook of cognitive-behavioral therapies.* New York: Guilford.

Butler, L., Miezitis, S., Friedman, R., & Cole, E. (1980). The effect of two school-based intervention programs on depressive symptoms in preadolescents. *American Educational Research Journal, 17*, 111–119.

Cicchetti, D., & Schneider-Rosen, K. (1986). An organizational approach to childhood depression. In M. Rutter, C. Izard, & P. Read (Eds.), *Depression in young people: Developmental and clinical perspectives.* New York: Guilford.

Cole, P., & Kaslow, N. (1988). Interactional and cognitive strategies for affect regulation: A developmental perspective on childhood depression. In L. Alloy (Ed.), *Cognitive processes in depression*. New York: Guilford.

Craighead, W., Meyers, A., & Craighead, L. (1985). A conceptual model for cognitive-behavior therapy with children. *Journal of Abnormal Child Psychology, 13,* 331–342.

DiGiuseppe, R. (1981). Cognitive therapy with children. In G. Emery, S. Hollon, & R. Bedrosian (Eds.), *New directions in cognitive therapy* (pp. 50–67). New York: Guilford.

Frame, C., Matson, J., Sonis, W., Fialkov, M., & Kazdin, A. (1982). Behavioral treatment of depression in a prepubertal child. *Journal of Behavior Therapy and Experimental Psychiatry, 3,* 239–243.

Guidano, V., & Liotti, G. (1983). *Cognitive processes and emotional disorders.* New York: Guilford.

Haley, G., Fine, S., Marriage, K., Moretti, M., & Freeman, R. (1985). Cognitive bias and depression in psychiatrically disturbed children and adolescents. *Journal of Consulting and Clinical Psychology, 53,* 535–537.

Hammen, C., & Zupan, B. (1984). Self-schemas, depression, and the processing of personal information in children. *Journal of Experimental Child Psychology, 37,* 598–608.

Ingram, R. (1984). Toward an information processing analysis of depression. *Cognitive Therapy and Research, 8,* 443–478.

Kanfer, F., & Hagerman, S. (1981). The role of self-regulation. In L. Rehm (Ed.), *Behavior therapy for depression: Present status and future directions.* New York: Academic Press.

Kaslow, N., Rehm, L., & Siegel, A. (1984). Social-cognitive and cognitive correlates of depression in children. *Journal of Abnormal Child Psychology, 12,* 605–620.

Kaslow, N., Tanenbaum, R., Abramson, L., Peterson, C., & Seligman, M. (1983). Problem-solving deficits and depressive symptoms among children. *Journal of Abnormal Child Psychology, 11,* 497–502.

Kazdin, A., Esveldt-Dawson, K., French, N., & Unis, A. (1987). Problem-solving skills training and relationship therapy in the treatment of antisocial child behavior. *Journal of Consulting and Clinical Psychology, 55,* 76–85.

Kazdin, A., French, N., Unis, A., Esveldt-Dawson, K., & Sherick, R. (1983). Hopelessness, depression, and suicidal intent among psychiatrically disturbed inpatient children. *Journal of Consulting and Clinical Psychology, 51,* 504–510.

Kendall, P. (1977). On the efficacious use of verbal self-instructional procedures with children. *Cognitive Therapy and Research, 1,* 331–341.

Kendall, P. (1982). Individual versus group cognitive-behavioral self-control training: One year follow-up. *Behavior Therapy, 13,* 241–247.

Kendall, P. (1985). Toward a cognitive-behavioral model of child psychopathology and a critique of related interventions. *Journal of Abnormal Child Psychology, 13,* 357–372.

Kendall, P., & Braswell, L. (1985). *Cognitive-behavioral therapy for impulsive children.* New York: Guilford.

Kendall, P., Reber, M., McLeer, S., Epps, J., & Ronan, K. (1990). Cognitive-behavioral treatment of conduct disordered children. *Cognitive Therapy and Research, 14*(3), 279–297.

Leitenberg, H., Yost, L., & Carroll-Wilson, M. (1986). Negative cognitive errors in children: Questionnaire development, normative data, and comparison between children with and without self-reported symptoms of depression, low self-esteem, and evaluation anxiety. *Journal of Consulting and Clinical Psychology, 54,* 528–536.

Lochman, J., Burch, P., Curry, J., & Lampron, L. (1984). Treatment and generalization effects of cognitive-behavioral and goal-setting interventions with aggressive boys. *Journal of Consulting and Clinical Psychology, 52,* 915–916.

Luria, A. (1959). The directive function of speech in development and dissolution. *Word, 15,* 341–352.

Luria, A. (1961). *The role of speech in the regulation of normal and abnormal behaviors.* New York: Liveright.

Mahoney, M. (1985). Psychotherapy and human change processes. In M. Mahoney & A. Freeman (Eds.), *Cognition and psychotherapy.* New York: Plenum.

Mahoney, M., & Nezworski, M. (1985). Cognitive-behavioral approaches to children's problems. *Journal of Abnormal Child Psychology, 13,* 467–476.

Matson, J., Esveldt-Dawson, K., Andrasik, F., Ollendik, T., Petti, T., & Hersen, M. (1980). Observation and generalization effects of social skills training with emotionally disturbed children. *Behavior Therapy, 11,* 522–531.

Mullins, L., Siegel, L., & Hodges, K. (1985). Cognitive problem-solving and life-event correlates of depressive symptoms in children. *Journal of Abnormal Child Psychology, 13,* 305–314.

Nolen-Hoeksema, S., Girgus, J., & Seligman, M. (1986). Learned helplessness in children: A longitudinal study of depression, achievement, and explanatory style. *Journal of Personality and Social Psychology, 51,* 435–442.

Petti, T., Bornstein, M., Delamater, A., & Conners, C. (1980). Evaluation and multimodal treatment of a depressed prepubertal girl. *Journal of the American Academy of Child Psychiatry, 19,* 690–702.

Rehm, L. (1977). A self-control model of depression. *Behavior Therapy, 8,* 787–804.

Rehm, L., & O'Hara, M. (1980). The role of attribution theory in understanding depression. In I. Frieze, D. Bar-Tal, & J. Carroll (Eds.), *Attribution theory: Applications to social problems.* San Francisco: Jossey-Bass.

Reinecke, M., Beck, A., & Stewart, B. (1990). Hopelessness, depression, and suicidal ideations among adolescent outpatients. Paper presented at the 37th annual meeting of the American Academy of Child and Adolescent Psychiatry, Chicago.

Schwartz, M., Friedman, R., Lindsay, P., & Narrol, H. (1982). The relationship between conceptual tempo and depression in children. *Journal of Consulting and Clinical Psychology, 50,* 488–490.

Sobel, H. (1981). Projective methods of cognitive analysis. In T. Merluzzi, C. Glass, & M. Genest (Eds.), *Cognitive assessment.* New York: Guilford.

Stark, K., Kaslow, N., & Reynolds, W. (1987). A comparison of the relative efficacy of self-control and behavioral problem-solving therapy for depression in children. *Journal of Abnormal Child Psychology, 15,* 91–113.

Swanson, H. (1985). Effects of cognitive-behavioral training on emotionally disturbed children's academic performance. *Cognitive Therapy and Research, 9,* 201–216.

Urbain, E., & Kendall, P. (1980). Review of social-cognitive problem-solving interventions with children. *Psychological Bulletin, 88,* 109–143.

Vygotsky, L. (1962). *Thought and language.* Cambridge: MIT Press.

Weisz, J. (1986). Contingency and control beliefs as predictors of psychotherapy outcomes among children and adolescents. *Journal of Consulting and Clinical Psychology, 54,* 789–795.

Winnicott, D. (1958). *Collected Papers.* London: Tavistock.

SUGGESTED READINGS

Braswell, L., & Kendall, P. (1988). Cognitive-behavioral methods with children. In K. Dobson (Ed.), *Handbook of cognitive-behavioral therapies*. New York: Guilford.

DiGiuseppe, R. (1988). A cognitive-behavioral approach to the treatment of conduct disorder children and adolescents. In N. Epstein, S. Schlesinger, & W. Dryden (Eds.), *Cognitive-behavioral therapy with families*. New York: Bruner-Mazel.

Emery, G., Bedrosian, R., & Garber, J. (1983). Cognitive therapy with depressed children and adolescents. In D. Cantwell, & G. Carlson (Eds.), *Affective disorders in childhood and adolescence: An update*. New York: Spectrum.

Kendall, P. (Ed.) (1991). *Child and adolescent therapy: Cognitive-behavioral procedures*. New York: Guilford.

Meyers, A., & Craighead, W. (Eds.) (1984). *Cognitive behavior therapy with children*. New York: Plenum.

15

Child Sexual Abuse

Esther Deblinger

Anthropological evidence suggests that child sexual abuse has been a persistent and widespread problem for thousands of years. Historically, however, attempts to raise public awareness concerning this problem have been met with disbelief and public disdain. Most notable was Sigmund Freud's attempt to enlighten his colleagues at the Vienna Society for Psychiatry and Neurology in 1896 with his presentation of the "Etiology of Hysteria." This paper outlined the seduction theory, in which he linked childhood sexual assault to adult mental illness. Not surprisingly, the paper was not well received, and Freud himself abandoned the theory in an apparent effort to avoid alienation by his skeptical and disapproving colleagues. Later, he developed a theory that seemed to be a more palatable and acceptable explanation for his patients' descriptions of childhood sexual assaults. Freud's Oedipus-complex theory not only gained wide acceptance but became the foundation for what would become a dominant force in Western psychology: psychoanalysis (Summit, 1989).

Freud's reversal fueled society's denial of child sexual abuse and continues to encourage skepticism regarding children's often painful and delayed disclosures. However, the mounting empirical data clearly support Freud's original beliefs about the prevalence and psychological impact of childhood sexual assault. The data suggests that child sexual abuse not only is highly prevalent, but appears to have a devastating impact on the psychological functioning of the victimized children (Deblinger, McLeer, Atkins, Ralphe, & Foa, 1989). Moreover, recent studies suggest that many sexually abused children suffer posttraumatic stress symptoms (McLeer, Deblinger, Atkins, Foa, & Ralphe, 1988). These symptoms can be quite persistent and can disrupt the child's emotional, cognitive, and behavioral development. Thus, for the sexually abused child, treatment is imperative. Since research suggests that child therapies are generally more effective when combined with parent interventions, the case study belows offers guidelines for working with the sexually abused child as well as the child's nonoffending parent.

CASE REPORT

The patient—Jenny, a 7-year-old girl—was attending a regular second-grade class at Wright Elementary School when her teacher, Mrs. Hall, reported a suspicion of sexual abuse to the local child protection agency. While Jenny was doing very well academically, Mrs. Hall was concerned about the patient's growing mood swings and her repeated touching of her genital area. Jenny's teacher felt compelled to call the child abuse hotline when Jenny described a picture she was drawing as follows: "That's

Esther Deblinger • Center for Children's Support, University of Medicine and Dentistry of New Jersey—School of Osteopathic Medicine, Stratford, New Jersey 08084-1505.

Comprehensive Casebook of Cognitive Therapy, edited by Arthur Freeman and Frank M. Dattilio. Plenum Press, New York, 1992.

Daddy and me; we're playing with Daddy's peepee, but we can't tell Mommy. It's a secret."

Initial Intake

Comprehensive evaluations in cases of suspected child sexual abuse aim to achieve several interrelated goals, including (a) evaluating the validity of the sexual abuse allegation and (b) assessing the psychological impact of the alleged abuse on the victim and his or her family. The evaluation will not be discussed in detail here; the assessment process, particularly with regard to "validation," is highly complex with suspected child sexual abuse cases and deserves more discussion than is feasible in the current chapter. Thus, readers are referred to de-Young (1986), Faller (1984), Kelly (1985), and White, Strom, Santelli, and Halpin (1986) for discussions and guidelines for interviewing and evaluating suspected cases of sexual abuse.

In this case, a comprehensive evaluation was conducted over the course of four sessions. Background information was provided by the child's mother, teacher, and pediatrician, and pertinent medical, school, child protection, and law enforcement records were obtained. During these sessions, Jenny and her mother were interviewed individually. The patient's father, Sam, declined an invitation to participate in the evaluation on the advice of his attorney. The impact of the alleged abuse on the victim's psychological functioning was assessed by means of direct observation, and standardized measures. The measures administered to the child included the Child Depression Inventory (CDI) (Kovacs, 1983), the Spielberger State-Trait Anxiety Inventory for Children (STAIC) (Spielberger, 1983), and the Harter Social Support Scale for Children (Harter, 1985). The patient's mother, Nancy, completed the Child Behavior Checklist (CBCL) (Achenbach, 1991) and agreed to keep a daily record of problem behaviors that were identified as targets for behavior change. These included angry outbursts, public masturbation, avoidance behavior, and nightmares. Nancy also completed the Symptom Checklist-90-Revised (SCL-90-R) (Derogatis, 1983) as an assessment of her own personal level of distress. Finally, the patient's teacher, Mrs. Hall, completed the Teacher's Report Form (TRF) (Achenbach, 1991), providing a profile of Jenny's school behavior.

Background

Nancy and Sam were 18 years old, recent high school graduates, and unmarried when Jenny was born. While they married shortly thereafter, their relationship difficulties ensued almost immediately. While Nancy had a fairly large circle of friends in high school, she lost contact with many of them after graduation. Both Nancy and Sam became increasingly socially isolated as they struggled with financial and parenting stressors. Sam began losing his temper over relatively mundane incidents and became more and more abusive. A particularly severe incident of domestic violence prompted Nancy to leave her husband when Jenny was approximately 6 years old. At that time, Jenny and her mother moved in with the maternal grandmother (Jenny's maternal grandfather and stepgrandfather had passed away before she was born).

When Nancy went to court several months later to obtain child support, she also suggested a bimonthly visitation schedule, to which Sam agreed. For a while, the bimonthly weekend visits seemed to go very well; Jenny clearly looked forward to seeing her father. However, approximately six months later, Jenny resisted going for her regularly scheduled visit. Nancy attributed her daughter's reluctance to an argument Jenny had witnessed between her parents two weeks before. Thus, she encouraged Jenny not to be angry at her father and insisted that her daughter go for her visit. Jenny returned from the weekend visit seemingly angry at everyone.

Two weeks prior to this intake, Nancy received a call from the patient's teacher, Mrs. Hall. Mrs. Hall explained that she called the child protection agency because she was concerned that Jenny may have been sexually abused by her father. Nancy was sure there had been some sort of misunderstanding, but she cooperated with the investigation fully. The child protection agency conducted a joint investigation with the prosecutor's office. The child protection agency referred the patient and her mother for a psychological evaluation and treatment following their substantiated finding of inappropriate sexual contact between Jenny and her father.

Interview With Mother

The patient's mother, Nancy, initially reacted to the allegations with disbelief. She, however, clearly exhibited concern for her daughter's health and welfare and slowly demonstrated increasing acceptance of the sexual abuse allegations over time. In retrospect, Nancy indicated that she had been noticing changes in her daughter's behavior, including noncompliance, public masturbatory behavior, nightmares, increasing fearfulness, and dramatic mood swings. Nancy, however, never considered the possibility of sexual abuse as the underlying cause for these behaviors. In fact, aside from Jenny's reluctance to visit her father on just a few occasions, Nancy believed that they had a very good father–daughter relationship.

At the time of the intake, Nancy was employed as an office manger for a small business. She denied suffering any medical problems or substance abuse difficulties, but indicated that she was experiencing mild to moderate anxiety symptoms. In addition to reporting domestic violence experienced during the course of her marriage, Nancy revealed a history of child sexual abuse perpetrated by her stepfather when she was between 8 and 12 years of age. She indicated that the abuse initially consisted of fondling only, but escalated to almost daily vaginal intercourse. While she never disclosed the incidents as a child, Nancy had shared her sexually abusive experiences with a counselor she saw for a brief period shortly after separating from her husband. She acknowledged that she continued to have nightmares about the abuse she suffered over 15 years ago. Nancy indicated that she was considering returning to therapy, as she wanted to avoid getting involved in another abusive relationship.

According to Nancy, Sam held a managerial position for a local department store chain. Nancy was unaware of any medical, psychiatric, or substance abuse difficulties suffered by Sam. She also noted that he never revealed any history of child sexual abuse, although he acknowledged suffering many physical beatings administered by his alcoholic father. Nancy indicated that although Sam rarely drank alcohol, when he did he exhibited a violent temper. He, however, was always very apologetic after these abusive episodes. Sam, in fact, seemed to be both overly dominant toward and dependent on his wife.

Interview With Child

Jenny was a petite child and appeared shy and withdrawn at the first meeting. Nevertheless, she separated from her mother for an individual interview with no difficulty. Nonabuse-related issues were discussed with Jenny initially to gather baseline data on her verbal and affective abilities and to establish rapport. Abuse-related questioning and discussion were introduced gradually. During free play and neutral questioning, Jenny was generally relaxed and cooperative. She, in fact, seemed to enjoy playing with the sexually-detailed dolls. However, when abuse-related questions were posed, she became highly anxious and avoidant. Jenny suddenly lost interest in the dolls, broke eye contact, and physically hid under my desk. After playfully coaxing Jenny out from under the desk, I repeated my questions. Her initial abuse-related disclosures were brief and accompanied by anxious affect. Additionally, like most children her age, Jenny was not able to provide an elaborate description of the course of events but was able to respond to basic questions, including what, where, when, and who. It should also be noted

that Jenny exhibited sexualized behavior during free play with both male and female dolls and was able to demonstrate the allegedly abusive interactions with her father using the dolls. Based on Jenny's verbalizations and demonstrations, the inappropriate sexual contact appeared to involve manual stimulation and genital-to-genital contact. Jenny also indictated that her father told her not to tell her mother about their games. She expressed ambivalent feelings about him, indicating that sometimes she loved him, while at other times he made her mad. Although initially she was very hesitant, Jenny ultimately described the allegedly abusive interactions with her father in a clear, consistent, and emotionally and developmentally appropriate manner.

Conclusion

Overall, the conclusions of this evaluation were consistent with the findings of the child protection agency, indicating a high likelihood of inappropriate sexual contact between the patient and her biological father, Sam. Additionally, Jenny's symptom profiles were consistent with DMS-III-R diagnoses of post-traumatic stress disorder and oppositional disorder. Nancy did not appear to be suffering any major psychiatric disorder, but she was clearly experiencing anxiety and coping difficulties. Cognitive-behavioral therapy requiring the participation of both mother and child was recommended. Initially, Jenny and her mother would be seen individually on a weekly basis for approximately two to three months. Joint sessions would be initiated some time thereafter, depending on Jenny's and her mother's progress.

Treatment

Individual Parent Sessions

The initial parent session was devoted to reviewing the evaluation findings, presenting the rationales for treatment, building rapport, and gathering information. I explained to Nancy that the parent sessions would provide information and skills training to help her cope with her emotional reactions as well as her child's emotional and behavioral responses. I emphasized that while a counselor could provide some therapeutic assistance, she would ultimately be her daughter's most important therapeutic resource, now and long after therapy terminated. I further explained that the healing process would only be initiated during Jenny's individual sessions. As Nancy became more comfortable with abuse-related discussion, she would be encouraged to participate as a cotherapist in joint sessions with her daughter. The rationales for the treatment techniques (e.g., relaxation and abuse-response skills training, gradual exposure) to be used in Jenny's sessions were also provided. While emphasizing that therapy would be difficult for Jenny because the processing of sexually abusive experiences could be painful, I explained that repressing these thoughts and memories could lead to even more damaging long-term consequences, including dysfunctional thought patterns and post-traumatic stress symptoms that could interfere with Jenny's development. Thus, Nancy was forewarned that although her daughter might complain that the sessions were distressing, she would need to encourage Jenny's continued attendance.

During the early stages of therapy, the parent sessions focused on addressing Nancy's cognitive and emotional responses to the discovery of her daughter's abusive experiences. As therapy proceeded, Nancy learned behavior management and communication skills that would assist her in coping with her daughter's difficulties.

I encouraged Nancy to share some of her initial emotions and reactions upon learning about her daughter's disclosure of child sexual abuse. As we talked, dysfunctional thought patterns were identified and educative feedback was provided to correct Nancy's misconceptions and to mediate her negative emotional reactions. For example, Nancy's tendency toward personalization seemed to be producing extreme feelings of guilt for not having prevented the abuse from happening. Information concerning the prevalence and secretive nature of child sexual abuse seemed to temper Nancy's exaggerated sense of responsibility. Nancy also revealed experiencing feelings of anger toward her daughter for not telling her sooner. Together we developed a list of the reasons Jenny may have chosen not to tell; moreover, we identified the positive aspects of her eventual disclosure to her teacher, Mrs. Hall. At the end of the session, Nancy was given an information sheet about child sexual abuse. It provided a general overview of the prevalence, characteristics, and psychological impact of child sexual abuse as well as practical advice for parents who suspect their child has been abused. Nancy agreed to review the information and prepare questions and/or concerns for the next treatment session.

This assignment proved to be more difficult for Nancy than anticipated. During the next session, noting that she had been feeling very down that week, Nancy reported that she could not read the information sheet because she feared it would be too upsetting. After discussing the powerful impact thoughts can have on one's mood (cognitive therapy model), Nancy was asked to share the saddest thought she had experienced during the past week. As the tears rolled down her face, Nancy explained that she had been obsessed with the idea that her

daughter would have to go through all that she had gone through as a child. Nancy described her secretiveness and aloofness as a child and her constant fear that others would find out about her sexual interactions with her stepfather. Nancy was quickly overwhelmed with emotions and would only discuss her personal sexually abusive experiences briefly.

With some encouragement, however, Nancy was able to describe how her daughter's circumstances differed from her own. Nancy began by indicating that she was older (8 years old) when she was abused and that the perpetrator was her stepfather, not her biological father. She needed some prompting before she began acknowledging other differentiating factors that would clearly have a positive influence on Jenny's long-term adjustment, including the patient's early disclosure and the maternal support she was receiving. Nancy's cognitive tendency toward overgeneralization from her experience to her daughter's was discussed. In addition, information and research that strongly suggests that maternal support can positively influence a sexually abused child's adjustment was emphasized with the intention of increasing Nancy's sense of empowerment and reducing her feelings of helplessness. The remainder of the session was spent reviewing the information sheet and discussing the feelings that the information provoked. Methods for positive coping were suggested and practiced (e.g., relaxation skills and sharing feelings with supportive others). In preparation for discussing her daughter's behavior problems, Nancy was asked to begin reading *Families* by Gerald Patterson (an excellent parenting book, ordered from Research Press, Champaign, IL).

By the next session, Nancy seemed to be coping more effectively. She had turned to close family members for assistance, and to her surprise, they were quite supportive. Nancy also had done the assigned reading. She was, in fact, anxious to learn appropriate ways to respond to her child's problem behaviors. The goal for this session was to help Nancy understand her daughter's behaviors in terms of how they are learned and how they are maintained. It was explained that children learn from all their experiences—good experiences, bad experiences, even sexually abusive experiences. The basic principles of social learning were presented to explain the development of both positive and negative behaviors. Jenny, like all other children, learned behaviors from many different sources and people, including perhaps her father, the perpetrator of the abuse. It was explained that problematic behaviors learned during the course of the abuse could be unlearned and replaced by more positive behaviors; children, in fact, may be more resilient because they are so receptive to new learning experiences. Three basic methods of learning were reviewed: observational learning, associative learning, and instrumental learning (learning from consequences).

With some prompting, Nancy was able to identify the learning mechanisms underlying several positive behaviors exhibited by her daughter. Similarly, the patient's abuse-related behaviors were demystified by establishing that the same learning mechanisms seemed to be responsible for their development.

Next, we examined the learning mechanisms that seemed to be responsible for the maintenance of Jenny's abuse-related difficulties. Nancy was encouraged to examine her interactions with her daughter by identifying their antecedents, behaviors, and consequences. This method allowed Nancy to recognize the patterns that seemed to be maintaining her daughter's problematic behaviors.

When reviewing Nancy's daily log, it appeared that the frequency and intensity of the patient's angry outbursts were increasing. Thus, we agreed this would be the first behavior problem we would tackle. For the next session, Nancy would keep a daily record of the interactive patterns (i.e., antecedents, behaviors, and consequences) associated with Jenny's angry outbursts. In addition, Nancy agreed to read Chapters 3 and 4 in *Families*.

During the seven sessions that followed, behavior management skills—including ignoring, differential attention, shaping, and effective commands and instructions—were introduced, particularly as they applied to the management of Jenny's angry outbursts. Nancy was initially resistant; she insisted that these methods would not be appropriate or therapeutic for her daughter. She expressed particular concern about the "cruelty" of ignoring Jenny's angry outbursts. With conviction and indignation in her tone, Nancy asked, "Don't you think Jenny has a right to be angry?" As we slowly examined Jenny's patterns of throwing tantrums, it became apparent that some of the tantrums had little or nothing to do with the abuse she had endured, but instead were simple bids for attention. Moreover, we talked about the long-term consequences of expressing anger in outbursts and tantrums, particularly in the context of peer interactions at school.

Nancy was reassured that the intent of these methods was not simply to eliminate troubling behaviors, but to help Jenny replace them with more effective means of satisfying her needs and/or expressing her emotions. Not only would Jenny learn to express her feelings during her individual sessions, but Nancy would be reinforcing these efforts on a consistent basis at home. Although initially skeptical, Nancy agreed to give the behavior management skills a try. She, however, was warned that an "extinction burst" might occur in response to her initial ignoring of Jenny's outbursts. We joked that Nancy should be prepared to turn up the volume on her Walkman as the outbursts got louder and not to succumb to the temptation to give in at the height of the tantrum.

Individual Child Sessions

To encourage Jenny's sense of control, she was often given a choice as to whether she preferred to have her session before or after her mother's time. Early on, Jenny almost always sent her mother in first. During Jenny's initial therapy session, rapport was developed and a treatment rationale geared to the patient's developmental stage was provided. I explained to Jenny that she would be asked to talk about things that might be upsetting because if she continued to talk about them, it would make her feel better in the long run. She would also learn some skills that would help her deal with troubling problems or situations that might arise in the future. Convincing Jenny that therapy would be worthwhile was not easy. Her facial expressions were very revealing; this was the last place she wanted to be.

THERAPIST: Jenny, did you ever have nightmares and wake up really scared that a monster was in your closet or under your bed?

JENNY: Sometimes I get scared of monsters.

THERAPIST: Sometimes when children are scared of monsters in their closets, they try to hide under the covers or run away from the monster. Do you ever do that, Jenny?

JENNY: I hide under my pillow.

THERAPIST: This usually makes children more afraid. But when children take the covers down, turn on the light, and look in the closet, they find out nothing bad happens and soon feel better. What do you think, Jenny? (I patiently waited for a response, allowing Jenny to set the pace.)

JENNY: (after a long pause) Maybe you're right.

THERAPIST: Even though you may be scared to do that at first, every time you face the monster and nothing bad happens, you will start to feel less scared and less upset. That's why even though it may upset you to talk about the secret games, we are going to try to talk about them. It may be hard at first, but each time you see that nothing bad happens when we're talking, you will start to feel better. You will start to feel less scared and less upset. Does that make sense to you, Jenny?

JENNY: Yeah, I think so.

Rationales like this were provided repeatedly throughout the course of therapy as encouragement for Jenny to overcome her avoidance and continue to confront her abuse-related memories and fears.

During the first phase of therapy (which lasted four sessions), a comfortable and consistent therapeutic environment was established in which Jenny could begin to build skills that would assist her in the recovery process. Through modeling, shaping, and role-playing, Jenny learned communication and relaxation skills. Jenny seemed to enjoy particularly the meditative breathing exercises and the guided imagery that aided her in undergoing a transformation from the tense "tin soldier" to the relaxed and floppy "scarecrow." These skills not only enhanced her sense of control and confidence, but seemed to assist her in coping with the gradual-exposure sessions. The directed, structured exposure sessions were aimed to encourage Jenny to confront gradually her abuse-related fears, thoughts, and memories. Alternative methods of addressing abuse-related issues, however, were always offered (e.g., talking, reading, playing, story telling, or writing letters, poetry, or songs) in order to allow the patient to maintain a sense of control. Moreover, throughout these sessions Jenny received educative and therapeutic feedback and was encouraged to express her emotions and concerns more openly.

Jenny's individual sessions generally began with nonabuse-related play or conversation. Jenny and I began one early session by looking at a magazine together and labeling the emotions the children in the pictures seemed to be exhibiting. Next, we role-played situations in which embarrassment, anger, frustration, and so forth might be experienced, thereby enhancing Jenny's ability to express emotions effectively. Aware of her enthusiasm for doll play, Jenny was later offered the sexually detailed dolls to assist her in expressing the feelings she experienced while playing the "secret games" with her father. Jenny exhibited a strong negative reaction and insisted on throwing the dolls out of the therapy room. I explained that other children liked playing with the dolls, and that they might get lost in the hallway. Thus, Jenny was encouraged to bring the dolls into the therapy room, but she was allowed to put them anywhere she chose within the room. Jenny agreed and placed the dolls in the corner facing the wall. She was then given a choice of drawing or reading a storybook. Jenny chose reading, and with minimal assistance she in fact read the book *It's My Body* by Lory Freeman. As Jenny read, I asked questions relating to the material in the book. Jenny showed some increased anxiety but responded to the general questions posed (e.g., "Does anyone ever tickle you that way? Did you ever feel that way?"). She clearly made an effort to respond to these questions, but fell silent when asked specific questions relating to the "secret games." Still, she was given a great

deal of praise and encouragement for reading and responding to some of the questions posed (i.e., shaping). The conversation then turned to more neutral topics so that by the end of the session, Jenny was feeling comfortable and appeared composed.

During the three sessions that followed, skills training and education continued until Jenny seemed ready to process her own abusive experiences. She was clearly showing less hesitation and greater ease in talking about her fears and discontinued the practice of putting the dolls in the corner. Thus, I suggested that Jenny show me the secret games that she played with her daddy, using the sexually-detailed dolls. Jenny appeared upset by this suggestion and carried the dolls to the corner. However, before placing them down, she held the adult male doll and punched him for several seconds. Jenny was asked if she was angry at the doll and was encouraged to express her anger by talking to the doll rather than punching or throwing the doll. I modeled verbal expression of anger by telling another doll, "I'm angry at you because you called me a name and hurt my feelings. Don't do that anymore." Jenny imitated this response, but addressed her doll as "daddy." I encouraged her to talk to her daddy about the secret games and tell him how the games made her feel, but Jenny remained silent as tears welled up in her eyes.

THERAPIST: Seems like you are pretty sad, Jenny. Can you tell me why you are crying?

JENNY: I am not crying!

THERAPIST: Well, if you feel like crying, it is OK. Remember, we talked about how good it is to talk about how you feel. Can you tell me how you are feeling right now?

JENNY: (letting out a deep breath and allowing the tears to flow) I am sad, and I am mad at my dad.

THERAPIST: Tell the daddy doll how you are feeling.

JENNY: (looking at the doll) Why did you play those games? Now I can't see you anymore, daddy. (crying quietly and after a pause) Why did my daddy make me play those secret games?

THERAPIST: That is a hard question to answer, Jenny. Why do you think your daddy played those games?

JENNY: He plays because he wants to; he likes the secret games.

THERAPIST: You are probably right, Jenny. That makes a lot of sense. Your daddy played those games because he wanted to, even though he probably knew secret games were not OK.

JENNY: Do all daddies play secret games?

THERAPIST: I am glad you asked me that, Jenny. Some daddies play secret touching games with their children.

JENNY: Like my daddy did?

THERAPIST: Yes, but most daddies don't play these games with their children, because they don't want to or because they know it is not OK. Does that make sense to you?

Jenny seemed to understand, but continued to ask questions that appeared to clarify further her understanding of "not OK" touching. Interestingly, she seemed to have at least partial answers to many of her questions, but clearly needed reassurance and confirmation about what she was thinking.

Throughout the remaining five child sessions, Jenny was consistently encouraged to share the details of her abusive experiences as well as the associated feelings and thoughts. To assist her in this process, I offered her many alternative methods, including talking, drawing, doll play, and reading. For Jenny, letter writing seemed to work the best. She wrote or dictated letters to her father, her mother, her teacher, and even the children of the world. Through these letters and discussions, Jenny was increasingly able to confront her most disturbing memories, thoughts, and feelings while also receiving therapeutic and educative feedback.

Joint Sessions

During the final phase of therapy, joint sessions were initiated. Role-playing exercises were used to rehearse Nancy's participation in these sessions as a cotherapist. The joint sessions would help her develop the skills to be an effective therapeutic resource for her daughter once therapy terminated. By the 10th session, Jenny was no longer complaining of nightmares, and her angry outbursts had diminished dramatically. Nancy was clearly sold on behavior management techniques and was anxious to apply them to the patient's sexualized behaviors, which seemed to be gathering momentum. Nancy was experiencing a growing sense that Jenny was timing these displays to cause her mother the greatest discomfort.

As we examined the interactive patterns associated with Jenny's public masturbation, it appeared that the antecedents or settings for these episodes varied dramatically (from the home to fine restaurants). The consequences, however, were more predictable. Nancy consistently reacted with one of two patterns. In public, she made quiet, deliberate, but desperate efforts to redirect the patient's behavior with what amounted to rewards (ice cream, spur-of-the-moment stops in toy stores, etc.). At home, unable to control her frustration, Nancy launched into loud, emotional lectures about respect and decency that seemed to stem from her fear that the behavior might be a precursor to promiscuity. As we talked, Nancy recog-

nized that she was inadvertently providing a great deal of positive reinforcement for Jenny's masturbatory behavior. Even the lectures, as negative as they seemed, satisfied Jenny's desire for attention.

Interestingly, while Nancy had lectured Jenny many times about respect and decency, she had never spoken with her daughter openly and calmly about masturbation or other sexual issues specifically. Nancy, in fact, was not initially encouraged to talk with her daughter about the patient's sexual abusive experiences, as she tended towards extreme emotionality and catastrophizing. These reactions may have modeled ineffective coping and may have inadvertently reinforced Jenny's anxiety and avoidance behaviors early on. During the course of therapy, however, Nancy seemed to process her personal reactions to her daughter's sexual abuse and was coping more effectively. She in fact had sat in on several of her daughter's sessions during which we initially reviewed abuse-response skills and Jenny had later disclosed some of her abusive experiences to her mother. Nancy responded with calm acceptance, praising her daughter's efforts toward disclosure. Still Nancy seemed to have some concerns about her ability to talk openly about masturbation with her daughter. After discussing Nancy's values and expectations concerning masturbatory behavior, we invited Jenny in for a joint session. Before initiating a discussion concerning masturbation, we briefly reviewed and praised Jenny's retention of the abuse-response skills learned.

THERAPIST: Good, Jenny! You told us about "not OK" touching. Now let's talk about "OK" touching. Jenny, is it okay to touch your own "gina" [vagina]?
JENNY: Yes, it's okay. (looks over at her mother) No, maybe, no, I don't know.
THERAPIST: Well, what do you think, Mom? Is it OK for someone to touch their own "gina"?
(Recognizing that Nancy looked confused, I nodded my head yes.)
MOTHER: Yes, it's okay to touch your own gina. I touch my gina when I wash myself in the shower.
THERAPIST: What about you, Jenny, do you touch your gina?
JENNY: Yes, I wash my gina, too. I touch my gina a lot; it tickles when I touch it. I like it so much I can't hardly stop.
THERAPIST: It sounds like sometimes you touch your gina to wash it, and sometimes you touch it to make it tickle.
JENNY: It tickles right here. (points to her vaginal area)
THERAPIST: Many people touch their gina or peepee because it feels good or makes them tickle; that's a

special kind of touching that has a big name. It's called masturbation. Can you say that word, Jenny?

JENNY: Mas-a-bation.

THERAPIST: Good. Masturbation is when someone touches their own gina or peepee because it feels good. That's OK touching, but it is important to know some of the special rules about masturbation.

JENNY: Is that OK, Mommy?

MOTHER: Yes (looks at the therapist, seemingly in desperate need of assistance), but let's learn the rules.

THERAPIST: Masturbation is something that is OK for people to do in private when they are by themselves. So it is OK to touch your gina or to make it tickle when you are alone in a private place. It is not OK to tickle your gina when you are with other people or in a place that is not private. Jenny, do you have a private place where you can be alone?

JENNY: Where?

MOTHER: You have your own room, Jenny. That's a private place.

JENNY: Can I touch my gina in my room?

MOTHER: Yes, that's OK, but you can't do it in the kitchen, living room, or anywhere else.

THERAPIST: Can you explain the rule for your house, Nancy, a little bit better? Speak more slowly and tell us what "it" is and where can you do it?

NANCY: (smiling and carefully, slowly choosing her words as we had role-played earlier) It is OK for people to tickle their ginas or peepees when they are in their own rooms alone. People do it . . . they tickle their ginas because it feels good, and that's OK. The special rule tells us that it is not OK to tickle your gina in public or where there are other people around, but it is OK to tickle your gina when you are in your room with the door closed for privacy.

JENNY: But what about the special rule, mom?

THERAPIST: Can you tell me the special rule now, Jenny?

JENNY: Didn't you hear?

THERAPIST: Yes, but I'd like to hear it from you.

JENNY: It is OK to tickle your gina when you are in your room alone.

SUMMARY

During the final therapy session, the standardized measures used during the evaluation phase were readministered, and the findings were discussed. Jenny and her mother each had participated in 10 individual sessions and 5 joint sessions. While all their difficulties had not been resolved, Jenny showed marked improvement on all self-report measures (i.e., the CDI, STAIC, and Harter scales) with the exception of trait anxiety. Similarly, Nancy's completion of the Child Behavior Checklist and the daily log revealed striking decreases in Jenny's originally targeted problem behaviors. Nancy's personal level of distress as measured by the SCL-90 also showed some improvement.

While Nancy was quite encouraged by these findings, she was reminded that she and Jenny had many hurdles yet to face. It would be a year or more before the child sexual abuse allegations would be heard in criminal court, and the legal outcome was highly uncertain. Jenny's father, Sam, continued to insist on his innocence and would likely press for renewed visitation and/or custody if a not-guilty verdict was handed down. I indicated that these events could lead to some relapse of symptoms. Moreover, I explained that as Jenny progressed through each developmental stage (e.g., adolescence), new abuse-related issues and concerns could arise. Thus, while we applauded Jenny's achievements, we reviewed the skills (e.g., abuse response and emotion expression skills) and identified resources (e.g., booster sessions, support groups, victim/witness assistance) that could be tapped for therapeutic assistance in the future. Jenny had a good start, but she and her mother would need to practice their skills and utilize the available resources to continue the healing process.

REFERENCES

Achenbach, T. M. (1991a). *Manual for the Child Behavior Checklist/4–18 and 1991 Profile*. Burlington, VT: University of Vermont Department of Psychiatry.

Achenbach, T. M. (1991b). *Manual for the Teacher's Report Form and 1991 Profile*. Burlington, VT: University of Vermont Department of Psychiatry.

Deblinger, E., McLeer, S. V., Atkins, M. S., Ralphe, D., & Foa, E. (1989). Post-traumatic stress in sexually abused, physically abused and nonabused children. *Child Abuse and Neglect, 13*, 403–408.

Derogatis, L. R. (1983). *The SCL-90-R Administration, Scoring and Procedures Manual-II*. Baltimore: Clinical Psychometric Research.

deYoung, M. (1986). A conceptual model for judging the truthfulness of a young child's allegations of sexual abuse. *American Journal of Orthopsychiatry, 56*, 550–559.

Faller, K. C. (1984). Is the child victim of sexual abuse telling the truth? *Child Abuse and Neglect, 8*, 473–481.

Harter, S. (1985). *Manual for the Social Support Scale for Children*. Denver: University of Denver.

Kelly, S. J. (1985). Interviewing the sexually abused child: Principle and techniques. *Journal of Emergency Nursing, 5*, 234–241.

Kovacs, M. (1983). *The Children's Depression Inventory: A self-*

rated depression scale for school-aged youngsters. Unpublished manuscript.

McLeer, S. V., Deblinger, E., Atkins, M. S., Foa, E., & Ralphe, D. (1988). Post-traumatic stress disorder in sexually abused children. *Journal of the American Academy of Child & Adolescent Psychiatry, 27(5)*, 650–654.

Spielberger, C. D. (1973). *Preliminary manual for the State-Trait Anxiety Inventory for Children*. Palo Alto, CA: Consulting Psychologists.

Summit, R. C. (1989). Hidden victims, hidden pain: Societal avoidance of child sexual abuse. In G. E. Wyatt & G. J. Powell (Eds.), *Lasting effects of child sexual abuse* (pp. 39–60). Newbury Park, CA: Sage.

White, S., Strom, G. A., Santelli, G., & Halpin, B. M. (1986). Interviewing young sexual abuse victims with anatomically correct dolls. *Child Abuse and Neglect, 4*, 519–529.

SUGGESTED READINGS

Berliner, L., & Wheeler, J. R. (1987). Treating the effects of sexual abuse on children. *Journal of Interpersonal Violence, 2(4)*, 415–434.

Clark, L. (1985). *SOS! Help for parents*. Bowling Green, KY: Parents Press.

Deblinger, E., McLeer, S. V., & Henry, D. (1990). Cognitive behavioral treatment for sexually abused children suffering post-traumatic stress. *Journal of the American Academy of Child and Adolescent Psychiatry, 29(5)*, 747–752.

Friedrich, W. N. (1990). *Psychotherapy of sexually abused children and their families*. New York: W. W. Norton.

Patterson, G. R. (1975). *Families: Applications of social learning to family life*. Champaign, IL: Research Press.

16

Bulimia Nervosa

David M. Garner

OVERVIEW

In recent years there has been extraordinary interest in cognitive therapy for eating disorders. Treatment reviews in this area indicate that cognitive therapy has been the subject of the majority of empirical evaluations, with results indicating that it is particularly effective for bulimia nervosa (see Garner, Fairburn, & Davis, 1987). At this stage, support for its use with anorexia nervosa rests largely on clinical evidence, since no controlled trials of efficacy have been published. The reason for this probably relates to the fact that the treatment of anorexia nervosa is usually a complicated and lengthy process involving the need for weight restoration as well as the integration of inpatient and outpatient phases of care.

PRESENTING COMPLAINTS AND BACKGROUND INFORMATION

Mary is a 29-year-old computer programmer who lives with her husband and two children, a girl (age 8) and a boy (age 5). She is 5'4" tall and weighed 155 pounds (mild obesity, defined by a weight 20% higher than age-

David M. Garner • Department of Psychiatry, Michigan State University, East Lansing, Michigan 48824-1316.

Comprehensive Casebook of Cognitive Therapy, edited by Arthur Freeman and Frank M. Dattilio. Plenum Press, New York, 1992.

and height-adjusted weight norms) at initial assessment. She sought treatment because of binge eating and self-induced vomiting occurring at least three times daily for over a year. She reported that she did not remember any days in the past six months in which she had not binged and vomited at least once. At least once a week, she added, she would binge and vomit 15 or more times in a day. The types of foods consumed on a binge usually consisted of those typically prohibited from her diet, such as desserts and other sweet foods that were high in fat content; however, she would also often binge on other foods that were not proscribed from her daily diet. Binge-eating episodes usually involved consuming more than 1000 calories of food before vomiting; however, she also described vomiting after eating small amounts because of feeling "guilty" or "bloated." She also reported abusing laxatives, taking between 5 and 10 Ex-Lax tablets daily. There was no reported history of diuretic, alcohol, or drug abuse.

Mary described herself as having been very concerned about her weight for as long as she could remember. She stated that she was a "fat" child and adolescent. Reportedly, her mother pressured her continually to lose weight, often seeking help for her daughter from various specialists and weight loss programs during the childhood and adolescent years. Mary could not remember a time when she had not been on a diet. Her typical pattern was to restrict her eating during the week and then binge on weekends. She indicated that her episodic bingeing began early in adolescence, but that the vomiting and laxative abuse had not begun until about five years before she sought treatment. At first, vomiting was infrequent, occurring usually less than once a month and following a particularly large binge-eating episode.

Mary's weight had fluctuated widely since adolescence; the highest was 200 pounds approximately three years ago. When she married at 19 years of age, her weight fluctuated around 130 pounds. Following the birth of each of her two children, her weight escalated by about 20 pounds. Her lowest weight since the birth of her second child was 145 pounds; this occurred about a year and a half prior to treatment, following the completion of one of the popular very-low-calorie diet programs. The diet program involved consuming a liquid formula of just over 400 calories a day for about three months, followed by the gradual reintroduction of conventional foods. This resulted in a 55-pound weight loss, and improved mood that lasted for several months. Mary then gradually began deviating from the maintenance diet of 1,200 calories a day, and despite extraordinary efforts to hold her urges to eat in check, she began slowly gaining weight while experiencing a marked return of the binge eating.

Mary was the eldest of five children raised in a middle-class home. Her mother was a high school teacher, and her father was a librarian. Mary described her mother as moderately obese and chronically struggling with her own weight. She was also described as extremely energetic, devoted, and competent at her job. Mary indicated that she admired her mother tremendously for her ability to raise five children and perform so well in her job. According to Mary, her father was not obese but "had a big stomach from drinking too much beer." He was shy, quiet, and described as much happier with books than with people. He had, however, taken an active role in child rearing, and Mary described a warm relationship with him.

Mary reported a history of excellent academic achievement from grade school through college, where she had majored in computer sciences. At the onset of treatment, she was a supervisor with considerable responsibility in a computer software firm. Her husband knew about her binge eating and self-induced vomiting and felt that it was related to the stresses of her job. He reportedly felt that she could stop if she exercised willpower, and that this was the one area of her life that she simply could not control. Mary had become increasingly depressed about her eating disorder during the six months prior to treatment, found little pleasure in her work or family, and sincerely wondered whether life was worth living. She said that she had not seriously considered suicide, primarily because she felt that it would be unfair to her children.

ASSESSMENT AND DIAGNOSIS

The initial evaluation as well as ongoing assessment of the eating-disorder patient may be divided into two broad areas. The first relates to attitudes toward weight and shape, as well as symptoms that are fundamental to the eating disorder. The second is aimed at the various psychosocial factors that may predispose toward or maintain the eating disorder. Accordingly, the initial assessments should cover several key areas, including (a) weight history; (b) attitudes toward weight and shape; (c) the presence, frequency, and duration of bingeing and vomiting; (d) details of weight-losing behaviors such as dieting, exercise, abuse of laxatives, diuretics, and appetite suppressants; (e) complications, such as swollen parotid glands, edema, paresthesia, and erosion of dental enamel (cardiac and metabolic functioning should be evaluated by a physician familiar with the complications of eating disorders); (f) psychological state, with particular reference to depression, anxiety, and personality features; (g) impulse-related behaviors; (h) social and family functioning; (i) reasons for seeking treatment; and (j) motivation for change. The relevance of each of these areas is discussed in detail in the articles suggested for reading at the end of this chapter. The interviewer should be familiar with specific questions or probes aimed at assessing eating-disorder symptoms (Garner & Parker, 1993).

The clinical features and background information that shape the approach to treatment are best derived from a clinical interview; however, psychometric evaluation with standardized psychological tests is also recommended. The Eating Disorder Inventory (EDI) is a widely used self-report measure that provides standardized scores for psychological dimensions commonly associated with anorexia nervosa and bulimia nervosa (see Garner, 1991). Mary had markedly elevated EDI subscale scores on drive for thinness, body dissatisfaction, bulimia, ineffectiveness, and perfectionism. Other self-report instruments indicated that she was experiencing moderate to severe depression, anxiety, and interpersonal sensitivity. Personality testing indicated that Mary had an obsessional style, with some evidence of poor impulse regulation and was suggestive of a possible borderline personality disorder.

INITIAL INTERVIEWS (MONTH 1 OF TREATMENT)

There are a number of general treatment principles and issues considered central to cognitive-behavioral therapy with eating disorders. These include (a) giving special attention to the therapeutic relationship, (b) enhancing motivation for change, (c) using a directive style, (d) following a two-track approach (the first pertains to issues related to weight, bingeing, and vomiting; the second addresses beliefs and thematic underlying assumptions that are relevant to the development and maintenance of the eating disorder), (e) recognizing and addressing ego-syntonic symptoms, (f) differentiating starvation symptoms from primary psychopathology, and (g) enlisting special strategies to normalize eating and weight. Since these have been described fully in previous publications (see Suggested Readings), they will be only briefly touched upon here to the extent that they pertain to the case material presented.

Much of the initial interview with Mary was devoted to obtaining detailed information related to attitudes and behaviors pertaining to the eating, dieting, and weight control practices outlined earlier. Mary indicated that she wanted to find a way to stop bingeing and vomiting because she felt that her symptoms were ruining her life. They had begun to interfere with her functioning at work: she would get up each morning with a firm resolve not to engage in a binge-eating episode but would then leave work and go to the fast-food area in a local mall to binge. She would then vomit and come back to work feeling depressed and hopeless. Mary also indicated that she wanted to gain control of her eating so that she could meet her weight goal of 130 pounds. Mary was asked for specific details of food eaten for all meals, snacks, and binge episodes for the past week. Mary's explicit objective was to limit her daily food intake to less than 1,000 calories. Except for a binge, she would only permit herself foods that had "healthy" and calorie-sparing connotations.

Mary conceptualized her binge eating as relating to an "addiction" to certain foods, particularly those that were high in sugar content. She also said that she would binge in response to stress or when she was feeling other emotions (such as boredom, anxiety, and anger). She also reported that her relationship with her husband had not been very rewarding over the past several years. She complained that he had seemed to become more distant and less interested in the family, and had left her to try to deal with the responsibilities at home in addition to major commitments at her job. Mary's husband had initially been very supportive of her dieting attempts but had become increasingly discontented with her recent failure to gain control over her binge eating.

After the above information had been gathered and other areas explored as outlined above, the therapist provided an initial formulation, a detailed overview of particular psychoeducational material (Garner, Rockert, Olmsted, Johnson, & Coscina, 1985), and specific recommendations for managing the eating-disorder symptoms. The initial formulation was as follows:

THERAPIST: You have really been helpful in answering an incredible number of questions. I would like to give you my initial impression of what I think is going on. The issues that are likely contributing to your disorder can be divided into two broad areas. The first relates to a host of possible background factors that could be important in the development and the maintenance of your eating disorder. Also, there may be things that have gone on in your distant or immediate past that have contributed to emotional difficulties, and it may turn out that they only tangentially relate to your eating disorder. If this is the case, these areas should be taken seriously and addressed because they are important in their own right.

It is important to leave the door open to the exploration of potential sources of psychopathology, since the initial formulation and the educational material to be covered next emphasize cultural factors as the most parsimonious determinants of the eating disorder. The patient needs to be reassured now and repeatedly throughout the course of treatment that serious consideration will be given to other issues that emerge as fundamental to the eating disorder, as well as those that really are best considered as functionally autonomous.

THERAPIST: (continuing) The second relates to the fact that there is good evidence that many eating-disorder symptoms are the direct result of dieting and weight suppression. Clearly, your attempts to control your weight have been a major theme for you for many years. Your mother was quite determined to have you lose weight. You have devoted an extraordinary amount of effort and thought to weight control over the past two decades. This makes complete sense, since you have grown up in a culture that has placed you under enormous pressure to diet in order to maintain a thin body shape. These cultural ideals have been reinforced by the multibillion-dollar-a-year diet industry that obviously has had a major stake in convincing women that they need to lose weight. This has been further reinforced by the strong and consistent messages from the health professions warning of the risks associated with obesity. I want to take a few minutes to review some specific points.

The therapist then reviewed the evidence that substantiates the following points described in detail by Garner et al. (1985):

1. In the past several decades, women have been victims of a tragic set of standards for physical appearance that have placed them under intense pressure to diet to meet the social expectations for thinness.
2. Generally speaking, body weight resists change. Weight appears to be physiologically regulated around a set point, a weight that one's body tries to "defend." Significant deviations from this weight result in a myriad of physiological compensations aimed at returning the organism to the set point.
3. Dieting is a relatively ineffective method of weight control because it usually goes against these biological determinants of weight.
4. There are marked interpersonal differences in these set points; some people are naturally heavier, and some naturally thinner. Most women's "natural weight" is well above the current ideal for physical attractiveness.
5. Bulimia, as well as certain distressing biological and social changes, may be linked to chronic dietary restriction.
6. Bulimia and vomiting become an escalating or vicious cycle, since vomiting allows the dieter to give in to her desire to eat without the fear of the caloric consequences.
7. The gradual return to the weight that one's body "prefers" leads to the gradual reduction of these symptoms, including the tendency toward binge eating.

These points have to be covered with sensitivity to resistance or fear that they might generate. Periodic statements such as "Does this make sense so far?" or "How do you feel so far about what I have said?" and being attuned to nonverbal signs of anger, fear, anxiety, and withdrawal are particularly important in pacing the presentation of the educational material. If the patient balks at any point, the source of concern should be identified and explored. It may be necessary to proceed more slowly or to curtail the educational mode of discussion temporarily while attempting to deal with emergent issues.

The use of an educational approach has several major advantages. First, there is intrinsic value in clarifying misunderstandings related to bodily functioning and weight control. Second, the suggestion that certain symptoms and behaviors may be logically derived from cultural pressures on women to diet, rather than being purely psychogenic in nature, may diminish potential untoward effects associated with psychiatric labeling. Third, sometimes educational material can provide the basis for testing and refining beliefs that drive symptomatic behavior. For example, if convincing evidence is presented on a point such as "Laxatives do not produce malabsorption," then other assumptions behind continued use of laxatives must be explored.

THERAPIST: I want to give some special attention to your use of laxatives. You have told me that you use laxatives, but what I would like to know is what it is specifically that you think that laxatives do for you—why exactly do you use them?

MARY: I use them to get rid of the food.

THERAPIST: When you say "get rid of the food," what do you mean?

MARY: It makes the food go through you faster so that you do not gain weight from the calories.

THERAPIST: You mean that you think that the calories will not be absorbed?

MARY: Yes.

THERAPIST: OK, I think that there are some things that you should know about the way that laxatives work.

The therapist then reviewed the studies (see Garner et al., 1985) indicating that laxatives appear to "work" not by creating malabsorption but rather by altering fluid balance through their influence on electrolytes.

The purpose of this interchange is to lay the groundwork for the recommendation that the patient begin to discontinue the use of laxatives. One of two things will usually happen: In most cases, the patient will discontinue using the laxatives without a great degree of difficulty. In others, there will be varying degrees of resistance to abandoning the laxative abuse; in such cases, it is important for the therapist to explore in detail the beliefs that are responsible for the resistance to change.

MARY: I don't think that I can stand the feeling of gaining weight once I stop taking the laxatives, even if it is just water [catastrophizing].

THERAPIST: Well, let's look at the alternatives. Either you try to give them up and allow your body to straighten out its water balance system, or you must take them for the rest of your life, since to some degree you have habituated to them.

MARY: They give me a sense of security. I get so anxious if I go without them for more than a day. I also get so bloated that I think I will explode.

THERAPIST: There are two issues here. First, you do not sound as if you have given yourself enough time off the laxatives to learn that, after a period of rebound, your body will sort out its water balance very well. It is getting over the initial two weeks or so that is the real hurdle. The second relates to the issue of security.

Laxatives don't work. They give you a *false* sense of security because they have become a way that you can "undo" the effects of a binge. In fact, because you have them at your disposal, they may even license you to binge because you have something to use to "get rid of the food." But as we have reviewed, they only change your water balance, they do not negate the caloric effects of the food.

MARY: OK, I will try, but it is terrifying. I won't be able to go on if my weight goes up. Everyone will notice my weight change, and I could not stand it if someone noticed or even commented on the change [catastrophizing, overgeneralization, selective abstraction].

THERAPIST: If it is frightening and you still maintained your resolve to abstain from laxatives, it would be a real sign that you are doing something different—that you are making genuine headway toward recovery [reframing, practicing alternative behaviors in response to the same affective stimulus]. I wonder if others really are that concerned about the change [decentering]? Do you notice changes in other people's weight from week to week?

MARY: I really don't notice small changes in others, but I might notice a large change. What if my weight goes up really fast?

THERAPIST: This may be a time to consider yourself and your welfare first rather than put other people's opinion first. You have suffered enormously because of your eating disorder, and I wonder if others have really had any more investment in your weight than you have had in theirs. There is an element of flattery in considering that others really care about things like your weight, but once you realize that others are really not that interested, it is liberating.

MARY: I know that the main reason that I binge eat is in response to stress at work and at home.

THERAPIST: Maybe you can tell me a bit more about how your binge eating is caused by stress.

MARY: Every time I am under stress at work, I seem to binge eat. The binge eating is an excuse for not having to deal with the stress in a more appropriate way.

THERAPIST: It is very likely that stress precipitates binge eating, and it is important for us to talk further about the sources of stress in your life, because these may very well reflect serious problems. However, it is important to recognize that binge eating is also closely linked to dieting and weight suppression attempts. It is possible to experimentally produce binge eating in people who do not have any apparent preexisting psychological aberrations simply by having them restrict their dietary intake [this was followed by a review of the evidence]. You may want to consider why binge eating is apparently so much more common in women these days than in men. This probably relates to the fact that dieting is endemic to women today, and this relates to the inordinate pressures on women in our culture to be thin. If stress rather than dieting were the primary *cause* of binge eating, then we should really expect an epidemic of binge eating on Wall Street these days!

During initial sessions, Mary was encouraged to keep self-monitoring records of her eating, bingeing, vomiting, laxative abuse, mood, circumstances surrounding eating, and eating symptoms. After the first session, her bingeing and vomiting declined dramatically. She vomited twice in the next three weeks and did not vomit thereafter during the course of treatment. She reported subjective "binges" (consuming amounts of food that were not objectively large outside of planned meals) about once a week, but was able to inhibit her subsequent urges to vomit or take laxatives. She did not take any laxatives after the first session and gained about five pounds in the first week. It was explained that this large weight gain was probably related to rehydration after discontinuing the laxative abuse. Mary was encouraged to begin consuming as close to 2,000 calories a day as possible, as this amount allowed her to have "nondietetic" meals and snacks each day. After the third week of treatment, Mary's weight remained relatively stable for several weeks, and then she gradually gained another five to seven pounds over the entire four-month course of treatment.

SUBSEQUENT SESSIONS (MONTHS 2 THROUGH 4)

After the first month of treatment, most of Mary's eating symptoms were under control. Rapid treatment response is not unusual for patients receiving cognitive-behavioral therapy for bulimia nervosa, although many patients may require prolonged treatment (see Garner et al., 1987). The remainder of Mary's treatment focused on consolidating early improvements and on factors (inferred from comments Mary made about her body weight) that were considered to increase her risk for relapse. Time was also spent on exploring Mary's background in detail (e.g., experiences in her family of origin, possible trauma such as emotional or sexual abuse, past relationships, current relations with her husband and children) in order to understand fully the context for her system of current beliefs about eating and her body. Many times, a systematic evaluation of the patient's current and past functioning reveals major sources of emotional distress that may not directly relate to the eating disorder but that have been dismissed previously as not justifying treatment in their own right. Obviously, these areas are just as appropriate for cognitive interventions as those specifically related to the eating disorder.

Although Mary was able to accept the fact that she must temporarily adopt a "nondieting" eating pattern in order to overcome her binge eating, she continued to engage in extraordinary self-disparagement because of her weight. Her concerns about her weight escalated as it slowly increased over the course of treatment. Bulimia nervosa patients at a statistically normal weight who complain about "feeling fat" at least theoretically could be provided with objective evidence to confront this "distortion"; any potential salutary effect of this type of evidence has little effect for those who are objectively overweight.

A major theme in Mary's treatment involved providing her with a rationale for not dieting in the face of her obesity. She maintained that her current weight (a) was inappropriate given the recommended weights for her age and height, (b) was unhealthy, (c) had negative social consequences, and (d) was inherently loathsome and thus contributed to her low self-esteem. Moreover, eating 2,000 calories a day and including certain good-tasting foods was inconsistent with much of the advice that she had received in the past during various weight loss programs delivered by health professionals. A theme repeatedly emphasized throughout treatment involved helping Mary alter certain disparaging assumptions regarding her own weight and obesity in general. The following is an example of a typical interchange, in which several cognitive techniques were employed.

MARY: I am pleased that my binge eating has improved, but I hate my weight. I am fat, and I weigh much more than I should. Just look at any weight chart.

THERAPIST: It is important that your binge eating has improved, and I think that this may be directly linked to the changes that you have made in your eating patterns. With regard to your weight, there are a number of real problems with weight charts, not the least of which is that they fail to take into consideration that body weight, like other physical and psychological attributes, is distributed normally in the population (draws a bell-shaped curve on the blackboard). We readily accept that intelligence, grades in school, height, heart rate, reaction time, and many other traits are distributed in the population so that most people fall somewhere around the average, but that it is expected that some people naturally are situated at the extremes. We may have some degree of control about where we fall with

regard to some of these traits, but this is often limited by things that we have no control over. There is more and more evidence that genetic factors play a major role in weight, and given your personal and family history, your "natural weight" is probably higher than the population average—so is your intelligence. It is absurd that we still depend upon weight charts that are some variation on average weights, to draw inferences about what a given individual should weigh. Can you imagine how ridiculous this type of formula would be in trying to establish "recommended heights"?

MARY: Yeah, but you can't do anything about height. You can change how much you eat.

THERAPIST: This may be true, but there is increasing evidence that in our culture, where there is ready access to good-tasting foods, genetics plays a major role in the expression of obesity [the therapist goes on to review some of this evidence; Garner and Wooley, 1991]. There is also convincing evidence that obese people do not eat more than the non-obese [ditto].

MARY: You mean that I am going to have to accept being fat all of my life. I can't stand it; I will never give up hope that I can be thinner. (crying) Being fat is disgusting. Everybody sees you as lacking self-control, having no self-respect, being incompetent. If there is agreement on any point in our society, it is that "thin is in" and fat people are only rationalizing if they say that their weight is OK.

THERAPIST: I can understand why you are so upset. The level of prejudice that is felt toward obesity is tremendous; it is one of the few remaining socially sanctioned forms of prejudice today. What is tragic is that you have spent most of your life loathing an attribute that has been part of you. You have been a victim of a particularly pervasive social stereotype about weight that has virtually required self-rejection. What is important to recognize is that you have a choice about believing or rejecting that self-defeating prejudice.

MARY: How can I reject something that everyone believes?

THERAPIST: First, is it true that *everyone* believes it?

MARY: Well, maybe not everyone, but most people do.

THERAPIST: Popularity has never been a particularly good index of the legitimacy of an idea. Do you have any beliefs or practices that you value greatly, but that are shared by only a small minority of the population?

MARY: Well, not really.

THERAPIST: For example, I remember you telling me that you had some pretty militant feelings about civil rights issues a few years ago that were pretty unpopular with your family.

MARY: I guess maybe you are right.

THERAPIST: In fact, obese people today form a minority group that is discriminated against in many ways. I wonder if some of the views that you have had about obesity have not been inconsistent with the highly humane values that you have applied to other minority groups.

MARY: You are right, but I have a long way to go to believe it.

THERAPIST: You have made a very good start. Believing it is a gradual process.

Challenging current cultural prejudices related to fatness without inadvertently attacking the personal values on which the patient bases self-esteem is a delicate task requiring thoughtfulness, a trusting therapeutic relationship, and a sense of pacing that is only crudely illustrated in case dialogue. Also, the "persuasive" cognitive style (like that illustrated above) has certain disadvantages over the Socratic method. Nevertheless, when the beliefs being challenged are highly culturally syntonic and support a distortion or self-defeating attribution, it may be necessary to draw upon evidence from highly credible sources such as scientific studies and to use more forceful methods in order to counteract the popular but self-defeating assumptions.

In the last month of treatment, Mary's eating symptoms were completely under control. She reported no urges to binge or to engage in dieting behaviors. Most of the last month was spent continuing to address her negative feelings about obesity. She was able to recognize that her disparagement of her own shape was based on assumptions about obesity in general that were inaccurate, arbitrary, inhumane, self-defeating, and inconsistent with her other principles for viewing human worth. She expressed considerable anger toward the fashion and dieting industries for promoting superficial standards for judging women's self-worth exclusively in terms of physical appearance. Mary was able to see that her mother's view of her obesity was an important factor in determining the strength of conviction about weight control that had led to her repeated attempts at weight loss. She was able to see how her early family environment had provided a window through which cultural values had been viewed and magnified. She was able to make headway at decoupling her self-esteem from her weight. Mary's anger gradually transformed into determination to organize a small group of like-minded women to engage in small-scale lobbying efforts directed toward diet advertisers who portray emaciated women as attractive and who suggest that permanent weight loss is a realistic goal.

SUMMARY

Mary responded very favorably to cognitive-behavioral intervention that emphasized establishing normal eating patterns by (a) increasing caloric intake to appropriate nondieting levels, (b) spacing meals so that food was consumed throughout the day rather than just in the evening, (c) gradually incorporating "forbidden foods," and (d) inhibiting urges to diet or engage in weight-controlling behaviors. These behaviors and their maladaptive alternatives are clearly linked to beliefs, underlying assumptions, and complex meaning systems. These had to be thoroughly addressed in order to optimize the durability of the new behaviors.

More emphasis was placed on controlling dieting than controlling bingeing, since the dieting efforts were conceptualized as the primary cause of the urge to binge. Challenging underlying assumptions related to dieting and obesity was the primary focus of treatment. However, more general themes related to self-esteem, family of origin relationships as they related to attitudes toward eating and self-definition, and current sources of job stress. Mary was abstinent from bingeing and vomiting after the first month of treatment. At one-year follow-up, she reported no disturbed eating patterns, and the improvements in general psychological functioning had been maintained.

DISCUSSION

Illustrating cognitive therapy for eating disorders using the case study format has the primary advantage of providing concrete examples of actual interventions, giving life to otherwise sterile theoretical accounts of treatment. Unfortunately, the case study format has a number of disadvantages that are particularly important in illustrating the treatment of eating disorders. It has repeatedly been emphasized that eating disorders are multidetermined and present with a myriad of associated forms of psychopathology. The case presented here demonstrates only one set of presenting problems, underlying assumptions, application of the method, format for delivery, duration of treatment, and resolution among a wide array of possibilities. Mary did not present with other primary psychopathology in addition to her eating disorder; it became evident that the psychological distress that she did report was secondary to her chaotic eating patterns. There are many bulimia nervosa patients whose presentation and course are not so straightforward, although the use of the cognitive techniques outlined here and elsewhere may still be quite effective.

The above case illustration could unwittingly convey the impression that simply recognizing a flawed underlying assumption is sufficient for change, whereas in most instances, there is a tremendous amount of creative redundancy required to essentially relearn a more accurate or adaptive system of thinking. Effective cognitive interventions can be brief in some cases, but for others they assume a lengthy course. Individual, group, or family therapy formats each may be advantageous for certain patients, or they may be combined in some instances. For some patients, inpatient treatment is necessary to normalize eating and weight, to interrupt bingeing, vomiting, or laxative abuse, to treat complications, and occasionally to disengage the family from destructive interactional patterns. Although there are many areas of overlap in treatment for anorexia nervosa and bulimia nervosa, there are important differences. Many of the nuances of treatment go well beyond the scope of the preceding case presentation but have been described in detail elsewhere (see Garner & Bemis, 1985; Garner & Rosen, 1990). The account of the style, course, and content of treatment for the case presented above should be understood with the limitations of the case study format in mind.

REFERENCES

Garner, D. M. (1986). Cognitive therapy for bulimia nervosa. *Annals of Adolescent Psychiatry, 13*, 358–390.

Garner, D. M. (1991). *Eating Disorder Inventory-2 professional manual*. Odessa, FL: Psychological Assessment Resources.

Garner, D. M., & Bemis, K. M. (1982). A cognitive-behavioral approach to anorexia nervosa. *Cognitive Therapy and Research, 6*, 123–150.

Garner, D. M., & Bemis, K. M. (1985). Cognitive therapy for anorexia nervosa. In D. M. Garner & P. E. Garfinkel (Eds.), *Handbook of psychotherapy for anorexia nervosa and bulimia*, (pp. 107–146). New York: Guilford.

Garner, D. M., Fairburn, C. G., & Davis, R. (1987). Cognitive-behavioral treatment of bulimia nervosa: A critical appraisal. *Behavior Modification, 11*, 398–431.

Garner, D. M., & Parker, P. (1993). Multimodal assessment of eating disorders. In T. H. Ollendick & M. Hersen (Eds.), *Handbook of child and adolescent assessment*. Boston: Allyn & Bacon.

Garner, D. M., Rockert, W., Olmsted, M. P., Johnson, C. L., & Coscina, D. V. (1985). Psychoeducational principles in the treatment of bulimia and anorexia nervosa. In D. M. Garner & P. E. Garfinkel (Eds.), *Handbook of psychotherapy for anorexia nervosa and bulimia*, (pp. 513–572). New York: Guilford.

Garner, D. M., & Rosen, L. W. (1990). Anorexia nervosa and bulimia nervosa. In A. S. Bellack, M. Hersen, & A. E. Kazdin (Eds.), *International handbook of behavior modification and therapy* (2nd ed., pp. 805–817). New York: Plenum.

Garner, D. M., & Wooley, S. C. (1991). Confronting the failure of behavioral and dietary treatments for obesity. *Clinical Psychology Review, 11*, 729–780.

SUGGESTED READINGS

Fairburn, C. G. (1985). Cognitive-behavioral treatment for bulimia. In D. M. Garner & P. E. Garfinkel (Eds.), *Handbook of psychotherapy for anorexia nervosa and bulimia* (pp. 160–192). New York: Guilford.

Garner, D. M. (1988). Anorexia nervosa. In M. Hersen & C. G. Last (Eds.), *Child behavior therapy casebook* (pp. 263–276). New York: Plenum.

Garner, D. M., Rockert, W., Davis, R., Garner, M. V., Olmsted, M. P., & Eagle, M. (in press). A comparison between cognitive-behavioral and supportive-expressive therapy for bulimia nervosa. *American Journal of Psychiatry*.

Garner, D. M., Garfinkel, P. E., and Irvine, M. J. (1986). Integration and sequencing of treatment approaches for eating disorders. *Psychotherapy and Psychosomatics, 46*, 67–75.

Garner, D. M., (1992). Psychotherapy for eating disorders. *Current Opinion in Psychiatry, 5*, 391–395.

17

Obesity

Andrea Karfgin and David Roth

INTRODUCTION

The cognitive approach to obesity has experienced a profound evolution over the past quarter century. Working from a 1960s operant framework, practitioners, utilizing state-of-the-art techniques, focused primarily upon modifying eating-related behaviors, propitiously arranging the consummatory behavioral environment, and judiciously orchestrating contingencies for weight and behavioral change. Self-monitoring of eating behaviors and their situational context was in vogue during these early years. With the cognitive revolution in clinical psychology came significant additions to the core treatment regimen for obesity. Clients learned how to assess and correct the maladaptive thinking that directly contributes to the etiology and maintenance of obesity. Cognitive restructuring, guided imagery, self-instructional training, goal setting, self-reinforcement, and problem solving are but a few of the interrelated, cognitively based procedures that have been incorporated into preexisting behavioral programs.

Over the past five years, a new series of advances has taken place. Now we have a truly comprehensive cognitive-behavioral therapy for obesity. Our clients are taught the ABCs of good nutrition; some may in fact be placed on a low-calorie diet. The importance of life-style change—and particularly the meaningful incorporation of exercise into one's day-to-day existence—is stressed. The value of social support, whether in the form of Overeaters Anonymous, family therapy, or peer encouragement, is widely recognized. Moreover, obesity is no longer treated as a distinct entity without biopsychosocial roots. Our clients are not shunted into a prepackaged program, but instead are evaluated by medically and psychologically sophisticated providers who aim to individualize therapy. A patient's history of abuse, low self-esteem, marital problems, hypothyroid disease, and so forth is assessed and addressed. What follows is a case description that details the use of a comprehensive multimodal, cognitive-behavioral treatment for obesity.

CASE REPORT

Sheila was a 48-year-old mental health professional and mother of two grown children. At the time of her initial psychiatric contact, her medium-sized 5'8" frame was supporting a weight of 260 pounds. Although she had recently gained 40 pounds, she had little understanding of the internal and external forces contributing to this weight gain. She felt out of control and described herself as "at wit's end."

An intelligent and articulate woman, Sheila realized that her lifelong struggle with obesity was more than a

Andrea Karfgin • Coordinator, Dissociative Disorders Program, Sheppard Pratt Hospital, Towson, Maryland 21204. David Roth • Inpatient and Outpatient Eating Disorders Program, Sheppard Pratt Hospital, Towson, Maryland 21204.

Comprehensive Casebook of Cognitive Therapy, edited by Arthur Freeman and Frank M. Dattilio. Plenum Press, New York, 1992.

battle for willpower. She believed that her dysfunctional eating patterns were a somatic manifestation of powerful psychological events. Prior "uncovering" therapies had not been effective in the management of her eating behavior. On the advice of her friends and through her own research, Sheila opted for a trial of cognitive therapy. She reasoned that this orientation would help her identify those thoughts, feelings, and behaviors that contributed to her ongoing cycle of weight loss and gain with concurrent fluctuations in self-esteem and mood.

BACKGROUND

Sheila was born and raised in the deep South, the second of three daughters and "a Great Dane in a litter of Pekingese." Her 4'10" petite mother most likely suffered from recurrent unipolar depression and somatization disorder and, more frequently than not, orchestrated the family activities from her "sickbed." Her father was a traveling salesman and baseball fanatic whose limited caregiving abilities were consumed by his fragile and demanding wife. Sheila experienced her parents' devotion to each other from the distance of an observer and—as she was identified as the "big, strong, healthy" child—found herself unable to secure their care and attention. When Sheila was approximately 7 years old, she discovered that chocolate candy bars could fill a profound social-emotional void in a way that nothing else could.

By age 10, Sheila could no longer hide the effects of sneaking money from her mother's purse to purchase sweets from the neighborhood confectionery store. Now 30 pounds overweight, she was forced to wear adult-sized clothes that clearly set her apart from her classmates. She was often the focus of playground taunts against which she felt defenseless. Moreover, Sheila believed she deserved the rejection of others as a natural consequence of her greedy and willful behavior. She gradually withdrew into her studies and herself, mindful that if she only could lose 30 pounds, she would again be accepted by the other children.

Attempting to adjust to the social environment of senior high school, Sheila began her first diet. Through her own resources, she located a pediatrician who placed her on a 900-calorie diet that was supplemented with "diet pills" (most likely amphetamines). Sheila was told that her chronic sadness, low self-esteem, and social isolation would disappear if she was thin and looked like the other girls. Within six months, her weight had stabilized at 150 pounds and, with the help of the pills, was maintained at this level throughout high school. Her mood and self-esteem, however, failed to improve. Because Sheila had

spent much of her late childhood and early adolescence alone, she felt unequipped to manage the attention her new body image incurred. She told herself, "If only they knew what I had looked like before and what is really under the surface, they wouldn't like me," or "I don't deserve to be liked. I'm not really in control—I'm only thin because of the pills," and sometimes, "I don't want to be friends with them now; they should have liked me when I was fat. I'm still the same person."

Despite her academic success, Sheila rejected college and married the first man who proposed to her. She immediately gained 20 pounds in what she viewed as a celebration of being accepted into the adult world. Two children and 35 additional pounds later, she consulted a hypnotist who facilitated a relatively rapid 45-pound weight loss. Unfortunately, the self-management portion of this program was insufficient to sustain the weight loss. Sheila returned to her former eating habits and deprecatory self-statements. Her husband reinforced Sheila's overvalued belief that weight determined self-esteem and social worth when he left their 15-year marriage.

Sheila clung tenaciously to the belief that happiness only could be attained through weight loss and marriage. She began a fad diet and lost nearly 100 pounds, thereby bringing her weight to about 140 pounds. Did her mood improve because she was finally "normal" weight? Absolutely! She met and married a new man, a health-conscious academic who encouraged her to return to school and to join him in amateur athletic competition. Sheila took this opportunity to attain her college degree. Predictably, Sheila binged her way through college. Being unable to cope effectively with academic stresses, social pressures, and the toll that both can take on self-esteem, Sheila turned to food. Consequently, Sheila's weight bounced back to 240 pounds.

Over the following 10 years, her eating patterns vacillated between excessively restrictive and grossly out of control. She joined the diet circuit—becoming a member of Overeaters Anonymous, receiving "diet shots," taking cellulose and appetite suppressants, using diuretics, and joining the usual assortment of fad diet programs. Every attempt at weight loss was first productive, yet within one to three years, all eventually resulted in relapse. As the years passed, Sheila's youthful optimism became transformed into demoralization and despair. Ultimately, these 10 years of yo-yo weight loss and gain reaffirmed Sheila's dysfunctional negative self-evaluation, sense of dyscontrol, pessimism, and belief that social worth only comes with thinness.

Finally, as Sheila's second marriage began to disintegrate, a new perspective took shape. Sheila thought it possible that weight loss was not simply a matter of finding the right diet, but perhaps related to the beliefs she held about herself and relationships. She thus called requesting evaluation and treatment of what we came to identify as an atypical eating disorder.

INITIAL ASSESSMENT

The evaluation and initial treatment plan for Sheila developed over a three-session sequence. During the first session, a complete history was taken that included previous therapy experiences and comprehensive weight history. Although Sheila had previously been in treatment, her weight-related problems were never accorded a primary therapeutic foci. Rather, Sheila was told that as she progressed in treatment, her bingeing would abate on its own. Disclosure of her actual weight and eating habits caused significant anxiety. Sheila could not discuss this material without perceiving it as evidence that she was a bad person, and moreover, Sheila believed that she was setting herself up for rejection by sharing this information. Sheila completed the Beck Depression Inventory (BDI), Michigan Alcohol Screening Test (MAST), and Minnesota Multiphasic Personality Inventory (MMPI) as part of the evaluation. Finally, at the conclusion of the first session, she was given an Impulsive Monitoring Form (IMF) and instructed in its use.

The IMF is a variant of the standard record of dysfunctional thoughts (see Figure 17-1). Sheila's relative lack of introspective ability and failure to internalize responsibility for her eating disorder indicated that a moderated introduction to cognitive therapy principles and techniques would be the wise course to follow. Her first assignment, therefore, was to record those situations in which she was aware of feeling out of control and wanting to binge. She was to try this task for a week and return her log at the next evaluation session.

Sheila returned for the second session with three completed IMFs representing 36 instances when she thought about bingeing. Collaborative review of these logs revealed that Sheila felt out of control and like bingeing when she was in the following three distinct situations: alone, with her husband, or in stressful encounters at work. Sheila's initial reaction to the task was to discount its informational value and remind herself of the scores of previously failed attempts to diet. Therapeutic differentiation of this regimen from past treatment and diets was sufficient to override Sheila's early pessimism. Moreover, Sheila's inherent curiosity was brought into the fray by the discovery that bingeing was related to discernible affective and interpersonal events, such as family disagreements or sudden changes in mood.

Results of psychological screening instruments indicated an absence of severe symptomatology or psychopathology, but both her BDI score of 22 and MMPI profile revealed a moderate degree of affective impairment. Sheila's scores on the MAST placed her in a high-risk category for alcohol abuse. Sheila corroborated these psychometric findings; she reported that thoughts about money, health, and weight reliably elicited dysphoric affect. She had been using alcohol on a semiregular basis (three times a week) to manage these emotions. Toward the end of the session, Sheila was trained to use the IMF to identify the thoughts and feelings underlying her impulses to binge.

At the third and final assessment session, Sheila tentatively turned in a partially completed IMF. Whereas she had previously experienced success in her self-monitoring of situations and associated binge impulses, the addition of recording thoughts and feelings brought into focus how difficult it was for her to gain access to affective and cognitive material. For example, she noted an incident when, after receiving a telephone call, she found herself frantically searching the refrigerator for food. Her motivation for this behavior was unclear. At first she could only recall a pleasant conversation with her husband and had no clue as to why this incident would precipitate a binge. On closer examination, however, Sheila remembered her husband's purpose for calling was to report an angry exchange with his boss. She then remembered a sudden burst of anxiety and thoughts of, "He will lose his job and we'll be out in the street. There is no one to take care of me, and I can't care for myself." In response to these thoughts and the associated anxiety, she headed for her primary coping and self-soothing resource—ice cream.

As she tentatively reported this behavior, Sheila noted a rising feeling of embarrassment and thoughts of, "My therapist thinks I'm a pig. I'm going to get yelled at for this." In the silence that followed, her therapist inquired into what Sheila was thinking. When she communicated her fears, she was able to reality test by noting her therapist's supportive, comforting, and anxiety-relieving manner. She was able to tell herself that her therapist "was neither abusive or neglectful." In fact, Sheila commented, "I hope that my therapist will be as reliable and calming as food."

This clinical exchange served as a springboard for illustrating the connections between situations, emotions, cognitions, and bingeing. Moreover, Sheila learned that certain interpersonal interactions could be as soothing, or more so, than food. At the end of session 3, Sheila and her therapist collaboratively developed a long-range treatment plan. This plan included initial weight stabilization,

Activity	Thought	Feeling	Binge	
			b	c
a				

a=date   b=urge rated from 1-10   c=binge completed

Figure 17-1. Impulse monitoring form.

with a goal of weight loss into a realistic range given her height, age, biology, and weight history. It was decided that effective weight management meant that Sheila's low self-esteem, recurrent depression, and maladaptive interpersonal orientation needed to be addressed.

BEGINNING TREATMENT

Sheila's enthusiasm for therapy quickly diminished upon making a commitment to begin. She noted an increase in anxiety before the next few sessions and feared she had placed herself in an untenable position by revealing to friends and family her intent to confront her eating problems. It became clear that Sheila's decision to diet activated a cluster of latent, maladaptive beliefs. Sheila collected a list of associated cognitions that largely explained her resistance to dieting. Attributes were added to and deleted from this list over the course of therapy. Below is a representative sample:

- I must start to diet now! I can't allow myself any slack.
- I must stay on the diet every day without fail until I reach my goal weight range.
- People will be disappointed in me if I can't get started. People might even reject me.
- I shouldn't be scared about dieting. What a *wimp* I am.
- I have to be able to get back into my "small" clothes or this won't be worth it.
- Only if I starve myself will I be able to lose weight (and I *don't* feel like starving).
- What if I fail? People will know how truly incompetent I am.
- Why should I lose weight for people who only care about my body?

Using this list, Sheila worked on formulating more realistic expectations for herself, therapy, and dieting. As mentioned above, Sheila had agreed to stabilize her weight at its current level. To accomplish this, Sheila required greater caloric intake than she willingly allowed herself. In consultation with a staff nutritionist, using a rule-of-thumb figure for weight maintenance of 10 to 12 calories per pound of body weight, Sheila agreed to follow a 2,500-calorie American Diabetic Association (ADA) food-exchange diet plan. This plan distributed total daily caloric intake over three meals and snacks; it also allowed for a wide selection of foods from the six major nutritional groups. Sheila expected that she could comply with the ADA dieting regimen without experiencing deprivation.

During the next four months of therapy, cognitive-behavioral interventions fundamentally focused upon teaching Sheila the rudiments of cognitive restructuring and helping her to acquire behaviorally oriented skills for coping with urges to binge. While she was "knocking at the door" of potent, affect-laden early maladaptive assumptions (EMAs), it was felt that she needed to have a definitively stronger alliance with her therapist and a true grasp of adaptive, growth-promoting coping skills before deep uncovering work could be attempted. Even though Sheila had been in a myriad of diet programs, she was surprisingly unacquainted with standard behavioral strategies. By using the IMF, Sheila quickly picked up the concept of appetitive behavior as the end point of an array of internal and external stimuli. She actively solved problems of how to minimize food cues in her home, to avoid supermarkets when at high risk, to keep herself from becoming overly bored, to eat only in the kitchen, to slow down her pace of eating, and to engage in specific alternative activities when feeling an urge to binge.

Sheila had become quite proficient at using the IMF to identify recurrent cognitions that led to heightened urges to diet and frequent episodes of bingeing. It took time, a bit of therapeutic persuasion, and a considerable amount of interpersonal surveying for Sheila to develop a constructionistic formulation about her thinking. Her recognition that beliefs were not immutable representations of reality fell into place after polling friends about their attitudes toward significant topics such as fat, domineering men, and educated women. Not only did she discover diversity, but she also found that she could assertively challenge and promulgate changes in some of these beliefs.

By synthesizing cognitive and behavioral strategies, Sheila became increasingly adept at adaptively managing her interpersonal and intrapsychic life. For example, Sheila frequently binged while waiting for her family to return home. At these times, she felt lonely and disconnected from people; she believed that only food could satisfy her cravings. An assignment was developed to test the hypothesis that only eating could reduce the tensions Sheila felt when home alone waiting for her family. The following is an excerpt from one of Sheila's sessions.

SHEILA: I can't seem to stop bingeing when I'm alone.

THERAPIST: Can you describe what you're feeling and how you're thinking at these times?

SHEILA: Nothing comes to mind right now.

THERAPIST: Let's try to recreate one of those experiences by using focused imagery. Sit back and relax yourself as best as you can. OK; I want you to recall the last time you were home alone and binged. Describe what you see.

SHEILA: Well, it's about 9 p.m., my husband [Dick] said he'd be home from an errand about 30 minutes ago. I'm beginning to feel hurt and desperately alone. I get up from my chair and head toward the refrigerator. I'm beginning to feel relief as I open the freezer door. I reach for a quart of ice cream and . . .

THERAPIST: Wait one moment. Slow yourself down. Can you imagine yourself putting the ice cream away and telling yourself, "It's always going to be available, but right now I'm going to sit down and identify what's really behind my feelings"?

SHEILA: OK, done. On my way to the den I find myself thinking, "Dick isn't here because he no longer loves me. In fact, how can anyone care about such a fat slob like me?" I feel a huge hole in my stomach and need to fill it with food.

THERAPIST: We've talked about how you *selectively overattend* to your weight and inaccurately *minimize* your importance to others. Take us, in your mind, over to your photo album, and let's fill up on the caring that really exists in your life.

(Sheila and therapist reminisce about pleasant times she's had with other people.)

SHEILA: Well, I'm not feeling very hungry any more. I guess I misjudged how people feel about me. It feels good to know that people care. I haven't spoken to Jane in a while, and I think I'll call her on the bedroom—not kitchen—phone.

During these four months, Sheila became quite versatile at using delay strategies coupled with cognitive restructuring and experiential self-enhancement on an in vivo basis.

MIDDLE PHASE

Around the 20th session, Sheila noted a shift in her attitude about weight loss and stated that she felt ready to diet. She remembered that a 10-pound loss was a reasonable start. Attitudinal changes were necessary to achieve this goal. When she found herself thinking, "Yes, but you still have 90 pounds to lose," she countered with "I may choose to lose as much as that, but for now I only wish to lose 10 pounds." She also felt driven by a perfectionistic attitude of "in order to be successful, I have to follow my diet perfectly every hour of every day." She coped with this belief by reading the following from an index card that she carried in her pocketbook: "I'll try to diet each day, but if I choose, I will allow myself planned times to be off the diet."

Sheila's initial weight loss was achieved by adjusting her maintenance diet of 2,500 calories to 1,200 calories. She began an exercise program of three days of strenuous exercise each week plus 20 minutes of walking two days a week. In Sheila's case, strenuous exercise was defined as 30 minutes of aerobic exercise including jogging, cycling, or an exercise class. Her family physician concurred that this was a medically safe dieting regimen.

She continued to complete a weekly IMF and, with the reduction in calories, became cognizant of a familiar cognitive and affective pattern elicited by serious dieting. Once in a weight loss mode, she disattended to the experience of hunger and its precipitants until the urge to binge became so intense she felt compelled to act on it. The precipitants of the urges to eat ranged from biological (e.g., late-day blood glucose decline secondary to daytime fasting, fatigue, premenstrual periods) to psychological (e.g., anger, frustration, loneliness). Her work, therefore was to *increase* her awareness of pertinent moods and thoughts and, thus, to enhance her capacity to control maladaptive eating behavior. Once Sheila's attributions about the cause of her hunger were corrected, she became better able to take appropriate and self-enhancing action (e.g., taking a nap, eating an orange, expressing her feelings).

After successfully losing 10 pounds, Sheila assessed her motivation for continuing to reduce her weight and decided that she was sufficiently in control of her eating behavior to consider a more strenuous diet. Largely attributable to obesity, Sheila had developed both hypertension and type II diabetes. Therefore, because of these medical concerns, she decided to pursue a more aggressive weight loss regimen. After considering the advantages and disadvantages of a number of weight loss programs, a very-low-calorie diet (VLCD) was instituted under her doctor's care.

The VLCD required her to consume five liquid-formula "meals" per day—with no choices, and no options except for flavor. Sheila's confidence in her ability to contain her impulses outweighed her trepidation about 13 weeks of not chewing solid food. Psychotherapy sessions at this juncture served to help her grieve about the loss of normal food and to support her through a period of deprivation. Sheila actively reminded herself about the positive consequences of a VLCD: (a) Fasting made it easier to avoid overeating by not needed to choose or prepare food; (b) results would be quick and dramatic; (c) there would

only be one "intense" episode of dieting in her new commitment to a healthier life-style; and (d) the time usually spent shopping for, cooking, and eating meals could be applied toward other self-indulgent activities (she loved massages). Sheila was frequently able to sustain her motivation to diet by reviewing these consequences.

Sheila's competence with cognitive-behavioral techniques continued to advance. Weaning herself from the IMF, she devised a more elegant recording system using a diary format. In her diary she tracked her weight, cognitive distortions, and coping strategies. She had become skillful in utilizing these methods in individual sessions and was therefore ready to change from individual therapy into a specialized psychotherapy group that was composed only of obese, eating-disordered individuals. This group provided a forum in which members worked on interpersonal issues and supported each others' weight loss efforts. Common negative self-evaluations were addressed and corrected in the empathic atmosphere of the group. Group members shared their experiences of mourning weight loss, fearing failure, contending with family resistance to change, struggling with body-image disparagement, and began a cautious reevaluation of self-worth.

Sheila's transition into the group went smoothly. A majority of the group members were in the early stages of weight loss. Sheila was an active group member; she brought her diary to group meetings to share examples of her most difficult moments while dieting. She often polled the group to check out others' strategies and how their difficulties were handled. She utilized the group setting to make public commitments about weekly goals, and the group helped her to set realistic standards in both interpersonal and dietary spheres. The group also contracted to walk together for 30 minutes after each session.

Within six months, Sheila lost 80 pounds. For 13 weeks she complied with the fast, then she slowly integrated food into her diet. Her loss on the fast totaled 60 pounds, and she continued to lose as she ate "real food" along with the supplement. However, food for her was no longer "user friendly." She began to overfocus upon urges to eat and deviating from her dieting protocol. She interpreted urges to binge as a sign that she was indeed a failure. Sheila repeatedly came to group and tearfully reported that she was a fraud and she would never be able to live and eat as a normal person.

The group helped her to weather this crisis. Members confronted Sheila's overgeneralizations and pointed out the catastrophizing that was typical of her. To Sheila's credit, she listened carefully to what the group was saying. Members took a problem-solving orientation; they suggested that Sheila identify binge-engendering situations, and the group then role-played a range of coping responses that had been effective for them. Also, they reminded her that a relapse did not represent a failure but, in fact, an opportunity for growth and self-learning.

Essentially, the middle phase of this therapy was characterized by profound weight loss. Group psychotherapy was introduced as an integral part of the overall treatment plan. The secretiveness, isolation, and stigma of binge eating were brought to light in the group and understood as problems shared by many. As group cohesion developed and members opened up, Sheila recognized that shame and embarrassment about one's body and eating behavior was a common experience. Such sharing enabled Sheila to become more self-accepting. She felt valued by the group for her insights, sense of humor, and genuine altruistic contributions. She finally realized that her social worth was determined by more than her physical stature. Her weight stabilized within her goal range of 170 to 180 pounds.

LATTER PHASE

Although Sheila's weight and mood continued to reflect the success of her treatment, Sheila felt that the changes in her body had occurred faster then the changes in her thinking. At this point, panic began to set in. She believed others expected more of her at this lower weight. She felt pressured to be more social, more energetic, more in control. But more than anything else, she feared relapse.

Sheila's husband also feared the changes that were occurring in her life. He began to bring hot fudge sundaes home, ostensibly as a special reward for Sheila's success. Arguments about innocuous issues escalated into major battles. Sheila initiated midnight forays to the kitchen for pretzels and popcorn. She stopped recording in her diary. She came to group and apprehensively reported a slow but steady weight gain. With the help of the group, she realized that her successful weight loss had precipitated an unexpected change in the marriage: Improvement in her self-esteem produced more assertive behavior and a greater investment in her work and career. Her husband, unprepared for these changes, interpreted Sheila's behavior as the first steps towards an impending separation.

In group sessions, Sheila asked for suggestions as to how to deal with her husband.

SHEILA: Now that I'm not fat, you would think Dick would be more loving and supportive. Instead I think he's trying to sabotage my diet. Why would he do this? I don't think he really loves me!

JANICE: I think you should get out before you gain everything back.

DON: Wait a minute, Janice. That's so all or nothing. There must be a reason why this is happening. (to Sheila) What makes you think he doesn't love you?

SHEILA: If he loved me, he wouldn't make dieting harder by bringing me everything that I love to eat.

DON: Seems to me that may be his way of saying, "I love you, and I'm scared of losing you." When I first lost a lot of weight, my wife did the same thing. I got to goal weight, and she started cooking everything I liked. We started to fight about it all the time. The group suggested we try a marriage counselor to help us through that time. We did and it helped. Maybe you and Dick need to see someone together.

Sheila and Dick began marital counseling to open a dialogue about their adjustment to her changes in appearance, attitude, and behavior. Several interrelated themes emerged. Sheila strongly believed that "if he loved me, he wouldn't, one, tempt me with food; two, leave me alone when he knows I'll eat; three, dump all the responsibility of the house and children on me; [or] four, drink as much as he does." Given Dick's behavior, Sheila concluded, "Dick doesn't really want me to be thin. He's holding me back so that he won't be threatened by my success."

Dick's perception of their marital problems had been predicted in the group. He believed that Sheila wanted out of the marriage. He assumed that Sheila's renewed interest in sexuality was a reflection of a secret affair that she was having. Men were viewed as interested in her because she "wore" a new body.

Sheila used her cognitive therapy skills in marital therapy. "Where's the evidence," she asked, "that I'm interested in someone else?" Dick allowed that he may have misinterpreted Sheila's behavior. With Sheila's help, he became proficient at cognitive techniques, realizing that his contribution to their marital problems could be traced to selective attention to sexual cues, mind reading, and prolific use of arbitrary inference. When confronted by the evidence that Sheila loved him and was committed to the marriage, Dick concluded that his fears were unfounded. As a result, he felt more supportive of Sheila's efforts, more willing to look at her complaints, and less intent on sabotaging her diet.

Sheila was able to empathize with Dick's position. She recognized that Dick was feeling insecure. His behavior was an unproductive way of holding onto what seemed like a deteriorating relationship. Together, they agreed that there were nonfattening, nondestructive methods to demonstrate their continued caring for each other.

In therapy, the couple role-played reassurance-seeking communications and reactions. They generated a list of "caring" behaviors that could be exchanged when either wished to communicate affection for the other. In this context, Sheila's sexual approaches were reframed as a way of sharing her love with Dick.

As the marital crisis resolved, Sheila's increased anxiety abated, and her bingeing ceased. In weekly group sessions, Sheila reported relative marital harmony. After problem solving with the group, she placed herself back on the ADA diet learned earlier in treatment, and within a month returned to her goal weight range. Sheila maintained her weight within this range for six months, then terminated group therapy.

FOLLOW-UP

One year after terminating therapy, Sheila remains at the high end of her goal weight range. Over this time she had a few telephone conversations with her individual therapist; contacts were largely precipitated by the crisis of weight gain. Standard relapse-prevention interventions were effected, and each crisis quickly passed. Sheila currently maintains a journal to help her recognize and cope with ambient stress, and she uses Weight Watchers to obtain a dietary handle on incipient weight gain. She remains dedicated to exercise, working out at a local gym three times a week. Sheila and Dick are still married, and they take nightly walks together. Sometimes, Sheila suggests that they go out for ice cream.

SUGGESTED READINGS

Brownell, K., & Foreyt, J. (1986). *Handbook of eating disorders: Physiology, psychology, and treatment of obesity, anorexia, and bulimia*. New York: Basic Books.

Stuart, R., & Jacobson, B. (1989). *Weight, sex, and marriage*. New York: Simon and Schuster.

Kirschenbaum, D., Johnson, W., & Stalonas, P. (1987). *Treating childhood and adolescent obesity*. New York: Pergamon.

Polivy, J., & Herman, P. (1983). *Breaking the diet habit*. New York: Basic Books.

18

Cocaine Abuse

Aaron T. Beck, Fred D. Wright, and Cory F. Newman

COGNITIVE MODEL OF DRUG USE

According to the cognitive perspective, the way in which people process information in specific situations determines their affective, motivational, and behavioral reactions. Information processing is shaped in many instances by the relevant beliefs that become activated in these situations. Certain individuals with a vulnerability to drug abuse have specific beliefs that are activated under particular circumstances and, consequently, enhance the likelihood of continued drug use (i.e., stimulate craving). Idiosyncratic beliefs such as "cocaine makes me more social" represent this vulnerability and are assumed to be activated in certain provocative situations.

Beliefs about cocaine use can change or become more complex over time. At the time of initial use, the patient might have *anticipatory beliefs* such as "it's fun to do this; it's okay to try it once." Then, as a result of some type of dependency (either physical or psychological), he or she may then develop the *relief-oriented belief* "I need cocaine in order to function; I can't continue without it." This notion can lead to the stimulation of or increase in craving or exciting belief. At this point, a *facilitating* or

permissive belief may come into play ("I deserve it," or "It's all right").

Contradictory Beliefs

In the various stages of cocaine use the patient can have two conflicting sets of beliefs, such as "I should not use cocaine" versus "It's OK to use this one time." Each belief can be activated under different circumstances or at the same time. The balance of the valences (strength) of each belief at a given time will influence whether the patient will use or abstain when exposed to a drug; for instance, where the drug-taking or permissive belief is activated, the abstinence belief may be deactivated.

Activation in High-Risk Situations

Drug-taking beliefs are typically activated in certain high-risk circumstances; these circumstances can be external or internal. Examples of high-risk *external* circumstances are a peer group using cocaine, or contact with a drug dealer or a certain section of town. *Internal* circumstances include various emotional states—such as depression, anxiety, or boredom—that can trigger drug-using beliefs and, consequently, craving for the drug.

Drug dependency may be conceptualized as representing the final effects of the activation of the cluster of the aforementioned beliefs. Treatment is aimed at modifying each of the categories of beliefs: anticipatory, drug seeking (craving), and permissive/facilitating (see Figure 18-1).

Aaron T. Beck, Fred D. Wright, and Cory F. Newman • Center for Cognitive Therapy, Department of Psychiatry, University of Pennsylvania School of Medicine, Philadelphia, Pennsylvania 19104.

Comprehensive Casebook of Cognitive Therapy, edited by Arthur Freeman and Frank M. Dattilio. Plenum Press, New York, 1992.

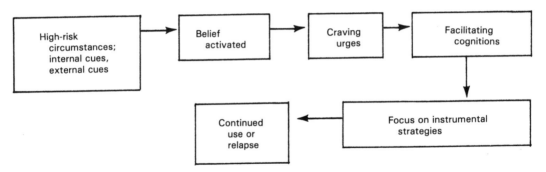

Figure 18-1. Drug–taking activation in high–risk circumstances.

When they are not in a stage of craving, patients are often able to recognize the disruptive effects of the drug on their lives. However, once the drug-taking beliefs are activated, a "cognitive blockade" reduces awareness of or investment in the long-term consequences of drug use and increases focus on immediate instrumental strategies (e.g., where to get money to buy drugs). As these beliefs become hypervalent, the relevant beliefs about the drawbacks of drug use become attenuated or even inaccessible (see Figure 18-2).

In the above example, the patient's belief (which was activated when he attended a party) centered on anticipation of relief from feeling sad. Other examples of relief-oriented beliefs are "There is only one way for me to cope with the pain," "I can't stand the withdrawal symptoms," and "I feel better knowing it's there."

Anticipation of pleasure is another category of beliefs. For example, a patient with a five-year history of cocaine use reported having a dream about using cocaine. Upon awakening, he "felt high." Next, he started daydreaming about the last time he used cocaine. This experience in turn activated the belief, "Life is more fun when I use," and was followed by the automatic thought, "Man, I love this stuff." His attention then focused on checking to see whether he had enough money to buy cocaine. A permission-giving belief was also activated ("There is no harm in this").

It should be noted that the belief about the harmlessness of drug taking stemmed from a more complex set of beliefs. The patient believed that since he only snorted cocaine and used it intravenously, he could not be addicted, and he saw himself as being safe from addiction provided he did not smoke crack. One of his typical permissive thoughts was, "I'm glad I don't smoke crack."

Beliefs activated		Automatic thoughts
"Life is more fun when I use."	→	"Man, I love this stuff."
"There is no harm in using this stuff."	→	"I'm glad I don't smoke crack (instead of snorting coke)."

TREATMENT

Cognitive therapy of cocaine abuse is a structured, collaborative, directive, problem-oriented treatment based on the cognitive model of substance abuse. The major thrust is to help patients discover, examine, and modify dysfunctional cognitive-behavioral processes that elicit and maintain their problem.

There are eight aspects of treatment: (a) conceptualization of the problem, (b) collaborative relationship, (c) motivation for reducing drug dependency (craving), (d) patient formulation of the problem, (e) setting goals, (f) socializing the patient into the cognitive model, (g) cognitive-behavioral interventions, and (h) relapse prevention (Beck, Wright, & Newman, 1990).

In the case to be described below, two of these approaches will be illustrated: reducing craving and using imagery.

Motivation for Reducing Drug Dependency

Motivation becomes an important factor in the treatment of substance abuse. In the first phase of treatment, it is imperative to facilitate the patient's understanding of the various advantages/disadvantages of using and not using

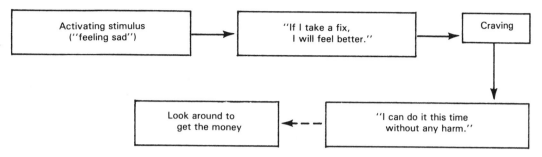

Figure 18-2. "Cognitive blockade" and drug–taking activation.

cocaine. This material can be used later to help motivate the patient during critical situations and can also be used as an intervention between the urge to use drugs and the consummation of this desire.

Teaching patients to cope with craving is one of the most important goals of treatment. Resurgence of craving contributes to treatment dropout and causes relapse after long periods of abstinence. The therapist must understand each patient's specific, idiosyncratic perception of the craving experience. Then, through a series of refined cognitive therapy techniques that focus on craving, permission giving, and instrumental behavior, patients learn to modify the cognitive-motivational-behavioral sequence and thus are better able to cope with their urges.

It is best to pursue the patient's craving experience by focusing on and identifying the "hot cognitions" while the patient is actually experiencing the craving. Craving can be triggered in the office by a number of methods, such as induced imagery, films of people using cocaine, and exposure to cocaine paraphernalia.

Induced imagery is often a powerful method to provoke craving. The patient, for example, is asked to imagine the last time he or she used cocaine and then to describe the imagined scenario in vivid detail. The therapist indicates that he or she will try to evoke the kinds of thoughts and/or images that precede and accompany the urge to use drugs. The steps in production of imagery are illustrated below:

1. The patient is asked to remember the events that led up to a recent drug-using incident.
2. The patient is then asked to image the event and to describe the setting, sequence of events, feelings, and thoughts in specific detail—as though the event were happening *right now.*
3. As the images are described, the patient is asked to indicate to the therapist when the cravings are aroused and to describe them.

4. As the patient begins to feel the craving sensations, the therapist asks him or her to relate the thoughts that preceded or are currently coexisting with these feelings.

This procedure helps the therapist and patient to understand better the images and thoughts that put the patient at risk for drug use, and to begin to formulate rational responses that can be tested for efficacy in reducing the cravings.

Still another powerful method is *exposure* in the office; where the patient sees, holds, and examines cocaine-using paraphernalia. This method can trigger strong craving reactions associated with "hot cognitions" (automatic thoughts or images) and activation of drug-using beliefs such as "the craving will always be there" or "I can't handle the urges."

The case described below illustrates the techniques of listing advantages and disadvantages and using imagery to enhance the craving experience. In this case, the interview focused on reducing the individual's investment in taking cocaine and helping to integrate the notion that he would gain more from giving up the habit than from sticking to it.

A 30-year-old, unemployed white male ("Cal") was referred by his probation officer because of addiction to cocaine. (Because of the need for confidentiality in drug abuse cases, this case is disguised in such a way as to prevent identification.) Cal most commonly used the drug during the daytime when his housemates at the halfway house were out working or looking for jobs. Characteristically, when he went out to get high, he would dress as if for a job interview (i.e., jacket and tie) so that no one would be able to detect his real intentions. Typically, "feelings of hopelessness and boredom" precipitated his urge to take the drug.

Some of his typical automatic thoughts accompanying his urge to use cocaine were:

- "Those guys are going somewhere, I don't have a chance."
- "I might as well enjoy today."
- "It's a lonely existence."

With induced imagery, the therapist guided the patient through circumstances leading to the experience of the urge to get high. The patient acknowledged that when he gets the craving, he doesn't care about the consequences of his drug habit; he "just has to get some money somewhere." The therapist used Socratic questioning to elicit the following advantages and disadvantages:

Advantages to giving into the urge
- "I can smile, laugh."
- "I would feel good about myself for an hour or two."
- "I would have a pleasant unreality."

Advantage of *not* giving into the urge
- "I can stay at the halfway house."
- "I can get a job."

Advantages of a job
- "Have something to fill my days rather than just sitting around and feeling sorry for myself."
- "Have pride in my own accomplishment."
- "Have my own place and some privacy."
- "Improve social life—have women friends over."

This excerpt from an early interview illustrates the procedure of eliciting the advantages and disadvantages of yielding or not yielding to the craving for a high.

THERAPIST: Cal, could you tell me a little bit about what your difficulty is in terms of drug taking?

PATIENT: The difficulty is not being able to stop, basically. That's what it comes down to.

THERAPIST: And what's your life situation?

PATIENT: The worst part is that I am unemployed, which doesn't help.

THERAPIST: And you are staying in a group facility?

PATIENT: Yeah. I better be honest with you. Got a lot of time on my hands and, you know, it's the only thing I've got that does anything for me. Pretty downgrade discouragement and everything. There is too much time on my hands, you know.

THERAPIST: And you feel bored as well as discouraged?

PATIENT: Yeah. That's a good way to describe it, actually pretty useless and bored.

THERAPIST: Now, Cal, can you remember the most recent time that you used drugs? Do you remember what the situation was?

PATIENT: Yeah. I can remember.

THERAPIST: When did this take place?

PATIENT: Well, I'm kind of hesitant to mention it, but I know some people—I'm not going to mention where they are, but small contacts, and it's within a bus or subway ride away. It's easy to get to. And it was like about a week ago, less than a week ago, and it was during the day and that's the time when most of the guys in the house either are working or they're out looking for work. I was supposed to be looking for work, and I took a little detour to my old contacts.

THERAPIST: You started off here in the house, and what was happening to you in the house?

PATIENT: Getting ready, putting on a jacket and tie to go out. Had an interview set up, but I didn't have much hope for it. So I was just getting my jacket and tie on, and I already knew I wasn't going to go through with the interview. I already knew what I was going to do instead. Of course, I didn't say anything. It would be stupid to say anything because I was just getting back in trouble again. So I just went through with it, like I was going out for the interview. But I didn't.

THERAPIST: Now just prior to putting on your jacket and tie, what were your feelings and what was going through your mind right then?

PATIENT: It was sort of like, "What's the point of going out looking for a job when it's not going to work out for me anyway? Nothing ever works out for me, so I might as well get loaded and enjoy today anyway."

THERAPIST: So your thoughts were, "What's the use of looking for a job that's not going to work out for me . . . Nothing is going to work out for me . . . I might as well get loaded." [Note: By repeating the patient's words, the therapist increases the sense of reciprocal understanding and also targets some beliefs for later examination.]

PATIENT: Slightly. Hey, it's a little bit of happiness. It's just something. Better than nothing.

THERAPIST: And then at that point you went out and you put on your necktie and jacket.

PATIENT: Yeah. I had to put them on; I had to make the show. If I go out just looking like I am going out to hit the streets, people in the household, they are wise to that stuff. They're like, "Cal, you are supposed to go out for an interview today. What about these clothes? Are they appropriate for your interview?" I would get the third degree, and they would know my stuff and they would know what I was doing. Did not want any of that hassle, so I figured just put the jacket and tie on and leave the house like everything is cool, and then just do what you want to do anyway. That's what I did.

THERAPIST: OK, so that was one experience. Now I thought I heard of an experience where you were sitting around with the other men and you were feeling bored.

PATIENT: Well, that happens a lot. That's not just the last time. That's happened a couple of times.

THERAPIST: What happened those times? Can you give me the details of that?

PATIENT: We have a game room—pool table, Ping-Pong table, a lot of books, magazines, sports magazines, TV; a lot of guys hang out there after hours and kind of shoot the breeze. And when I'm in there, I mean, when I first got into the halfway house, it was like a nice place to go and just talk to some people and play some Ping-Pong. Now I've been there for about three weeks and it just bores the hell out of me. And I see guys that are coming in new, they were guys I was with before and they already left. New guys coming in, I don't even want to talk to them. I'm just thinking that they are going to find a job before I find a job, and everyone is coming in, leaving, coming in, leaving, and I am just staying there and I am just rotting away, so I don't talk to nobody now. I just kind of sit there and stare in space and feeling about as bored as you can feel. I'm really, like, antsy.

THERAPIST: And it was under one of those conditions that you then decided to . . .

PATIENT: Yeah. Picked up and left. And I knew where to go.

THERAPIST: When you got to where you went to go, what did you do?

PATIENT: Well, I had a little bit of money in my pocket. Not much. So I was only able to get a couple of hits. But there's a house where I know where there is 24-hours-a-day action.

THERAPIST: Well, let's take the second incident, if you might. Would you want to do a kind of role play with me on this? Kind of imagine that you are going through this again? Get the feeling as to what you were experiencing and what you were thinking at that particular time?

PATIENT: Reenact it, you mean?

THERAPIST: Yeah. See, what you try to do is kind of imagine the fact of the halfway house and sitting in front of the television, and you are getting these various thoughts that you told me about people coming and going and just rotting away. And one way in which we can help you to deal with these desires is to actually go through it and try to communicate to me just what you were feeling and thinking at that time. Just as though it were happening right now. Might you be able to do that? Just imagine now that you are back in that situation. I am going to ask you some questions to help you get into the role. Cal, where are you right now? [Note: By inducing imagery, the therapist gets the patient to relive the situation. By bringing the experience to life, as it were, the therapist gains a better grasp of the patient's

experience and also can utilize this state of heightened arousal as a vehicle for modifying beliefs.]

PATIENT: Sitting in the corner and got my head down like I've got now, and I can hear the TV on, and I can hear some guys laughing and yelling from the things happening at the pool table.

THERAPIST: Right now, you can hear them laughing over at the pool table. They seem to be having a good time.

PATIENT: They're clowning around.

THERAPIST: They're clowning around. And what are you feeling right now, Cal?

PATIENT: Real depressed.

THERAPIST: And what are you thinking?

PATIENT: Those guys are happy. They are going somewhere. They are making something of themselves. They are going to succeed. I don't have a chance. I don't have a prayer.

THERAPIST: "I don't have a chance. I don't have a prayer." What else is going through your mind?

PATIENT: Might as well enjoy today, while you've got a chance. Might as well do what you can just to get loaded. Get high. There's no tomorrow anyway; might as well enjoy today.

THERAPIST: And how do you see your current situation right now?

PATIENT: Back in this remembering? My current situation?

THERAPIST: How do you see yourself?

PATIENT: Like I said before, I'm rotting away. I'm just rotting away in this house. I'm good for nothing, doing nothing. I don't want to put myself out there again. I don't think I can make it work. I can't see getting a place by myself again, some run-down place. Making seven dollars per hour someplace.

THERAPIST: You can't see yourself getting such a job?

PATIENT: It's just existing. It's lonely and just existing. It's backbreaking. It's no way to live.

THERAPIST: It's lonely. It's just existing. It's backbreaking.

PATIENT: And what's the point of doing it?

THERAPIST: Are you feeling an urge right now?

PATIENT: Yeah.

THERAPIST: Now as you are sitting here in my office, you are also feeling an urge?

PATIENT: Yeah, I am. And it's very depressing stuff we're talking about.

THERAPIST: Now what is your urge? Why don't you follow through right now with your urge?

PATIENT: You mean leave the office?

THERAPIST: Follow through with it mentally.

PATIENT: Oh. You'd think you wanted to talk through eventually. Well, it just means making sure I've got enough money for a bus or a subway, or if I'm real desperate, I'll walk the four miles. I've done that before. When I'm in this state, I don't care who knows or . . .

THERAPIST: So you just don't care.

PATIENT: I just get up and walk out. Usually if I'm thinking of anything, I'm thinking of just getting a few bucks for just a bus back and forth. I'll bum it off somebody. I'll trade some cigarettes for it.

THERAPIST: You have the urge, but does the urge then mean that you should go out and do something about it since you have the urge?

PATIENT: Well, I think it's the only way I'm going to, it's the only way to not be depressed. It's the only way to help myself.

THERAPIST: You feel you should do this as a way of getting over the depression?

PATIENT: Yes. That's a pretty fair summary.

THERAPIST: You feel it's OK to do that?

PATIENT: Well, I don't know if it's OK, but you know, when you are desperate you do things that aren't OK because that's all you can do. So I figure, you know, I'm desperate. What else, what other choices do I have?

THERAPIST: So you see yourself as running away, not getting anywhere, people coming and going, you're at a dead end, you're desperate, and this is the only thing that can neutralize the depression maybe and give you some satisfaction. Now what do you think right now, as you have the urge, what do you think of the advantages of giving into the urge? [Note: The state of arousal is the best state in which to consolidate new patterns of thinking; this is a form of state-dependent learning. Hence, the therapist proceeds to an evaluation of the advantages and disadvantages of using.]

PATIENT: Well at least for a little bit of time, just for an hour or two, I can smile and laugh. I can think I'm hot shit for a change. Most of the time I feel like I'm nothing.

THERAPIST: So most of the time you feel like you're nothing, but for an hour or two you can feel like you are hot shit.

PATIENT: Yeah. I mean it's totally false. Totally like an unreal illusion, but you don't care when you are in it. You think you are tough and you think you are smart and you think you can do anything you want and the reality is just the opposite. So, I like a little unreality for an hour or so.

THERAPIST: So the advantage is it gives you unreality for an hour or two, you think you are tough, and you smile.

PATIENT: Yeah. That's a big advantage. That's a pretty big advantage compared to most everything else in life.

THERAPIST: Now what's the advantage for not giving into the urge?

PATIENT: Well, it's hard to see advantages, except for not risking getting kicked out of the house or having some of the counselors get down on my case. I don't have to worry about the urinalysis going dirty.

THERAPIST: So one advantage is you can stay in the house.

PATIENT: Without getting hassled. Without someone saying, "Hey, Cal, where the hell were you?"

THERAPIST: So you can stay in the house. Eventually you might get kicked out of the house?

PATIENT: That's a possibility. I'm pushing my luck.

THERAPIST: Now you say that you haven't been able to get and keep a job. If you got off the stuff, what are the probabilities you can get a job and keep it?

PATIENT: Well, everyone keeps telling me that I have a good chance. Sometimes it's just hard to see that, because sometimes I just don't think it's worth it to work so hard for so little, with so little enjoyment. So I think maybe, I mean, in reality I could do the job. I could keep a job and stay clean, but sometimes I don't know if I want to do that, because that's just being depressed and bored plus working day in and day out. [Note: At this point, the therapist decides to elicit the advantages of a job. Somehow one gets into a bog—a negative bias—when one is out of a job, about what the real advantages are.]

THERAPIST: Now, Cal, other people have jobs, right? And most people, by and large, do like to work. What do you think are some of the reasons why people do take jobs?

PATIENT: If they are good at something and they take pride in their work, then that's pretty good. We've got a couple guys in the house who are, like, really experienced carpenters, and they've done some really good work and they take pride in their work. And when they are clean, when they're straight, they really get a lot of satisfaction in their work. There's another guy who's an expert mechanic. I mean this guy is well-known, and if he's straight, people come and have him rebuild engines of things. He can rebuild even a powerboat engine. This guy is amazing. And so, there's a pride involved.

THERAPIST: Let's see, suppose you got a job, would it be manual labor, or . . .

PATIENT: I suppose it would have to be, which doesn't pay very well. Even if you are in a union of some sort, it's pretty difficult.

THERAPIST: Now what would be the advantage? What could you see would be the advantages of you having a job?

PATIENT: Something to do, something that I can have,

something to do with my days, instead of just sitting around and feeling sorry for myself.

THERAPIST: So it would fill in your days, in preference to just sitting around feeling sorry for yourself.

PATIENT: Right, right.

THERAPIST: What other advantage?

PATIENT: Well, when people ask what I do, I can tell them something instead of feeling like I've been a jerk.

THERAPIST: You can tell them something instead of feeling like a jerk.

PATIENT: That's one of the toughest parts, when people ask what I do and I have to tell them I'm in between jobs.

THERAPIST: You can imagine yourself having a job, and somebody asked you what you did, and you then were able to say you were working at such and such a place. How do you think that would make you feel?

PATIENT: At least I could look them in the eyes and talk.

THERAPIST: So you'd have some self-respect.

PATIENT: Yeah. I suppose a little bit.

THERAPIST: Now what other advantages are there to having a job?

PATIENT: I could pay some rent. I could move out of this halfway house, have my own place, have some privacy for a change.

THERAPIST: OK, so you could move into your own house and have some privacy.

PATIENT: Well, now an apartment. Privacy. That's important to me.

THERAPIST: See. Now don't stop here. What are the advantages of having . . . so what are the advantages of having privacy?

PATIENT: I can calm down a little bit. I get really annoyed with lots of noise in the house and people always hassling me about leaving things behind, and not cleaning up after myself, and hassling me about my schedule and hassling me about coming to this class we have on time, hassling me about things I say that they don't like, just hassles, hassles, hassles. I don't get any peace and quiet.

THERAPIST: So having your own apartment could give you peace and quiet.

PATIENT: Right.

THERAPIST: What would that do to your nerves?

PATIENT: It will be good. Because then if I want to be with somebody, it's my own choice. So I could just kind of kick back and watch a game on TV and read a newspaper maybe and just have things the way I want them.

THERAPIST: You could watch TV.

PATIENT: Watch what I want to watch, not to fight.

THERAPIST: And read a newspaper without being has-

sled. You said you could have somebody over there.

PATIENT: If I wanted to call up a friend of mine or my brother or somebody and just kind of shoot the breeze and maybe watch a game, I can do it at my place when I want to.

THERAPIST: You could have some male friends over.

PATIENT: Now that you mentioned male friends, if I wanted to go out socially with women, I have a place to come back to and not a halfway house, which definitely kind of ruins your social life.

THERAPIST: Would having a job help you to go out with women?

PATIENT: Well, it would be still not the greatest because I'm not exactly rolling in money, but at least I would have a place to myself.

THERAPIST: You would have more money with a job than you have right now?

PATIENT: Oh, yeah. Definitely. No question about it.

THERAPIST: So you would have a better chance of going out with . . .

PATIENT: Yeah, that's a big advantage.

THERAPIST: And if they asked you what you did?

PATIENT: I wouldn't be too proud, but at least I'm employed. Women, if they hear you are out of work, it's like they think, "Another deadbeat is going to be a leech on me. Forget it. Dump this guy." I've heard that before. I don't want to be a leech.

THERAPIST: Now, Cal, our time, unfortunately, is running out, but I would like you to think of some of these things. I would like to review them. How important is having an apartment to yourself? You look at the different things, for example, being able to watch the TV when you want to watch it. Is that a source of satisfaction?

PATIENT: Yeah.

THERAPIST: Reading a newspaper when you want to? Is that a source of satisfaction?

PATIENT: Yeah, definitely.

THERAPIST: Is being free of all the hassles that you are having in the house? Is that kind of an important relief to you? Being able to have your brother and some other male friends over?

PATIENT: All those things. It would be great.

THERAPIST: Would that be satisfying to you?

PATIENT: Yeah. I'd say so.

THERAPIST: And having women over? Would that be satisfying?

PATIENT: Definitely.

THERAPIST: Being able to tell people, look them in the eye, tell them you have a job?

PATIENT: All those things. I guess the point you are making is that if I stay off the stuff I can get that.

THERAPIST: There are satisfactions. Number one is relief from all the hassles you are going through. So, in terms of your nerves, that's something. Now in terms of depression, you have all these other sources of satisfaction, which could add up. And then in terms of having respect for yourself, you could get all that. Now would you be giving up two illusory hours after you have taken something?

PATIENT: I don't know if I would need illusory, whatever the word you used.

THERAPIST: Two hours of illusion?

PATIENT: I don't know if I would need that if I was able to do the things you just talked about. I don't think about those things. I just get too depressed. I don't even think about that stuff.

OUTCOME

Having helped the patient recognize the advantages of abstaining from drugs, the therapist then provided the patient with coping tools. At their next appointment, they made flash cards of corrective thinking for the patient to use when he experienced depression, a precipitant of his drug-seeking behaviors. The therapist was persistent in his level of intervention but also listened to the patient (i.e., gave him opportunities to complain). Both factors facilitated the patient's willingness to take the therapist seriously. Although the patient's drug addiction was longstanding, the persistent intervention at the levels of his craving and drug taking and of his hopelessness and depression ultimately enabled him to kick the habit.

REFERENCES

Beck, A. T., Wright, F., & Newman, C. (1990). *Cognitive therapy of cocaine abuse*. Philadelphia: Center for Cognitive Therapy.

SUGGESTED READINGS

Beck, A. T., Wright, F. D., & Newman, C. F. (1990). *Cognitive therapy of cocaine abuse*. Philadelphia, PA: Center for Cognitive Therapy.

Beck, A. T., & Emery, G. (1979). *Cognitive therapy of substance abuse*. Philadelphia, PA: Center for Cognitive Therapy.

Beck, A. T., Freeman, A., & Associates (1990). *Cognitive therapy of personality disorders*. New York: Guilford.

19

The Older Adult

Dolores Gallagher-Thompson and Larry W. Thompson

INTRODUCTION

This case is about a 66-year-old Caucasian woman who was widowed three years prior to starting therapy, after having been a caregiver for a spouse with Alzheimer's disease. Her presenting concerns involved very negative views and fears about her retirement, which had happened about a year prior to seeking treatment. This situation seemed to be exacerbated by her tendency to devalue herself due to her socioeconomically deprived background earlier in life. Mrs. A. also reported two other problems: (a) intense feelings of distance from her grown children, and (b) worries about her health. She had both hypertension and arthritis, but these were under good medical control. Her worries seemed more focused on what could happen in the future in terms of declining health if she had a stroke, a fall, or some other event that could cause a decrement in her functional ability. She began therapy with a diagnosis of primary major depressive disorder, and after 30 sessions of individual treatment was no longer clinically depressed. She maintained these gains consistently over a two-year follow-up period with no relapses, despite additional life stressors during that time (e.g., family emergencies).

BACKGROUND INFORMATION

Mrs. A., a 66-year-old widow, had been retired for one year from her career as an executive secretary at the time of entering therapy. She was reasonably groomed, although mildly overweight, and shy and withdrawn in relating to staff during the assessment process. She had been a caregiver for five years for her husband, who had had Alzheimer's disease, and had been widowed for three years upon seeking treatment. She had four grown children—one son and three daughters, two of whom lived nearby. Initially, she described conflict with all of them because they "didn't turn out like I wanted them to."

Mrs. A. described two prior episodes of depression earlier in life related to negative circumstances (the son's psychological problems, and her husband's diagnosis of Alzheimer's disease), but she had not sought treatment either time because she did not believe it would work. She described herself as basically well-adjusted throughout adulthood, although she recognized that from childhood on, she had felt somewhat inadequate compared to other people because of coming from a blue-collar background with "none of the advantages that people here take for granted." She also barely completed high school, and this caused her some problems in the affluent community in

Dolores Gallagher-Thompson and Larry W. Thompson • Older Adult and Family Research and Resource Center, Division of Gerontology, Stanford University School of Medicine and Gerontology, Stanford, California 94305 and Geriatric Research, Education, and Medical Center Veterans Affairs Clinical Center, Palo Alto, California 94304.

Comprehensive Casebook of Cognitive Therapy, edited by Arthur Freeman and Frank M. Dattilio. Plenum Press, New York, 1992.

which she lived and had worked. She had moved to that area with her husband, who was a successful businessman and a good provider for the family. However, she described a great deal of tension at different times in the marriage because of significant differences over child-rearing practices: She demanded higher achievement from the children, and he was more easygoing.

From her description of how each child "turned out," three appeared to be at least moderately successful in the sense of having stable jobs and/or average family situations, with only the son having had a serious drug and alcohol problem and being in and out of substance abuse programs at different points in Mrs. A.'s life. She perceived his "failure" as reflecting on her and deepening her lifelong sense of inadequacy. She acknowledged that since her husband's death, she was very lonely and socially isolated, and probably overdependent on her nearby children for emotional support. She made the initial contact with our center with some trepidation because of her son's experiences as an inpatient in a very confrontive therapeutic community, along with her feeling that she would probably not be a "good client" since she wasn't well educated enough.

ASSESSMENT AND DIAGNOSIS

The initial assessment consisted of a Schedule for Affective Disorders and Schizophrenia (SADS) (Endicott & Spitzer, 1978) interview conducted by a trained clinical psychologist. Based on the data obtained, Mrs. A. was diagnosed as being in a current major depressive episode. Her history indicated that she had experienced two distinct prior episodes, but there was no indication of a chronic depressive (dysthymic) condition. She was also queried for signs of a concomitant personality disorder and was found to have marked features of an avoidant personality disorder (DSM-III-R; American Psychiatric Association, 1987), though this assessment was difficult to make because of the strong depressive overlay that influenced how she reported experiences and perceptions over her lifetime.

Following this assessment, she was interviewed by a geropsychiatrist who, with the patient's permission, had spoken to her primary care physician prior to the appointment in order to be familiar with Mrs. A's health history and current medication regimen. The psychiatric evaluation confirmed the initial diagnoses, ruled out suicidal ideation, and reviewed her medications and health status. Mrs. A. was taking a nonsteroidal anti-inflammatory drug for her arthritis and a diuretic for her hypertension. She

appeared to understand how to take each medicine, and her physician reported that she was compliant with the regimen. He thought there was minimal possibility that her depression was being caused or exacerbated by her medication. The psychiatrist agreed with this evaluation once he had seen the patient and integrated the various bits of available information.

The psychiatrist also discussed with Mrs. A. his understanding of her depression and the pros and cons of participating in this research project, as opposed to seeking treatment from a clinic or a private practitioner in the area. Mrs. A. seemed relieved that she was judged to be an appropriate patient for the study and eagerly accepted the invitation to participate. She signed a consent form indicating that she understood what the research project entailed and then completed a set of several self-report measures of distress, such as the Beck Depression Inventory (BDI; Beck, Ward, Mendelson, Mock, & Erbaugh, 1961) and the State-Trait Anxiety Inventory (STAI; Spielberger, 1983). Following this initial evaluation, follow-up assessments were conducted regularly at three- to six-month intervals for a period of two years following completion of therapy. All follow-ups used the SADS-Change interview (SADS-C; Spitzer & Endicott, 1977)—which does not go into prior history of depression but focuses on a here-and-now assessment of affective status—along with the BDI, the STAI, and other measures that were repeated at each assessment point to assess progress more closely. The general purpose of this research project was to compare the effectiveness of several different modalities of psychotherapy in the treatment of late-life depression.

Mrs. A. was randomly assigned to cognitive therapy. She did not select this treatment but expressed some satisfaction upon learning that it was the type of treatment she would receive (versus behavioral or psychodynamic therapy), because she'd always believed that her thoughts affected how she felt about things. However, she was skeptical that she could change at her age. She indicated that if she did not feel she was making progress after a month or so had passed, she would terminate therapy so that "the spot can be used for someone else in greater need." Yet her initial diagnosis had been major depressive episode and her initial BDI score was 43, putting her in the severe range of self-reported depression. Her STAI scores were above the 75th percentile for both state and trait anxiety. Taken together, these data strongly suggested a person in significant distress who was experiencing a combination of depressive and anxious symptoms but tended to under estimate their severity. The latter is very common among older adults who grew up in an era where "keeping a stiff upper lip" was a highly valued behavior (Cavanaugh, 1990).

At our weekly clinical staff meeting, the input of the treatment team was solicited to form the case conceptualization; this information was then shared with the primary therapist to guide her in starting the treatment program. This is our usual practice, with the understanding that the primary therapist will usually modify the case conceptualization over time as more information becomes available. The initial formulation was based on the idea that Mrs. A. was experiencing a reactive depression subsequent to the multiple losses she had experienced. First, she had been a primary caregiver for a very disabled husband with Alzheimer's disease. It is well-known that such a situation is extremely stressful, and that many caregivers experience significant psychological problems as a result of the constant burden of the role (Gallagher, Rose, Rivera, Lovett, & Thompson, 1989; Zarit, Reever, & Bach-Peterson, 1980). Second, her husband had died not long ago; evidence from both the research and clinical literatures points out that loss of a spouse is the single most significant stressor one can experience at any age (Parkes, 1987) and that older persons are likely to have a very difficult time adapting to this event, with depression and health problems as common negative outcomes (Lund, 1989). Third, Mrs. A. had retired from her busy position as an executive secretary about one year prior to seeking treatment—undoubtedly, yet another major loss. This loss was further aggravated by an absence of preretirement counseling and the possibility that she had not fully mourned the death of her husband.

Thus, it seemed to us that her normally adaptive coping strategies were quite overwhelmed by this chain of events, leading to the development of significant depressive symptoms. On another level, it seemed reasonable to expect that prior conflicts with grown children could reappear in the wake of this reaction, along with reactivation of earlier feelings of low self-esteem. Thus, therapy was judged to require a minimum of 20 sessions at the outset. Following the standard evaluation at that time, it was agreed that some additional sessions would probably enable her to make progress with schema work and to have time to address maintenance-of-gains issues.

TREATMENT

Mrs. A. actually received 30 sessions of individual therapy. Initial treatment goals were (a) developing her understanding of how her depression arose and explaining to her that therapy would involve developing skills to help her cope with her changed world; (b) specifically, how to adapt better to retirement, including examining her thoughts about the situation and what it meant and also analyzing her activities to determine if new behaviors needed to be added; (c) examining conflicts with her adult children in more depth, with the aim of increasing positive interactions; and (d) if time permitted, examining her early beliefs that fostered her sense of inadequacy, with the goal of challenging these beliefs and freeing her from some of these long-held ideas. No specific goals were set regarding health concerns, since these seemed to be adequately dealt with by the primary care physician, to whom Mrs. A. was repeatedly referred when health or medication questions arose. It should be noted that Mrs. A. participated in setting these treatment goals and was a very willing participant in therapy throughout the process, despite her initial belief that she was not well educated enough to benefit from therapy.

The structure of therapy was such that the first four sessions were spent socializing this client into therapy and helping her understand how her depression arose and was being maintained. Sessions 5 through 9 focused on helping her adapt better to retirement; sessions 10 through 17 were spent on relationship issues involving the adult children; sessions 18 through 26 dealt with the schema work; and finally sessions 27 through 30 were devoted explicitly to termination issues and maintenance of gains.

Therapy began with the therapist, a female psychologist in her 30s with about five years' experience with older adults, sharing her conceptualization regarding Mrs. A's depression—specifically, that it resulted from the multiple losses she had experienced, beginning with the loss of time and of some aspects of a life for herself as her husband's Alzheimer's disease progressed (although she still maintained her demanding full-time job). That was followed by his actual death, which, although she had several years to prepare for it, was nevertheless a severe loss. Then Mrs. A. had apparently decided to retire from her job, expecting that this would relieve her stress but not anticipating how empty and lost she would feel without any sort of regular schedule and with no one apparently needing her. Mrs. A. wept frequently during these first few sessions as she thought about these cumulative losses, and she voiced hope that she could get over her depression once she had dealt with them more adequately. The therapist reassured her that cognitive therapy would do exactly this by focusing on the cognitions and behaviors that were maintaining the current depression. Homework at this stage consisted of the client learning how to record her daily behaviors on an activity log, along with writing down her frequent negative thoughts (called "mistakes in thinking," rather than distortions) so that she could see what her recurrent themes were and how often they were repeated in her mind. She used the standard Dysfunctional Thought Record (DTR) for this (see Burns, 1989, for sample forms), beginning with the triple-column technique. Below is one example of Mrs. A.'s early DTRs:

- *Situation*—At home alone in the evening, having dinner
- *Thoughts*—Is it always going to be like this? When will I have adults other than my family in my life again? I'm very cut off from other people right now.
- *Feelings*—Lonely, sad, depressed

It was helpful to have Mrs. A. rate the extent to which she believed each thought, along with the intensity level of each of her different feelings, but this took some time for her to learn how to do because she tended to see most aspects of her life in all-or-none terms and so had difficulty describing her thoughts and feelings in shades of gray. Once she saw these shadings, she began to challenge her thoughts more and so advanced to the next column of the DTR for homework. This coincided with moving into the next problem area (at session 5), namely, adapting better to her retirement. At this point, several techniques were particularly helpful to this client in learning how to challenge her negative thinking effectively; examples follow.

1. *Examining the evidence*. As noted above, Mrs. A. was also keeping an activity log in the first four weeks of therapy. By really reviewing what she was doing, she was able to challenge thoughts like "I never do anything fun anymore," "I have no one to go out with," and "I'm just wasting my time these days."

2. *Developing experiments to test out her beliefs about herself and her current life-style.* Mrs. A. believed that she had to be busy in order to be happy; since she wasn't busy (in the sense of a full-time job or caregiving activities), she concluded that she was both lazy and ineffective. A series of experiments was used in order to challenge these beliefs, including a discussion of activities that formerly made her feel good—such as cooking for family, going to lunch with friends, and watching certain TV shows—and planning for how she could begin to do these activities again. She was also asked to predict the amount of pleasure she expected to get from each and then rate her actual pleasure. Since none of these activities involved "keeping busy" in the usual sense of the term, she was then able to challenge the thought that paid employment was essential to her sense of well-being.

Automatic thought	Cognitive disortion	Adaptive response
"If I don't work for a living, or continue to be a caregiver, I am ineffective."	All-or-none thinking	"I can feel good about myself if I'm doing things I enjoy; it just takes practice."

3. *Reattribution of the reasons for her retirement.* At first, Mrs. A. described these reasons in terms of her "giving up" on life and being "too old and tired" to continue working. She did not see any of the potential rewards of retirement, particularly since she had the interrelated thought of "I must be working all the time in order to feel I am of value." So she was asked to think about other reasons why people (in general) retire and how others she knew thought about their situation. This variation on Burns's (1989) "double standard" technique was helpful to her and led to her asking herself the question, "What is wrong with me that I don't see this as a positive step in my life?" She was able to generate a host of positive expectancies that applied to others; she then realized she *was* tired, partly as a result of her years of caregiving and her coping with her husband's death. She was able to reframe this into the thought, "I deserve more in life than just working all the time. My husband provided well for me, plus I have my own retirement income, so what is holding me back from moving into this new phase of my life?" This reattribution (from blame to a more balanced view of her life) led to a generally more positive attitude about her current living situation. This in turn permitted therapist and client to move on into the next problem area: relationships with her adult children.

Sessions 10 through 17 were focused on her overgeneralizing about her children. Because her son had turned out badly did not mean that (a) she was a bad mother "through and through," or that (b) her other three children were failures. Mrs. A. was not easily convinced regarding her son; she clearly took responsibility for his substance abuse problems and felt that they were caused by family dynamics, particularly frequent tension and open conflict between herself and her husband regarding child-rearing practices. She described her husband as very permissive and herself as the taskmaster. She felt she had more control over how the daughters were raised, but was less confident regarding her son and so often "gave in" to her husband's approach. This was causing her a great deal of guilt and shame, and it seemed to be interfering with her ability to relate appropriately to any of her children (each of whom was at least 30 years old).

To help put this in perspective, Mrs. A. was asked to examine the evidence regarding child-rearing practices in the United States at the time her son was small. She went to the library, where she read some old Dr. Spock books on the subject and was reminded about how parents were then encouraged to be permissive and easygoing with their children. She read other books about peer pressure, addiction, and related subjects; these helped her gradually come to the conclusion that parents in general cannot be held totally responsible for how their children turn out, whether the outcome is very good or very bad. She also began to challenge her labeling of her son as "bad" because of his problem and seemed to be able to take a less harsh view of him. This, along with reduced self-blame, enabled her to reestablish contact with him after several years of significant emotional distance between them.

Once this was accomplished, it was relatively easy for Mrs. A. to discuss what she wanted from her daughters currently in terms of a relationship, and then to take needed behavioral steps to implement this. For example, she realized that they tended to avoid her after she made remarks that could seem critical about their child-rearing practices. Through role-playing, Mrs. A. learned to modulate her remarks and to be more active in arranging pleasant events with her daughters. This was most easily accomplished with the one who lived close by; for the out-of-state daughters, this meant arranging special trips, sending cards and gifts on occasion, and doing regular telephoning. Once she initiated these behaviors, her daughters responded in a very positive way. This in turn enabled Mrs. A. to challenge the thought that she was a bad parent and to begin to see herself as a likable person with relatively healthy family ties.

By this time, therapy was up to about session 18. Therapist and client discussed whether it would be useful to do some schema work next (versus termination). Mrs. A. was very motivated to continue in therapy, since she was beginning to see (on her own) that many of her strongly held beliefs had their origins in childhood or early adulthood. Through use of the downward-arrow technique, she quickly saw that many of her distorted thinking patterns were tied into early experiences that led her to develop an inadequate self-perception and low self-esteem.

CLIENT: If I let people get to know me, they will see how ineffective I am. After all, I came from a blue-collar family and barely finished high school.
THERAPIST: Supposing that happened; what would it mean to you?
CLIENT: Well, if they saw I couldn't do things as well as

I put on I can, and that I didn't go beyond high school, they would think I wasn't as good as them.
THERAPIST: And if that were true, why would that be so upsetting?
CLIENT: People would see me as inferior.
THERAPIST: Well, assume that happens. Why would that be so upsetting?
CLIENT: That would just be more proof that it really is true that I'm inferior. I'd feel terrible because it would show that even though I tried to overcome my upbringing, I never really have.
THERAPIST: And if it is true that you haven't fully risen above your early life circumstances, what does that mean to you now?
CLIENT: That I am truly inadequate and there is no hope for me.

This example illustrates how the downward-arrow technique revealed several of her core beliefs that clearly were implicated in her depression and, if not challenged, would predispose her to future episodes of depression when new events occurred that triggered the inadequacy schema. To help Mrs. A. work with this schema, techniques described in Young (1990) were used. First, she was asked to review the evidence in its support and play "devil's advocate" by defending the schema to the therapist. She was asked to make the best case she could in support of the schema and to give as many examples as possible to validate it. This she could easily do. Then Mrs. A. was asked to examine the supporting evidence critically and see if there was any other way to view the same information. Finally, she was asked to detail as much evidence as she could to contradict the schema.

For example, in support of the schema, Mrs. A. came up with, "my parents were poor and did not encourage me to pursue much in the way of education; they did not encourage me in much, actually, so it was hard for me to gain confidence in myself." Then, when examining the evidence, she saw that much of her thinking was a direct reflection of her parents' attitudes about life. They valued financial and other forms of success very highly and were frequently pushing her very hard to achieve. Although Mrs. A. was of at least average intelligence, she was not a genius, and so early on she learned that her successes weren't enough. She was unable to please her parents fully, despite trying her best to do so in the one arena she could (schoolwork). This is where she acquired the "work ethic" so strongly; it was an attempt to gain approval and make up for the underlying feelings of inadequacy.

Finally, Mrs. A. challenged the schema by reviewing what she had actually accomplished in her life—which was substantial, once she took the time to think about it carefully and to write it out in detail. For example, she had adjusted to a very upscale environment, married a successful man, raised several children well, obtained employment and progressed in her career over a number of years, and now was financially well off enough to be able to retire and have leisure time. She had also survived the death of her husband and was slowly putting her life together again. This kind of review enabled her to see herself as a strong person who actually coped quite well with most of life's pleasures and its pains. This loosened up the schema considerably, so that after about nine sessions of work on it, she was trying out a new schema: that of the "good coper."

The final four sessions were spent on termination and maintenance-of-gains issues. Regarding termination, Mrs. A. was sad about the regular sessions ending and was feeling insecure that she could continue to help herself, by herself, in the future. It was pointed out that she could return to the center if circumstances warranted it, and that she did not necessarily have to be in the throes of a major depression again in order to seek help. In other words, she was given permission to return even with "lesser" problems and was reminded that she could probably tackle them as effectively as she had this round of difficulties. Mrs. A. was also asked to review possible triggers for future depressions and to make a plan for how to assess their intensity and how to decide what to do. She was then asked to select a particularly distressing incident that was likely to occur in the future and to discuss in detail how she would handle it. Finally, she made notes in her "survival guide" notebook about these discussions; it was pointed out to her that otherwise, she might forget some of the material learned (particularly specific techniques used), so having some written material was part of the preventive approach. Therapist and client also expressed their thoughts and feelings about having worked together (the therapist modeled this for the client, so that she would feel safe doing it). The door was left open for future contacts, with the statement that "self-understanding is never finished."

After 20 sessions and again at the conclusion of therapy, Mrs. A. was interviewed by an independent clinical evaluator in our setting; she also completed the self-report questionnaires each time. At both assessment points, she was judged to be free of any significant depressive symptoms on the SADS-C interview. Her BDI score was down to a 3 or 4, where it remained steadily for about the last six weeks of therapy. This is clearly in the nondepressed range. Her STAI scores were also within normal limits. In short, from a number of perspectives, this client had made significant change in about six months of

treatment, to the point that she was no longer symptomatic. This improvement was maintained over two years of periodic follow-up, despite the fact that she developed some new health problems that limited her mobility somewhat. One of her daughters also had severe marital problems and became divorced, which distressed Mrs. A. considerably but did not lead to another depressive episode. We learned that she has kept up her activities in the community and, in general, seems to be a quite well-adjusted, functional older adult with normal problems in living.

SUMMARY

This case illustrates how the principles and techniques of cognitive therapy were successfully used to treat a severe major depressive episode in a 66-year-old Caucasian woman whose depression resulted primarily from a series of negative life events. After a few initial sessions focused on socializing her into therapy, she became a very cooperative client, eager to learn more about herself and to modify her ways of thinking and perceiving. A number of specific depressogenic thinking patterns were dealt with, including negative ideas about herself in retirement, conflicted relationships with her adult children (based on unrealistic expectations), and examination of long-held beliefs of personal inadequacy. Successful therapy methods included regular use of the Dysfunctional Thought Record (progressing from the triple-column technique to completion of all five columns); application of such cognitive skills as examining the evidence, making reattributions when possible about events; and learning to think in shades of gray (to counteract her tendency to think in all-or-none terms). Behaviorally, she engaged in a number of experiments designed to help her test out some of her beliefs about how families behave in general. She also learned to increase her participation in pleasant activities, both by herself and with other friends and family members.

A critical ingredient of success in this case was Mrs. A's compliance with homework, especially in the early stages of therapy, when she may not have fully understood why homework was so important. Given her sensitivity about her educational background and her feelings of inadequacy stemming from her upbringing, it is a credit to the skill of the therapist that homework was given in as nonthreatening a manner as possible. Mrs. A.'s success over time indicates that she learned a number of the skills taught in therapy and was able to apply them to other potentially depressogenic situations that occurred after therapy ended.

DISCUSSION

This case is typical of the kind of older client who seeks psychotherapy as a remedy for his or her distress. While many older persons go first to their primary care physician (rather than to a mental health worker, because of stereotypes about mental illness), most will accept a referral for counseling or therapy if they are reassured that this does not mean they are "crazy" and if an adequately trained individual is available to work with them (Cavanaugh, 1990). However, due to negative stereotyping of old age that occurs during the training of most mental health professionals (even today), the latter is not so easy to find. Yet increasing availability of continuing education programs about aging and mental health, along with an ever-increasing number of clinical and research reports indicating that older adults can and do respond well to psychotherapy in many forms, suggests that this picture is changing rapidly. This will be facilitated by the recent federal decision to include psychologists and clinical social workers as recognized service providers in the Medicare system, which means that many mental health services will now be reimbursed, thus making it possible for larger numbers of elders to participate in psychotherapy than has ever been the case historically.

In this final section, we would like to present some of the common problems or concerns that many mental health practitioners experience when attempting therapy with older adults. These are presented in greater detail, with additional case examples, in Thompson, Davies, Gallagher, and Krantz (1986) and Thompson, et al. (1991); the main points are abstracted here due to space limitations.

First, the typical older adult's lack of experience with therapy makes it difficult for him or her initially to engage in treatment, so time for socialization to therapy needs to be included in the treatment plan. This would be the case with any underserved minority group, particularly one with a lower level of educational attainment. Second, it is essential that the practitioner routinely contact the client's medical doctor in order to clarify issues of diagnosis and to gain support in the therapy endeavor. For example, in Mrs. A.'s case, antidepressant medication was contraindicated because of the medication regimen she was already on. Unfortunately, this is very common in the over-60 age group. It should also be noted that many older adults do not tolerate well the common antidepressant medications because of extensive and/or troublesome side effects, such as orthostatic hypotension, urinary retention, constipation, and dry mouth (Fitten, Morley, Gross, Petry, & Cole, 1989). Because of this, they often discontinue medication against their physician's advice; yet depression does not

tend to remit easily in older persons, so that in such instances, it remains essentially untreated. The primary care physician needs to be consulted for another reason: Sometimes older adults are misdiagnosed as depressed when in reality they have a tumor or another problem that needs medical (not psychosocial) care. Given that many kinds of cancer can mask as depression, it is critical to not assume a psychosocial origin to the problem in the absence of an up-to-date medical evaluation.

Let us assume that you have gotten the older adult to commit to some amount of therapy, and that you are reasonably convinced that the problem is one that psychotherapy in general—and cognitive therapy in particular—can address. You then need to take several specific steps to engage the older client in treatment. First, you need to be aware of sensory limitations and to adjust yourself accordingly. Most older persons have significant vision and hearing problems but are too embarrassed to reveal them openly, so misunderstandings can easily occur if no inquiries are made. It is also a good idea to try and be flexible when the client becomes ill and cannot make it to the office for his or her scheduled appointment. It is often necessary in such instances to see older clients in their homes or in the hospital. This type of flexibility in scheduling is generally very much appreciated by the older adult.

Second, it must be emphasized that therapy is a *learning experience*, and is not intended to change the personality or to change other people. In order to bring about maximal learning, clients need to have material presented in a multimodal fashion (e.g., hearing it said, writing it down themselves, and possibly reviewing a tape of it in between sessions). Many older adults are fearful that they cannot really learn anything new; others are pleased that therapy will have this type of activity in it. In any event, it is important to do all that you can to enhance learning. It is also important for therapists to remember that memory problems are common in persons over the age of 60. Typically, short-term or recent memory is slower and/or less efficient than it was. This means that you need to repeat and reemphasize important concepts and techniques so that they will become encoded properly in the older client's memory. Also, use of aids such as notebooks, flash cards, Post-It notes, and the like can make a substantial difference in how well the older client will remember topics in therapy.

A related issue is whether or not (and when) to include family members in the therapy endeavor. We have done this on a limited basis but would suggest that it be considered in each case, particularly when the older adult is living with other family members who have potential to help the client either overcome or maintain his or her depression. Issues such as confidentiality are extremely important in these instances, along with the family members' personal issues about what is happening to their relative. A great deal of tact is needed when family members are involved. We would recommend keeping the interaction very task oriented in order to gain their support for the older client's improvement.

A final issue pertains to the importance of the therapeutic relationship for the depressed and often isolated older adult. This relationship can sometimes turn into one of dependency on the therapist unless attributions for change are clearly credited to the client. Increased self-efficacy perceptions should be a goal of all cognitive therapy with older persons. Along with this, thought needs to be given to how best to terminate therapy. Many older persons prefer to keep the door open rather than experience an abrupt termination. Our experience indicates that this is generally a good approach, since it will permit the older person to seek help again more readily. Another way to handle this is to taper off sessions gradually over a period of several weeks or months, rather than doing it abruptly. For some older persons, this gives them enough time to practice their newly gained skills in a myriad of situations, thus increasing their confidence, while giving them a supportive person to report to about their experiences.

In brief, older adults can and do respond very well to time-limited cognitive therapy for such problems as depression, anxiety disorders, and caregiver stress. Very little modification of either the form or content of therapy is needed, except for the points noted above and some others discussed in Thompson et al. (1991) that serve to alert the therapist to some special needs of older adults. We have found that if they are treated with respect and with the expectation that they can learn and improve, very significant change can and does frequently occur.

ACKNOWLEDGMENTS. This work was supported in part by several grants from the National Institute of Mental Health, including MH43407, MH40041, and MH37196. The authors also wish to thank the many older adult patients whose experiences have permitted them to learn so much about psychotherapy in later life.

REFERENCES

American Psychiatric Association. (1987). *Diagnostic and statistical manual of mental disorders* (rev. 3rd ed.). Washington, DC: Author.

Beck, A. T., Ward, C., Mendelson, M., Mock, J., & Erbaugh, J. (1961). An inventory for measuring depression. *Archives of General Psychiatry, 4,* 561–571.

Burns, D. (1989). *The feeling good handbook: Using the new mood therapy in everyday life.* New York: William Morrow.

Cavanaugh, J. C. (1990). *Adult development and aging.* Belmont, CA: Wadsworth.

Endicott, J., & Spitzer, R. (1978). A diagnostic interview for affective disorders and schizophrenia. *Archives of General Psychiatry, 35,* 837–844.

Fitten, L. J., Morley, J., Gross, P., Petry, S., & Cole, K. (1989). Depression: UCLA geriatric grand rounds. *Journal of the American Geriatrics Society, 37,* 459–472.

Gallagher, D., Rose, J., Rivera, P., Lovett, S., & Thompson, L. W. (1989). Prevalence of depression in family caregivers. *Gerontologist, 29,* 449–456.

Lund, D. (Ed.). (1989). *Older bereaved spouses: Research with practical applications.* New York: Hemisphere.

Parkes, C. M. (1987). *Bereavement: Studies of grief in adult life.* Madison, CT: International Universities Press.

Spielberger, C. D. (1983). *Manual for the State-Trait Anxiety Inventory.* Palo Alto, CA: Consulting Psychologists Press.

Spitzer, R., & Endicott, J. (1977). *The SADS-Change Interview.* New York: New York State Psychiatric Institute.

Thompson, L. W., Davies, R., Gallagher, D., & Krantz, S. (1986). Cognitive therapy with older adults. *Clinical Gerontologist, 5,* 245–279.

Thompson, L. W., Florsheim, M., DelMaestro, S., Gantz, F., Gallagher-Thompson, D., and Bryan, H. (1991). Cognitive/behavioral therapy for affective disorders in the elderly. In W. Myers (Ed.), *New techniques in the psychotherapy of older patients* (pp. 3–19). Washington, DC: American Psychiatric Association Press.

Young, J. E. (1990). *Cognitive therapy for personality disorders: A schema-focused approach.* Sarasota, FL: Professional Resource Exchange.

Zarit, S., Reever, K., & Bach-Peterson, J. (1980). Relatives of the impaired elderly: Correlates of feelings of burden. *The Gerontologist, 20,* 649–655.

SUGGESTED READINGS

All of the following are suitable for professionals who wish to gain more knowledge about mental health, depression, and aging; the third and fifth are also appropriate for lay readers.

Blazer, D. (1990). *Emotional problems in later life: Intervention strategies for professional caregivers.* New York: Springer.

Brink, T. L. (Ed.). (1986). *Clinical gerontology: A guide to assessment and intervention.* New York: Haworth.

Burns, D. (1989). *The feeling good handbook: Using the new mood therapy in everyday life.* New York: William Morrow.

Fry, P. S. (1986). *Depression, stress, and adaptations in the elderly: Psychological assessment and intervention.* Rockville, MD: Aspen.

Mace, N. L., & Rabins, P. V. (1991). *The 36-hour day: A family guide to caring for persons with Alzheimer's disease, related dementing illnesses, and memory loss in later life* (rev. ed.). Baltimore, MD: Johns Hopkins University Press.

20

Inhibited Grief

Frank E. Gantz, Dolores Gallagher-Thompson, and John L. Rodman

INTRODUCTION

Losses of all kinds are extremely common in the lives of older adults, with spousal bereavement being the most common (see Cavanaugh, 1990). Spousal loss is more common for women; over half of all women over age 65 are widows, compared to only 15% of men of the same age. Other types of losses—such as friends moving away or dying, loss of income through retirement, loss of physical health or one's functional capabilities, and so on—are more common among older adults, although they occur less frequently in younger segments of the population as well. Note that, according to several prominent researchers in the field, loss of a child may be the most painful type of bereavement one can experience (Oster-

weis, Solomon, & Green, 1984), and loss of a spouse may be more difficult for younger than for older persons (Parkes, 1987).

A comprehensive and insightful volume on various types of bereavement, and how they were coped with by persons of different ages and socioeconomic strata, was compiled by Osterweis et al. (1984). In it, the authors stress the importance of viewing grief as a lengthy process of adaptation, an experience from which most eventually recover adequately. Yet it should not be overlooked that reactions such as failure to grieve (a delayed or inhibited response), excessive grief that persists for many years, or grief complicated by clinical depression will generally require professional intervention regardless of age. Osterweis et al. (1984) do not discuss the utility of cognitive therapy per se in these instances— partially because the therapy was relatively new at that time and little had been written in the cognitive literature about treatment of grief. But their review of other forms of psychologically oriented treatment (e.g., psychodynamic) supports the point that therapy can be extremely beneficial. Abrahms (1981) has written one of the few cognitively oriented chapters for treatment of grief reactions, focusing on identification and challenging of the common negative thoughts experienced by persons undergoing bereavement. In this chapter, we believe we have gone beyond her work and demonstrated how an integrated cognitive-behavioral approach, oriented around helping a client complete the common "tasks" of grieving, can be successfully used with an older adult.

Frank E. Gantz • Psychology Service, Veterans Affairs Medical Center, Salisbury, North Carolina 28144.   Dolores Gallagher-Thompson • Older Adult and Family Research and Resource Center, Division of Gerontology, Stanford University School of Medicine, Stanford, California 94305 and Geriatric Research, Education, and Clinical Center, Veterans Affairs Medical Center, Palo Alto, California 94304.   John L. Rodman • Department of Psychiatry, The Ramsey Clinic, St. Paul. Minnesota 55101-2595. This work was done at Stanford University and was supported in part by several grants from the National Institutes of Mental Health, including: MH43407 (Gallagher-Thompson), MH40041 (Yesavage), and MH37196 (Thompson).

Comprehensive Casebook of Cognitive Therapy, edited by Arthur Freeman and Frank M. Dattilio. Plenum Press, New York, 1992.

IDENTIFYING INFORMATION

Mr. G. was a 67-year-old semiretired man with the equivalent of 18 years of education. He had no prior experience in psychotherapy, and did not report any history of psychological difficulty prior to the death of his wife, who died a year earlier after a long battle with a chronic illness. They had met while he was in the service, and had been married for 35 years. In addition to having developed a family real estate business together, they had raised three children, all of whom had moved elsewhere to pursue career and family goals. The client still maintained active contact with the children, as well as with the many friends he and his wife had developed over the years.

ASSESSMENT AND DIAGNOSIS

As part of our normal intake procedure, a clinical psychologist conducted a careful diagnostic interview using the Schedule for Affective Disorders and Schizophrenia (SADS; Endicott & Spitzer, 1978). A diagnosis of minor depressive disorder was obtained using these criteria, with primary complaints including depressed mood (worse in the evenings), self-reproach, and appetite disturbance (with a weight loss of 10 pounds since his wife's death). Mr. G. scored a 10 on the Beck Depression Inventory (bordering on the mild clinical range), and a 9 on the Hamilton Rating Scale for Depression (mild mood disturbance). (The latter is an interview instrument and is more specific for physiological correlates of depression, which may account for the difference in classification.) The diagnosis was modified to include inhibited grief, since this better described the client's condition and because his depressive symptoms were understandable sequelae of his bereavement.

TREATMENT

Early Phase (Sessions 1 Through 5)

Mr. G. was seen for a total of 18 sessions over a period of about one year. This lengthy duration was in part due to the fact that the client traveled a great deal during this time. The first three sessions focused (in chronological order) on (a) eliciting a history of his wife's death and his reactions to it; (b) obtaining a history of their relationship; and (c) educating the client about the cognitive-behavioral (CB) model, using didactic presentation and pertinent readings. Once these objectives were accomplished, therapeutic work focused directly on his clinical complaint.

Immediately following the death, Mr. G. reported that he had coped well, which further exploration revealed meant that he was extremely active. As time moved on, however, he began to feel "stuck" and, as he put it, he needed "something to get [him] over the hump". The therapist hypothesized that this high activity level could represent a form of avoidance. Therefore, he began having Mr. G. make systematic observations regarding his activity level and mood, and attempted to correlate this information with the client's avoidance of loss issues. This self-monitoring technique, called the Daily Mood Monitor, involves a retrospective rating of the day's average mood (1 being very sad, to 9 being very happy) with space to record events related to the obtained mood rating. Although Mr. G. did not always comply with this assignment, valuable information was acquired, and the client was made more conscious of his hectic pace of life.

In addition, to facilitate the client's understanding of the grief process, a reading on Worden's (1982) "four tasks of mourning" was presented at the end of the third session. These four tasks are:

1. Accepting the reality of the loss
2. Working through the pain of the loss
3. Adjusting to an environment in which the deceased is missing
4. Withdrawing emotional energy from the deceased and reinvesting it in new relationships

Unlike stages, these tasks are considered to overlap and to be accomplished somewhat in tandem. Therapeutically, this psychoeducational intervention reduced some of the client's confusion about the grief process and where he was "stuck." More importantly, it provided the client and therapist a conceptual framework within which to focus their work.

Sessions 4 and 5 were spent discussing this material and identifying the degree to which Mr. G. had accomplished each task. By the fourth session, it was determined he had completed task 1 (accepted the death's reality), and had started task 3 (adjusting to the environment without Jane). On the other hand, he was clearly avoiding task 2—experiencing his profound loss. When discussing his wife's death in session, for example, he displayed little emotion. Although he had cried for her, he did so only the day after she died, and then only alone. Given this avoidance, it is not surprising that he was failing to form any new relationships (task 4). A clinical decision was therefore made to approach slowly the issue of experiencing his pain. The initial "task work" emphasized task 3 (adjusting to the environment without the deceased).

Socratic questioning and guided discovery were used to help Mr. G. identify the roles his wife fulfilled within their marriage and how he could now get these needs met in alternative ways. The client possessed strong problem-solving skills and excelled with this task. For example, his wife had played an integral role in their real estate business. The client gradually assembled a team of consultants who essentially provided the same functions. This behavior was seen as adaptive, since it allowed the client to continue to stay active in real estate. The client's difficulties with accepting the pain of the loss and reinvesting energy in new relationships (tasks 2 and 4) were collaboratively explored and hypotheses were generated during this time, but no interventions were implemented.

A second major issue addressed early in treatment (sessions 3 through 5) involved the client's guilt feelings. These feelings were related to his perceptions of how he handled his wife's medical condition and the fact that he was not present at the moment of her death. Mr. G. believed he had allowed valuable time to elapse—two to three weeks that could have been used to treat her more aggressively and possibly prolong her life—in an effort to let his wife maintain more control over her care. Through Socratic questioning and examination of the lack of evidence for his belief "If I'd intervened earlier, she could have lived longer," Mr. G. was able to view his behavior much more realistically. His guilt about not being present at the moment of death was addressed in similar fashion during session 4. However, unlike the previous issue, significant guilt feelings remained to be resolved later (as will be seen).

Meanwhile, his progress with other tasks of grieving was continuously monitored. By session 5, Mr. G. was able to use the Daily Record of Dysfunctional Thoughts (DRDT) in session to overcome his guilt and anxiety about asking a longtime female friend to accompany him on a trip to Canada to visit mutual friends. Socratic questioning about this issue revealed that Mr. G. believed that his behavior would be frowned upon by friends who had known them as a couple and possibly be seen as evidence that he didn't really love his wife. These thoughts were addressed and more adaptive thoughts developed, which appeared on the DRDT (see Figure 20-1).

Recall that the client had early on equated high activity with good coping. The trip to Canada had been planned for some time, but evidence accumulated during treatment tended to confirm the therapist's hypothesis that activity equaled avoidance. In the collaborative spirit of CB therapy, he shared this hypothesis with Mr. G. before the trip, resulting in the following dialogue:

THERAPIST: We've looked over the tasks, and we seem to agree that you've coped on a practical level with certain aspects of the void you experience with Jane

dying . . . But then there is the emotional level of the void and my feeling is you haven't *quite* done all the work in that—

CLIENT: (interrupts) What do—what do you mean? Uh—I'm not quite with you there?

THERAPIST: Okay . . .

CLIENT: In other words, uh—(smiling) I'm not graduated from your class yet? (chuckles)

THERAPIST: I'm just wondering if this very high level of activity is—

CLIENT: (interrupts) I'm interested in what you have to say, because if I'm intentionally or unintentionally doing things to cover up that, I want to get that through with.

THERAPIST: OK, but what I'm planting here is a seed. I'm wondering if this very high level of activity is your way of coping with some of the pain of the loss and the loneliness. And it's not for me to judge whether you are or not . . . I don't think these activities are *only* to avoid the pain of the loss. It's not black or white. But there may be another level you aren't aware of, and I want to raise your consciousness about a *possible hypothesis* . . . and you can determine the validity of this for yourself.

CLIENT: OK. I'll keep that in mind.

It was at this point, due to his trip abroad, that there was a two-month hiatus from therapy.

Middle Phase of Treatment (Sessions 6 Through 12)

The middle phase of treatment was characterized by continued work on the hypothesis raised before the trip. The therapist, for example, pointed out that earlier in therapy, the client revealed that he had not really cried after his wife's death and had quickly become involved in a very busy schedule. Specifically, within a few months of her death, the client was traveling extensively and was busier than ever before. These behaviors were gently presented with observations of the client's lack of emotional expression when discussing his wife's death in the sessions. At first, Mr. G. adamantly denied there was any relationship between these factors, asserting he had largely dealt with the emotional consequences of her death. However, the therapist persistently raised the issue, and by the 10th session, the client reported a significant change in his experience.

CLIENT: You know, I—as we left the last meeting, something just popped out of me. I don't know if you caught it or not. I said, "I haven't spent enough time with her." And I think I've been so involved with the

Figure 20-1 Daily Record of Dysfunctional Thoughts

Situation	Automatic Thoughts	Emotion(s)	Adaptive Responses	Outcome
Describe the event or experience leading up to your unpleasant emotions; be as specific as possible.	Write down your negative thoughts and/or negative self-talk that occurred in connection with the event or experience just described. Rate your degree of belief in the thoughts or self-talk; from 0% to 100%.	Write down what you are feeling (sad, anxious, angry, etc.). Rate degree of emotion, from 1% to 100%.	Try to challenge your negative thoughts or self-talk. Think about: What is the evidence for the idea? What are its pros and cons? Can I think of an alternative? Then write down these counter-thoughts. Rate your degree of belief in these new thoughts, from 0% to 100%.	Re-rate your belief in automatic thoughts, from 0 to 100%. Specify and rate your emotions *now*, from 1% to 100%.
Date				
Thinking about asking Martha to go with me to Joe & Cindy's party.	I shouldn't be looking at female companionship this soon after Jane's death.	Guilt (50%)	*Should statement*—Who says I shouldn't? It has been almost a year since Jane died. Where is the time limit set in stone?	Guilt (15%)
	My friends will think I didn't really love her.	Anxiety (50%)	*Mind reading*—I can't know what they'd think. Plus those who really know me know I loved her very much.	Anxiety (10%)

Note: Ratings for beliefs in thoughts: 0% = not at all; 100% = completely. For degree of emotions: 1% = a trace, 100% = the most intense possible.

other things, I'm gonna have to, uh, just sit down and do some of the things that—uh—well, one, in her will that she wanted me to do and, two . . . maybe just concentrate on grieving a little more. Does that make any sense? I feel like I've thought a lot about her, but, uh—there's something that I have to do. I don't know exactly what it is yet.

THERAPIST: Maybe we can discover that together.

CLIENT: Yeah. I just feel like I haven't spent enough time with her. Does that make any sense?

THERAPIST: Well, what do you mean exactly by "haven't spent enough time with her"?

CLIENT: I guess, uh—not really thinking that much about her and letting these other things really crowd in. I just don't quite understand yet.

THERAPIST: So, maybe spending more time in terms of just not being really busy . . .

CLIENT: Yeah . . .

THERAPIST: . . . and allowing yourself to focus on her more emotionally?

CLIENT: Yeah. I feel—feel sort of guilty, like I sort of shoved her aside too fast. I need to spend more time with her.

This shift in Mr. G.'s perspective was crucial and marked a period of significant therapeutic movement. The primary intervention focused around the use of what Worden (1982) has called "linking objects." These are objects (photographs or memorabilia) that are meaningfully linked to the deceased, and exposure to which evokes strong emotions in the survivor. In behavior therapy terms, of course, this is known as "flooding," and there is evidence that exposure to such stimuli is essential to overcoming a distorted grief reaction and the avoidance coping underlying it (Callahan & Burnette, 1989). The rationale for using the linking objects was explained, and the client agreed to participate in this aspect of treatment.

First, relaxation training was initiated, not only to lay the groundwork for the linking-objects (or modified flooding) procedure, but to give Mr. G. an alternative response to "staying busy." Meanwhile, it was found that he not only had photos and letters from his wife, but audiotapes and videotapes of them together. Under conditions carefully planned in advance with the therapist, Mr. G. began to review these items several times over a monthlong period. He began by exposing himself to photographs, reminiscing about their shared activities. He then progressed to reading letters and eventually watched videotapes of them together. His reactions were processed in session. The intervention was quite successful, and it enabled the client to experience his powerful feelings of loss in a controlled and gradual way. Unlike previously, it

was also noted that Mr. G. would become visibly moved in therapy—he would shed tears, or his voice would crack.

A second intervention that facilitated a more complete acceptance of his wife's death was helping him to focus on what he missed about her, as well as what he did not miss about her. The latter issue was tedious at first, but assisted in reducing the cognitive process of idealization that had in many ways kept her alive for him. For example, he was eventually able to admit that he was relieved that he would not have to continue to worry about Jane's chronic physical illness, nor deal with some of her other, more idiosyncratic foibles that had irritated him. Mr. G. later reported this intervention was instrumental in helping him to obtain a more balanced (i.e., positive and negative) memory of his wife.

Overall, largely through his work with linking objects, the client was able to initiate and work through the emotional pain associated with his wife's death. Interestingly, as he began to deal more directly with the pain of the loss, Mr. G.'s activity level decreased dramatically, confirming the hypothesis first proffered by the therapist in the early phase of treatment.

Final Phase of Treatment (Sessions 13 Through 18)

By the final phase of treatment, the client was making significant progress in accepting the pain of the loss. The focus of therapy gradually shifted to task 4, and forming new emotional bonds (not necessarily romantic) was identified by both therapist and client as the next developmental step in the process. As with his gains in other areas, the client's movement on this task was graduated and stepwise. Although this progression was largely contingent on his ability to work through the pain and begin to let go of his wife, at various times during treatment, the client's movement toward completion of task 4 was facilitated by collaborative exploration of underlying dysfunctional attitudes that served as cognitive obstacles. Once these thoughts were addressed, the client rapidly progressed to a higher level of interpersonal intimacy and emotional bonding with male and female friends, including the serious consideration of romantic relationships.

In addition to developing new and/or deepening existing relationships, the client's unresolved guilt regarding his absence at the moment Jane died (unsuccessfully discussed early in therapy) was also deliberated. This issue was particularly painful for Mr. G. because he had just been relieved at her bedside by his son after two consecutive days and nights. As the reader may recall, initially, his guilt responded poorly to a DRDT intervention. Further discussion and definition of his emotions revealed that he actually felt regret over not being able to tell his wife certain things prior to her death, rather than guilt per se. Thus, one important outcome of this dialogue was that the client came to relabel his emotional experience in a more accurate manner. To deal with these regrets, Mr. G. was asked simply to express his unspoken thoughts to Jane in a letter, which he did. The letter was then sealed in an envelope, and the client mailed it to himself. After having done this, the client reported no longer feeling guilt or regret surrounding his "unfinished business."

Termination of therapy with this gentleman, particularly given the nature of the case, was carefully planned. As he began forming increasingly significant bonds with friends, the issue of ending treatment was raised. The end point of therapy was jointly agreed upon, and once designated, the therapist regularly commented on the number of sessions that remained. Mr. G. was encouraged to share both positive and negative thoughts and feelings about the course of treatment. He was specifically asked what he thought he would lose with the ending of therapy (i.e., of the therapeutic relationship). Finally, treatment gains, as well as *how* the gains were achieved, were systematically reviewed to help the client identify himself as the main agent of change. Shortly before the end of therapy, he became romantically involved with a woman and later that year married her, two years after his former wife's death.

A four-month follow-up evaluation conducted by an independent clinical psychologist using the SADS revealed that Mr. G. had no diagnosable psychological disorder. There were no residual symptoms of depression, and his scores on both the Beck Depression Inventory and on the Hamilton Rating Scale for Depression were zero.

Summary

Overall, this case was extremely successful. By the end of 18 sessions of CB therapy, the client had completed a significant amount of grief work. A central ingredient in the outcome was the clear conceptualization provided by Worden's (1982) model. This provided the client with a framework within which to understand his grief and specific tasks on which to focus. These features provide a good fit with the collaborative approach of CB therapy, and thus, the model is favored at our center. We also draw heavily in our grief work on the suggestions of Abrahms (1981) regarding how to identify and challenge common dysfunctional thoughts associated with grieving. In the present case, the DRDTs and the Socratic questioning of the therapist helped to alleviate some of the client's guilt while leading him to examine the hypothesis of avoiding his grief. In terms of working through the grief, the modified use of flooding was, without question, of major importance. Similarly, the development of a realistic im-

age of the deceased using cognitive techniques enabled the survivor to move on in life without being bound by idealized memories.

DISCUSSION

This case was presented because it bears on several important points. First, it illustrates how well a collaborative cognitive-behavioral approach works with older adults. Second, it demonstrates how complicated grief reactions can be successfully facilitated within a relatively short-term structured framework. Third, it highlights how both cognitive and behavioral interventions are necessary to facilitate an individual's grief process. In this case, as with most complicated bereavement, exposure to stimuli associated with the deceased and the eliciting of strong emotional reactions were crucial to successful treatment. Similarly, one's cognitive process plays an important role in the adaptation to the loss of a loved one. In our view, a balanced or "realistic" memory of the deceased is a desirable outcome of therapy—a memory including the kinds of strengths and weaknesses inherent in any human being. This issue has not, to our knowledge, been explicitly addressed by other scholars in the field of grief.

The reader might ask if this approach would be successful with younger bereaved persons or with older widows (who are greater in numbers). Our experience indicates that the basic approach outlined above is indeed appropriate in such instances. For example, the second author has treated numerous younger and older widows using time-limited cognitive-behavioral therapy and found that the majority respond very well. In general, bereaved women tend to be more emotionally expressive, with the most common problem being grief complicated by clinical depression. Their most frequent cognitions include thoughts that "life is not worth living without [the spouse]" and "I can't go on alone." Their distress can appear overwhelming, and support and encouragement (as well as referral to ancillary self-help programs) may help clients gain emotional stability more rapidly. For many widows, the option of remarriage is not available due to their circumstances. For example, a widowed younger woman with children is often unable to find time or resources to search for a new mate; an older widow may find too few options in terms of men close to her own age. Nevertheless, while demographics may influence longer-term adaptation, the therapeutic process is much the same.

Besides depression, a very common complication of bereavement in women is a significant level of anxiety (Parkes, 1987), which may make participation in therapy difficult. In our experience, it may be necessary to have a client evaluated for anxiolytic or antidepressant medication for a short time at the onset of therapy in order to encourage the client to make the commitment to therapy. However, along with others in the field (see Osterweis et al., 1984), we do not recommend long-term usage of medication in the treatment of grief.

Finally, the point should be made that not all bereaved persons respond well to cognitive-behavioral therapy. Some may develop intensified grief reactions that may seem almost psychotic in nature and intensity. For these clients, we recommend longer-term therapy and/or brief hospitalization to help restore and maintain reality testing. In addition, somatic complaints are common among bereaved individuals. Such complaints should not be assumed to be benign and can represent serious health problems (see Osterweis et al., 1984; Parkes, 1987) that require medical attention. If multiple symptoms are present, it is wise to refer the client for a medical evaluation.

REFERENCES

Abrahms, J. (1981). Depression versus normal grief following the death of a significant other. In G. Emery, S. Hollon, & R. C. Bedrosian (Eds.), *New directions in cognitive therapy*. New York: Guilford.

Callahan, E. J., & Burnette, M. M. (1989). Intervention for pathological grieving. *Behavior Therapist, 12*(7), 153–157.

Cavanaugh, J. C. (1990). *Adult development and aging*. Belmont, CA: Wadsworth.

Endicott, J., & Spitzer, R. L. (1978). A diagnostic interview: The Schedule for Affective Disorders and Schizophrenia. *Archives of General Psychiatry, 35*, 837–844.

Osterweis, M., Solomon, F., & Green, M. (Eds.). (1984). *Bereavement: Reactions, consequences and care*. Washington, DC: National Academy Press.

Parkes, C. M. (1987). *Bereavement: studies of grief in adult life*. Madison, CT: International Universities Press.

Worden, J. W. (1982). *Grief counseling and grief therapy*. New York: Springer.

SUGGESTED READINGS

Kushner, H. S. (1983). *When bad things happen to good people*. New York: Avon.

Lewis, C. S. (1961). A grief observed. London: Faber & Faber.

Rando, T. A. (1984). *Grief, dying and death: Clinical interventions for caregivers*. Champaign, IL: Research Press.

Tatelbaum, J. (1980). *The courage to grieve*. New York: Harper & Row.

21

Schizotypal Personality Disorder

Ruth L. Greenberg

"They're laughing at me, Mrs. Greenberg!"

Perhaps I had never guessed, in the early years of our relationship, the depth of Elsie's fear and the breadth of her dysfunction. She entered therapy in despair, hurtling from rage to depression, then mired in terrified self-doubt. At 37, she had taken a 15-year journey around the mental health system, not omitting a several-month stay in the custody of a state hospital. A newly equipped cognitive therapist, I thought I could shape her up and ship her out, a model of socialization and employability.

It was a supervisor who, after hearing of Elsie, sobered me up. "If you can get her to talk to another person at the boarding house, that will be a miracle," he said. Of course, he was right. Did he know Elsie was afraid to wear a hat, or open a window, or read a book, or that the fear of talking to a neighbor could preoccupy her for weeks at a time?

Elsie struck one immediately as bizarre. Her fear of strangers was so extreme that she took no chances on inadvertent eye contact, but regulated her gaze by rotating her entire head, so that frequently she appeared to be observing something on the ceiling or in the corners of a room. She walked with a wide stance and a heavy, deliberate step, as though she needed at each moment the reassurance of feeling an expanse of ground beneath her. When she did interact with people, she had a tendency to assume dramatic expressions that she seemed to keep on her face just a little bit too long.

Elsie presented an unusual profile for a patient at the Center for Cognitive Therapy in Philadelphia. She had not worked for many years, and lived on public assistance. She had temporal lobe epilepsy and was being treated with anticonvulsant medication. There were paranoid psychotic features to her condition, which seemed to merit a diagnosis of schizophreniform disorder as well as schizotypal personality disorder. Antidepressant and antipsychotic medications had been only minimally helpful to her. She was markedly isolated, interacting regularly only with her father and a single friend. It was difficult to find areas of strength!

Still, we were able to specify some goals appropriate for cognitive-behavioral intervention. After many years of what has become a long-term therapeutic relationship, I believe I can identify the operating principles and techniques of a therapy that eventually allowed Elsie, if not vocational success or a sparkling social life, at least to live with a far more generous measure of emotional comfort— and to talk to the people down the hall.

Ruth L. Greenberg • Center for Cognitive Therapy, Department of Psychiatry, University of Pennsylvania School of Medicine, Philadelphia, Pennsylvania 19104.

Comprehensive Casebook of Cognitive Therapy, edited by Arthur Freeman and Frank M. Dattilio. Plenum Press, New York, 1992.

BACKGROUND

Elsie was the only child of a loving, but passive, mother and an authoritarian father who seems to have fit the criteria for paranoid personality disorder. A shy and fearful child, she was deeply attached to her mother and reluctant to be separated from her. She was only marginally successful at school. At age 13, she began to experience neurological symptoms; however, temporal lobe epilepsy was not diagnosed until she was 17 years of age. Elsie managed to graduate from high school and to become engaged, for a short period, to a young man in the neighborhood who seems to have been passive, socially avoidant, and sexually naive. The relationship foundered, apparently because Elsie's fears precluded normal relationships with her fiancé's family; her lack of sexual interest probably also contributed to the difficulties. Elsie also succeeded in working for a few years before she became disabled by severe psychiatric disturbance. Shortly after, while Elsie was institutionalized, her mother was killed in an automobile accident. Once Elsie was discharged to a halfway house, her struggle to live independently began.

CORE ISSUES

Elsie's psychosocial development appears to have been profoundly affected by the development of a neurological illness and her family's reaction to it. By age 13, Elsie already knew she was different from her peers and that she was having unusual experiences, but for several years she was not given an adequate medical explanation for symptoms or appropriate treatment. She seems to have come to perceive her symptoms as a representation of some deficiency at the core of herself, a sign of inferiority and unacceptability. Elsie had also to contend with the seizures themselves. While I will not describe the seizures here (see Benson, 1986; Fedio, 1986, for such detail), I will note that Elsie not infrequently experienced lapses of consciousness, after which she feared she had done something bizarre that she could not remember, but which others had observed. Indeed, it appears that she sometimes grimaced, performed repetitive movements, spoke incoherently, or even picked up merchandise in stores during these episodes.

Elsie's parents appear to have reacted to her emerging difficulties by attempting to protect her, but also conveyed the idea that her condition was shameful and must be kept secret. They encouraged her to trust only family members, and to follow her father's authoritarian rules and precepts; her father, in particular, disparaged her ability to solve problems on her own. When Elsie's neurological illness was diagnosed, her parents refused to disclose it to neighbors and relatives, so that Elsie could not explain to others why she behaved strangely at times, why she could not drive a car, and so on. Elsie became convinced, with some reason, that others mocked and talked maliciously about her. At a more tacit level, she believed she was incompetent, inferior, and vulnerable to harm.

Cognitive therapy with Elsie revolved around the gradual modification of three beliefs and their behavioral corollaries: (a) "I am incapable of taking care of myself"; (b) "Others will hurt me, mock me, take advantage of me, or deprive me of help"; and as a result, (c) "Grave harm may befall me at any time." Elsie's strategy for coping with the world as she saw it was to remain isolated, mistrustful, and dependent on her aging father (who frightened and intimidated her, and gave her ongoing lessons in dependency and paranoia). When acutely threatened, Elsie would become hostile, belligerent, and noncooperative.

ASSESSMENT AND TREATMENT

Elsie was referred to the center by a relative who had read about cognitive therapy in a newspaper account. Formal assessment of her case consisted of the standard intake procedure at the Center for Cognitive Therapy, an elaborate combination of interviews and questionnaires that included such instruments as the Beck Depression Inventory (Beck, Ward, Mendelsohn, Mock, & Erbaugh, 1961), the SCL-90 (Derogatis, Rickels, & Rock, 1976), and the Hamilton Anxiety Rating Scale (Hamilton, 1959). However, the more crucial assessment—the formulation of core issues and appropriate long-term treatment strategy—took place over the first few weeks of treatment. It coincided precisely with the beginnings of my attempt to establish a relationship, which in turn consisted of an attempt to provide initial symptom relief using principles of short-term cognitive therapy (Beck, Rush, Shaw, & Emery, 1979).

Initial Maneuvers

Elsie's presenting problems included depression, rage, and mistrust, and some of the last item was directed toward me. I doggedly followed the routine of structuring sessions, from setting a simple agenda to asking for feedback at the end, hoping that the establishment of an unvarying routine would help to define me in Elsie's eyes as a benign and predictable figure, rather than the threatening authority she seemed to fear.

Capsule summaries, another classic structuring device, also proved helpful. Again, despite Elsie's frequent displays of hostility and occasional refusals to speak, I stoically adhered to a routine of periodically summarizing my understanding of what she was telling me. I believe this technique allowed her to see me as someone who tried actively to understand her—without judgment. Later, she told me that what was important was that "you believed me."

Whenever possible, I used capsule summaries to emphasize the presence of thought content associated with the storms of disturbing affect Elsie experienced. "So, when you were feeling depressed, you had the thought that it was all over for you?" Using this approach, as well as explicit instruction, I gradually conveyed the basic ideas of cognitive therapy. I learned through trial and error (though mostly error) that keeping the presentation clear and simple, and the pace steady and slow, reduced the chance of misunderstanding, misinterpretation, and mistrust.

After a few sessions, I was able to teach Elsie to complete a Dysfunctional Thought Record. For a woman who had had so little experience of success throughout her life, the mastery of a basic task of therapy proved a moving experience. The technique also provided an outlet for a previously unrecognized hypergraphic tendency—which others, I learned much later, have associated with temporal lobe epilepsy (Stevens, 1988). Elsie, it turned out, loved to write. Although she never became especially adept at independently challenging automatic thoughts, she did find relief in recording the troubling situations, emotions, and thoughts. Writing seemed to reduce her sense of being overwhelmed by affect. Over time, she also came to expect that with my help, she would come to see things differently.

Feeling better, Elsie began to show more of her personality. She could be grateful, amiable, and funny, and had a gift for mimicry. Laughter consolidated the growing bond between us.

Identifying Cognitive Distortions . . .

My initial goal had been simply to teach Elsie a technique that would help her cope with her extremes of affect. After several weeks, we had also collected reams of thought content, and some general patterns had begun to emerge.

Elsie, it developed, was prone to three main types of cognitive distortion. The first, and most obvious, was a type of *personalization* error, in which she saw herself as the target of others' behavior. When a physician changed her appointment time and then appeared with his neck in a brace, she thought he had donned the brace "for my benefit," so that she would not realize he was giving her second-class treatment, assigning her appointment less priority than others. More typically, she would think that fellow bus passengers, shoppers behind her in a grocery store checkout line, residents of her boarding house, were talking, whispering, or laughing . . . about *her*.

Elsie also tended to *minimize* her own capacities. She thought she would be unable to find a new address, or if she found the building, to locate the correct room. If she had more than one appointment in a week, she thought she would be unable to keep them straight. She imagined that if she spoke to someone, she would find herself confronted by intrusive questions ("Where do you live?") with which she would be unable to cope. In her own mind, she was also the utterly helpless victim of government agencies, driven to hostile noncompliance. When given the radical suggestion that she might try simply explaining herself to the officials involved, she would shriek desperately, "I can't—they won't believe me!"

Finally, Elsie *catastrophized*: "I'll die"; "I'll be put in jail." When unsteady because overmedicated, "I won't be able to walk; I'll fall and be hit by a car." If someone yelled at her, "She'll kill me." Catastrophizing, when linked to personalization errors, produced paranoia. For example, if a neighbor mentioned that she had seen a mouse, Elsie would form a mental image of mice overrunning her room and become frightened. "That woman is trying to scare me," she would then conclude. Elsie lived in a malevolent, unmanageable, dangerous world.

It is worth noting, though, that Elsie also tended to *idealize* the rare person with whom she felt safe. She would seize upon that occasional friendly doctor or mental health worker as a source of pleasure and protection, interest and caring. Inevitably, that person would at some point fall short of providing the perfect secure haven of Elsie's fantasies. The bright savior would become the dark depriver, and Elsie's fear and mistrust would be reinforced.

. . . And Challenging Them

Elsie learned to identify some of these types of distortion, and began to appreciate the possibility that her perceptions and interpretations might not accurately reflect reality. She came to be able to say, "It's just my thoughts, Mrs. Greenberg," or "It's coming from my cognitive set!"

Challenging Elsie's thoughts and beliefs was made, at every possible opportunity, a matter for demonstration and experiment, rather than persuasion. Elsie learned best through concrete observation. Our alliance worked best when I collaborated with her to devise tests of troublesome ideas.

It was imperative to devise some test of Elsie's frequent perception that others were laughing at her or whispering about her. I had first to teach her something about the nature of inference—no small task in itself. By drawing on everyday examples, I managed to convince her that some statements were true, others might be true, and some were untrue; and that the closer a statement was tied to what could be sensed directly through sight, smell, or hearing, the more likely that others (such as myself) would agree that it was true. One afternoon, we stroked desks, kneaded and smelled leather office upholstery, in an attempt to agree on some notion of what constitutes "reality"!

Next, we defined what we would both accept as evidence that others were laughing at her. I insisted the "evidence" must comprise things I, too, would observe in the same situation. Generally, Elsie was fairly sure she had actually heard the sound of laughter, so tests had to address the question of what the laughter was *about*. (Years later, Elsie began to ask herself whether the laughter of people many feet away would actually be as loud as the laughter she was "hearing.") Knowing she liked movies, I asked Elsie how an actor would make it clear that he was laughing at another character. Elsie clasped her hand over her mouth, pointed, rolled her eyes, and guffawed. That performance provided our list of criteria against which to test the automatic thought, "They're laughing at me!"

Soon Elsie agreed that most such instances fell into the category of "might be true." I trained her, then, to consider alternative explanations for others' laughter. I looked for ways to make *her* laugh, for example, by telling her jokes or recounting stupid things I had done (the latter was a no-miss tactic). I had her read names aloud from the telephone book until she got bored and tired and conceded there might be people besides herself in Philadelphia who might evoke a chuckle or two. I sometimes convinced her to return to a location to see if people continued to react to her in a troubling way. Once, I asked the clinic secretary to join us in a session; we quizzed her together on her interpretation of the giggling that had rippled through the waiting room the previous hour (admittedly, this technique could have backfired). At last, Elsie began to see that these situations could be interpreted differently.

Finally, we attacked the problem in its existential belly: "So what if they are laughing at you; so what?" Catastrophic predictions ("They'll hurt me!") were repeatedly tested and repeatedly proved false. Elsie began to accept the idea that she might sometimes be an object of curiosity, but that generally others meant her no harm.

An interview might go something like this.

ELSIE: I can't go back to the supermarket anymore.

RUTH: Why not, Elsie?

ELSIE: I'm scared! I got scared there!

RUTH: Can you tell me what happened there?

ELSIE: A woman was whispering about me. She said, "I wish she'd hurry up!"

RUTH: What went through your mind then?

ELSIE: (starting to cry) She'll beat me up!

RUTH: And how much did you believe that, Elsie?

ELSIE: A hundred percent! I still believe it a hundred percent!

RUTH: Let's try to test that thought. First of all, are you sure you heard it? Do you think I would have heard it if I had been there?

ELSIE: Yes, I'm sure, I heard it.

RUTH: All right. Could she have been talking about someone else?

ELSIE: I don't think so, but there *were* other people there.

RUTH: Well, OK. Let's say she was talking about you. What was the evidence she intended to hurt you?

ELSIE: I was really scared!

RUTH: Remember your feelings and thoughts tell us something about *you*, not about her. To find out about *her* we have to use observation. What did you see or hear that suggested she was going to hurt you?

ELSIE: She just whispered, what I told you.

RUTH: She didn't raise her fist, or tell you she was going to beat you up?

ELSIE: No. There was no evidence.

RUTH: Elsie, have you ever felt impatient waiting in line? What do you do about it?

ELSIE: Sometimes I stand on one leg, then I stand on the other leg.

RUTH: How often do you beat the other people up?

ELSIE: You know I never would, Mrs. Greenberg!

RUTH: Then why do you think someone else would?

ELSIE: (With relief) Well, maybe I was wrong! Maybe she could just be impatient! Actually, she didn't hurt me!

RUTH: OK, so let's look for some reasons why you are pretty safe in the supermarket. How often do you hear of people getting beaten up in the supermarket line?

ELSIE: Never. People wait in lines all the time. They must get used to it.

RUTH: Sure, they wait in lines all the time. And traffic jams. And there is another reason . . . It's against the law to beat people up.

ELSIE: It is? I didn't know that. You really helped me, Mrs. Greenberg!

Elsie's concurrent participation in group therapy at a community mental health center provided many occasions on which to address such issues.

RUTH: What are some reasons why people in the group would be unlikely to hurt you even if they are angry at you?

ELSIE: I don't know any.

RUTH: Well, you were pretty upset about some things that were said in the group. Why don't you hurt the other members?

ELSIE: I'd be too scared! They wouldn't like me!

RUTH: Don't you think they realize that others won't like them if they often do hurtful things?

ELSIE: (brightening) I never thought of that! My father always said you couldn't trust anybody. He always said people were planning to hurt him.

RUTH: That seems to be how you got some of these ideas, doesn't it? Now think about it. How often did your father have the thought that others would hurt him?

ELSIE: Every day.

RUTH: And how many times did others actually hurt him?

ELSIE: Never! They never did!

RUTH: Why do think that is?

ELSIE: Maybe he was wrong! Maybe he had all-or-nothing thinking, too—"If someone doesn't smile and say 'Hi!', then he's going to hurt you!"

RUTH: That is how you learned to think, and you're beginning to learn to think a little differently.

As Elsie lost bits of her fear, I began to learn the many ways it had tormented her. She had been afraid to wear a hat in winter, because others might think it looked wrong and mock her. She had been afraid to open windows in summer, lest she hear sounds of talk and laughter. Recently, she had been emboldened to try new things, and she found herself full of gratitude and cautious optimism. She relaxed in the waiting room and began to chat and joke with clinic staff. A gregarious side to her personality emerged.

Increasing Self-Efficacy

As we progressed, exercise upon exercise was devoted to enlarging Elsie's sense of her own capabilities. To test this music-lover's belief that she could not find places on her own, I had her search for every record store listed in the central Philadelphia business directory. I taught her to record her appointments on a calendar, and if she felt overwhelmed by forthcoming obligations, to cover over with paper each calendar day but the present. At a more advanced stage, when she had many obligations (vocational day program, neurological tests, Social Security office, etc.), I showed her how to write each one on an index card, then line up the cards in the order she needed to attend to them. As time went on, I gave her less and less help and simply acknowledged her growing ability to care for herself. Little by little, she was able to let go of her dependence on her father, and a good deal of related fear and distress.

In the course of therapy, Elsie made a remarkable discovery—that she could read! She had greeted with astonishment and anxiety my suggestion that she read books such as *Feeling Good* (Burns, 1980) and *A New Guide to Rational Living* (Ellis & Harper, 1975). She had thought, she told me, that reading was something "other people" did. We dispensed with that notion quickly. Books became new friends, a source of comfort, wisdom, and pleasure.

Elsie also profited by acquiring some skill in regulating distance between herself and others. Her previous tactic had been to restrict contact to those few people with whom she felt reasonably safe and to avoid others, sometimes to the extent of avoiding shared bathrooms and showers. She feared not only that others would hurt her, but that they might want too much contact and closeness. She believed, of course, that she could not control the amount of closeness she offered.

Again, this was a matter for practice and experiment. We role-played possible responses to others' inquiries about her, responses that ranged from nondisclosing (e.g., politely change the subject, give a very general answer) to minimally disclosing. I instructed her in normalizing eye contact, demonstrating that she could always reduce eye contact if she felt it was necessary. I used all my powers to convince her that she retained her free will even if she related to people, that she did not have to subjugate herself to their wishes. She remains dubious about this notion, and has yet to succeed in extricating herself from an overextended conversation with her garrulous neighbor—though I have offered her a *Vogue* magazine if she does.

Most important, perhaps, we weighed the advantages and disadvantages of complete isolation. Together, we observed that Elsie's paranoia tended to increase with extreme isolation and also with very frequent contact. She seemed to feel best when she steered a consistent middle course and felt in control of the degree of closeness she offered. When less fearful, she also behaved in a less bizarre, erratic manner and provided fewer reasons for others to react to her in ways she found unpleasant or threatening.

Similarly, we developed alternatives to behaving with hostility and belligerence when acutely threatened. I offered myself as a role model, and would tell Elsie little stories about how I had dealt with an unfriendly neighbor or a conflict with a friend. Often, these made a strong impression; Elsie would find herself thinking, "Mrs. Greenberg wouldn't let that woman scare her!" Further, I guided her through the new experience of working out difficulties in a cooperative manner, and thus developed evidence that this is the preferable course. After much hard work, and after acquiring many new skills, Elsie has begun to tell me she no longer thinks she is inferior to others.

RUTH: You can walk tall, and hold your head high; right?

ELSIE: Right.

Outcome

I accepted long ago that my responsibility was not to reconstruct Elsie, but to help her achieve and maintain a higher level of functionality and a lower level of emotional distress. Currently, although her symptoms wax and wane, she rarely experiences the depths of despair, rage, or terror that she did when therapy began. She does not work, but participates in a job-readiness program and does so with gradually increasing comfort, freedom, and social effectiveness. While she still becomes frightened by her neighbors at times, she is no longer continually preoccupied with the thought that they intend to harm her.

I believe our relationship itself has a stabilizing function for Elsie; I have "been there" for her so long and so consistently that her trust in me usually remains solid when trust in others has badly eroded. In this special position, I am able far more quickly to guide her to new perspectives about others' intentions and, when necessary, my own. By having her trust, I have also been able to intervene on her behalf, on occasion, with agencies and hospitals. Possessing needed information and understanding, I have sometimes been able to help resolve problems that might actually have imperiled or disadvantaged her.

Cognitive therapy may have offered some unique advantages in the management of Elsie's complex diffi-

culties. Our practical focus, our love of directed learning experiences had an impact on Elsie that more exclusively verbal therapies had not. Perhaps our emphasis on self-help skills allowed her to feel less vulnerable in the therapeutic relationship, and thus more able to trust. I know that I, and the staff at the Center, provided models of accepting and caring that she had not previously experienced. We must have assured her, at some level, that such things were possible.

REFERENCES

Beck, A. T., Rush, A. J., Shaw, B. F., & Emery, G. (1979). *Cognitive therapy of depression*. New York: Guilford.
Beck, A. T., Ward, C. H., Mendelson, M., Mock, J. E., & Erbaugh, J. (1961). An inventory for measuring depression. *Archives of General Psychiatry, 4*, 561–571.
Benson, D. F. (1986). Interictal behavior disorders in epilepsy. *Psychiatric Clinics of North America, 9*, 283–292.
Burns, D. (1980). *Feeling good*. New York: New American Library.
Derogatis, L. R., Rickels, K., & Rock, A. F. (1976). The SCL-90 and the MMPI: A step in the validation of a new self-report scale. *British Journal of Psychiatry, 128*, 280–289.
Ellis, A., & Harper, R. A. (1975). *A new guide to rational living*. N. Hollywood, CA: Wilshire.
Fedio, P. (1986). Behavioral characteristics of patients with temporal lobe epilepsy. *Psychiatric Clinics of North America, 9*, 267–281.
Hamilton, M. (1959). The assessment of anxiety states by rating. *British Journal of Medical Psychology, 32*, 50–55.
Stevens, J. R. (1988). Psychiatric aspects of epilepsy. *Journal of Clinical Psychiatry, 49*, 49–57.

SUGGESTED READINGS

Beck, A. T., Freeman, A., and Associates. (Eds.). (1990). *Cognitive therapy of personality disorders*. New York: Guilford.
Hall, J. (1989). Chronic psychiatric handicaps. In K. Hawton, P. M. Salkovskis, Kirk, J., & D. M. Clark (Eds.), *Cognitive behaviour therapy for psychiatric problems: A practical guide*. Oxford: Oxford University Press.
Wallace, C. J., Boone, S. E., Donahoe, C. P., & Foy, D. W. (1985). The chronically mentally disabled: Independent living skills training. In D. H. Barlow (Ed.), *Clinical handbook of psychological disorders: A step-by-step treatment manual*. New York: Guilford.
Young, J. E. (1990). *Cognitive therapy for personality disorders: A schema-focused approach*. Sarasota, FL: Professional Resource Exchange. (To order, call 813–366–7913.)

22

Borderline Personality Disorder

Ralph M. Turner

Historically, persons diagnosed as borderline personality disordered (BPD) have been considered difficult, if not impossible, to work with for therapists of all theoretical orientations. This classification of patients actually was derived from the notion that there exists a psychopathological disorder having features common to both psychotic disorders and what used to be called the neurotic disorders (the anxiety disorders and some types of depression).

Although numerous psychodynamic and biological treatment models have been promulgated, only recently have cognitive and behavioral theorists discussed and proposed treatment regimens for this diagnostic group (Linehan, 1987a, 1987b, 1987c; Turner, 1983, 1988, 1989). The principal reason for this neglect has been behavior therapists' opposition to the notion of personality structure and personality disorder. However, with the advent of DSM-III (American Psychiatric Association [APA], 1980) and its revision DSM-III-R (APA, 1987) and the development of explicit, reproducible criteria, this view has changed. Since specific symptoms and symptom patterns can be assessed, the condition is more amenable

to empirical investigation and cognitive-behavioral intervention.

The essential features of BPD involve cognitive, emotional, and behavioral dysfunctions. In the cognitive domain, there is a severe instability of self-image, a deficit in self-control abilities, and a lack of the capacity to maintain a consistent perspective about significant others. The most debilitating cognitive dysfunction, however, is the occurrence of micropsychotic episodes. Instability in the affective domain is also a typical feature. Dramatic shifts in mood involving depression, anxiety, irritability, angry outbursts, and impulsivity occur rapidly and often. The deleterious behavioral manifestations include recurrent suicidal gestures, self-mutilating behavior, drug abuse, or aggressive outbursts.

Under stress, BPD patients can decompensate and suffer short-lived dissociative or psychotic episodes requiring hospitalization (Pope, Jonas, Hudson, Cohen, & Tohen, 1985). Numerous studies have also shown a significant comorbid vulnerability for persons diagnosed with BPD for major depression (Charney, Nelson & Quinlan, 1981; Pfohl, Stangl, & Zimmerman, 1983; Shea, Glass, Pilkonis, Watkins, & Docherty, 1987) and anxiety disorders (Koenigsberg, Kaplan, Gilmore, & Cooper, 1985; Perry, 1988; Turner, 1987).

Ralph M. Turner • Adolescents and Families Treatment Research Center, Department of Psychiatry, Temple University School of Medicine, Philadelphia, Pennsylvania 19140.

Comprehensive Casebook of Cognitive Therapy, edited by Arthur Freeman and Frank M. Dattilio. Plenum Press, New York, 1992.

INTEGRATIVE COGNITIVE TREATMENT

The treatment approach for BPD patients developed by Turner (1983, 1988, 1989) and illustrated in this chapter is based upon a cognitive-behavioral orientation. It is an integrative approach, however, in that it incorporates aspects of a modern, cognitive, psychodynamic approach to the assessment of self-organization (Horowitz, 1988, 1989; Luborsky & Crits–Christoph, 1990). The inclusion of Horowitz's "configural analysis" method provides cohesion in the cognitive-behavioral assessment and treatment of BPD patients. It does so because it elucidates the tacit self-schema coupled to both the borderline's instability of self-image and the resultant interpersonal manifestations of this instability. Luborsky's "Core Conflictual Relationship Theme" method provides the basic data for the cognitive–dynamic approach. This integrative cognitive approach is called Dynamic–Cognitive Behavior Therapy (D-CBT).

The D–CBT treatment plan, however, adheres closely to the model developed by Beck, Rush, Shaw, and Emery (1979). It consists of (a) using didactic presentation to teach the patient to understand the role of both overt and covert cognitions and schemas in contributing to the problems in living; (b) teaching patients to discriminate and to observe systematically negative self-statements and images that guide feelings and behavior; (c) training the person in the essentials of problem solving, including problem definition, anticipation of consequences, evaluation of alternative strategies, and comprehending feedback; and (d) utilizing role-playing and rehearsal to engage the patient in the application of self-statements, the use of coping strategies, and problem-solving skills. In addition, this treatment approach makes use of imaginal techniques such as guided imagery and evocative flooding.

This chapter focuses on strategies for making a reliable diagnosis, assessment of both cognitive distortions and deep structured self-schemas and role-relationships models, and the application of a D–CBT program for the amelioration of BPD symptoms.

CASE ILLUSTRATION: BACKGROUND INFORMATION

The patient was a 29-year-old white female I will call Anne. Her presenting complaints were (a) angry outbursts; (b) getting along poorly with people; (c) emptiness, loneliness, and depression; (d) rapid mood swings involving depression, anger, and anxiety; (e) vacillation between periods of taking care of herself and periods of letting herself go; (f) episodes of wrist slashing; and (g) lack of a sense of identity at home or work—made more difficult by several years of unemployment and

marriage difficulties. Anne claimed she did not love her husband, but that she needed him to take care of her.

When Anne first came to treatment, she had just been released from a psychiatric hospital. The precipitant was a series of violent arguments with her husband. Anne had finally become outraged, lost control, and thrown dishes and furniture at him. She broke two lamps, and finally took a small kitchen knife and made nonlethal cuts on both of her arms. As these events transpired, a sense of despairing sadness mixed with panic swept over her, only to be followed by a chaotic state in which she was flooded by disconnected sequences of thought, felt frightened, was confused and disoriented to time and place, and became blocked in her attempts to communicate. Under pressure from her parents, she voluntarily admitted herself to the hospital; after 3 days she returned to her normal level of functioning. She was discharged after 10 days in the hospital with a diagnosis of BPD. Upon release from the hospital, Anne was referred to our treatment program for aftercare.

ASSESSMENT AND DIAGNOSIS

The first session was directed toward gathering background information and providing Anne with an overview of treatment. A treatment schedule of three times per week was established.

The second, third, and fourth sessions were devoted to conducting a formal diagnostic evaluation. Structured clinical interview instruments were used to enhance the reliability and thoroughness of the diagnostic process. Axis I diagnosis was made using the Structured Clinical Interview for DSM-III-R (SCID; Spitzer, Williams, Gibbon, & First, 1989). The presence of Axis II disorders was determined by use of the Personality Disorder Examination (PDE; Loranger, 1988) and the Diagnostic Interview for Borderlines (DIB; Kolb & Gunderson, 1980).

Anne responded positively to a sufficient number of questions in the major depression, anxiety, and drug abuse categories to meet criteria for all three disorders. The results of the PDE showed Anne met all eight criteria for the BPD diagnosis and five of eight criteria for histrionic personality disorder. The DIB results corroborated the BPD diagnosis.

The next assessment task was to develop an understanding of Anne's self-schemas and role-relationship model schemas. Such deep structured schemas are assumed to operate unconsciously, affect day-to-day information processing, and act as an integral part of cognitive feed-forward mechanisms (Mahoney, 1985) with regard to interpersonal relationships and self-image. In addition to the 10 categories of typical cognitive distortions described by Beck et al. (1979), individuals make errors in interpersonal judgement and self-esteem based upon their erroneous working models, or schemas of self and others. These schemas are learned during childhood and adolescence in response to real interpersonal threats and devaluations; however, when they remain as the preeminent working models for self and others in adulthood, interpersonal difficulties arise and self-understanding is distorted.

Assessing role-relationship schemas is an inferential process that involves careful review of session transcripts and a collaborative working relationship with the patient; details of the procedure are provided by Horowitz (1988, 1989) and by Luborsky and Crits–Christoph (1990). Session 5 and a review of the first four hours were used in determining Anne's self- and other schemas.

THERAPIST: You mentioned during our last session that you see yourself in two ways: well and not well. Can you tell me more about that?

ANNE: Well, actually, I don't know who I am. I seem to be different all of the time. I never know what I'll feel like, even five minutes from now. I'm just up and down like a roller coaster.

THERAPIST: What do you do to try to control your moods?

ANNE: Most of the time I'll get high and sleep. If I'm really feeling edgy, though, the only thing that helps is to call one of my boyfriends and have sex. That can make me feel better. Sometimes my husband . . . but then we always start fighting. It's always better if it is somebody I don't know. Then they don't know about all my problems, and I can act well.

THERAPIST: What do you mean?

ANNE: Well, if he doesn't know me he'll think I'm great, or at least normal. He'll think I'm pretty and sexy, and I can act like I want. And as long as I don't let him get close he can't control me, or hurt me by finding out what I am really like and leave me. But it doesn't really work. I can't act well long. I get tired and have to get somewhere . . . home . . . so I can just be myself again.

THERAPIST: What is it like when you don't feel like yourself in that kind of situation?

ANNE: Oh, I get dizzy, and feel like I am looking at my face in a mirror; only it doesn't really look like me. That's when the panic attacks come! Or, I just feel numb and scared. Sometimes I can get out of that feeling by telling the guy to tie me up and do the nastiest things he has ever wanted to do to a woman. Then, even if he thinks he is having fun, I know he won't want me. I can scare men!

THERAPIST: Is that what you really want?

ANNE: I don't know what I want!

THERAPIST: It sounds like you are saying that you do not want to be loved.

ANNE: Nobody loves me. Nobody ever has. My life is shitty! It always has been. Even my parents didn't love me.

THERAPIST: That still hurts you terribly bad.

ANNE: Wouldn't it you! I mean how many 16-year-olds' parents say they are going away on a vacation, put you up in the YWCA, and then not let you come home when they come back? Even then, they could tell I was worthless.

THERAPIST: You never say anything positive about yourself. You're sick, you're worthless, you're emotionally unstable, you're fake. Yet, you seem very nice to me.

ANNE: It's just an act. You don't really know me.

THERAPIST: Tell me, Anne, what would you like to be like? What do you wish your life was like? How do you wish a man would be with you?

ANNE: I wish . . . I want . . . What I wish is that I was an adult woman, in control, responsible, able to love. I want a man who is loving and caring . . . a real man. I don't want to feel just lucky to be loved. I wouldn't have any problems with my feelings, and I wouldn't have to worry about being left alone. I wouldn't have to feel so vulnerable.

From Anne's statements I was able to begin to understand her self-schemas and other schemas, as well as some of her irrational, automatic thoughts. Tables 22-1 and 22-2 provide a summary description of Anne's affective states and her predicted scripts for interpersonal interactions in each case. Again, there are considered to be deep structured (i.e., unconscious), automatic schemas.

Anne appeared to have two supraordinate self-schemas: well and not well. Fear of being vulnerable and too close motivated a defensive shift to the not-well schema, while fear of decompensating and being weak motivated a shift back to the well schema. Since she was caught in conflict between wanting love and caring and a belief that she was emotionally weak and worthless, she was constantly immersed in emotional shifting and instability.

Within the supraordinate self-schemas were nested self- and other schemas that reflected conflict regarding her wishes to be loved and cared for versus her fears of being abandoned. In addition, her pattern of emotional instability appeared to serve as a compromise defense, albeit a costly one, against becoming overwhelmed with the conflict. She could be plunged into derealization epi-

TABLE 22-1   Anne's Well Superordinate Schemas

Dynamic element	State	Self-Schema	Expected action schema	Other schema
Desired	Adult, genuine, responsible, in control, loved	Adult, loving woman	Expresses self lovingly ($\rightarrow$) ($\leftarrow$) Expresses love ($\leftarrow$) Anxious about abandonment	Caring, loving man
Dreaded	Severe depression and abandonment, grief	Vulnerable woman	Demands to be loved ($\rightarrow$) ($\leftarrow$) Anger, fear, abandons Grief and depression ($\rightarrow$)	Caring, loving man
Problematic	Depersonalization, loss of sense of self, panic stricken	Emotionally unstable woman	Sexual acting out and drug abuse ($\rightarrow$) ($\leftarrow$) Abuse Shame ($\rightarrow$)	Detached man
Compromise	Depressed and anxious, indecisive, lack of identity, lonely, bored	False, pretending woman	Acts as if charming adult ($\rightarrow$) ($\leftarrow$) Uses her Fatigues ($\leftarrow$)	Superior man

sodes in the best-case scenario or a chaotic, decompensated state in the worst-case scenario.

Many of Anne's typical cognitive distortion errors were also elucidated through this analysis. She was especially adept at all-or-nothing thinking, labeling, personalization, emotional reasoning, mind reading, fortunetelling, and disqualifying the positive.

Even at her strongest moments, Anne believed that any man she would try to love would eventually "see her for what she really was," "find her disgusting," and abandon her. This was the way it was and always would be. She felt it was desperately critical not to trust others.

TREATMENT

Session 6

Session 6 was spent orienting Anne to the cognitive psychological view of emotions. The therapist approached the session as a teacher with a lesson to impart.

The central concepts taught are discussed in the remainder of this section. First, intense negativistic thinking always accompanies episodes of anxiety, depression, or a sense of loss of control. The thoughts are the cause of the feelings, not the reverse. These thoughts are automatic and occur so rapidly as to be unconscious; they occur as self-statements or conversations we have with ourselves about what life events mean and what we should feel about them. Negative self-statements are so well understood by

cognitive therapists that they are classified into 10 distinctive types of cognitive distortions.

In addition, when growing up, people learn to have cognitive representations of themselves and others and beliefs about what will always happen in interpersonal transactions. These beliefs, too, are filled with distortions. The good news is that by learning to observe one's feelings and automatic thoughts and to identify cognitive distortions and false beliefs about oneself, an individual can then begin to correct these thinking errors and obtain emotional self-control.

The session was finalized by assigning Anne homework that involved reading sections 2 and 4 of David Burns's (1980) self-help book *Feeling Good*. These sections of the book explain the practical details of cognitive therapy and provide a valuable adjunct to treatment.

Session 7

The goals set for the seventh session were to expand upon the role of automatic thoughts and cognitive distortions in causing moods, and to teach Anne how to observe dysfunctional thoughts using a daily record. Anne, however, had other ideas about how the session should proceed. She showed me new cuts on her right arm, told me she had binged on drugs and alcohol over the weekend, and proceeded to describe how emotionally unstable she was feeling.

ANNE: Listen before you start with your therapy bullshit; I want you to know that I just don't care. I'm going

TABLE 22-2   Anne's Not-Well Supraordinate Schemas

Dynamic element	State	Self-Schema	Expected action schema	Other schema
Desired	Low self-esteem, anxiety and mild depression	Weak, helpless woman	Request caretaking ($\rightarrow$) ($\leftarrow$) Provides care, but controls Anxious over submission and vulnerability ($\rightarrow$)	Caring, loving man
Dreaded	Acute self-shame, despair	Worthless woman	Shows worthlessness ($\rightarrow$) Abandons/abandonment ($\leftarrow$) Depression ($\rightarrow$)	Caring, loving man
Problematic	Chaotic and decompensated	Sick woman	Decompensates to psychotic level of functioning ($\rightarrow$) ($\leftarrow$) Anger, grudging caretaker Anxious and depressed over shame ($\rightarrow$)	Superior man
Compromise	Rapidly shifting states of anxiety, depression, and elation with behavioral acting out.	Emotionally vacillating woman	As if interpersonal, contact ($\rightarrow$) ($\leftarrow$) Anger Distancing with shift to another man ($\rightarrow$)	Any man

to kill myself. I started to do it last night. That's where the cuts are from, but I decided I wanted to let you know it's not your fault. That's all. I have just got no reason to live. I'm, worthless, hopeless, and I . . . don't have any energy left. (starts to cry)

THERAPIST: Why are you feeling this way? What are you thinking about that suicide seems to be the only answer?

It was clear that Anne was responding from the self-image of the sick woman. She saw herself as weak, and her clarity of thought was severely impaired. She required firm and concrete support to face up to her problems in living.

ANNE: There's just no reason for me to keep going through this pain. And no matter what you or anybody else says, I've got a right to die if I want to.

THERAPIST: Listen, I don't care to disagree with you about suicide; that is something that is every individual's choice, and to be honest, I cannot really help you with that decision. I am not trained for that. That is something you talk with a minister or a theologian about. I am a psychologist. I can only help you with your problems in living. The problem for me is if you are not going to be here, I cannot work with you to help you solve your problems in living.

ANNE: So, you won't have to work with me any more. You won't have to waste your time on me. You'll be better off.

THERAPIST: Sounds as though you feel worthless.

ANNE: I am worthless; my whole life is worthless!

THERAPIST: OK, stop! Now, I want you to look at the thoughts automatically going through your mind associated with the statement I am worthless.

ANNE: Well . . . I don't know what you mean. Just I'm worthless and I should be dead.

THERAPIST: What are the reasons for that?

ANNE: Well . . . I . . . I . . . um, do everything wrong. I'm not nice. My parents didn't love me, nobody will ever love me. I'm not normal; I can't even control my feelings.

THERAPIST: That's good! Now you are taking the first step in solving your problems in living. You are beginning to identify the automatic thoughts that flash through your mind in an instant. At this point in your life, practically all of those automatic thoughts are false statements, illogical, and distorted.

I went on to utilize Anne's current crisis as a platform to teach her how use the three-column technique to monitor and identify the types of cognitive distortions she typically made. From there we began to practice positive counterarguments to her damaging self-statements. As we worked on countering her cognitive distortions, she stopped crying and began to work enthusiastically. Her mood improved dramatically; however, she still expressed doubts about her ability to really succeed.

During the next five sessions we focused only upon her daily record of cognitive distortions. The emphasis was placed on increasing her ability to use this technique to take self-control over her feelings.

Session 13

At this point, Anne had mastered the three-column technique; therefore, we could take the next step. This was to teach her about her self- and other schemas and to tie them into her automatic thoughts. The goal was to extend her understanding of how her cognitive processes guided her feelings and behavior at an even deeper level than her automatic thoughts.

The therapeutic strategy was a straightforward, educational one. I showed her my working model (Tables 22-1 and 22-2) of her role-relationship models and projected interpersonal scenarios. As I described how she functioned with regard to her various schemas, I also pointed out the surface-level automatic thoughts associated with them. I taught her to understand how her core interpersonal conflict generated the sequence of self-dynamics which produced both the rapid shifts in emotions and the experience of lacking a coherent sense of self.

Furthermore, it was pointed out that the core conflict was learned at a time when it was appropriate, but that she now projected it onto situations that were not appropriate. All of her self- and other schemas except her ideal schema were erroneous. They were simply errors in thinking.

The fifth week of therapy (sessions 13, 14, and 15) were spent helping Anne to understand these lessons. She continued to maintain her daily record as before.

Session 16

Once again, our attention was directed to self-monitoring. Now the emphasis was placed upon the patient observing her self- and other schemas as they were evoked on a day-by-day basis. In addition, she had to consider what adaptive alternative, rational, self- and other schemas were possible for each situation, as well as the emotions that would have resulted from the alternative scenarios.

Sessions 17 and 18 were spent enhancing Anne's ability to self-monitor her self- and role-relationship schemas. An example from a part of her daily record is presented in Table 22-3.

Session 19

Starting with session 19, the next six weeks of treatment were directed toward improving Anne's ability to stabilize and strengthen her "desired" self-schema. To accomplish this, we used a covert self-modeling technique.

The first step in this procedure involved teaching Anne meditative relaxation according to the instructions outlined by Turner (1991). Next, we took the most recent events Anne had recorded on her daily record of evoked self-schemas and wrote a scenario in which she thought, felt, and acted in accord with the rational, alternative schemas she had generated.

An example, using that part of her daily record presented in Table 22-2, is presented below:

> You are in your kitchen. You and Rich are sitting at the table drinking coffee. You are telling him you would like to work on your marriage and try to save it. As you talk, you look into his eyes and think to yourself that he cares for you; he just doesn't want to be used or hurt. You feel fully adult and worthy of love. You feel in control. There is no strong motion, just balance. You are aware of your vulnerabilities, but this situation is unlike any other you have ever been in. It is new. It will have its own outcome.

During this phase of the therapy, we addressed issues regarding Anne's relationships with men, friends, and family in this same way. In addition, we worked on stabilizing her self-schema during times when she was alone and during the process of finding a job.

SUMMARY

Intensive therapy (three times per week) with Anne lasted for a period of three months; then the schedule was shifted to once weekly for the next eight months. Currently, she is still continuing in these supportive-booster sessions to ensure that her gains are maintained. She is now working as a secretary, is reunited with her husband, and expresses that she has never felt so healthy in her whole life. There have been no micropsychotic episodes, wrist-slashing or other self-damaging behavior, or depersonalization episodes. Consequently, there has been no need to consider hospitalization.

Anne has shown a continual need to self-monitor her automatic thoughts in order to maintain stable emotions. Her investment in maintaining good cognitive hygiene is unusual, but I have certainly reinforced her for it. Additional work will be directed at enhancing her self-esteem and strengthening her resistance to depressive episodes.

The therapy techniques used in her case consisted of the traditional ones described by Burns (1980), plus covert self-modeling and the addition of the psychodynamic procedure of role-relationship model assessment developed by Horowitz and the Core Conflictual Relationship Theme method developed by Luborsky and Crits–Christoph. Furthermore, Anne and her husband have engaged in cognitively oriented marital therapy (Datillio & Padesky, 1990), which has markedly improved their relationship.

TABLE 22-3 Sample Daily Record of Self- and Other Schema Activation

Emotion	Events	Automatic Thoughts	Operative Self-Schema
Fear, anxiety, sadness	Talking with Rich about fixing up our relationship	"He won't understand me; he'll laugh at me; he'll think I'm weak. I don't know what I am saying or doing."	Emotionally unstable woman

Operative Other Schema	Alternative Self-Schema	Rational Other Schema	Resulting Emotion
"He is better than me. He will take advantage of me."	Worthwhile, adult woman Caring and in control	"He cares and loves me, but doesn't want to be used."	"Just OK." "No strong emotion." "I would feel balanced."

REFERENCES

American Psychiatric Association. (1980). *Diagnostic and statistical manual of mental disorders* (3rd ed.). Washington, DC: Author.

American Psychiatric Association. (1987). *Diagnostic and statistical manual of mental disorders* (rev. 3rd ed.). Washington, DC: Author.

Beck, A. T., Rush, A. J., Shaw, B., & Emery G. (1979). *Cognitive therapy of depression*. New York: Guilford.

Burns, D. D. (1980). *Feeling good: The new mood therapy*. New York: William Morrow.

Charney, D. S., Nelson, C. J., & Quinlan, D. M. (1981). Personality traits and disorder in depression. *American Journal of Psychiatry, 138*, 1601–1604.

Dattilio, F. M., & Padesky, C. (1990). *Cognitive therapy with couples*. Sarasota, FL: Professional Resource Exchange.

Horowitz, M. J. (1988). *Introduction of psychodynamics: A new synthesis*. New York: Basic Books.

Horowitz, M. J. (1989). Relationship schema formulation: Role-relationship models and intrapsychic conflict. *Psychiatry, 52*, 260–274.

Koenigsberg, H. W., Kaplan, R. D., Gilmore, M. M., & Cooper, A. M. (1985). The relationship between syndrome and personality disorder in DSM-III: Experience with 2462 patients. *American Journal of Psychiatry, 142*, 207–212.

Kolb, J., & Gunderson, J. (1980). Diagnosing borderline patients with a structured interview. *Archives of General Psychiatry, 37*, 37–41.

Linehan, M. M. (1987a). Dialectical behavior therapy for borderline personality disorder: Theory and method. *Bulletin of the Menninger Clinic, 51*, 261–276.

Linehan, M. M. (1987b). Dialectical behavior therapy in groups: Treating borderline personality disorders and suicidal behavior. In C. M. Brady (Ed.), *Women's therapy groups: Paradigms of feminist treatment*. New York: Springer.

Linehan, M. M. (1987c). Dialectical behavior therapy: A cognitive behavioral approach to parasuicide. *Journal of Personality Disorders, 1*, 328–333.

Luborsky, L., & Chrits-Christoph, P. (1990). *Understanding transference: The CCRT Method*. New York: Basic Books.

Loranger, A. W. (1988). *Personality disorder examination*. Yonkers, NY: D. V. Communications.

Mahoney, M. J. (1985). Psychotherapy and the human change processes. In M. J. Mahoney & A. Freeman (Eds.), *Cognition and psychotherapy* (pp. 3–48). New York: Plenum.

Perry, J. C. (June, 1988). *The natural history of anxiety symptoms in personality disorders*. Paper presented at the 19th meeting of the Society for Psychotherapy Research, Santa Fe, New Mexico.

Pfohl, B., Stangl, D., & Zimmerman, M. (1984). The implications of DSM-III personality disorders for patients with major depression. *Journal of Affective Disorders, 7*, 309–318.

Pope, H. G., Jonas, J. M., Hudson, J. I., Cohen, B. M., & Tohen, M. (1985). An empirical study of psychosis in BPD. *American Journal of Psychiatry, 142*, 1285–1290.

Shea, M. T., Glass, D. R., Pilkonis, P. A., Watkins, J., & Docherty, J. P. (1987). Frequency and implications of personality disorders in a sample of depressed outpatients. *Journal of Personality Disorders, 1*, 27–42.

Spitzer, R. L., Williams, J. B., Gibbon, M., & First, M. B. (1989). *Structured clinical interview for DSM-III-R*. New York: New York State Psychiatric Institute, Biometric Research Department.

Turner, R. M. (1983). Behavioral therapy with borderline patients. *Carrier Foundation Letter, 88*, 1–4.

Turner, R. M. (1987). The effects of personality disorder diagnosis on the outcome of social anxiety symptom reduction. *Journal of Personality Disorders, 1*, 136–143.

Turner, R. M. (1988). The cognitive-behavioral approach to the treatment of borderline personality disorders. *International Journal of Partial Hospitalization, 5*, 279–289.

Turner, R. M. (1989). Case study evaluation of a bio-cognitive-behavioral approach for the treatment of borderline personality disorder. *Behavior Therapy, 20*, 477–489.

Turner, R. M. (1991). Systematic desensitization. In V. E. Caballo (Ed.), *Handbook of behavioral therapy methods and training*, Madrid, Spain: Siglo XXI Editores de España SA.

SUGGESTED READINGS

Burns, D. D. (1980). *Feeling good: The new mood therapy*. New York: William Morrow.

Horowitz, M. J. (1988). *Introduction to psychodynamics: A new synthesis*. New York: Basic Books.

Horowitz, M. J. (1989). Relationship schema formulation: Role-relationship models and intrapsychic conflict. *Psychiatry, 52*, 260–274.

Masterson, J. F., & Klein, R. (1989). *Psychotherapy of the disorders of the self: The Masterson approach*. New York: Brunner/Mazel.

Mahoney, M. J. (1991). *Human Change Processes: The Scientific Foundations of Psychotherapy*. New York: Basic Books.

23

Narcissistic Personality Disorder

BACKGROUND INFORMATION

The "Little Prince," as he came to be known in supervision, was a "special" person who felt he was in danger of losing this status. He alternated between insisting on his need for (indeed, his right to) perfection in his life and immediate gratification, and his distaste with this in himself. The work conducted in therapy was characterized by his ongoing struggle to reconcile his idealized childhood image of himself with his need to grow and mature, and take on a more adult, less self-centered view of the world. His task, as he put it, was to "grow up and realize that the world won't come to a screeching halt if I die," and to learn to accept this.

Warren was 22 years old, in his first year of graduate business school, when he came for treatment. He presented with combined anxiety and depression surrounding difficulties in his adjustment to the new academic environment at a highly prestigious university. His ability to concentrate on his schoolwork, his sleeping pattern, and his social adjustment were all impaired as a result of his difficulties. At intake he reported extreme anxiety, doubts about his choice of business as a career (versus his first

love, drama), and extreme distress over being able to complete the semester's work and prepare for finals.

Warren had been in psychotherapy twice previously. At age 7, he was taken for therapy for "behavioral problems"—he would hit others and throw things when he did not get his way. Additionally, he was having problems with motivation in school (procrastination). He reported that the therapy did effect some changes in his behavior at that time, and that in addition he on his own "learned how to get what I wanted in other ways by being more manipulative and charming." A second therapy lasted from ages 13 to 17 for academic problems in school, characterized again by procrastination, and for the depression that resulted from his declining performance. He responded "yes and no" when asked whether this therapy had been helpful, elaborating that it did not provide much in the way of concrete improvements, but that he did enjoy the opportunity to talk about himself to someone. A characteristic he had observed in himself during both treatment periods was that he would try to "perform" for the therapist, attempting to impress him or her with his intelligence, charm, and insight.

Warren was born of Jewish descent in a northeastern city. Both parents were high achievers (father a highly successful physician, mother an attorney) who, he believes, only gave him attention and affection when he was performing well (i.e., achieving in school). His evidence for this included the fact that his relationship with them was very poor during the time he was having academic and disciplinary problems in high school, but vastly improved when he began doing better again in college. The

---

Donald A. Bux • Department of Mental Health Sciences, Hahnemann University, Philadelphia, Pennsylvania 19102.

Comprehensive Casebook of Cognitive Therapy, edited by Arthur Freeman and Frank M. Dattilio. Plenum Press, New York, 1992.

pressure he experienced from them throughout his school experience was quite high.

His educational history began with "exceptional" performance in elementary school, which then declined gradually throughout high school as the demands placed on him increased; he became, as he put it, "less and less exceptional." As a child, Warren recalled being told of how "special" he was, and that his early teachers (and a drama instructor) believed he was destined for greatness. This belief became a theme central to his self-concept. His explanation for this praise, however, was that he had some natural talent and the ability to be charming, and thereby he could win people over—thus, he believed that his "exceptionality" was simply by virtue of his personality, rather than a product of hard work. He had long held the dream of attempting a career in drama, expressing full confidence that if he did, success would simply "happen" to him. He was unable to consider the need to work hard or otherwise pay his dues in pursuit of this goal, nor could he seriously contemplate or prepare for the possibility of failure in this endeavor.

Warren reported a decline in his academic performance throughout high school. He also was involved in two disciplinary actions: once when he stole a student's coat that he had badly wanted, and a second time when he scratched a girl's car with his keys after she laughed at him in class. Although his academic achievement did improve in his senior year, he was expelled from school one month before graduation when he was caught cheating on an exam (which he did in order to ensure the highest mark in the class). His expulsion from school, he felt, was what led to his failure to qualify for admission to the university of his choice, which he had planned on attending since elementary school. This, to him, was a devastating blow. The quite reputable college he instead attended, and the honors he received there, still to him represented his failure to achieve his "fullest potential," and he thus devalued his experience and performance there. He also expressed the belief that he had faked his way through college, not believing he had worked for his achievements.

Warren described himself as obsessed with beautiful women. He reported a series of relationships that tended to start out with passionate interest and "lustful pursuit" on his part, but eventually died out when "something better came along." He typically became dissatisfied as a result of some imperfection in the woman. (His current girlfriend, for example, had gained five pounds since meeting him, which he said sometimes made him want to cry.) Otherwise interpersonally, he reported having developed very close friendships with several people since elementary school, but stated that these friendships typically ended when he discovered some "fatal flaw" in the other person, which it was impossible for him to overlook.

ASSESSMENT AND DIAGNOSIS

Warren was evaluated using a combination of self-report measures and the Structured Clinical Interview for the DSM (SCID; Spitzer, Williams, & Gibbon, 1987). The self-report scales used included the Beck inventories for anxiety (Beck, Epstein, Brown, & Steer, 1988), depression (Beck, 1972), and hopelessness (Beck, Weissman, Lester, & Trexler, 1974); the Cognition Checklist (Beck, Brown, Steer, Eidelson, & Riskind, 1987); the Self-Concept Test (Beck, Steer, Epstein, & Brown, in press); and the Dysfunctional Attitude Scale (DAS; Weissman & Beck, 1978). His diagnoses at intake (according to DSM III-R) were Axis I, adjustment disorder, mixed mood, with academic inhibition; Axis II, personality disorder, not otherwise specified (antisocial, histrionic, narcissistic, and passive-aggressive features).

On the Beck inventories, Warren indicated moderate levels of anxiety and depression. On the DAS, his responses revealed that his self-esteem was closely tied to others' opinions of him, as shown by his strong agreement with statements stressing the importance of this in determining his worth as a person. Further, he revealed that he set very high standards for himself, as indicated in his agreement with statements stressing the importance of success in life and in determining his self-worth. Thus were revealed the importance to Warren of obtaining recognition from others, and of being number one, both of which figured quite prominently in his history and his current adjustment disorder.

COURSE OF TREATMENT

Presenting Problems

Warren began his graduate program, as he stated it, "expecting to be at the top of the class, expecting to be number one, and I presented myself as such"—a goal consistent with the high standards he typically set for himself. This meant befriending those whom he saw as the best students in the class, and arranging study groups with them. However, he soon found himself falling behind these peers, in terms of his ability to keep up with the material, the quality of his participation in class, and his subsequent feedback from professors. Lacking any sense of his own ability to handle hard work (believing instead that he had charmed his way into graduate school), Warren began to see himself as inadequate and felt increasingly unhappy and anxious in his study group and in classes. His dichotomous way of thinking made it seem to him as though by *not* being number one as he had expected (or more importantly, not getting *recognition* for this from his peers and professors), he had failed miserably. By the time of intake, he had taken to skipping classes and looking for shortcuts in his workload, such as obtaining notes on readings from other students so that he would not have to do them himself, in order to alleviate his anxiety.

The danger in Warren's expectations for graduate school was twofold: As stated above, he saw success quite dichotomously; in addition, he did not enter school with the expectation of having to work hard. As a child, he had come to believe that he was exceptional simply by virtue of being himself, and that he would be successful without having to work very hard at it. Hence, in therapy he would complain frequently that business school was too demanding, unfair, and "a joke" (i.e., not representative of his true abilities). He resented the requirements imposed on him in courses, most notably the volume of work assigned, believing that these requirements were silly and beneath him.

Short-Term Interventions

Short-term goals for Warren included helping him get through his first round of final exams. This included standard cognitive-behavioral interventions: relaxation training, gathering automatic thoughts and generating coping statements, reducing his all-or-nothing thinking with regard to his academic performance (anything less than all A's represented failure to him), breaking his workload down into manageable parts, and briefly, thought stopping (to help limit his daydreaming and ruminations). Later, when his daydreaming recurred in the second phase of treatment, I suggested that he keep a journal of his thoughts. This helped to introduce more structure into his thinking, thus encouraging him to "get it all out" in the journal and improving his concentration on other tasks.

These interventions, along with some changes in his study patterns and the acquisition of a new study partner, helped Warren past the initial crisis, and he was able to negotiate finals relatively successfully. Most helpful of all to him was a set of coping statements generated in therapy, which he kept beside his desk while studying. Being someone who saw himself as a good friend to others, he particularly liked solving problems by asking himself the question, "What advice would you give yourself?" By the end of the semester, his anxiety and depression had dropped to normal levels. This phase of treatment ended when Warren took a hiatus from therapy for the winter holiday, returning about one month later.

"I Am Princely"

Beginning with the first session after the holiday (session 6), therapy began to focus on the underlying factors that contributed to the adjustment disorder. We began by setting goals for treatment now that the immediate crisis had passed. Warren stated as a goal for this next phase of treatment to become more patient with other people—for example, in traffic and while waiting in lines. In discussing this, he revealed his belief that he was special, or "princely," as the source of this impatience: "I guess I just think I'm too special to have to wait in lines." He went on to describe some of the background that contributed to this belief, including the history noted above. I asked Warren how he thought this belief may have related to his recent crisis in business school, and he revealed the fear that, while as a child he had been "truly exceptional" in school, he might now have to give up the notion that he was special given the decline in his relative standing in school. The downward-arrow technique was utilized to access the core meaning to Warren of not being special.

THERAPIST: What does it mean to you that you haven't lived up to your goals for school last semester [of being at the top of your class]?
PATIENT: I guess that I'm not as exceptional as I used to be. I used to be a truly exceptional student, I mean really tremendous; everybody thought I was going to win the world. Now I guess I'm just not as great as I was before.
THERAPIST: And what would happen if you weren't as exceptional as you used to be?
PATIENT: I guess I wouldn't be special.
THERAPIST: What does that mean to you?
PATIENT: Basically, I guess it means I haven't lived up to my potential . . . I guess it means I'm a failure.
THERAPIST: And your potential was . . .?
PATIENT: Like I said, to be really, truly exceptional. Now, I'm just average, nothing special.
THERAPIST: So by being average, you become a failure?
PATIENT: Well, it's like I'm torn between just trying to get through and not worrying about being on top, and really trying to be the best. But I'm always afraid that if I don't go for it, I'll see it as a failure later on.
THERAPIST: What meaning would it have for you to be a failure, as we've defined it here?
PATIENT: It would mean I'm lazy, and weak. Pretty pathetic, basically.

Warren's "potential", as he saw it, was what others thought he was capable of. As noted above, he had the experience as a child of being noted for "exceptional" potential, and thus received the message that he could do anything, that he was the greatest, but *without the accompanying message that it would take hard work to achieve success*. It was pointed out to him that whenever he found himself falling short of this impossible standard, he would attribute this "failure" to some flaw in himself (just as he would attribute every success to being "special"), rather than a result of the amount of effort he put in. At every point where he failed to meet his own expectations, therefore, he encountered a crisis: He had "failed" in high school (note that he entered therapy for the second time at age 13), "failed" in college (by not getting in where he had wanted to go), and now, again, he was "failing" in graduate school. The reason for Warren's extreme distress in business school, therefore, was the *meaning* for him of his academic difficulties—this triggered for him the fear that perhaps he was *not* special, but rather the opposite. Warren was quite pleased with this conceptualization, especially since it incorporated a fear he had been dealing with for years (i.e., that he might not be special).

The next several sessions dealt with this fear of losing his status as "princely." Warren generated a list of the advantages and disadvantages of his world-view that he was special:

Disadvantages

- Getting speeding tickets and having accidents [six accidents in the six years he had been driving]
- Setting myself up for disappointments when I fail to live up to my own standards
- I am devastated by women when they reject me
- Feeling lonely (because no one thinks like I do; no one understands me)
- Unable to feel good about myself without getting recognition from others
- It makes me an unattractive person
- Since I think things will just happen to me, I don't work hard

Advantages

- It will help me in my business career
- It feels good to feel special
- [from his adolescence] Thinking I am special makes me a deep person; not to see myself as special would make me shallow and fake

It was essential to investigate the advantages (as Warren saw them) of believing in his own specialness, as well as the disadvantages, in order to know what maintained his narcissism. The last two advantages listed above, in particular, allowed access to what he feared as the *alternative* to being special ("I am nothing; just a cog

in a wheel") and the fear of being inconsistent with himself at a younger age ("If I no longer think I am special, a 15-year-old Warren wouldn't like me.") De-dichotomizing Warren's thinking by generating options between these extremes was essential to the task of making therapy less threatening as we began to challenge some of his schemas. He was able to consider that there was some middle ground; specifically, that he might be special in *certain* ways without being reduced to a "cog." The next task of therapy was to examine in what other ways Warren's belief was dysfunctional.

Entitlement and the Need for Perfection

The theme dealt with during the majority of Warren's time in therapy concerned his belief that, by virtue of being special, he was entitled to special treatment and to have the best of everything. For him, this meant having perfection in his life, and getting immediate gratification of his desires (a need that was evident since his childhood when he first attended therapy). He had great difficulty tolerating not having his needs and expectations met. This theme arose in several contexts, both interpersonal and individual: in his relationships with women and friends, and in his need for material things.

Romantic Involvements

Warren raised this issue first in session 9, concerning his dissatisfaction in his relationship with his girlfriend. Although initially "obsessed" with Jeanne, Warren complained that he was no longer satisfied with the relationship because she was no longer perfect. He elaborated that although he told her he loved her, he in fact did not, and that he knew one day he would meet the perfect woman and thereafter have a perfect marriage. His recurring pattern had been to enter a relationship quite infatuated, only to grow increasingly disappointed as he discovered imperfections. He would stay in the relationship—because he "could not stand to be without someone"—until he had met someone new, and then he would end it. I attempted to challenge Warren's assumptions underlying this pattern via Socratic questioning:

THERAPIST: You told me before that Jeanne was "perfect" when you first saw her, but that she's not anymore. Why?

PATIENT: Aside from the fact that she's gained weight, I guess it's mostly because I'm not truly in love with her. I mean, I really care for her, and I'm fond of her, but I'm not in love with her.

THERAPIST: How do you know when you're in "true love"?

PATIENT: Well, it's like there are two kinds of love—romantic, idealized, forever love; and fondness, caring, affection, and attachment. I just don't feel real love with Jeanne.

THERAPIST: Have you ever felt that kind of true love?

PATIENT: Sure, I even felt it with Jeanne in the beginning, but it didn't last.

THERAPIST: Do you know of anyone else who has experienced it?

PATIENT: Yeah, lots of people.

THERAPIST: Did it last for them?

PATIENT: Yes, as far as I know.

At this point, we reached an impasse: Warren's belief in true love was quite firmly entrenched, and apparently was supported by reports from friends or family. This point of the discussion came at the end of session 10, and the subject was resumed in session 11. Here, rather than again attempt directly to refute Warren's belief in the perfect relationship, I decided to reason the consequences of his beliefs and relate it to our earlier discussions of his specialness:

THERAPIST: You've said that you feel like everything's in flux when you can't commit to your relationship with Jeanne. Tell me more about how that feels.

PATIENT: It makes me feel unhappy, and frustrated, and unsure of what's coming next. I also feel guilty sometimes about Jeanne, since I don't give her as much as I should. But I really think she's a lot better off than before she met me.

THERAPIST: What is the effect of your not committing to the relationship, in terms of what *you* get out of it?

PATIENT: It makes me hold back . . . I'm always thinking that it's not going to last. I guess I don't open up to her as much as I could.

THERAPIST: So, by not committing to the relationship and holding out for the perfect woman, you actually make the relationship worse for Jeanne, by not giving her enough, and for you, by making you unhappy and pulling back from her. Is that right?

PATIENT: [Affect shift] Yeah, I guess it is . . . but what can I *do* about it?

THERAPIST: What do you think?

PATIENT: I don't know . . . (long pause) I guess I just have to keep trying to find someone else.

THERAPIST: Do you think that's realistic for you, given what we've just discussed?

PATIENT: I know she's got to be out there somewhere; I just have to find her.

It is worth noting that this session contained an important opportunity that I overlooked until reviewing the session tapes much later—specifically, his affect shift during the above dialogue. A quick probe for automatic thoughts at this point may have gained access to his reluctance to give up perfection as an ideal, which would in turn allow the opportunity to restructure his underlying beliefs. This opportunity missed, however, Warren returned to his original rigid belief that "she's out there somewhere," and this went essentially unchanged through the remainder of therapy.

Materialism

The next theme in treatment arose in session 12. This concerned a particular manifestation of Warren's need for immediate gratification; specifically, his obsession with material things. He described how he had become "obsessed" with radar detectors over his spring break, seeking all the information available to him about them, and eventually buying the most expensive model available (which was more than he could afford). He was quite upset over this incident, not only because it resulted in his spending money he did not have, but also because it had led to a fight with his girlfriend. I asked him to recall his automatic thoughts, and he identified the overall themes of "I must have it now," and "It has to be perfect/the best." We then discussed these thoughts and their relationship to the other themes already discussed in therapy, and Warren was surprisingly quick to connect his impatience to have a radar detector to his belief that he is special and therefore entitled to immediate gratification. We further generalized this finding and related it to other sources of dissatisfaction in his life (such as his girlfriend and overall pattern with women). In session, Warren was able to generate a number of effective rational responses to his automatic thoughts:

- "You are an adult; behave like one. Only children have to have everything right away. Be mature: Maturity is good."
- "Look at yourself: what do you look like? It is unattractive to be impatient."
- "You make mistakes when you rush. Take your time and you won't end up spending money you don't have."
- "You make those around you unhappy when you get this way. Think about others!"

Novel in the content of these responses was Warren's ability to show some consideration of the effect of his behavior on others; in other words, empathy. It is equally interesting to note, however, the overall narcissistic quality of the statements. It was clear very early on in therapy that any amount of therapy would be unlikely to make Warren *not* narcissistic; rather, it would merely succeed in *moderating* some of its dysfunctional aspects, helping him to function more adaptively within his narcissism.

Friendships

Toward the end of our work together, Warren and I began to deal with his similar inability to tolerate imperfections in his friends. He described a recurring pattern where he made friends, became very close with them for a period of time (thinking he had found a "soul mate"), and then discovered some "fatal flaw" that made it impossible for him to continue the friendship. He related this again to his belief that he was special and entitled to a perfect life, in the form of assumptions such as "My life must be perfect for me to be happy," and "Only very special people can understand me." (Although not elicited in therapy, it is also likely that Warren held the belief that he needed to be with people he saw as perfect in order to enhance his own perfection. This is also one likely reason for his belief that he always needed a romantic interest.)

For homework after one session spent discussing this, I asked Warren to chart a time line of his significant friendships, and to list the reasons why these ended. It was difficult for Warren to see how his schema was in operation in specific instances: Although he was able to recognize that no person was perfect, and thus that any friend would have faults, Warren insisted that these people's particular faults were so "major" as to make them intolerable for him, and that he needed friends whose faults were less serious. In order to establish more firmly the connection between his schema and this pattern in friendships, and to drive home the effect of this pattern (the loneliness that resulted from his lack of friends), he was asked in session to describe in detail the course of a particularly important friendship:

PATIENT: [John] and I were the best of friends; we were both really *deep*. We really understood each other well, and could be really supportive of each other. He was probably my best friend ever. But the problem was, he was basically an unreliable person. He would forget to meet me when we had agreed to meet, or he'd always show up late, with these really flimsy excuses. I just couldn't stay friends with someone who I couldn't count on like that.
THERAPIST: And how do you feel about [John] now?
PATIENT: I think he was a great guy. I really valued his friendship. But it just couldn't work once I realized how unreliable he was.

THERAPIST: So for you, having a friend who was late for get-togethers, and who forgot things sometimes, was unsatisfying?
PATIENT: Yeah.
THERAPIST: What did you get that was positive from that friendship?
PATIENT: We could really *talk*. He had this incredible ability to think deep thoughts; like we could have the longest conversations about the meaning of life, and philosophy, and religion, and just about anything! I don't think I've ever had a friend I could relate to that way.
THERAPIST: But that wasn't enough to outweigh the fact that he was sometimes forgetful?
PATIENT: Well . . .
THERAPIST: I mean, it just seems kind of a shame to throw away all the good things you had with him. Do you ever miss that?
PATIENT: [Affect shift] Yeah, I feel lonely sometimes.
THERAPIST: You seem sad now.
PATIENT: I guess I miss having a friend like that.
THERAPIST: You wish you had a friend like [John] now?
PATIENT: I wish I could have done it differently. I feel like I may never have a friend like that again. I guess I never really realized how good a friend he was.

For a time, Warren appeared truly to understand the dysfunctional nature of his all-or-nothing thinking, expressing anger with himself for his attitude later in writing:

> God, I have such an ego. And because of that ego I set ridiculous standards for myself, my companions, my lovers. . . . Yes, maybe at best I'm even special. But I am still one of 5,000,000,000 people. Look at that number . . . I am one of many trillion people since the beginning of people, and many trillion more until we're done. I am only one. Not even two.

However, as mentioned above, Warren's central belief that perfection was in fact possible in friendships (and, in fact, in all areas of his life) was very rigid and did not easily yield to interventions, because this was such a central assumption around which he had organized his life. At the point in treatment where this issue arose, Warren had nearly finished school for the summer and was preparing to return home; thus, rather than begin the difficult process of pursuing this issue, it was jointly decided to leave it aside and instead deal with termination issues, maintenance, and relapse prevention.

Self-Aggrandizement

As we neared the end of therapy, Warren came to a session with another event about which he had been extremely upset, and that required some processing. This dealt with his need to impress people, a theme that heretofore had never been directly addressed. He reported that on his flight back to school from a weekend at home, he had sat next to a young woman to whom he lied in order to impress. He was quite upset with himself for his behavior, stating that "I used to do that all the time, but I thought I had stopped it"—referring to a long-standing pattern in college where he would attempt to win over women by charming them, impressing them with his intelligence or wealth, or by lying or otherwise "putting on airs" (such as wearing copies of expensive watches). Warren's automatic thoughts included:

- "I have to impress her"
- "I have to get her to like me"
- "I must be attractive to her"
- "If she isn't interested in me, I am worthless"

Warren believed that he would have to lie to the woman in order to *ensure* that he would impress her: He feared he would not be impressive on his own, but yet needed to impress her in order to maintain his self-esteem. He held the all-or-nothing belief that "I can make any reasonably intelligent woman be attracted to me." This left him open for potentially devastating consequences when, for whatever reason, he failed to attract a woman, since any evidence to the contrary of this belief would invalidate it altogether. Thus, he would be left with the only alternative—that he was unattractive. In discussing this conceptualization of the incident, Warren was able to see the dysfunctional nature of his grandiose assumption and saw the value in substituting a more rational alternative: "I am a good person, charming and attractive. Most women with similarities to me who are unattached and looking, given the opportunity to see me not at my worst, but not necessarily at my best, will be interested in me." Warren found this session to be particularly enlightening, and expressed a great deal of satisfaction in its outcome.

DISCUSSION

The major limitation of my work with Warren was time: in only 19 sessions, it would be unrealistic of the therapist to expect that successful modification of Warren's dysfunctional schema could be accomplished. In this limited time, we had a choice of either addressing in depth one problem aspect of Warren's schema and working toward change in this area, or dealing primarily with identifying the scope of the schema in all of its aspects. Warren's style in therapy was to raise a new, fairly major

problem issue nearly every week; in order to accommodate his need to manage so many concerns and yet maintain some focus overall, I decided to process each event or issue and help Warren to conceptualize it within the overall framework we were developing. Primary in therapy had been insight and understanding; the work of more fundamental adaptations in Warren's beliefs would be left for the future.

Several opportunities for more thorough work with Warren were overlooked. For example, Warren had difficulty reconciling his self of today with the self at a younger age: He feared that "a 15-year-old Warren wouldn't like me." A useful intervention here may have been to use imagery to create a dialogue between the 15-year-old Warren and the older, wiser, present-day Warren. In this dialogue, Warren would attempt to reason with himself that he knew more about life at 22 than he did at 15, and thus try to lessen the strength and validity of some of his childhood beliefs. This may have helped to loosen the hold that Warren's childhood beliefs had over him in the present, and make the prospect of restructuring them less threatening by putting himself in the position of being wiser (more mature, and therefore better) than he was at 15. Hence, what the 15-year-old Warren thought would not matter. This approach would make use of his narcissistic need to see himself as always "better than" something while effecting the subtle changes necessary to make his narcissism less dysfunctional overall.

As mentioned above, I did not directly challenge Warren's assumptions about marriage and romance. His belief in true and perfect love, while immature, was nevertheless quite powerful, and to refute this directly at the stage of therapy when it arose might have been too threatening. However, such a challenge may also have been quite effective if used later in therapy and in the context of a dialogue with an adolescent self. A confrontational, wake-up-and-smell-the-coffee approach would probably have been useful with this particular patient, since toward the end of treatment rapport was quite good. As mentioned above, another opportunity to intervene on the belief level was overlooked quite by accident during a dialogue on this subject in session 11.

A means toward addressing his all-or-nothing thinking style might have been found in his reaction to the dialogue in session about his past friendships. His reaction was typical in its extremity, carrying a very negative and self-punitive tone—as if to say, "You fool, you're not special at all! In fact, thinking you are makes you worthless!" Clearly, this was not the most adaptive response possible to a realization that his narcissism had some negative consequences. A discussion not only of how to correct his thinking in this one instance (as we did in a later session), but also pointing out this example's place in his overall thinking *style*, could have been useful.

SUMMARY

Warren's treatment lasted only a total of 19 sessions, the first five of which focused on short-term problem solving to help him through finals. In the interest of maintaining a focus on his immediate crisis, the personality features relating to his problems were not addressed at all during this phase. Upon his return to treatment, we began to investigate how a variety of underlying beliefs contributed to his difficulties in adjustment, as well as to other problem areas in his life. Primary among these were his belief that he was special, and the subsequent belief that he was entitled to have everything exactly as he wanted it: perfect. Although the bulk of therapy was spent discussing his expectation of and need for perfection, this belief remained largely intact by the time it was decided to begin termination. Warren was able to recognize some specific instances of when these beliefs became problematic, and to abandon some of his assumptions in favor of more realistic alternatives. As Warren was leaving town for the summer, no follow-up visits were arranged; however, it might be expected that he will reenter therapy at some time in the future when he enters a crisis at the challenge of another major assumption. Most predictably, he may finish school and move to California to pursue his longtime dream of a career in cinema, only to learn that his belief in his inevitable success was unrealistic. Or, marriage may challenge his belief in perfect love.

REFERENCES

Beck, A. T. (1972). Measurement of depression: The Depression Inventory. In A. T. Beck (Ed.), *Depression: Causes and treatment*. Philadelphia: University of Pennsylvania Press.

Beck, A. T., Brown, G., Steer, R. A., Eidelson, J. I., & Riskind, J. H. (1987). Differentiating anxiety and depression: A test of the cognitive content-specificity hypothesis. *Journal of Abnormal Psychology*, *96*(3), 179–183.

Beck, A. T., Epstein, N., Brown, G., & Steer, R. A. (1988). An inventory for measuring clinical anxiety: Psychometric properties. *Journal of Consulting and Clinical Psychology*, *56*(6), 893–897.

Beck, A. T., Steer, R. A., Epstein, N., & Brown, G. (in press). The Beck Self-Concept Test. *American Journal of Consulting and Clinical Psychiatry*, *2*, 2.

Beck, A. T., Weissman, A., Lester, D., & Trexler, L. (1974). The measurement of pessimism: The Hopelessness Scale. *Journal of Consulting and Clinical Psychology*, *42*(6), 861–865.

Spitzer, R. L., Williams, J. B. W., & Gibbon, M. (1987). *Instruction manual for the Structured Clinical Interview for DSM-III-R* (SCID, 4/1/87 revision). New York: Biometrics Research Department, New York State Psychiatric Institute.

Weissman, A. N., & Beck, A. T. (March, 1978). *Development and validation of the Dysfunctional Attitude Scale*. Paper presented at the 62nd annual meeting of the American Educational Research Association.

SUGGESTED READINGS

Beck, A. T., Freeman, A., & Associates. (1990). *Cognitive therapy of personality disorders* (Chaps. 4, 5, & 11). New York: Guilford.

24

The Schizophrenic Patient

Bruce N. Eimer and Arthur Freeman

Community mental health centers, university-based counseling centers, church-supported or governmental social service agencies, or psychiatric residency program sites are often the main training ground for therapists and counselors. These settings are often most needy of practicum students and interns to provide the services to the agency's clientele. These agencies are also the direct service providers for some of the most chronic and emotionally disturbed patients. The system provides several paradoxes: The most chronic, needy, and disturbed patients may get the least experienced therapists. The patients who are in need of long-term contact and a strong, ongoing therapeutic relationship are often limited to one year of treatment by an intern or trainee. There is, of course, the option of beginning again the next training cycle with a new therapist. This pattern, however, is becoming part of the more general service provision of psychotherapy as third-party payers and managed health care systems place limits on the number of sessions that consumers may have for therapy.

When treating unipolar depression with cognitive therapy as per the treatment outlined by Beck, Rush,

Shaw, and Emery (1979), a year is more than enough time to address the symptom distress and to work on schematic issues (Freeman, Pretzer, Fleming, & Simon, 1990). Similarly, anxiety and panic can be dealt with in a year (Alford, Freeman, Wright, & Beck, 1990; Beck, Emery, & Greenberg, 1985). The treatment of personality disorders and the psychotic states, however, requires a longer-term treatment, greater intensity and/or frequency of sessions, and the establishment and maintenance of a long-term therapeutic alliance (Beck, Freeman, & Associates, 1990; Greenwood, 1983).

In the present case, all of the negative factors were in place. The therapist was an intern placed in a community agency setting as part of his postdoctoral respecialization in clinical psychology, working under the supervision of a licensed psychologist and adjunct faculty member of the university. Given the limited time available for treating this patient by the dictates of the agency, limited goals were set so that the patient could get some sense of success in the brief therapeutic contact.

BRIEF HISTORY, BACKGROUND, AND PRESENTING COMPLAINTS

Doris was a 41-year-old unemployed, divorced black woman who first came to the community clinic in an acutely psychotic state, accompanied by her 33-year-old sister. Doris complained of hearing voices that were telling her to go to other people's homes. At one point, she reported a voice telling her that her aunt was harming

Bruce N. Eimer • The Behavior Therapy Center, Jenkintown, Pennsylvania 19046.   Arthur Freeman • Department of Psychiatry, Cooper Hospital/University Medical Center and Robert Wood Johnson Medical School at Camden, Camden, New Jersey 08103.

Comprehensive Casebook of Cognitive Therapy, edited by Arthur Freeman and Frank M. Dattilio. Plenum Press, New York, 1992.

Doris's parents, so Doris went to her parents' home with two bricks in her hand. Her sister reported that over the past four or five years, ever since an automobile accident, Doris's functioning had deteriorated markedly. Doris's view was that her problems predated the accident, though she was unclear as to how long the voices had been bothering her. Upon questioning, she denied any physical illness or substance abuse. The agency psychiatrist interviewed Doris and diagnosed her as evidencing "atypical psychosis" and prescribed Mellaril (50 mg BID, 100 mg HS).

Subsequent to the auto accident, Doris was seen and followed by a neuropsychiatrist. A CT screening, electro-encephalography, and periodic neurological examinations yielded negative results. The psychiatrist treated her with neuroleptic medication for about four years on an inter-mittent basis; his diagnosis was schizophrenia, paranoid type. He would diminish the frequency of the contacts when Doris showed a general remission of her symptoms and increase contact when her symptoms became more florid. He finally referred her to the community agency with the rationale that she needed more intensive and consistent treatment than he was able to provide.

When Doris first contacted the clinic, she was as-signed to work with Dr. M., a psychologist. They worked together for two months, at which point Dr. M. abruptly left the clinic to take a job in another city. Doris later described the therapy as "helpful." From Dr. M.'s notes, the therapy appeared to be directive and supportive, with a major focus on helping Doris to maintain compliance with her medication regimen. When Dr. M. left, Doris termi-nated her involvement with the agency.

She reappeared approximately two months later for medication and therapy. It was at this point that the present case study begins. At the initial session, Doris was en-couraged to build a problem list. The main issues on her list were (a) hearing disturbing voices; (b) vague visual disturbances; (c) aches and pains throughout her body; (d) feeling tired and "drained" all of the time; (e) being unable to relax; (f) conflict with her younger sister and niece (with whom she boarded); (g) social anxiety that prevented her from holding a job; (h) difficulty with sim-ple life chores (e.g., picking up her public assistance check); (i) being confused, troubled, and nervous; and (j) losing track of things. Given the extensive list, the thera-pist questioned Doris about how she presently coped with her many problems. She responded that she kept to her-self, avoided people, rested and napped a lot, stayed in her room and watched television, and avoided work because the voices became louder and more disturbing when she was around people. She also expressed her feeling that life was "very painful."

BRIEF FAMILY BACKGROUND

Doris was one of five children, having a younger sister (Lilli, age 33), a younger brother (Bob, age 35), an older sister (Ellen, age 43), and an older brother (Harold, age 45). Doris lived with her sister Lilli and her niece, Tanya (Lilli's 13-year-old daughter). Doris claimed she really loved her sister and her niece, but she and Lilli argued frequently because Doris believed that she just couldn't meet their expectations and so was "too much trouble." Doris's parents were both living in a different section of the city. She reported that although she also loved them very much as well, she had not had much contact with them since her divorce several years earlier. (She had been married for a brief time in her early 20s; she was unclear on exactly when.) Doris's sister Lilli had reported in their first clinic contact with Dr. M. that Doris had been mentally and physically abused as a child. Also, Doris reported that she and Lilli had always gotten along the best, and there was the sense that the family had put some subtle pressure on Lilli to take care of Doris.

EDUCATIONAL AND VOCATIONAL BACKGROUND

Doris was graduated from high school, where she studied secretarial skills. She lived at home with her parents after high school graduation but never held a steady job. She moved out when she got married; during the years of her marriage, Doris didn't work. She reported that following her divorce, she received financial help from various relatives and took various jobs to support herself. She worked on and off as a nighttime homemaker in various hospitals and state homes. She reported that the automobile accident had made her eligible for workmen's compensation in that the accident occurred while she was working. She reported that when she tried going back to work, she found herself unable to work because she would become very "emotional and upset."

More recently, Doris reported, she had been receiv-ing public assistance, food stamps, and money for medi-cal assistance. She had applied for Social Security disabil-ity income (SSI) but was refused benefits. She claimed angrily that she was determined to keep trying to obtain it, as it was her "due" inasmuch as she was not able to function like a normal person. How could she work, she questioned, when she experienced "blackouts" or fainting spells, was nervous and tense around people, heard them laughing and talking negatively about her, was very con-fused and disorganized, and experienced sensory distur-bances (which included hearing derogatory voices, watering eyes, blurred vision, excessive sweating, dry mouth, tingling and numbness, tension, headaches, aches and pains, dizziness, palpitations, stomach trouble, and fatigue)?

TREATMENT PLAN

Based on the history obtained, the presenting symptom picture, and supporting data contributed by projective personality testing, a treatment plan was drawn up. The problems that were identified in collaboration with the patient and the therapist's assessment and diagnostic impression formed the basis for setting goals. Table 24-1 lists the problems identified, goals set, and intended methods for attaining these goals. The diagnostic impression was Axis I, chronic schizophrenia, paranoid type; Axis II, borderline personality disorder. The following conceptualizations are based on the history, test data, and interview material.

1. *General sense of the world and her relatedness to the world (sense of reality, reality testing, and judgment).* Doris was quite fearful of the world and of the destructive potential of her own anger. She viewed the world as very threatening, and was therefore extremely guarded. She conducted herself interpersonally in a very stilted and rigid manner. She consistently misinterpreted social situations, and her behavior was marginally socially appropriate. She either deferred to others or had angry outbursts.

2. *Ways of dealing with conflict and her modes of coping (defensive functioning, regulation and control of drives, affects and impulses, control of stimuli).* Doris harbored a great deal of nonspecific social anxiety stemming from early negative schemas of failure, rejection, abandonment, and mistrust. She repeatedly transformed her vague, negative feelings into perceived threats. Her low threshold for alarm stemmed from her inability to view events as having both positive and negative aspects. Good impressions were totally and immediately erased by any negative feelings. Given her projected expectations that others harbored negative and hostile intentions toward her and her all-or-nothing thinking, she had only two responses—to withdraw or to retaliate. It is of little surprise that she found constant confirmation of her schema regarding the hostility of others. Doris's coping style was to do something, as opposed to thinking and planning things out; her lack of thoughtfulness and planning made her vulnerable to acting out her feelings in intense and unmodulated ways. At the same time, she appeared fearful that her pent-up emotions would make her "blow up."

Her low threshold also caused difficulty in managing stimulus input. She easily became overwhelmed and disorganized. Her self-representation was comprised of unintegrated, contradictory good and bad impressions. She viewed herself as a failure, worthless, unlovable, and untrustworthy, as well as abandoned, rejected, victimized, alone, and in pain. Others were viewed as cruel, insensitive, rejecting, abandoning, and untrustworthy. She was fearful of people, expected rejection, and avoided involvements.

3. *Cognitive capacities (includes thought processes and synthetic and integrative functioning).* Doris's attention, concentration, and memory were all seriously impaired. She reported "getting nervous with other people around," not being able to do more than one simple thing at a time, being very slow, and having difficulty remembering. She was very concrete and literal, though neurological examinations did not reveal signs of organicity (it probably would have been helpful to have done more extensive psychological testing, i.e., intellectual and neuropsychological assessments).

In terms of Doris's thought processes, she used peculiar language that was not validated by subcultural standards. Although her speech was coherent, it was generally pressured. She evidenced preoccupations with somatic complaints, depreciation of self and others, and anger. Also in the cognitive realm, Doris was a very poor scanner and organizer of stimulus input and easily became disorganized and confused. Her efforts at synthesizing the elements of situations and integrating disparate events were few (i.e., synthetic and integrative functioning), but when she did attempt to do so her efforts were poor. Her approach to the world was overly simplistic and economical. In addition, both ideationally and behaviorally, she was very rigid and inflexible. These characteristics could have been responsible for placing Doris repeatedly at risk for interpersonal confrontations, given a psychological set/response style of avoiding, rejecting, or ignoring stimulus complexity and ambiguity, thus placing her at odds with other's expectations.

4. *Ability to get along in the world/current level of adaptive functioning (autonomous functioning, mastery and competence, and self-preservation drive).* Doris was free of impairments of hearing, vision, speech, and motility. She was, however, impaired in her ability to be around people. She had a poor sense of self-efficacy; she was self-critical, rigid, and lacking in purpose and initiative. Her present performance was congruent with her negative perceptions.

The factors identified thus far contributed to Doris's hopelessness, and put her at risk for suicide. Her poor judgment and reality testing, tendency to act out, proneness to disorganization, social anxiety, social withdrawal,

TABLE 24-1 Treatment Plan

Problem	Goal	Means
Incapacitating social anxiety; inability to tolerate crowds	1. Patient will feel more comfortable in social situations 2. Patient will make small steps towards more social involvement	1. Establish relatedness with patient 2. Teach patient coping techniques such as distraction 3. Encouraging and reinforcing social activities 4. Exploring disturbances in relationships 5. Social skills training through modeling and behavioral rehearsal
Difficulty making decisions; very ambivalent	1. Patient will be able to make simple decisions and follow through on them	1. Therapist reassurance 2. Reduction of fears 3. Modeling and behavioral rehearsal 4. Provision of confidence in patient; unconditional positive regard and warmth
Hears derogatory voices, command hallucinations, and has delusions of persecution and control and ideas of reference	1. Patient will be better able to distinguish between fantasy and reality 2. Patient will raise her "alarm threshold"	1. Ongoing neuroleptic medication 2. Cognitive-prescriptive approach to "catch" the antecedents of hallucinations and delusions and vigorously dismiss them 3. Interpreting cognitive mechanisms 4. Explore underlying interpersonal conflicts 5. Validating partial insights; praising accurate reality testing 6. Encourage patient to collect evidence to build distrust of her own paranoia
Affective instability; intense, overwhelming anger	1. Better modulation of ways feelings are expressed 2. Patient will think before acting out; will take rage or disappointment as a signal to stop and think of alternatives and options 3. Better discrimination of "shades of gray"	1. Anger management training (e.g., pause technique, diversion, advantages and disadvantages, options) 2. Confronting disproportionate expressions of rage in the transference; making connections to current and past relationships; confronting "entitlement" 3. Therapist modeling responsibility for own aggressiveness 4. Therapist guiding patient to work on reducing her "indebtedness" to significant others
Tension; inability to relax	1. Patient will be able to utilize simple relaxation skills	1. Discovering pleasurable activities 2. Distraction and creative daydreaming
Disorganization and memory problems	1. Patient will keep track of daily, then weekly schedule 2. Patient will plan activities	1. Activity scheduling 2. Keeping a daily diary
Inability to maintain gainful employment	1. Development of enough confidence to seek work 2. Increase frustration tolerance 3. Will be able to hold onto job	1. Assess interests, aptitudes, strengths, and limitations 2. Explore job options in light of above 3. Making arrangements for training in simple job skills or mobilizing dormant capacities 4. Training in job search skills 5. Confidence building Discouraging all-or-nothing thinking 6. Modeling and role-playing
Conflicts with significant others	1. Patient will get along better with others—fewer blowups; better at saying "no"; better at making clear requests, communicating her needs 2. Increased self-acceptance	1. Exploring schemas of failure, abandonment, rejection, and mistrust 2. Encouraging acceptance of compromise 3. Modeling and role-playing socially appropriate means of working toward goals 4. Confronting "entitlement" 5. Interpreting aspects of the transference and linking to current and past relationships

guardedness, cognitive rigidity, limited problem-solving behavior, perceived limited options and alternatives, and sense of being overwhelmed by negative and powerful affective states were all contributing factors. These factors took on even more significance in light of her expressed suicidal ideation. While she never described a plan or intent, she would throw her hands up and say, "Say, Doc, maybe I should just end it all. It's too much to handle. What do you think?".

OVERVIEW OF TREATMENT

The course of therapy was based on the assumption that the chronic patient requires a treatment that is flexible and responsive to the patient's myriad needs and problems. Greenwood (1983) states,

> Given the "multimodal" pathology in these patients, it is important for the therapist to delineate an internally consistent view of the therapy process. This will allow the therapist to experiment with a wide range of techniques in an orderly and coherent fashion. Perhaps more so than with other patients, therapists must think "cognitive" and yet operate in a multimodal fashion in order to exploit opportunities for constructive change. (p. 186)

Treatment consisted of 21 sessions lasting over the course of approximately eight months. Termination was built into the therapy from the outset, as early on it was explained to Doris that this therapist was a psychology intern and would be leaving the clinic at the end of his training year. Doris indicated awareness and acceptance of this fact of life, stating that "doctors always come and go in clinics."

Arieti (1974) points out that the first stage in treatment needs to be devoted to establishing relatedness. He recommends that the therapist provide hearty doses of reassurance, communicate a sincere desire to understand and share in the patient's experiential world, demonstrate caring for and confidence in the patient, communicate warmth (also termed "unconditional positive regard"), and become actively engaged with the patient. Especially with the paranoid patient, these qualities and activities are important for reducing the patient's fears that would be aroused by close interpersonal contact. It was important to communicate to Doris that the therapist was trying to understand her. It was difficult, yet essential, that no comments initially be made about her self-defeating behavior, as these might be construed as intolerance or misunderstanding.

Reducing Doris's anxiety to its lowest possible level was always the aim. Comments were brief, simple, understandable, and directive, avoiding open-ended interpreta-

tions. It was essential to provide ample structure to supplement her lack of it and in order to ameliorate the negative therapeutic effects of her ambivalence. In addition, therapist comments were aimed at reinforcing her reality testing and encouraging her to reduce her heavy reliance on denial through the judicious use of personal disclosure on the therapist's part. In addition, given that attention to the nonverbal components of therapy is very important, the therapist tried to accentuate friendly nonverbal behaviors. Over the course of the first few months of therapy, Doris brought up material that covered all of the problems outlined in the treatment plan.

Despite the therapist's best efforts, on many occasions Doris expressed frustration at the therapist's inability to understand her limitations—"what I'm up against, Doc." For example, somewhere around the eighth session, she was discussing her financial difficulties. The therapist suggested jobs she might be able to obtain that would not interfere with her eligibility for SSI. She became very angry, and said that nobody really understood her, including the therapist, that he did not recognize the extent of her limitations in terms of work. At that point, the therapist thought it best to confront her anger directly and to point out what was happening in the session. The goal was to identify the stimulus for her rage (i.e., hot cognitions), and to attempt to deal with it in the session. However, given the pressures with which Doris was confronted by others to relinquish the "sick role," to deny her serious problems and the chronicity of her experiences of being misunderstood by others, the therapist opted to confirm her reality and convey understanding about why she was angry. He also accepted responsibility for perhaps expecting too much from her. When Doris calmed down, the therapist suggested that perhaps she expected too much from him, that he was only human and consequently did at times fail in sensitivity and empathy. This personal admission seemed to have a great effect on Doris, as she herself then generated the insight that perhaps the reason she got angry so often and so intensely was because she expected too much from people and "they never came through."

Over the next four or five sessions, a lot of time was spent on helping her reduce her social anxiety. The therapist taught Doris several techniques for coping with anxiety (e.g., distraction, positive coping self-statements, controlled or patterned breathing). He first modeled them and then rehearsed them during the sessions. They were then practiced as homework, and she reported her success or failure in practicing them at home. During these sessions, Doris discussed her distress when she heard the voices. She reported that although they diminished somewhat because of her medication, they did not go away. She believed that people were "having fun at my expense" and were saying terrible things about her. The therapist introduced the ideas of fear, negative expectations of others, the "listening attitude," hallucinatory experience, the self-referential attitude, and the notion of ideas of reference (Arieti, 1974). In addition to explaining these cognitive phenomena in simple terms, the therapist gave Doris specific techniques for breaking the cycle of distress (e.g., using positive self-statements, emphatically instructing the voices or thoughts to stop, and distracting herself with activities such as deep, rhythmic breathing).

A significant event occurred in the second half of the sessions: Doris was refused eligibility for SSI a second time. This became the central theme for the next four sessions. At this point, the therapist took on an advocacy role and coached her on the appeals process. He also completed the required forms that testified to her neediness and eligibility. During the next sessions, Doris brought up many instances of her failure, rejection, and being abandoned. She related these to the "joke" of not being sick enough for SSI.

Another issue that surfaced was the conflict with her sister and niece. Doris had great difficulty in accepting having both good and bad feelings toward them. She would either go far out of her way to please them or go into a rage and retreat into her room for several days. The therapist was quite directive and worked with Doris by instructing her in prosocial behavior.

The issue of the therapist leaving the clinic and the upcoming termination was the focus of the last four sessions. It was not a pleasant task, and one with which the therapist had difficulty. The therapist worked in supervision to examine options of continuing working with Doris, but for many reasons, this was not a reasonable goal. Doris was already agitated because of the SSI refusal, so that the impending ending of the sessions and having her start with another therapist was a source of additional stress. She was upset about the upcoming appeal and the ambiguity of the appeals process. The therapist tried to reduce the ambiguity of the process as much as possible by breaking it down into concrete steps. He also tried to reassure her (without instilling false hopes) that the majority of eligible applicants who are turned down for SSI win on appeal.

Doris, however, was only reassured during the period that the issue was discussed. Even during the same session, following having focused on another issue, she again would restate her fears of being denied in the appeal. She also expressed anger—at the system, at her family, and at the therapist. She accused him of being uncaring like all the rest of the world. She expressed hopelessness and ambivalence: "It's hopeless, Doc. Maybe I should just give up. What do you think, Doc? Is there any hope for me? Even you said the first time that people would wonder if I'm really sick. Am I sick, Doc?" The therapist to wanted to show empathy for her experience and at the same time reflect an accurate appraisal of reality. Thus, he addressed the last question first: "That's a loaded question, Doris. We both know how much pain you suffer—that's one of the reasons you have come to this clinic." This got around the confrontive aspect of her question, but it did not address the issue of providing a concrete basis for hope.

Falling back on something that often gives a basis for hope in oppressive situations, the therapist employed some humor and told her a story. Stone, Albert, Forrest, and Arieti (1983) recommend the use of jokes or humorous stories with schizophrenic patients as a potentially useful technique when their "meaning is highly relevant to the stage of psychic development at which the patient is currently situated, or has evolved in the past, on his way to a higher level" (p. 293). The story was about a man whose car has a flat tire on a lonely country road. He needs a jack. He sights a farmhouse off in the distance. First he thinks the farmer can lend him a jack, but as he trudges to the farm he thinks negative; maybe the farmer won't lend him his jack. Then, worse yet, he more negatively thinks: "maybe he'll charge me a pretty penny for it? The nerve of him!" His thinking gets more and more negative, and he gets more and more angry. Finally, exhausted, he arrives and knocks on the farmer's door. The farmer answers, and the fellow—by now angry and completely without any faith—punches the farmer in the face, saying, "Keep your damned jack!" This joke drives the point home that no matter how justified one's anger is, if one reasons from a false premise one is likely to have used up a whole lot of energy uselessly ("for naught").

Also, the therapist tried to make the point that Doris had struggled so far (trying to obtain SSI, to cope with "the forces" fighting with her will to hold a job, trying to trust people, having different therapists, etc.) that it would be a great shame for her to give up now. It would appear that this intervention had some of its intended impact. It seemed that some of the steam was lost from the intensity of her protests about how hopeless things were for her. Over the last sessions, she was reminded of the man and the farmer at strategic points as a shared metaphor, especially when she voiced ideas of hopelessness and rejection in response to her discussions of the therapist leaving and her picking up with a new therapist. In the last session together, she brought up the metaphor and said, "My new therapist is gonna be luckier than that old farmer, Doc. No punching for him, no punching for him . . . I'll see if he'll lend me that jack. We'll just have to see."

Session Transcript

What follows is a session from the early part of the therapy that illustrates the directive nature of the therapy with Doris. The initial interactions involve greetings and rapport. The first issue on the agenda is Doris's medication; she had been hurt in another auto accident when a truck hit the car in which she was riding. The agency psychiatrist wanted to meet with her briefly to discuss the synergistic effects of combined neuroleptics, anxiolytics, and pain medication.

THERAPIST: OK. Let me, let me see if Dr. G. is available for me to speak to for a moment before you leave, so that he can prescribe . . . well, you have pain medicine now?

PATIENT: Yeah . . . they gave it to me, he told me to take extra Moban.

THERAPIST: Who did?

PATIENT: Dr. G.

THERAPIST: Uh-huh.

PATIENT: When I saw him yesterday. He told me to take an extra one. I had taken an extra one on Sunday. And he put me on an extra one again. And he asked me if I was suicidal, had I been thinking about suicide . . . when I hadn't been. Not lately. Oh, and one other thing. What was the report on my EEG?

THERAPIST: (looking at case record) The report says that it's normal.

PATIENT: Oh. Did you read the whole report?

THERAPIST: Yes.

PATIENT: Oh.

THERAPIST: That's great, isn't it?

PATIENT: Yes. You said it would be, didn't you?

THERAPIST: Well, I said . . .

PATIENT: (interrupts) You kinda thought it would be.

THERAPIST: Yes, I thought it would be. I had a hunch.

PATIENT: Yeah.

THERAPIST: But it's good it was checked out. Now we no longer have to worry about it.

PATIENT: Well. . . . I was telling Dr. G. how close people are when there's a big crowd. The same thing that I told you.

THERAPIST: You get nervous.

PATIENT: And I want to run away.

THERAPIST: OK.

PATIENT: He had a word for it.

THERAPIST: Phobia?

PATIENT: No, he didn't call it phobia. I don't know what he said.

THERAPIST: Agoraphobia?

PATIENT: No. He said, when you wanna run away, it's a, it's a fear that I have. Of people, of crowds of people, like they're coming at me? So I said, do you know . . .

THERAPIST: (interrupts) Claustrophobia?

PATIENT: Yes. And the fear, too.

THERAPIST: Right.

PATIENT: And then he says, you know, I told him that you told me don't run away, try not to run away . . . how to try to get myself straightened out and not to be so afraid and so upset. I can try to talk to myself or talk out and, and stay with it, don't run away from it, like when I run out of line and run around? (brief pause) So he said, that's good if you can do that—you must, you know. I said that's what you had told me to practice. I said I was going to stay away as much as I can from a crowd of people . . . which you can't always do that, but I tried. So, so he was saying it's a, it's a, it's a fear and it's in you, it's like, like closing in on me, you know? And then I'm hearing like all kinds of voices that everybody can't be saying all bad about me, but I feel this when people are talking, there's a lot of talk going on . . . OK? (therapist nods) So, he was saying that I should try. I told him I hadn't been in a crowd with lots of people since I've been to see you. OK? So I will try it when I go back to the office to get my next check. You know that they've been on strike, don't you?

THERAPIST: At the state?

PATIENT: Yes. The state.

THERAPIST: DPA?

PATIENT: Yes. The state's been on strike, but they went back. When I go back it should be nice and crowded, because all of the people will be there to get their checks. So I'll be able to test myself on those long lines.

THERAPIST: When you start getting anxious . . . remember, that the fact that you're getting anxious is good because it will give you a chance to practice all of what you've learned.

PATIENT: From you?

THERAPIST: Right. Do you want to go over it again?

PATIENT: OK. Alright.

THERAPIST: Let's go over it again.

PATIENT: OK. When I'm in the line and I want to just run away . . . there's just so many people and stuff for me. I'm going to breathe slowly three times to myself. I just breathe and I say, "Doris, *stop.*" And then I try to stop.

THERAPIST: Stop what? What are you stopping?

PATIENT: (pause) I'm stopping running away.

THERAPIST: Good. You're stopping running away . . . what else? (pause) How about the thoughts?

PATIENT: Oh, I forgot.

THERAPIST: The bad thoughts. They're the ones that get you. How about the voices?

PATIENT: Yeah.

THERAPIST: First come the thoughts and then comes the voices. Isn't that the way that it goes?

PATIENT: Yes. Always first. The thoughts are first.

THERAPIST: I see.

PATIENT: But why is it always around a crowd of people? To me, it's always around lots of people.

THERAPIST: Does it have to do with losing control?

PATIENT: Maybe. Dr. G. says it's a fear.

THERAPIST: (later in session) We start to have all these bad thoughts about what could happen to us.

PATIENT: Yeah.

THERAPIST: (later in session) Think back to the times you hear voices. It's always preceded by bad thoughts, isn't it?

PATIENT: Yeah. Always.

THERAPIST: (later in session) So what I'm thinking is maybe . . . maybe we can stop the voices by stopping the thoughts.

PATIENT: You think I can just stop the thoughts myself just by using your method of what you told me to do. I understand what you're saying to do,, and I'm going to do it when I go to the office, that's my next crowd, that's next week. That's Monday. OK? Um . . . It'll be really crowded now, like always. It's really crowded. And you think it'll just make my mind, it'll clear my mind up some?

THERAPIST: Works for a lot of people.

PATIENT: Does it?

THERAPIST: Sure. I've used it with other folks, and it works for them. (brief pause) I don't know if it'll work for you for sure; it might take some practice. It might not work totally the first time.

PATIENT: Yeah. But I don't want to run away from everything. Where there's people, well, that's where I won't go.

THERAPIST: So, we'll, this is what you'll do. I'll give you this sheet of paper (therapist writes coping steps on paper). So breathe deeply three times.

PATIENT: I remember that.

THERAPIST: OK? And then, you'll say stop. . . .

PATIENT: (later in session) Yeah. OK, thanks a lot. (pauses) Now I won't see you for two weeks, but I still have to come here to see Dr. G.

THERAPIST: And if you have a problem. . . .

PATIENT: (interrupts) What do I do if I have a problem?

THERAPIST: When I'm away, if you have a problem, just call the clinic. . . .

PATIENT: And say what? What do you want me to do?

THERAPIST: And say that I'm, I'm, seeing Dr. Eimer, this is Doris O., and I need to talk to somebody. The secretary will find you somebody to talk to or she'll have somebody call you back, have that person call you

back to schedule an appointment. You know, if you really need to talk to somebody.

PATIENT: Yeah.

THERAPIST: (later in session) Do you like to read?

PATIENT: Yeah.

THERAPIST: So, bring a book with you.

PATIENT: Yeah.

THERAPIST: You can even bring a brook with you for when you're standing on line at the welfare office.

PATIENT: Yeah, I could, couldn't I?

THERAPIST: While you're standing there. I do that a lot. I stand on lines, I hate standing on lines. But, I stand there on line and I read my book, and I forget everything that's around me.

PATIENT: Yeah?

THERAPIST: Yeah.

PATIENT: Yeah. That's probably why a lot of people read on the buses and subways and all. Huh. Well, anyway, I could do that. I have books I can read. (Short pause). But, then again, that's the way I pass my time at this office.

THERAPIST: (later in session) Well, sure, you know, you told me at the very beginning of when we worked together that you would go off into your room and stay by yourself all day. Then you would start having bad thoughts and before you know it you'd start hearing voices.

PATIENT: That's right.

THERAPIST: Right?

PATIENT: And talking back to voices. That was the extent of what I was doing.

THERAPIST: You didn't have anybody else to talk to.

PATIENT: Yeah.

THERAPIST: Right!

Discussion of Session

The session began with a discussion of the patient's medication. Doris reported that the extra Moban helped. To avoid being placed in the position of dealing with the medication (which is not the therapist's area of expertise or concern), the therapist made an effort to have the patient confer with Dr. G., the psychiatrist. When Doris asked about the EEG, the therapist—having the report and having gone over it with Dr. G. earlier—shared the results of the medical evidence to reduce her fears of there being a neurological basis for her memory difficulties, light-headedness, and fainting. She had been notified earlier of the results of a CT scan and a neurological evaluation, both of which came out in the normal range.

Throughout the session, Doris was rather distractible. She tended to follow each thought that achieved focal attention in her mind at the moment. The therapist's goal was to decide when to keep her on focus and not let her wander, when to refocus her to something more pressing, and when to let her go. At several points in this session the therapist decided to let her go on, as she was bringing up an ongoing problem that was addressed in earlier sessions and was still of therapeutic interest: her social anxiety and great discomfort around other people.

It was always important to help Doris to find a label for her experiences in the interest of making the problems manifest, concretizing them, shaping the vague problems into workable therapeutic foci, and lastly, facilitating shared communication. This becomes clear as Doris, at several points, validated the "working alliance" and expressed her hope that she could cope better with her social anxieties and paranoia. She also stated her commitment to therapy by agreeing to practice a coping technique that the therapist had introduced in previous sessions. By verbalizing the idea of turning adversity into advantage (i.e., using the occurrence of the symptom as an opportunity to practice coping techniques), the therapist worked to reduce the possibility of failure. The problem is not to be avoided, but rather to be sought as an opportunity for mastery. It was interesting that Doris demonstrated rational thinking; this included positive self-talk for coping and "staying with" the uncomfortable situation—what to do and what not to do, and the long-term negative consequences of not following through with her plan.

The therapist suggested that Doris could use specific techniques to limit the voices. The reciprocal dialogue and the therapist's decision to use prescriptive techniques with Doris rested on adequate relatedness and contact having already being established. This is important with this type of patient, where one of the key goals is to validate selectively those actions, behaviors, and feelings of the patient that are consensually validatable. In other terms, this might be viewed as encouraging reality testing. It was important to offer Doris the possibility of decreasing the thoughts (i.e., quieting them down) versus an all-or-nothing stopping of the thoughts. Helping Doris avoid the dichotomous thinking (i.e., decreasing versus stopping absolutely) would have a greater probability of success. By directly or indirectly suggesting the notion of gradual versus all-or-none progress, the therapist can attempt to inoculate the patient against the stress of experiencing failure.

The therapist's choice of intervening by utilizing a simple, concrete story as a metaphor of Doris's problem was designed to assess Doris's ability to make the connection herself. A number of principles are relevant. First, insights that a patient generates herself (via "guided dis-

covery") are usually more meaningful than those that are told to the patient (Beck, Rush, Shaw, & Emery, 1979). Second, the use of stories as "teaching tales" has been shown by many seasoned therapists (e.g., Erickson) to have a profound influence on a patient, on both conscious and unconscious levels; in this way, suggestions may be "seeded" indirectly or positively. Third, the stories can direct the patient outwardly. Stories designed for this have an important utility of employing catchy, imagery-laden strategies with patients having a surplus of inwardly directed attention and distractibility. As he goes through this short, simple story, the therapist must continually monitor that the patient is attending. Telling the story in brief segments rather than one long story helps immeasurably. As the patient consistently and spontaneously affirms that she is following, the therapist goes on with the example. Actually, a reciprocal dialogue ensued; this indicated good collaboration, a necessary ingredient of any form of therapy. The therapist then uses inquiry to enable the patient to anticipate the consequences of employing the option of not acting or turning in the other direction. Doris then demonstrated an accurate anticipation of the likely consequences—an appraisal that the results will likely be negative.

The therapist used inquiry to help Doris better focus her attention. The use of the deep breathing acts as a distraction, and distraction or diversion techniques have clinically evidenced significant efficacy in reducing anxiety (Beck, Emery, & Greenberg, 1985).

A break in the therapy was going to occur shortly, as the therapist was going on vacation for two weeks. Doris had been prepared for this separation many sessions in advance. She appeared to be asking for reassurance that the loss would not be total, that she would still have someone to see and talk with. It was important for the therapist to make sure that Doris was comfortable with using the clinic in the event of a problem. It probably would have been better if the therapist had been more specific with Doris and informed her that if she needed to see someone, or in the case of an emergency, one of the staff people would definitely get back to her.

Often, the patient shared her perceptions with the therapist. Rather than not responding (which would have contributed to Doris's deficiencies in reality testing), the therapist needed to help her maintain her reality focus. Since many of her perceptions were distorted, the therapist wanted to help her to see that some of her perceptions were entirely accurate—providing consensual validation for her shaky reality testing. Arieti (1974) recommended validating "punctiform" insights, that is, praising partial insights. Doris would often share her confusion and her inability to trust her own perceptions. She also communicated her ongoing struggle to retain hope that things would improve.

SUMMARY

The present case is, we think, unfortunately representative of common practice. A new therapist is assigned to work with a chronic patient for a short time. Given the limits placed on the therapy, the goals of the therapy were developed to be met within the brief time parameters. By using a focused, directive, educational model, the patient was helped to begin to identify some of her distortions, and to respond more effectively to them. The collaborative relationship was useful in developing trust and confidence, and the patient ended the brief therapy with several skills that could be used in the next therapeutic encounter.

REFERENCES

Alford, B. A., Beck, A. T., Freeman, A., & Wright, F. (1990). Brief focused cognitive therapy of panic disorder. *Psychotherapy*, 27, 230–234.

Arieti, S. (1974). *Interpretation of schizophrenia*. New York: Basic Books.

Beck, A. T., Emery, G., & Greenberg, R. L. (1985). *Anxiety disorders and phobias: A cognitive perspective*. New York: Basic Books.

Beck, A. T., Freeman, A., & Associates. (1990). *Cognitive therapy of personality disorders*. New York: Guilford.

Beck, A. T., Rush, A. J., Shaw, B. F., & Emery, G. (1979). *Cognitive therapy of depression*. New York: Guilford.

Freeman, A., Pretzer, J., Fleming, B., & Simon, K. M. (1990). *Clinical applications of cognitive therapy*. New York: Plenum.

Greenwood, V. B. (1983). Cognitive therapy with the young adult chronic patient. In A. Freeman (Ed.), *Cognitive therapy with couples and groups*. New York: Plenum.

Stone, M. H., Albert, H. D., Forrest, D. V., & Arieti, S. (1983). *Treating schizophrenic patients: A clinico-analytical approach*. New York: McGraw-Hill.

SUGGESTED READINGS

Arieti, S. (1974). *Interpretation of schizophrenia*. New York: Basic Books.

Bellack, L., Hurvich, M., & Gediman, H. (1973). *Ego functions in schizophrenics, neurotics, and normals*. New York: John Wiley.

Freeman, A., Pretzer, J., Fleming, B., & Simon, K. (1990). *Clinical applications of cognitive therapy*. New York: Plenum.

Greenfield, J. G. (1984). *The psychotic patient: Medication and psychotherapy*. New York: Free Press.

Gunderson, M. H., Albert, H. D., Forrest, D. V., & Arieti, S. (1983). *Borderline personality disorder*. Washington, DC: American Psychiatric Press.

Stone, M. H., Albert, H. D., Forrest, D. V., & Arieti, S. (1983). *Treating schizophrenia patients: A clinico-analytical approach*. New York: McGraw-Hill.

25

The Patient with Multiple Problems

Jacqueline B. Persons

INTRODUCTION

The case presented here illustrates two points. First, although the controlled outcome studies of cognitive therapy for depression (e.g., Rush, Beck, Kovacs, & Hollon, 1977) focus solely on depressive symptoms, depressed patients typically have many problems. This patient had several, and treatment addressed them all. Second, the case formulation—the therapist's hypothesis about the patient's central dysfunctional attitudes—helped the therapist focus the treatment on central issues, no matter what problem was being worked on.

BACKGROUND INFORMATION

Susan grew up in a small town in the Midwest in a conflict-ridden home. She was the oldest of two children; her brother was three years younger. Susan's mother was a housewife; Susan reports that her father "wouldn't let" her mother work until Susan was in high school. Susan's father owned his own business and spent most of his time

there ("Work came first"). At one point, he lost his business and went to work for someone else, and during this period he had an alcohol problem ("He'd be blasted at lunch").

Susan's parents were dominating and critical, setting strict standards of appearance and behavior for Susan and berating her when she did not meet them. Her weight, which began to be a problem early in adolescence, was a particular focus of parental disapproval. Most attacks were verbal, but when she got particularly angry, Susan's mother would strike her. As a youngster, Susan felt oversupervised by her mother; however, when Susan was 14, her mother went to work and Susan felt abandoned ("She wasn't there").

Susan did well in school but hated it. She was especially unhappy in high school, where she felt nauseous in the mornings, fearing she hadn't done her homework properly and that she would be ridiculed by her teachers. Her father was quite strict, so she felt unable to participate in the social life the rest of her peers had; her weight, of course, interfered as well. Susan's father told her that if she became "lithe and lovely" he would buy her a car. She couldn't do it ("I never really tried after that").

After graduating from high school, Susan kicked around several junior colleges and vocational schools but was overwhelmed by each and unable to stick anything out. At age 22, her cousin invited her to come to San Francisco. When she arrived, she walked into the office where she has now worked for 13 years and was immediately hired as a secretary. She married her husband John, who also works as a secretary, 7 years later.

Jacqueline B. Persons • Department of Psychiatry, University of California, San Francisco, California 94143.

Comprehensive Casebook of Cognitive Therapy, edited by Arthur Freeman and Frank M. Dattilio. Plenum Press, New York, 1992.

ASSESSMENT AND DIAGNOSIS

Most assessment information was collected in interviews with the patient. In addition, I asked Susan to complete the Beck Depression Inventory (BDI; Beck, Rush, Shaw, & Emery, 1979) in the waiting room before each session.

Susan was referred by a plastic surgeon to whom she had gone seeking breast reduction surgery; the surgeon had refused to consider surgery until Susan lost 75 pounds. Susan told me this when she came but also said, "I need to lose weight, but that's not my problem." Susan was a bright, verbally quick and articulate woman, and even when quite depressed she displayed a quick (though frequently self-deprecating) wit. She was motivated to change and receptive to new ideas. An evaluation of her situation revealed several problems, which are detailed below.

1. *Depression.* Susan had a severe clinical depression. When I asked her to complete the Beck Depression Inventory (BDI) and bring it to the second session, we saw how depressed she really was. Her score was 36. She reported symptoms of dissatisfaction and boredom, feeling discouraged about the future, feeling like a failure, guilt, self-hate, self-blame, inability to cry, constant irritability, loss of interest in others, feeling ugly, difficulty getting anything done, fatigue, early morning awakening, loss of appetite, worry about physical problems, and loss of libido. She did not report sadness; Susan explained this by saying that she substituted anger for sadness. Several depressive symptoms (feeling like a failure, self-hate, self-blame, feeling ugly) reflect the theme of self-hate that became a focus of the treatment. Several weeks prior to seeking treatment, Susan reported that she had simply "stopped functioning" and gone to bed for about two weeks, feeling unable to do anything but not knowing why. When a letter came back from the post office because the stamp had fallen off, Susan felt overwhelmed and went to bed and cried.

2. *Obesity.* When Susan sought treatment, she was at her heaviest weight ever—almost 300 pounds. She couldn't given an exact figure because she was avoiding weighing herself. Susan said she had been heavy all her life, but that the latest weight increase occurred with the birth of her son six years earlier. Susan reported she had some sort of "mental block" against losing weight and spontaneously volunteered that this might be due to thoughts like "It doesn't matter. I'm married now. No problem."

3. *Marital difficulties.* Marital difficulties were not fully described at the beginning of treatment, as Susan was so overwhelmed with her depression that she could not see far beyond it. However, it was clear that the marriage was not doing well. Susan described her husband as bright and interesting but passive ("He tells me he married me to make his phone calls for him"). Susan seemed to take responsibility for her husband, the apartment, and the child as well as working full-time, and she felt quite resentful about this. She also reported in an offhand way that "he drinks too much beer"; later it became clear that John had a serious alcohol problem. The couple had no sexual relationship. She wanted to make plans to buy a house, but he would not participate, saying, "It will never happen anyway, so what's the point?"

4. *Job dissatisfaction.* Susan had been working as a secretary for 13 years. She did a good job and had friends at her office but was bored by the work. However, she felt unable to look for another job because "I don't know what I want to be when I grow up."

5. *Difficulties in relationships with her parents.* Susan did not describe this as a problem. However, it soon became clear that she was furious at her parents, particularly her mother, whom she described as "a barracuda." Susan felt extremely guilty about avoiding visiting and phoning her parents, but she felt abused and enraged (and guilty about having these feelings) whenever she did contact them.

Susan denied problems with drugs or alcohol, saying "Alcohol makes me sick." She had stopped drinking caffeine about two weeks before beginning treatment and reported feeling better as a result.

I formulated Susan's case by proposing a central dysfunctional belief underlying all of her difficulties (Persons, 1989). I hypothesized that her central dysfunctional belief was "I'm no good; if I accept myself the way I am and develop my own interests, I'll fail and be criticized and rejected." This idea I call the *self-hate* theme. Presumably, Susan learned to hate herself by internalizing the criticism she received from her parents. A second, closely related, belief was "My needs don't count; my job in life is to take care of others." This is the problem Young (1990) aptly labeled *subjugation.* Young describes clearly how the subjugation problem leads both to resentment about always having to care for others and to a lack of sense of one's own direction and interests in life. It seems likely that Susan learned this belief from her mother, who modeled it for her.

Both of Susan's core dysfunctional attitudes can be seen in the statement Susan's mother made to her when Susan's first child was born: "You can stop now—you've had your son." This amazing statement conveys two ideas: (a) the way you are (female) is unacceptable, and (b) the purpose of having a child is to get my (the parent's) needs met.

TREATMENT

The first three sessions were spent collecting a description of Susan's current problems and their history, as well as a full family, social, and medical history. In the second session, I explained to Susan that she was clinically depressed and that we needed to work on that before we could solve anything else. I also suggested antidepressant medication, but Susan didn't want to take medicine. I proposed that we reopen the medication discussion if she did not respond to the therapy; she agreed to this plan.

I view Susan's accepting my proposal that we needed to work on the depression before we could do anything else as one of the keys to the success of the treatment. I believe this treatment strategy was successful—and therapeutic—because it carried the implicit message "You are OK the way you are; you don't need to lose weight to be acceptable to me or to be happy." This message addressed Susan's central dysfunctional belief head-on, and she accepted it readily.

I began working on the depression by assigning Susan *Feeling Good* (Burns, 1980) to read, and we did some Thought Records in the sessions (see Beck et al., 1979; Persons, 1989). Susan was quite depressed, hopeless, and tearful at first but quickly established a good, open, trusting relationship with me. She did her homework and worked well and collaboratively during the sessions.

Early sessions focused on her continual self-blame and self-criticism (the self-hate theme). In session 5, for example, we worked in a structured way to elicit and respond to her negative automatic thoughts about the linoleum she had put in her bathroom. After doing this project, she reported feeling "nothing, tired, hungry, empty, and bored." Her automatic thoughts were "So what?," "It should have been done years ago," "It's just a drop in the bucket," "I made mistakes," and "If I eat, at least I'll be doing something useful." We developed the rational responses "It would have been nice if it had been done a year ago, but I wasn't ready," "Better something than nothing," "It looks 100% better and even smells good," "Even if I made mistakes, I learned something new," and "Eating is not really an accomplishment for me."

By session 6, Susan had shown the sharp initial drop in her BDI score that is typical of a good treatment response (see Figure 25-1). Susan began to feel excited about starting additional projects at home, and it even occurred to her that it would be good to spend some time on pleasure.

In sessions 7 and 8 we began talking about Susan's mother, who was scheduled to visit soon. Susan very articulately outlined the way in which she had spent many years fighting against her mother and her mother's criticisms and demands, but at the same time failed to develop a clear idea of who she (Susan) was and what *she* wanted for herself. Susan also reported, in a clear expression of the subjugation theme, "I have a hard time feeling I deserve to find out who I am."

When her mother arrived, Susan was able to gain some perspective, describing her mother as "a goofy old lady." She reported that she was enraged but able to refuse her mother's insistent request that Susan send a birthday card to her *mother's* friend. Susan reported that she had learned from me (although I did not teach it explicitly!) to tell herself "You're not a bad person," and that saying this to herself over and over helped her "survive" her parents' visit.

In session 11, Susan reported feeling less angry. She said, in her delightful way, "I'm saying 'remarkable' instead of f-words." We spent two or three tearful and painful sessions working on her overwhelming shame about her failures in junior college and technical schools. She was tearful when describing her perception that her parents "just wanted me to go away and be successful so they wouldn't have to be ashamed of me." She had never able to accept these failures—instead, she punished herself brutally and felt totally humiliated about them. We developed an analogy she found helpful: filmmakers who have huge flops but go on to be successful.

We spent several sessions working on her fears of undertaking projects (e.g., a haircut, more projects at home, ceramics) for fear of failing or not finishing. I also suggested that she read a book on assertiveness (to work on the subjugation theme). We worked on how guilty she felt when she missed a week of work due to illness (again, the subjugation theme).

By session 16, Susan's BDI was 11; she was feeling much better and was having fun with projects around the apartment. She began the session saying, "I know this is the time to think about starting to lose weight. I want a sex life." She raised this issue with her husband. Part of the problem here was *his* weight, and in discussing this she reported that he and his friends regularly drank huge quantities of beer—they had just spent the weekend drinking at a christening. She also reported that he drank heavily at football games and then drove home with their son in the car. I practically leapt out of my chair when I heard this, and stated in the strongest terms that she couldn't allow this any more.

From this point on—particularly until session 40, when John entered treatment for his alcohol problem—the alcohol issue was a central focus of therapy. I consulted with a colleague who had worked extensively with wives

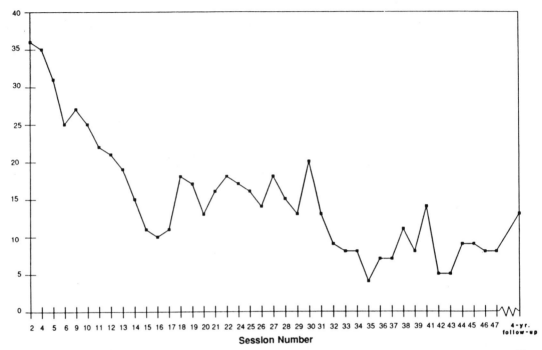

Figure 25-1. Beck Depression Inventory (BDI) Scores for the First 47 Sessions of Treatment and at Four-Year Follow-Up.

of alcoholics. She suggested, and I followed, a very active strategy: I advised Susan that if she could get herself to the position where she was committed to leave her husband if he did not stop drinking, then she could wait for (or precipitate) a crisis and issue an ultimatum, and he would probably stop; however, she couldn't threaten to leave unless she was fully prepared to do it. She wanted the marriage and was frightened of losing him, but I pointed out how dependent on her he was and suggested that he was unlikely to leave. I made a contact with an alcohol treatment specialist who suggested that when Susan was ready and the time was right, the four of us (Susan, John, myself, and the alcohol specialist) should meet to get John into treatment. With this overall strategy in mind, Susan and I worked patiently to boost her resolve and confidence and to wait for a "crisis" to bring things to a head.

The following session, Susan's BDI had nearly doubled (18). She was becoming increasingly aware of the alcohol problem: "I've been denying there is a problem for a long time. They've been doing it since he was 15." She had told him to stop drinking and planned to throw away all the liquor in the house and to attend Al-Anon with a friend. I congratulated her on these initiatives.

She came to the next session (number 19) saying, "I've been real sad." And indeed, she had marked "2" on

the sadness item on the BDI for the first time ever. She reported, "I didn't go to Al-Anon and I'm still denying, 'Maybe he's not an alcoholic.' " Her husband had not had any alcohol for eight days but was scheduled to go camping next weekend, an activity she feared would inevitably lead to drinking. I encouraged her to attend Al-Anon.

The next session, she was feeling better (her BDI was 13) and had started a Weight Watchers program. Her husband did go camping and drink, but did not drink and drive. She had agreed to his request that on the next camping trip he could drink 6 beers a day—a reduction from his usual 12 or more. By session 25, she was being more assertive about John's drinking. The session focused on a camping trip the couple was planning, this time together. She reported that usually he packed beer in a cooler. She decided that if he did this, she wouldn't go camping (he didn't). She had set aside $1,100 of her own earnings in a separate bank account, and this felt good.

In session 26, Susan reported that John was not drinking. However, she felt off balance because her parents were planning to visit. We returned to the self-statement that helped her when they last visited ("I'm not a bad person"). We also agreed that as a homework assignment, Susan would shave her legs. Susan reported that if she did something to improve her appearance, her mother commented, "What does it matter if you got a haircut if you're fat?" We worked on the idea that Susan could challenge her mother's attitude and improve her self-esteem by treating herself *as if* she were valuable—that is, by shaving her legs. Shaving her legs became a theme of the therapy and a regular homework assignment.

In session 30, Susan's BDI jumped to 20. John had had "a lot of beers" over the weekend, and she had stopped going to Weight Watchers and stopped shaving her legs: "I've lost it. You told me I would." I had prepared her for a setback, and that seemed to help her take the first step to regain her equilibrium. We spent the session getting back on the track, with homework assignments to shave her legs and write in her journal.

Susan came to her next session having done her homework and feeling better (her BDI was 13). She had made herself go to a play instead of making the usual excuse, "No, I'm fat." Over the next few sessions, Susan continued to improve but reported that John was drinking a little; she planned to confront him about this, but so far had not.

In sessions 34 and 35, Susan reported, "I am *pissed*." We worked on her anger at herself about overeating (this was probably a mistake—we should probably have been focusing on anger at John about drinking). In session 36, Susan felt angry at me for not paying careful attention to what she had said about overeating last session. She responded to this anger by overeating, as she did when she felt angry at her mother ("I'll show you—I can do what I want!"). However, after a couple of days, she saw what she was doing and stopped. She accepted a referral to a modified protein-sparing fast program (but didn't go). In session 37, Susan reported that John took a cooler of beer to his sister's wedding. Now the focus of the treatment began to shift from the weight issue to the alcohol issue, where it belonged.

Session 38 was an important one. Susan had been feeling excited about plans to lose weight and find a new job. Then she had a dream of an old boyfriend, which frightened her ("If I lose weight I'll become promiscuous"). This fear was exacerbated by her awareness of feeling bored by her husband, who drank too much on Sunday while watching the football game, and so was unavailable to her ("What's the use of doing all this if my family won't stay together?").

Session 40 was an emergency session held the day after Susan called, panicky and upset, because John had come home hours later than expected, drunk, from a football game. She was ready to confront him, so I booked an appointment with the alcohol specialist for the following week.

We had a therapy session on the morning of the evening of the big pow-wow. John had agreed to come to the appointment that evening. She acknowledged, for the first time, that he had beaten her more than once when drunk and that he had suffered injuries himself that required emergency-room visits. She had told him that the marriage was over if he didn't stop drinking.

At the evening meeting, John was passive—reluctantly agreeing to treatment, looking like he did so only because he felt backed into a corner. However, he agreed to enter a month long outpatient treatment program that included Antabuse and AA, with the first meeting to be held the subsequent evening.

At session 42, Susan reported that John went to treatment, but that she had had to drive him to the first meeting. She attended the family meetings and found them useful; we worked on her automatic thought "If he gets himself together, he won't want me." Her parents had visited, and she reported, "I'm relaxed around my parents." This was a first. A couple of sessions later, Susan reported that she and John had had a big fight and he didn't respond by getting drunk; this was another first.

Susan began session 46 saying that she wanted to take a college course in English but was quite anxious about it, fearing that she'd start and not finish, that she'd hate it, she'd fail, and she wouldn't fit into the desks. We did a Thought Record (see Beck et al., 1979, p. 403; Persons, 1989, p. 128) on this issue; one of the responses was a suggestion that she go to the classroom ahead of time to see if she fit in the desks. She found this suggestion helpful—and did fit! The next sessions focused on her difficulty in following through with the course, with some time spent on emotional turmoil raised by a visit from her parents. A few sessions later, she began attending Overeaters Anonymous (OA).

By session 53, Susan felt very good. John continued to abstain from drinking, she was doing well in her course and attending OA, and she reported that "shaving my legs is now automatic." At this point, our treatment focus moved to couples issues. Susan and John had difficulty working together; she tended to dominate, and he responded by becoming passive. Although I recommended couples work, Susan did not follow through. I announced my pregnancy at this point, saying I would need to take a 10-week maternity leave in about 12 weeks. In my thinking about the break in treatment, I was guided by my case formulation. I had proposed that Susan's central belief was "I'm no good; if I accept myself the way I am and develop my own interests, I'll fail and be criticized and rejected." This formulation suggests the possibility that Susan might feel criticized or rejected by my leaving. Although I probed for this type of reaction, Susan did not report it. I had also viewed Susan as having a subjugation problem, which cause Susan to be more aware of *my* needs than of her own. This formulation is perhaps consistent with Susan's request that I send her a birth announcement; however, I agreed to do this.

In session 58, Susan reported missing two classes due to the flu and was contemplating dropping the courses. I encouraged her to hang in and worked with her to choose a topic for her term paper. Her homework assignments were to go to the library and to outline the paper.

In session 61, Susan listed several successes. She had finished her term paper, she had met with a career counselor, she and John painted a bathroom together, and she had lost 30 pounds. In session 63, Susan reported that John had handled a holiday without drinking. Susan felt less overwhelmed than ever before by career ideas that required AA or BA degrees. She bought some new clothes in smaller sizes. At this point, I was seven months pregnant, and we reviewed our plan for terminating in five sessions. Susan seemed comfortable with this plan.

In session 64, Susan described functioning very well during a trip to visit her family on the occasion of her maternal uncle's funeral. She learned that he had died of cirrhosis at age 60 and felt angry that her mother didn't want anyone to know this. Susan noticed for first time that her father "got mean" after his usual two drinks in the evening. Her brother was drunk when he telephoned his parents. Susan felt angry, more aware than ever of how much alcohol abuse had cost her.

In session 66, Susan reported that she and John went on a camping trip and he didn't drink ("like the camping trip of my dreams!"). She admitted to feeling a little anxious about my leaving.

Susan continued to do well. In the last three sessions, she reported some anxiety about coping without me, but said she expected to do OK; I told her I expected that, too. We scheduled an appointment for 10 weeks later, following my maternity leave.

We did meet as scheduled 10 weeks later, and Susan had continued to make progress. She was not depressed, she was excited about a flower-arranging class, and John had not been drinking. She had lost 50 pounds and reported, "My legs are always shaved now." She felt she wanted to discontinue treatment, that she was working well on her own.

Susan's request to terminate her therapy raised an important question. Should I encourage Susan to stay in treatment longer, or support Susan's plan to terminate at this point? I found it useful to refer to the case formulation to guide my decision about how to handle termination.

A case could be made that although Susan had solved many of the problems on her problem list (she was no longer clinically depressed and had done some significant work on her marriage and her sense of herself as awful), she had plenty of work still to do. The major unsolved problem was her weight; although she had lost 50 pounds, Susan still weighed about 250 pounds. In response to Susan's suggestion that she terminate treatment, I might have suggested that she stay in therapy until she lost more weight and consolidated her other gains.

I could also choose to support Susan's plan to terminate and strike out on her own, even though she wasn't "perfect." In view of Susan's formulation, I believed that a major goal of her therapy was to learn to accept herself the way she was. This view of the therapy guided my decision to support her plan to terminate treatment even though she was still quite obese. Therefore, I supported Susan's plan to terminate, but encouraged her to schedule one more final session to ease the transition. In this session we reviewed the treatment, focusing particularly on what she had accomplished and how she would know if she needed to come back.

SUMMARY

This was a long treatment, with a series of stages. We worked first on Susan's depression, then on the marital issues, and finally on the weight and vocational issues. We worked on Susan's difficulties with her parents whenever this issue came up, generally when they visited. At the end of treatment, Susan was doing quite well: She was not depressed; she had lost 50 pounds; her husband had not had a drink for nearly a year, and they were interacting in a more collaborative way; she was having fun exploring vocational issues; and she coped with her parents better.

Nearly four years after the treatment ended, Susan completed a BDI by mail and we met for a 30-minute telephone follow up interview. Susan had continued to do well in all areas except weight. She did not describe herself as depressed, although her BDI score of 13 indicated some dysphoria. Perhaps the best way to think about this is to view Susan as having "double depression." She began treatment with an acute depressive episode superimposed on a chronic dysthymia. The treatment alleviated the acute depression, but not the dysthymia. Susan felt she coped well with her negative moods. She reported mood fluctuations but said, "I'm aware of the telltale signs [of depression]. As soon as I start to feel down, I shave my legs." She said she had not had a recurrence of depression like the one we had worked on in therapy. This is impressive in view of evidence that 30% of depressed patients experience a relapse during the first year following an episode (Lewinsohn, Hoberman, Teri, & Hautzinger, 1985).

Susan had given birth to another baby and had regained all the weight she lost; she weighed 294 pounds. She had recently begun attending Overeaters Anonymous, though sporadically. She had gone back to the surgeon, saying, "I'm never going to lose that weight, so let's just do it." The surgeon had agreed, so Susan had the breast reduction surgery and said she was "pleased." Susan's going ahead with the breast reduction surgery can be viewed in two ways. First, it can be viewed as evidence that she was unable to accept herself as she was and needed surgery to try to modify herself in some fundamental way. Second, the surgery can be seen as evidence that Susan was no longer willing to accept the idea that she couldn't have what she wanted because she was fat. From this point of view, Susan's assertiveness with the plastic surgeon and her decision to go after what she wanted can be viewed in a positive light.

John had continued not to drink, though Susan suspected he drank occasionally on camping trips. She remarked, "I haven't found out about it yet, but if I do, I know what to do." She reported the marriage was doing "I think fine—we fight and then we laugh." The couple had bought a small house. Susan was still working as a secretary, though now with more responsibility, essentially serving as office manager in a small office. She had been exploring her lifelong dream of being a librarian but realized that it meant earning less money than she was currently making, so she was investigating other options. "I'm career searching, having fun. I still don't know what I want to be when I grow up." She had taken several community college courses, receiving A's and B's, and was working toward an AA degree. She had learned to say to herself, "All I have to do is finish what I do." Susan claimed things with her parents were unchanged. However, she observed, "My conflicts with them provided me with lots of material for my writing class!"

DISCUSSION

Overall, this treatment was quite successful. A key to the success of the treatment, in my view, was its focus on the case formulation: Susan's view of herself as unacceptable, awful, ugly. This issue was a theme of the therapy throughout, even though the sessions focused on many varied problems. I found the formulation to be particularly helpful in guiding my handling of the weight issue and the decision to terminate treatment.

Much of the success of the treatment also stems from the strengths and assets Susan brought to treatment, as well as the hard work she did. Although her early environment was abusive in some respects, it must also have had a number of positives, as Susan presented with a core of strength and confidence in her ability to function independently that made it fun to work with her and contributed enormously to the success of the therapy. Although she was angry at her parents, she didn't insist on holding on to this anger or punishing them for their faults; instead, she was willing to take responsibility for herself and move ahead with her life. This case was one of those "easy" ones in which I frequently felt I didn't need to do much— Susan did most of the work.

REFERENCES

Beck, A. T., Rush, A. J., Shaw, B. F., & Emery, G. (1979). *Cognitive therapy of depression*. New York: Guilford.

Burns, D. D. (1980). *Feeling good: The new mood therapy*. New York: William Morrow.

Lewinsohn, P. M., Hoberman, T., Teri, L., & Hautzinger, M. (1985). An integrative theory of depression. In S. Reiss & R. Bootzin (Eds.), *Theoretical issues in behavior therapy*. New York: Academic Press.

Persons, J. B. (1989). *Cognitive therapy in practice: A case formulation approach*. New York: Norton.

Rush, A. J., Beck, A. T., Kovacs, M., & Hollon, S. (1977). Comparative efficacy of cognitive therapy and pharmacotherapy in the treatment of depression outpatients. *Cognitive Therapy and Research, 1*, 17–38.

Young, J. (1990). *Cognitive therapy for personality disorders: A schema-focused approach*. Sarasota, FL: Professional Resource Exchange.

SUGGESTED READINGS

Beck, A. T., Rush, A. J., Shaw, B. F., & Emery, G. (1979). *Cognitive therapy of depression*. New York: Guilford.

Burns, D. D. (1980). *Feeling good: The new mood therapy*. New York: William Morrow.

Persons, J. B. (1989). *Cognitive therapy in practice: A case formulation approach*. New York: Norton.

26

Working with Gay Men

Kevin T. Kuehlwein

INTRODUCTION

This chapter will offer a basic model for the use of cognitive therapy with men who are struggling to better understand and integrate their same-sex sexual orientation. Its aim is to aid the expansion of a man's social, behavioral, and self-identity to include more positive feelings and actions consonant with his sexual and affectional attraction to men. This chapter will take the reader through the course of a simulated case and will present reading suggestions for gay men in therapy and/or their therapists. Although it is presented in largely linear fashion, the therapeutic focus with this population (as with others) would likely oscillate between the delineated stages as gains were solidified. The examples in this chapter are based on gay men I have known and worked with clinically, but do not represent any one person. (The approach could probably easily be applied also to lesbians but because of my own limited experience on this account, I purposely focus here on the population with which I have worked most closely.) The word *heterosexism* is used here to refer to the valuing of heterosexual over homosexual behavior and orientation, rather than the more common

term *homophobia*, because of the latter's imprecise meaning. The chapter assumes a basic knowledge of Beckian (Beck, Rush, Shaw, & Emery, 1979; Beck & Emery, 1985) cognitive therapy principles.

All gays with a positive self-image probably go through a cognitive restructuring process that is somewhat similar to, if less intentional, than the one presented here. At their own pace, they alternately learn about people and aspects of the gay subculture and then integrate this new information, revising their beliefs and ideas about themselves, others, and their sexuality. One possible advantage to using the present model is that it can replace with a quicker and more reasoned approach the slow, more haphazard individual one that most gays follow on their own. The therapy approach also offers the important addition of a constant, supportive person providing an important anchor as the client explores and experiences aspects of how his own evolving identity and the gay world intersect or differ. The therapist not only helps the client make sense of what he sees and hears, but also provides an important, nonpartisan reality factor that may often be missing for the client. The therapist can further demonstrate and/or model support for the client's emerging sexuality and self-identity, either as a positive gay or lesbian role model or as a supportive straight man or woman able to accept the client's orientation in a matter-of-fact way.

Below is a common presentation of a man coming in for therapy: A gay college freshman with incidental pubertal homosexual experiences came into treatment with dysthymia, low self-esteem, and social inhibition. He felt defective with regard to people around him, especially to

Kevin T. Kuehlwein • Center for Cognitive Therapy, Department of Psychiatry, University of Pennsylvania School of Medicine, Philadelphia, Pennsylvania 19104.

Comprehensive Casebook of Cognitive Therapy, edited by Arthur Freeman and Frank M. Dattilio. Plenum Press, New York, 1992.

men who appeared popular on campus with women and other men. He envied their seeming confidence and imagined they had few, if any, social problems or self-doubts. He reported the following automatic thoughts: "I'll never have a relationship," "I don't want to be gay," "No one else here is gay," "I'll always be lonely," and "I will lose all of my friends if they find out I am gay."

INITIAL RAPPORT: ACCEPTANCE OF THE CLIENT'S SEXUALITY

One aspect of early therapy is that the client (due to internal heterosexism) is likely to have automatic thoughts about the therapist's ability to accept his gay feelings and behavior (or to make the assumption that the therapist could not be gay). The therapist could respond to the former in the following way.

THERAPIST: You seem a little reluctant to reveal much of your dating and sexual life. I wonder if you have some concerns about this.

CLIENT: Well, I don't know. I'm not sure how much I can tell you.

THERAPIST: OK. Without going into details of what these issues are, what are you worried *might* happen if you told me?

CLIENT: Well, I don't know how you'd react.

THERAPIST: OK. So you don't know *for a fact* how I'd react. Am I right in assuming that you *think* I might react negatively and so you're holding back just to be safe?

CLIENT: Yeah, I guess I am.

THERAPIST: So what sorts of emotions are you feeling as you're thinking those thoughts?

CLIENT: Well, that I don't want to tell you.

THERAPIST: OK, we'll note that down as a thought, but what *feelings* are you having connected with that thought?

CLIENT: I guess I'm worried and a little nervous.

THERAPIST: Hmmm. How do you think you'd feel if you knew that I'd really understand and *not* react negatively at all?

CLIENT: I'd feel a lot better.

THERAPIST: Would you also be more likely to share these thoughts?

CLIENT: Sure.

THERAPIST: OK. Here's a good example of how your thoughts affect your mood and behavior. Notice how if you think of one thing you get nervous and hold back (draws sequence on paper), whereas if you think another thing you feel more comfortable and maybe more

likely to talk about yourself (draws parallel sequence). It's not surprising that you picked a negative reading of the situation, even though you don't know for a fact how I'd react. That's very common in people who come in to see me. Now let's look at the evidence you have about what my reaction would be . . .

In this way the therapist could demonstrate caring, concern, and interest in the client's presenting problem while socializing him into the model. Without pushing the client to reveal material prematurely, the therapist gently illustrated the cognitive therapy approach while gaining the client's trust in terms of respecting his boundaries, yet also showing how one can explore a situation without judging. Naturally, the requirements of confidentiality are especially important to make clear when working with this population due to overconcern about adverse consequences of disclosure.

ASSESSMENT OF CLIENT'S BELIEFS AND SOCIAL ENVIRONMENT

A critical part of working with the client was to assess the current state of his beliefs, as well as the kinds of messages he got about himself, sexuality, and homosexuality. In this way the therapist was able to develop a conceptualization that could help explain the blocks to self-acceptance by the client. The following aspects of the origins of internalized heterosexist messages were explored: where (e.g., religion), when (i.e., at what age), from whom, how frequently, and the meaning attributed to gay sex and/or orientation by important figures in his life. For example, a respected but heterosexist elder would likely have a greater impact on him than a political candidate espousing the same negative message. Likewise, a parent who views gays merely as missing out on some of life's joys would transmit a more positive message than one who saw gays as mentally disordered.

An early homework task to investigate some of these beliefs involved the client writing down lists of free associations about homosexuality and heterosexuality. What he brought back was very informative about his assumptions and acculturation. He believed that once he embraced his gay sexual orientation, many avenues would be forever closed to him (e.g., children, a close relationship with family or friends). He also had some fears that being gay meant some very specific things, to the point that he would have to change his behavior radically (e.g., wear makeup, dress like a woman, go into certain areas of employment). Essentially, there were two major categories of items about being gay: giving up various positively valued experiences, and having to engage in negatively valued behaviors, roles, and vocations, which closely paralleled the stereotypes of larger society. Items about heterosexuality largely involved stability of and access to positively valued experiences (e.g., child raising, relationships).

The client was then asked what the evidence was in favor of or against these ideas. Once the client was asked to think of specific examples, he was able to list a wide variety of heterosexual men who in fact did not live up to these positive images, as well as a short list of gay men he had heard of who did not seem to conform to his negative images. The client was also asked whether he could explain the mechanism by which having sex with men would *inherently* deprive him of the formerly elucidated positive experiences or propel him *inevitably* toward the latter ones. A similar exercise was done in examining the guarantees of positive experiences he had associated with a heterosexual orientation. The therapist then asked the client to summarize the point of the exercise so as to ensure that the client had understood and assimilated the intended lesson. The client was able to see that his assumptions of what it meant to be gay and straight might in some cases be distorted. At this point, the client experienced a great deal of relief and began to accept more seriously the idea that his view of what it meant to be gay might be based greatly upon incorrect information he had grown up accepting uncritically.

The therapist presented these negative ideas as similar to automatic thoughts with possible negative biases. A copy of the client's initial list of what it meant to be gay was kept and dated, and this was compared at various times in therapy with his evolving views. This gave concrete evidence to the client of the shifts in his attitudes toward himself and gay orientation during the course of therapy.

EXPLORING MYTHS AND IDEAS ABOUT SEXUALITY

Because of the above exercise, the client was able to see the utility of putting his previous beliefs about homosexuality on hold, considering them tentative and unproved. The therapist suggested investigating the truth of these beliefs together, using logic, hard data, and any personal experiences the client might have during therapy. The client was educated first as to the varying levels of "evidence" (Newman, 1989) that people often use in supporting their ideas: high (based on objective, unambiguous data), medium (based on ambiguous data; possible biased by unwarranted conclusions), and low (no good data; based on assumption or hunch alone). We wrote down many of the ideas he had heard about homosexuality and began to sort them into these groupings. Where there was a low level of evidence, he was encouraged to seek out higher levels of evidence on the same point.

The client noted that the preponderance of information he had heard had been negative toward homosexuality, but that the quality of this evidence was in many cases questionable and that he had also heard some things about it that had been positive or neutral, many of these from reputable sources. For ongoing homework, he consciously sought out and wrote down in a notebook counterexamples to his negatively biased beliefs. As he amassed counterexamples, he began to be more aware of the breadth of the possibilities ahead for him, and his mood improved greatly.

Escalation Fears

Another concern early in therapy was something like "If I'm gay, it'll escalate and I'll have no control over it." This seemed to boil down to two related assumptions: that how he acted was (or would be) out of his control, and that there were some aspects to being gay that inevitably pushed people toward some identical outcome. We dealt with this by exploring how long he had been attracted to males (ever since he could remember) and whether he had been in control of how much of his gay identity he had revealed to others. He admitted that none of his family or heterosexual friends knew, due to his strict control on what he told them and how he misled them about romantic liaisons with women. We also explored whether all gays he knew or knew of were uniform in their demeanor or dress. He agreed they were not, citing Rock Hudson, who had for years been able to hide his sexuality from most of America successfully. Another tack was to explore the alleged mechanism by which these feared changes must occur, which he was unable to identify.

These explorations subsequently reassured him visibly and seemed to show him that there was no necessary or uncontrollable speed involved in exploring his gay identity; that he could do this at any pace that was comfortable; and that being gay did not imply any one particular type of person, behavior, or look. The therapist also explicitly agreed with the client's stated autonomous goals not to give in to the expectations of others (heterosexuals or gays) of behaving in certain ways with respect to his sexuality. The therapist suggested that the expression of the client's sexuality and relational orientation was the *client's* decision, regardless of what pressures he received to behave in certain ways.

Religious Concerns

Because of the client's religious background, he had gotten some negative messages from the church about homosexuality also. These the therapist tried to put into historical context, noting that the Christian church had shifted its beliefs over the years substantially—that some beliefs commonly held today (e.g., that the earth revolves around the sun, rather than the sun around the earth) were considered heretical (and even punishable by death) hundreds of years ago. Following is a sample interchange.

THERAPIST: What leads you to believe that homosexual behavior is "bad?"

CLIENT: Well, the church says it's bad, so it must be bad.

THERAPIST: So if the church declares something bad, then it's bad?

CLIENT: Yeah.

THERAPIST: Is the church allowed to change its mind over time?

CLIENT: I don't know; I guess so.

THERAPIST: So if the church changes its mind, where does that leave you? It was bad at one point, but all of a sudden the very same thing is not bad?

CLIENT: (looking puzzled) I don't know.

THERAPIST: Let me ask you this. Does the earth go around the sun or the sun go around the earth?

CLIENT: The earth around the sun.

THERAPIST: So far as you know has it always been that way?

CLIENT: Yeah. So?

THERAPIST: Did you know that by making that statement hundreds of years ago in Italy you would have been burned at the stake for speaking against official church teachings?

CLIENT: Really?

THERAPIST: It's true. Galileo had to take back under threat of torture what he said about the earth going around the sun. How does this information fit in with your idea about the church being the ultimate judge of what's right?

CLIENT: Ummm.

THERAPIST: Is it possible that the church might change its mind on this, too, in the future, or that some things might be OK even though the church currently speaks against them?

CLIENT: Uh, yeah, I guess so.

THERAPIST: OK. Here's another point: Which of the two *appears* to the observer to travel around the other?

CLIENT: The sun, because it rises and sets.

THERAPIST: Right, so if you were just going by what *appears* to be correct, you'd actually be wrong, wouldn't you?

CLIENT: Yeah, I guess I would.

The client was not wholly convinced by this one exchange, but repeated attention to examples of how the church and/or society had shifted its position on the correctness of various beliefs and acts over the centuries seemed to soften his negative self-judgments. Good analogical examples used here were the disdain for, cognitive distortions about, and even attributions of evil to left-handed people, Jews, blacks, and even the early Christians by other groups at various times in history. Left-handed people were for him a particularly apt group for comparison because of the parallel assumption throughout various historical periods that left-handed people were "sinister" and should change to writing "normally" (i.e., normally for right-handed people). He acknowledged, because of his own left-handed brother, that these people wrote normally *for them*. (See the bibliotherapy section below for more sources of helpful materials and analogies.)

CONSOLIDATING A POSITIVE GAY IDENTITY

Seeking Out More Objective Outside Reading Materials

As a therapist, I believe greatly in the educative and healing power of bibliotherapy—the reading of materials that may effect positive cognitive change in the client. When working with gay men, incidentally, these need not be cognitive therapy focused. Often, helpful materials (particularly at the beginning of therapy) are those that are autobiographical journeys from self-deprecation to self-acceptance. I have found that clients often identify readily and easily with the characters in these nonfiction or fiction texts. This step can be a very significant process in therapy, enabling the client to entertain multiple perspectives and vicariously foresee hope and progress through the characters' own developmental movement. Nonfiction autobiographical materials also have the advantage of providing proof to the otherwise skeptical client that others have successfully negotiated this often daunting-looking path. Similarities and differences the client notes can also be informative issues to discuss in therapy.

Many texts are available for these purposes, most of which demonstrate the process of going through difficult times and triumphing over them through more effective coping brought about by increased experience and wisdom. Other good texts can be those with a historical and/or cross-cultural flavor, high-lighting the quite considerable shifts over time in how the majority has viewed, tolerated, or encouraged homosexual acts in different times in places. Kinsey, Pomeroy, and Martin (1948) and Churchill (1967) are particularly helpful in their emphases on norms. This exploration is all in the spirit of gathering evidence for rational adaptive responses to automatic thoughts, assumptions, and beliefs.

Linking with Positive Values

The therapist had elicited early on in therapy many of the more adaptive values and beliefs held by this client that could usefully be juxtaposed with his internal heterosexist ones to provide maximum disequilibration (and therefore internal momentum for cognitive change). For example, the client prided himself on integrity and honesty in other areas of his life, which was not in accord with his lying and covering up about his orientation. This lack of congruence was used to facilitate his gradual movement toward appropriate disclosure of his orientation to trusted others. In this way, he was able to view not his homosexuality per se as a problem, but his lack of integration of his own positive values across different domains of his life.

Sexuality and Coming Out as a Continuum

The therapist also gently fostered the client's thinking about sexuality in shades of gray, rather than in all-or-none terms. Since the client was attracted to the occasional woman, this approach helped to reduce the confusion he felt about these feelings. One homework assignment involved his looking up the figures for admitted sexual attraction in males in the Kinsey et al. (1948) study. He was greatly surprised to discover the large number of males with same-sex sexual attraction, and more amazed to find out the percentage of males who had acted on these feelings. He even noted that the famous Kinsey Scale of 0 (equal to exclusive heterosexual interest and behavior) to 6 (equal to exclusive homosexual interest and behavior) was itself a helpful example of thinking in shades of gray in an area where many people think quite dichotomously. This research enabled him to feel much less alone with his feelings and more hopeful of finding others with whom to forge relationships. He also began to reduce his own sense of stigma for being "so different" from other males by realizing that his feelings were much more common than he had realized and that some of his friends were statistically likely to have had and/or acted on same-sex feelings of attraction.

Also related to this was his increasing awareness that he had ultimate control over how much he decided to reveal his orientation to others (i.e., "come out"). He was able to shift to a less dichotomous position here also. He

realized that he could come out to as few or as many people as he wished, tell people only some aspects about his dating life, not come out in certain situations at all, or pursue a middle course of coming out only to selected people and only after testing the waters by allowing people to get to know other, less controversial and possibly more assimilable aspects of him first. The key point was for him to make this disclosure or lack of it more of a conscious, voluntary decision, rather than one determined by unreasonable, unspoken, and unexamined fears. He also soon realized that his therapist was not pushing him to "tell the world," but would be there to help him assess in a realistic way the advantages and disadvantages of self-revelation in each circumstance (including the risks of people he told telling others whom he would choose not to tell). This further increased his sense of self-control and his trust in the therapist.

It was also helpful for him to explore the idea that his gay orientation was only one aspect of his personhood; that he had not lost those many other aspects of himself that he considered important parts of his personality. He was further able over time to see that he alone had control over the amount of importance he attached to the gay aspect of his identity.

Comfort Hierarchy

Following the above exploration of his fears of escalation, the client used a technique to rank (in a manner similar to a desensitization hierarchy) various gay-related activities by the anxiety he associated with them. The client listed a number of activities engaged in by some gay people, and was told that we would together evaluate whether his desire to do them might change over time as he became more comfortable with himself. The client drew up a list of activities ranging from those easily in his grasp to those he "would never do." In some cases, items low on the list were also represented at higher levels because of slightly altered circumstances (e.g., going into a gay bar alone versus with a bunch of people he knew; going into a gay bar in his city versus one in a more distant city).

The client compiled a detailed list and was encouraged to attempt an activity near his current comfort level. Predictions about the experience and his possible emotions during it were noted beforehand and compared with actual data later. This was set up as a no-lose situation, so that if he came back with data that confirmed his negative predictions, this could be seen as possible evidence that the activity might be one that he would not choose to engage in, but now from a position of actual knowledge and informed choice rather than just vague, possibly distorted impressions and fear. What the client found was that most of his predictions about these experiences were not borne out. This gave him more courage to try experiences ranked higher on the scale, since he saw that he might be wrong about some of the assumptions that inhibited his trying these actions as well.

This experiment was repeated numerous times during the course of therapy, always with the same components of comparing predictions with actual experiences. Repeated disconfirmation of negative expectations helped chip away at his entrenched ideas regarding gay sexuality and behavior.

Evidence Sifting About Attitudes of Family and Friends

It was also important to sift the truth from the feared fantasies about the heterosexism of people around him whose opinions he valued highly. This was presented in two ways: to help him predict their responses to his orientation if and when others found out, and to help him distinguish the quality of evidence he was using to assess others' attitudes about gays (see the earlier discussion regarding levels of evidence). One way he did this was by listening more carefully when the subject of homosexuality or gay issues came up around him. Generally, people were more neutral or positive toward gays than he had suspected. He also noted that those who were critical of gays were often intolerant in other areas; therefore, he began to see their negative reactions less as indictments of him (a personalization error) and more as a reflection of themselves. He was also able to gauge roughly people's attitudes toward homosexuality by extrapolating from their opinions on other controversial ideas (e.g., abortion, religion, politics, race). This was visibly relieving to the client, enabling him to feel a better sense of control and predictability over others' reactions by better anticipating them. Information gathered about this was later used as a guide as to whom to approach safely (and in what order) with the news that he was gay.

MEETING AND MIXING WITH OTHER POSITIVE PEOPLE: DEVELOPING A BETTER SOCIAL NETWORK OF GAY AND HETEROSEXUAL FRIENDS

An important aspect of therapy was to induce the client gradually to explore contact with other gay people and aspects of the gay subculture. By means of the "comfort hierarchy" idea mentioned above, the therapist took care to introduce the client only to as much as the client could assimilate, and to experiences that were less likely to confirm negatively biased beliefs that stood in the way of his self-acceptance. The client was able to expand his social network by meeting gay people through groups that met for other purposes, yet had an implicit or explicit social component as well. These are especially common in larger cities, but often exist in nonmetropolitan areas as well. The groups cover such areas as religion, politics, language, sports, social service, and music.

The client learned of a running club, for example, which he began to meet with, and there he was able to mix socially with other gay men and lesbians in an environment where there was low social pressure and where he could regulate the amount of socializing he did. As he became more comfortable with his gay identity, he also noted that he was able to befriend heterosexuals to whom his sexual orientation did not matter. This he did first by meeting heterosexual people who already knew gay people (those with gay relatives, friends, or acquaintances). Naturally, he did not hesitate very long in revealing his orientation to these people, since he had good reason to believe they would accept him as he was.

COMING OUT TO OTHER PEOPLE: ASSISTING THE PROCESS

When the client has begun to establish a firmer, more positive grasp of his own evolving identity as a gay man, it may be time to help him inform others, if this is a goal of his. As mentioned above, it was helpful to have a rough sense of which people around him were most likely to be supportive and understanding. Often the client finds it better first to tell a person who is likely to be gay himself or herself. This can help establish a connection with a larger social network as well as increase greatly the amount of correct information the client receives about homosexuality.

The client and therapist did some role-playing exercises to rehearse various approaches to telling others about his orientation. These were audiotaped and then played back for the client and therapist to critique. In this way, different styles of delivery and word choice could be attempted and modified before the real event. The therapist and client also took turns playing both sides of a feared fantasy (i.e., negative outcome) interchange wherein his news would not be well received. By this method, the client's confidence and skill at handling difficult situations effectively were built up. Standard communication and assertion techniques were utilized (e.g., teaching the client to defuse attacks via empathy). Empathy and patience were fostered by placing into context possible negative reactions of others (e.g., by exploring how long it had taken the client himself to accept his orientation) and by acknowledging the false beliefs his parents were likely to hold that might interfere with their being pleased about the news.

SUMMARY

Cognitive therapy, because of its emphasis on examining and correcting negatively biased, maladaptive assumptions, is uniquely suited to assist clients in accepting and dealing more adaptively with their same-sex sexual orientation. It requires little modification from standard techniques, but the therapist using it for this issue would be well served by familiarizing himself or herself with some of the recent literature on gay sexuality and history.

Basically, the process involves the client exploring new behaviors and testing old assumptions. It aims to increase the client's knowledge about himself and his sexual orientation so he can make more informed choices than in the past. This process is greatly assisted by his seeking out less biased sources of data (e.g., books and real gay/lesbian individuals) as well as examining and then reducing his own negative biases from faulty information processing. The course of therapy is likely not to be precisely linear, as described above, but rather to oscillate between outlined stages. Cognitive therapy can be an important step in helping gay men to live more fully up to their potential in all spheres of life. It will likely be increasingly used with this population as its unique contribution to gay men's mental health is recognized.

REFERENCES

Beck, A. T., & Emery, G. (1985). *Anxiety disorders and phobias: A cognitive perspective*. New York: Basic Books.

Beck, A. T., Rush, A. S., Shaw, B. F., & Emery, G. (1979). *Cognitive therapy of depression*. New York: Guilford.

Churchill, W. (1967). *Homosexual behavior among males: A cross-cultural and cross-species investigation*. Englewood Cliffs, NJ: Prentice-Hall.

Kinsey, A. C., Pomeroy, W. B., & Martin, C. E. (1948). *Sexual behavior in the human male*. Philadelphia: Saunders.

Newman, C. F. (1989). Where's the evidence? A clinical tip. *International Cognitive Therapy Newsletter*, 5(1), pp. 4, 8.

SUGGESTED READINGS

Borhek, M. (1983). *Coming out to parents: A two-way survival guide for lesbians and gay men and their parents*. New York: Pilgrim. (Superb book for anyone by a mother whose strong religious beliefs initially made her react negatively to her own gay son; especially good regarding grief, religion, and the parents' point of view.)

Brown, H. (1976). *Familiar faces, hidden lives: The story of homosexual men in America today*. New York: Harcourt Brace Jovanovich. (An autobiographical book by a physician. Has good chapters on religion, psychiatry, and parents.)

Churchill, W. (1967). *Homosexual behavior among males: A cross-cultural and cross-species investigation*. Englewood Cliffs, NJ: Prentice-Hall. (Good for skimming; pretty exhaustive.)

Fairchild, B., & Howard, N. (1989). *Now that you know: What every parent should know about homosexuality*. New York: Harcourt Brace Jovanovich. (Written by parents.)

Fox, J. (1984). *The boys on the rock*. New York: St. Martin's. (Great novel for gay men about coming out.)

Hobson, L. (1975). *Consenting adults*. New York: Doubleday. (Excellent semiautobiographical novel—and 1980s telemovie—about the author's own struggle to understand her son's homosexuality. Good for parents or clients.)

Kinsey, A. C., Pomeroy, W. B., & Martin, C. E. (1948). *Sexual behavior in the human male*. Philadelphia: Saunders.

Kopay, D., & Young, P. D. (1988). *The David Kopay story*. New York: Donald Fine. (Excellent book about the first American professional football player to go public with being gay.)

McNaught, B. (1988). *On being gay: Thoughts on family, faith, and love*. New York: St. Martin's. (Excellent essays, many autobiographical, on religion and other topics.)

McNeill, J. (1988). *The church and the homosexual* (3rd ed.). New York: Putnam. (Excellent book by a Catholic priest; addresses many of the thorny theological issues.)

Miller, N. (1989). *In search of gay America: Women and men in a time of change*. New York: Atlantic Monthly. (Fascinating reportage of gay life even in remote regions of the United States.)

PFLAG, P. O. Box 24565, Los Angeles, CA 90024, 1-(800) -4FAMILY. (Stands for Parents & Friends of Lesbians & Gays, a national group. Call or write for a chapter near you.)

Reid, J. (1973). *The best little boy in the world*. New York: Putnam's. (Good autobiographical first book.)

Silverstein, C. (1977). *A family matter: A parents' guide to homosexuality*. New York: McGraw-Hill. (Good book for parents or clients; excellent chapter on the changing views and perspectives of medicine and psychiatry on this issue. Also touches on some religious aspects.)

Warren, P. N. (1974). *The front runner*. New York: Bantam. (A good gay male love story about an athlete.)

Weinberg, G. (1983). *Society and the healthy homosexual*. New York: St. Martin's. (A very readable, but somewhat more psychological book.)

27

Working with Gay Women

Janet L. Wolfe

Even with the advent of the women's liberation movement, women continue to flood our therapy offices in a ratio of two to one as compared with men. Most frequently, they present us with psychological disorders linked to powerlessness: feelings of inadequacy, chronic low self-esteem, guilt, depression, and anxiety. These symptoms are a natural by-product of women's being steeped from childhood in the idea that their worth and happiness should derive from living for and through others (usually men and children).

While lesbians struggle with the same interpersonal and intrapersonal issues as nongay women, they also experience concerns uniquely related to living in a society that is both homophobic and heterosexist. The popular viewpoint—in the United States and most other cultures—is that a lesbian is "sick" or "perverted"; someone who couldn't get a man, who hates men, or perhaps wants to *be* a man. She is viewed as someone to be feared, pitied, cured, ostracized, or even locked away.

Consider that lesbians are also women, and we have an awesome case of double jeopardy. As a *woman*, she is (to others and often to herself) a second-class citizen. As a *lesbian*, she has a double "hex." Being known as a lesbian can have truly negative consequences: rejection by friends

Janet L. Wolfe • Institute for Rational-Emotive Therapy, 45 East 65th Street, New York, New York 10021.

Comprehensive Casebook of Cognitive Therapy, edited by Arthur Freeman and Frank M. Dattilio. Plenum Press, New York, 1992.

and family, ridicule, hostility, altered relationships with work colleagues, or worse—loss of children or job or physical punishment. Even for a heterosexual woman, to be called (or even risk being called) a lesbian is to strike terror in her heart, often serving as an effective deterrent to her becoming more assertive or trying to make it to the top of her field or to consider having an intimate relationship with a gay woman.

COMING OUT

To "come out" is the process of deciding to love women fully and to be comfortable with that decision. To come out is an act of great courage: it is choosing what you believe to be good over what society tells you is good, and choosing to stop leading a double life and remaining invisible over continuing to reap the many rewards of cultural acceptance.

A lesbian usually chooses to come out because of a desire to maintain her personal integrity and achieve more freedom—to end the fragmentation, lying, and other behaviors that have diverted her energies away from her emotional, intellectual, and professional growth. Coming out is a process that continues over time (as new people come into her life or as her surroundings change) and continues to require courage (as she never knows what the response of others will be).

It takes a tremendous amount of emotional fortitude to live happily and self-acceptingly as a lesbian today. In light of the fact that women have been injected with a double dose of internalized self-hatred (she's a second-class citizen because she's a woman, a freak because she chooses not to pair with men), the task is an especially monumental one. A cognitive-behavioral therapist who is highly sensitized to the issues of being homosexual in a heterosexist society (including having worked on her own homophobia), can be a powerful coach and ally in helping the woman-identified woman move successfully along her chosen path. A good consciousness-raising experience for the heterosexual therapist to understand this process is to close her eyes and see herself telling someone in her life that she is a homosexual.

The treatment model used in this case is rational-emotive therapy (RET). First articulated by Albert Ellis in 1955, RET is the pioneering cognitive-behavioral therapy. RET posits that it is the individual's "shoulds"—especially the demands for approval, success, fair treatment, and comfort—that lay the groundwork for most emotional disturbance. These demands lead to "awfulizing" about not getting what one "needs," "I-can't-stand-it-itis," and the tendency to damn oneself and/or others. Through learning to analyze problems by means of RET's ABC framework, clients can acquire (usually within relatively few sessions) a problem-solving method for working through a seemingly inextricable tangle of emotional and behavioral problems. The diagram in Figure 27-1 illustrates RET's ABC theory of emotional disturbance.

A major difference between RET and other cognitive-behavioral therapies—such as those of Beck, Mahoney, and Meichenbaum—lies in its heavy emphasis on therapists' looking for clients' dogmatic, unconditional *musts* and differentiating them from mere *preferences*. Two of the most important and useful concepts developed by Ellis that derive from this emphasis on people's absolutistic demands for love, approval, success, and comfort are those of *ego anxiety* (arising from fear of failure and rejection), and *discomfort anxiety* (which involves fear of fear and fear of discomfort).

CASE STUDY

Ellen was a 26-year-old administrative assistant seen for a total number of 6 individual and 15 group therapy sessions at an outpatient psychotherapy clinic. She had grown up in the Midwest and moved to the East with her family as a teenager. She had several months of therapy at her university's counseling center at age 19, when she experienced anxiety and depression triggered by difficulties in completing her coursework and choosing a major. She had subsequently dropped out of college in her junior year and begun to work at a series of secretarial jobs. At the time she entered therapy with me, she was working part-time and going to school part-time to complete her undergraduate pre–med degree.

Highly attractive and outgoing, Ellen had dated males throughout her high school and college years and had lived with a male student for several months. She reported that although she had enjoyed her boyfriend's companionship in many ways, the relationship had not been particularly fulfilling sexually or emotionally. In addition, she complained that her boyfriend had not been very empathic when she was upset about school, nor very willing to work on problems in their relationship when they had a disagreement. After having spent many tearful and draining hours trying to communicate with her last two boyfriends, she had eventually come to feel as though she was "trying to draw blood from a stone."

Joining a women's consciousness-raising group the second semester of her sophomore year, coupled with her discovery that she tended to have far better times with her women friends than she had with her boyfriends, led her to experiment sexually with one of the women she had grown close to in her women's group. Although this particular relationship ended after a few weeks and was followed by a brief "dalliance" with another woman, Ellen began to realize that she felt significantly more emotional and sexual connection with women than with men. For the past year, Ellen had been steadily dating Maggie, a nurse. Ellen had recently come out to her mother and stepfather, who were quite disturbed over it and refused after one meeting to allow Maggie to enter their home or to participate in any family events. This was made especially difficult by the fact that Ellen was currently reliant on her parents' financial help in order to finish college. From being "Queen of the May" in high school, Ellen had now become an outcast, a *persona non grata*.

When Ellen began therapy with me, she was experiencing intermittent depression and anxiety about her coming out and about being able to complete her pre-med requirements and get into medical school. Ambivalent about being in therapy—lest it reinforce her parents' idea that she was emotionally disturbed—she tended at times to bristle at any therapeutic interventions that suggested in any way that her thinking might in some way be dysfunctional. (Given the fact that she was in rational-emotive therapy, this at times made the going rough!) On the positive side, however, it afforded frequent opportunities to use in-session material to illustrate how she got herself upset when the world didn't treat her the way she wanted.

At intake, the client enumerated the following as her therapy goals:

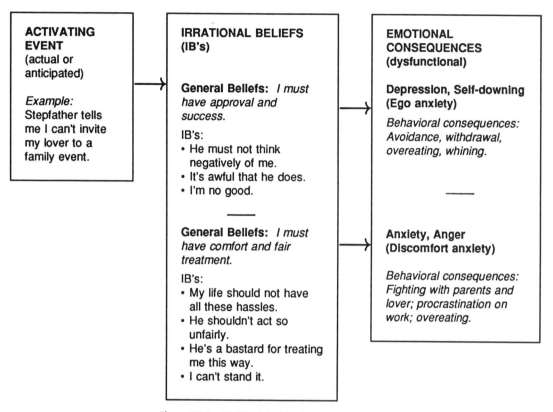

| ACTIVATING EVENT (actual or anticipated)

Example: Stepfather tells me I can't invite my lover to a family event. | IRRATIONAL BELIEFS (IB's)

General Beliefs: *I must have approval and success.*
IB's:
• He must not think negatively of me.
• It's awful that he does.
• I'm no good.

————

General Beliefs: *I must have comfort and fair treatment.*
IB's:
• My life should not have all these hassles.
• He shouldn't act so unfairly.
• He's a bastard for treating me this way.
• I can't stand it. | EMOTIONAL CONSEQUENCES (dysfunctional)

Depression, Self-downing (Ego anxiety)
Behavioral consequences: Avoidance, withdrawal, overeating, whining.

————

Anxiety, Anger (Discomfort anxiety)

Behavioral consequences: Fighting with parents and lover; procrastination on work; overeating. |

Figure 27-1. ABC Model of Rational-Emotive Therapy

• To become better able to handle the stresses of living as a lesbian in a largely heterosexual world
• To increase academic self-confidence and decrease procrastination on writing papers
• To decrease food bingeing when anxious or depressed
• To decrease self-downing over how long it had taken her to complete her undergraduate degree

Following a history taking and problem assessment, the remainder of Ellen's first session was spent in orienting her to the ABC model. This was done by my writing out a diagram (see Figure 27-1) that contained her feelings, thoughts, and behaviors in response to a recent event in which her stepfather had verbally attacked her. I then gave her this diagram to take home so she could begin to see the connection between her irrational beliefs and their emotional and behavioral consequences. I emphasized to Ellen that she could eventually learn to apply this problem-solving model to just about any of her problem situations—whether they involved negative societal reactions to her homosexuality, academic pressures, or the urge to overeat.

As part of her socialization to therapy, I explained that between-session homework assignments would be a vital part of her therapy; that the more she worked on turning around the thoughts leading to her emotional overreactions, the more quickly she would be able to start *feeling* better as well as doing better with her life goals. I also emphasized that the goal of therapy was not to get rid of all negative feelings, but rather to learn—by de-escalating her shoulds to preferences—to begin to experience more appropriate feelings (such as sadness, regret, disappointment, or annoyance) when her desires were not fulfilled.

Ellen's second session focused on two different problem situations: anger at her parents' refusal to acknowledge her female lover and at their frequent comments about Ellen's "abnormality," and feelings of inadequacy when writing papers or when criticized by a work supervisor. From an analysis of the major dysfunctional emotions, cognitions, and behaviors that seemed to cut across these problem areas, the following revised RET treatment plan was jointly developed by the therapist and client.

Behavioral Goals

1. Learn to communicate more assertively rather than aggressively with parents and others who rejected her sex-love choice.
2. Decrease perfectionism and resultant procrastination in completing school assignments.
3. Decrease food bingeing and at least maintain (rather than increase) weight.

Emotional Goals

1. Decrease depression and hopelessness over her academic and social difficulties.
2. Decrease anger and low frustration tolerance over people's prejudice against homosexuality.
3. Decrease anxiety about writing papers.

Cognitive Goals (thoughts to decrease)

1. "I shouldn't have to struggle so much; life shouldn't be so hard (e.g., my parents shouldn't hassle me about my love life; teachers shouldn't give me such difficult assignments; it's terrible I have to work and go to school and have so little money; my lover shouldn't pressure me to have sex when I'm so exhausted)."
2. "My family and society must approve of everything I do (e.g., I must always write great papers; if I don't I'm no good; I'm not smart enough, too undisciplined; I just don't have what it takes to get through school)."
3. "Because I've messed up so much in the past, I must continue to do so; I'm hopeless."

Since most of Ellen's problems centered around awfulizing about the discomfort and unfairness of the world (causing anger and low frustration tolerance) and self-downing when she did not do as well as she wanted or get the approval she wanted (resulting in depression), the above sequence of irrational beliefs—and their emotional and behavioral consequences—was explained to her. Beginning with the first session, she was shown how she could fit any of her problem situations (whether they involved negative societal reactions to her homosexuality, academic pressures, or the urge to overeat) into this problem-solving model. The following is a transcript excerpted from her second session.

Excerpt from Session 2

CLIENT: I'm really pissed off at my parents. They're insisting that I go to my cousin's wedding. I said I wouldn't go unless Maggie could come with me, and they absolutely blew up. But I'll be damned if I'll drag along some token male. So for two weeks we've barely been speaking to each other. And now I feel *really* guilty!

THERAPIST: No question but that these situations can become sticky, and I can certainly appreciate how frustrating it is to have your partner excluded from a family event. I gather you're feeling pretty angry. Is there anything else you're feeing?

CLIENT: Yeah, I'm feeling really bummed out—depressed, I guess. It just seems that whatever I do, I'm never really going to fit in. I'm sick of the constant hassles.

THERAPIST: When your parents came down on you about forbidding you to bring Maggie to the wedding, what were your thoughts?

CLIENT: That they have no right to tell me, at age 26, who I can take to a wedding; and that they should be more supportive, especially after all I've been through trying to get through school.

THERAPIST: Do you see the "should" behind "they have no right to criticize me"?

CLIENT: Well, they shouldn't! Do you mean to tell me that you think it's OK for them to hassle me?

THERAPIST: It's not OK. It's a pain in the neck! And there's no question it would be *preferable*—in terms of your relationship with your parents and with Maggie—if they didn't give you such a hard time. Let's try an experiment, shall we? If you really believed it would be *preferable* if your parents and society disapproved of your lesbianism, as opposed to believing it was an awful thing they *must* not do, how do you think you'd feel?

CLIENT: Well, I still wouldn't like it.

THERAPIST: No reason you should like it or feel happy about it. My guess is that you'd still feel some negative feelings—say, disappointment or mild frustration—but not rage and depression. But when you escalate a *preference*—it would be preferable if my family didn't hassle me—to an absolutistic must—they must not—you're generally going to feel fairly emotionally disturbed, angry, enraged, then get into even more difficulties with your family and feel guilty about that.

CLIENT: Yeah—every time I get upset, they use it as further proof that I'm emotionally disturbed and that's why I'm a lesbian!

THERAPIST: So let's see if we can dispute some of these shoulds and awfulizings. First, where is it written that people must not be prejudiced?

CLIENT: Well, a hell of a lot of people are; so I guess there's no law. But it's really awful that they cause so much pain to people. Do you know my stepfather calls Maggie "hairy legs"?

THERAPIST: They do act badly at times and cause hassles. But you have far more control than you allow yourself over the amount of pain and disturbance with which you react to these hassles. Now is it really awful and intolerable, on the same level as being tortured to death or having a child die? Or just a first-class pain in the neck?

CLIENT: Well, I guess if you put it that way . . . but I can't *stand* it when they keep pressuring me about Maggie.

THERAPIST: You obviously don't like it—and there's no reason you should. But you *are standing* it. The trick is to learn to stand it with less upsetness.

CLIENT: Why should *I* have to work on changing, when it's my mother and stepfather who are so bigoted and upset?

THERAPIST: Well, I agree it would be nice if they were less bigoted and upset. But, unfortunately, neither of us controls the universe. They may or may not be interested in changing their feelings and behavior. But by changing your *own* overly upset reactions to them, you will, first, feel better, and second, stand a better chance of their taking you more seriously and accommodating better to your life-style choices. Or, at least, they won't be able to accuse you of being a nut case when you start yelling at them about excluding Maggie from the family. (pause) Let's try an experiment—some rational-emotive imagery. Close your eyes, and imagine yourself having dinner with your parents and their berating you about bringing Maggie to the wedding; and really *get into your feelings* of upsetness—feel very angry, very enraged about your parents, and the hassles of being a lesbian in a straight world. Can you get into those feelings?

CLIENT: You bet. I feel just the way I did the other night—absolutely enraged and depressed.

THERAPIST: Now, with your eyes still closed, imagine the same event and feel only frustrated and disappointed, but not depressed and enraged. Keep working at imagining the same situation, but only feeling *mildly negatively* about their behavior. Let me know when you're able to achieve that.

CLIENT: (after about two minutes, opens her eyes) Well—it sure wasn't easy, but I did finally manage to get to the point where I wasn't feeling so upset.

THERAPIST: What was different in your head?

CLIENT: I told myself that I don't like their having this kind of attitude toward me, but they're screwed up. And that although I really don't like it, I guess I can stand it. Like you said last week, it's a hassle, not a horror. Now, if only I could really believe that!

THERAPIST: If you really keep working on it—both in imagery, and in actual situations where your parents or others attack you unfairly—you can learn to make yourself considerably less enraged. But I suspect there's some tie-in with your depression here, too. You say you really believe yourself that homosexuals are not defective or pathological. If you really believed it as strongly as you say, do you think you would get so angry at others' disapproval? Or does their criticism somehow add to your general feelings of defectiveness as a human being?

CLIENT: On some level, I think you're right. But if just about everyone's rejecting you, it's hard to feel good about yourself. Don't we need other people's approval to some extent to feel OK about ourselves?

THERAPIST: Most of us prefer to be liked and approved by most significant others, and are disappointed or moderately frustrated when we're not. But I think in your case you also feel somehow downgraded, and as a result, get furious at those who seem to be putting you down. But if you refused to buy into the belief that if they think less of you, it *makes* you less, you're much less likely to feel downgraded or hopeless. Do you see that?

CLIENT: Intellectually, yes—but emotionally, I still feel pretty depressed when my parents or professors criticize me.

THERAPIST: Intellectual insight usually means that once in a while, you weakly tell yourself, "Just because they think I'm bad doesn't make it true." But the *majority* of the time, what you're really telling yourself is, "Yes, if they think badly of me, there must be some truth to it— I am defective, less worthwhile and less normal than other human beings."

CLIENT: Yes, I guess that is what I really believe. But how do I change?

THERAPIST: You can work at developing emotional muscle much in the same way as you do physical muscles: by practice! Each time you find yourself becoming angry or depressed at your parents' rejection of your homosexuality, ask yourself the following questions: One, where is it written they *must* not have society's antihomosexual prejudice? Why *must* they approve of everything I do? Two, is it really awful that they treat me this way? Can I really not stand it? Three, does it really make them lousy, rotten parents? Four, how does their criticism of me make me a less worthwhile human being? You can also feed yourself some positive self-messages: "Even if I have a nonnormative sexual orientation that many people may erroneously believe is sick, I'm still OK. I have a right to choose my sexual partners. By the same token, others have a right to disagree with my choice, even if I don't like the way they do it.

CLIENT: I guess feeling OK about myself is going to be an uphill battle. I feel so inadequate academically, and my parents' putting me down in the one area where I feel good about myself—my relationship—just seems so unfair.

THERAPIST: Life isn't easy. As Albert Ellis, the founder of RET, says, 'Life is spelled H-A-S-S-L-E.' But by learning not to feel put down when others criticize you or you fail to live up to your own expectations, and by refusing to fall into the trap of 'poor me, life is so hard,' you can greatly decrease the amount of misery—rage, low frustration tolerance, depression—you experience in response to life's hassles. (pause) Now let me suggest two homeworks for you to do this week.

CLIENT: Homework! As though I didn't have enough work to do. Why does everything have to be so hard?

THERAPIST: Are you perchance telling yourself yet again that 'it's *too* hard . . . poor me that life is such a grind?'

CLIENT: Yeah. (grinning) Something like that.

THERAPIST: And when you think that, how do you feel?

CLIENT: Pretty depressed and anxious.

THERAPIST: Well, one of your homeworks—the cognitive, or self-talk, one—is to continue to dispute the idea that the world shouldn't be so unfair. That I shouldn't have to work so hard to be happy, shouldn't have parents who pressure me to get married, shouldn't have to work at my therapy. Your *behavioral* assignment is to assertively, rather than aggressively, let your parents know that while you understand their concern over your sexual orientation, you feel frustrated and sad at their nonacceptance of Maggie into their life.

(Note: We rehearsed for this dialogue by first role-playing it during the sessions, with coaching and feedback by the therapist.)

Discussion

While the target problem introduced by the client was her anger and depression over her difficulties in living in a "straight" world, the session focused on the dysfunctional beliefs that underlay not only this problem but other

"activating events" dealing with unfairness or criticism or discomfort. Thus, the groundwork was laid for helping her increase her frustration tolerance in other areas of her life.

Four more individual sessions were held with the client, following which she was put into an RET women's group. During the third through the sixth sessions of individual therapy, work continued to focus on the themes of low frustration tolerance/anger and self-acceptance. In the area of self-acceptance, situations brought up included self-downing over her weight, feelings of inadequacy about how long it was taking her to get on a career track (as she would not be completing her BA until age 27), and anxiety about an important class presentation.

In the area of frustration tolerance, situations dealt with included bingeing when anxious about schoolwork, procrastination on completing assignments (which resulted in considerable fatigue and irritability with her lover, due to last-minute all-nighters), and anger at not being able to be as open as she'd like to be with work colleagues and classmates about her lesbian relationship.

In each session, we continued to dispute the beliefs underlying her disturbance. Typical examples of self-downing/depressive cognitions included:

- "I am fat and ugly because of my current weight."
- "I am lazy and stupid."
- "I will never be happy or successful."

In line with RET principles, Ellen was shown that it was invalid to equate any single trait or behavior (e.g., her weight or performance on a class presentation) with her entire worth, and that just because she had had difficulty in completing school in the past didn't mean she could not succeed in the future. As a result of the disputation of irrational beliefs during each session, new rational countermessages were arrived at that she was then instructed to spend at least 10 minutes a day working on reinforcing. These new self-messages included:

- "Even though I have flaws and make mistakes, I'm still OK. ı am a worthwhile person with many good qualities who is doing the best she can."
- "I don't like my excess body fat, but it does not make me an ugly and disgusting person."
- "Even if my presentation did not go very well, there's no evidence that I'm a stupid person who can never complete my degree and function in my profession."

Irrational beliefs identified as leading to low frustration tolerance and anger included the following:

- "I can't stand all this hard work I have to do. I must have some comfort, so I'm going to eat all this candy even though it's going to make me fatter."
- "Poor me. Life should be easier; I shouldn't have so much to contend with. My lover shouldn't be complaining about my having so little time for her when I'm so busy and hassled already."
- "Not only am I hassled because I'm a lesbian, but I don't have the option that a lot of married women do of quitting my job and being supported by my husband so I can go to school full-time."
- "It's awful to be hassled by men on the street."

Disputation of these irrational beliefs—done in session as well as on self-help homework forms—resulted in the formulation of new, rational countermessages. These included the following:

- "I wish my lover didn't put additional demands on me now that I'm so exhausted, but it's a hassle, not a horror. She's not a louse for doing so; she's just expressing her own needs."
- "Even though I may not have some of the benefits that some heterosexuals have, I still have many advantages in my relationship (not the least of which is mutual love and respect and a lot of emotional and sexual satisfaction)."
- "I don't like being hassled on the streets by men, but I can stand it. This isn't Camelot; it's a highly screwed-up world. People who act badly are not rotten. They're just—like me—FFHB's (fallible, fucked-up human beings)."

Behavioral assignments given during sessions 2 through 6 included the following:

1. Invite sister and brother-in-law to dinner hosted by you and your lover, and discuss with them your concern about some of the friction with parents caused by the lesbian relationship. Suggest that they, in turn, host a dinner for your parents and you and your lover.
2. Continue to try to express yourself assertively—rather than aggressively—with your parents when they criticize you.
3. Do one nice thing a week for your parents.
4. Stand in front of the mirror each day and state three positive things about yourself.
5. When anxious about schoolwork, do a relaxation technique (such as listening to music or a relaxation tape, or going for a walk) instead of bingeing on sweets.

6. Go to a restaurant with your lover and hold hands without awfulizing or self-downing about other people's "dirty looks."

Ellen had made considerable progress by the end of six sessions in decreasing some of her frustration and depression over her heavy workload, parental and societal discrimination, and failure to do perfectly well at school and at maintaining her desired weight. Moreover, because she was no longer getting so angry and upset at her parents, they had begun to attack her less about her "emotional instability" and had actually accepted an invitation to dinner with her sister, brother-in-law, her lover, and herself—stating for the first time that although they wished that she would settle down and lead a "normal life" with a man, they would try to accept her choice as long as it made her happy and would no longer exclude her lover from their house and from selected other family activities.

Finally, she had also made progress in countering some of her demands for perfection in her schoolwork, as a result of which she was up-to-date on most assignments and completing her pre-med requirements with A's and B's. As a result, she was feeling considerably less "stressed out" and fatigued, and her periods of depression and hopelessness had decreased significantly in frequency, duration, and intensity.

At this point, she was put into an RET women's group co-led by her individual therapist, partly for economic reasons (it was significantly less expensive than individual therapy) and partly for the purpose of getting more "laboratory" practice in dealing with interpersonal issues. The following is a transcript of her participation in her third session with the group that illustrates how the same cognitive themes keep coming up.

Excerpts from Group Therapy Session

ELLEN: I'm feeling uptight about this weekend. Maggie and I are going to this dinner party for several of my chemistry classmates, and it's such a bummer because I'm gay and can't just look forward to having a nice relaxing time, like other couples.

KATHY: I understand that it is more uncomfortable—when everybody's probably in heterosexual pairs—to be with a woman. And I don't mean in any way to discount that it is hard. But it can be uncomfortable to be single at a coupled event, or with a man that people might disapprove of. So what are you telling yourself to make yourself not just apprehensive, but really anxious? [Note: The RET group therapy model involves having the members all serve as "adjunct therapists," focusing especially on helping each other to identify and dispute irrational beliefs leading to upsetness about events in their lives.]

ELLEN: (angrily) I thought that in a women's group, of all places, people could understand how difficult it is for a lesbian in this society. But all I'm getting is, "Well, your experience is no different from anyone else's!" I come here to get support; I shouldn't have to put up with this kind of crap here!

JUDY: You really didn't seem to hear what Kathy said.

ELLEN: Sure I did. "There's no difference between being gay and straight at a dinner party. It's all in my head."

THERAPIST: Let's take a look at what's happening here. Even though Kathy did acknowledge the special difficulties of being with a same-sexed partner at a professional social event, you didn't hear what you apparently had hoped to hear, and consequently got angry. Now what "shoulds" were going through your head when Kathy responded to you?

ELLEN: (still angrily) That women should be more sympathetic to other women and not trivialize how hard it is for a lesbian. And that's a *rational* belief, as far as *I'm* concerned: They *should* have been more sympathetic.

THERAPIST: And what happened when you thought this, and got angry?

ELLEN: I let Kathy know in no uncertain terms how I felt, that's what. And what's more, I think this group sucks, and I have no intention of staying in it.

THERAPIST: That's certainly an option, and I can understand your wanting to get away from people whom you think are treating you unfairly. But can you think of some *disadvantages* of opting out of the group now?

ELLEN: Well, I suppose I'm going to get these kinds of reactions all the time; so maybe I can get more practice in dealing with them? But that sounds like a lousy reason to me.

SUSAN: If it were just going to add another hassle to your life, without any benefit in return, I'd agree with you; it wouldn't be a very good reason. But here we can look at our reactions as they occur and figure out better ways to handle *emotionally* what we don't like, as well as better ways to *respond* to people when they don't act the way we'd like. So how about giving us a chance to try to help you feel less anxious about the dinner party? We are on your side, even though you may not perceive that we are!

ELLEN: (reluctantly) OK. So I'm telling myself that it's rotten that I'm going to have so much harder a time at this dinner party than the rest of the guests; that I might

have to inhibit myself somewhat with Maggie so I don't make them uptight . . . and . . . heck! That's just not fair!

SUSAN: And the world *should* be fair—right? We all know how very fair and nonbigoted this world is, don't we? (looks at other members, who chuckle)

ELLEN: What am I supposed to do, think it's funny?

KATHY: I'm sorry if you felt we were laughing at you, Ellen. No, it's not funny to feel like the odd woman out, or to possibly be thought of by some of the guests as a freak. But neither is it awful and intolerable. Our laughter was not at your situation, but at the ludicrousness of our philosophy when we demand that this world— which *is* unfortunately full of unfairness—absolutely *should not* be full of unfairness!

JOYCE: Ellen, we're not saying the *events* in your life are the same as they are for heterosexuals—clearly there are lots of special stressors you're having to face. What we *are* saying is that you have the power to choose how disturbed you get about them.

THERAPIST: And by changing your belief to "it's unfortunate—but not terrible, awful, or intolerable," you can greatly decrease the amount of discomfort you'll feel at the dinner party, not to mention a lot of your anticipatory anxiety and anger. Another *behavioral* choice you have is not to go to the dinner party, or to go alone—but then you're joining with society's prejudices, rather than confronting them and trying as best you can to have an enjoyable social life despite your sexual orientation.

ELLEN: I see what you're saying. It makes sense to go to the party and try to enjoy myself and not feel too upset. But I still can't help feeling pissed off that the women here weren't more sympathetic.

THERAPIST: Perhaps they weren't as sympathetic as you would have liked. But sometimes, saying things to each other like "Poor you, it really *is* awful" may temporarily help you feel better, but it's really reinforcing your awfulizing philosophy. And sometimes the most compassionate thing we can do here is to help each other change our misery-producing philosophy *about* life's discomforts and hassles. Or, as they say in Alcoholics Anonymous, "Grant me the courage to change what I can change, the serenity to accept what I can't change, and the wisdom to know the difference." By the way, Ellen, can you see how your reaction here to the women was in fact quite similar to what you tell yourself when a professor criticizes your writing, or your lover isn't as nurturant as you'd like?

ELLEN: You mean, my "It's awful, they shouldn't treat me this way . . . poor me" shtick? (laughs somewhat sheepishly)

THERAPIST: That very one! How are you feeling right now about the group's reaction?

ELLEN: Well, I'm still a little frustrated, but I don't feel as angry as I did before.

THERAPIST: And your thoughts about the members who didn't respond the way you wished they would?

ELLEN: I guess they're just FF*HH*B's.

KATHY: I beg your pardon?

ELLEN: Just fallible, fucked-up *heterosexual* human beings! And I'll just have to try to focus on the good stuff I can get here, as long as it outweighs the negatives, and try to use this as one of life's golden opportunities to practice frustration tolerance—as if I didn't have enough already!

THERAPIST: A good approach!

CONCLUSION

At no time in therapy was Ellen's sexual orientation challenged. The evidence seemed to indicate clearly that her sexual identity was a freely chosen expression of what felt most natural and rewarding to her. To allay any residual doubts she had about her sexual orientation, we applied rational criteria to her choice: It was clear that it (a) was more gratifying than painful (despite society's prejudice); (b) was not harming herself or others; and (c) was not obstructing progress toward a commitment to some other field of endeavor.

This is not to imply that the ramifications of a lesbian life-style did not present special dilemmas not normally faced by heterosexuals. Indeed, numerous such situations became the focus of therapeutic work. These included:

- Deciding which friends and family members to come out to, and how to present it to them
- Dealing with her upsetness at her failure to speak up in a group where antihomosexual remarks were being made
- Anxiety about a recent short haircut she feared made her look "dykey"
- Deciding how much physical expression to risk in public (e.g., kissing her lover goodbye on the lips at the airport)

- Deciding how far to assert her rights to attend family functions with her lover when she risked losing the financial support her parents were providing her with

In each of these situations, we first worked on reducing her emotional disturbance *about* the practical problem (her anger, guilt, self-downing, or anxiety), then did an analysis of the various options for *handling* the practical problems—making certain to include in the analysis special variables related to being gay (e.g., potential societal discrimination and the importance of good support networks). Finally, we had her role-play with group members better ways of handling various interpersonal situations.

Rather than viewing her diagnosis as "homosexuality" (thankfully, one no longer recognized as a pathological category in the *Diagnostic and Statistical Manual* of the American Psychiatric Association), assessment was made in terms of dysfunctional cognitive, emotive, and behavioral patterns, be they connected to situations particular to her lesbian identity or other situations having nothing to do with it. In turn, treatment focused on helping her identify and change faulty cognitive schemas that led to disturbance when others, the world, and she herself failed to live up to her expectations.

SUGGESTED READINGS

For professionals:

Boston Lesbian Psychologies Collective. (1987). *Lesbian psychologies*. Urbana: University of Illinois Press.
Walen, S., DiGiuseppe, R., & Wessler, R. (1980). *A practitioner's guide to rational-emotive therapy*. New York: Oxford University Press.

For clients:

Darty, T., & Potter, S. (1984). *Women–identified women*. Mountain View, CA: Mayfield.
Ellis, A. (1988). *How to stubbornly refuse to make yourself miserable about anything—yes, anything!* New York: Carol Publishing/Lyle Stuart.

28

Marital Therapy

Norman Epstein

Although the concepts and methods of cognitive-behavioral therapy initially were developed for application with a variety of disorders of the individual client, in the past decade marital theorists, researchers, and therapists have extended the range of cognitive-behavioral therapy to encompass dysfunction in interpersonal relationships. A hallmark of cognitive-behavioral marital therapy is that it focuses not only on the internal cognitive processes and affective responses of each member of a relationship, but also on the unique pattern of behavioral interactions between partners that are both the results of, and the stimuli for, those internal processes. The cognitive-behavioral marital therapist pays attention to the complex interplay of cognitive, behavioral, and affective responses that occur during a couple's interactions (Baucom & Epstein, 1990). Consistent with a systems-theory conceptualization of marital relationships (see Leslie, 1988), it is assumed that a particular couple's problems are due to the unique combination of those two partners' intra- and interpersonal responses.

At present, clinical interest and publications concerning cognitive-behavioral marital therapy (CBMT) have grown more rapidly than empirical research on cognition in marriage, but there is already an encouraging body of research findings supporting theoretical and clinical claims. For example, studies have demonstrated that spouses' cognitions about their relationships are associated with their current *and* future levels of marital discord (see reviews by Baucom & Epstein, 1990; Bradbury & Fincham 1990; Fincham, Bradbury, & Scott, 1990). Furthermore, the initial outcome studies of CBMT efficacy have indicated that its cognitive restructuring and behavioral interventions have comparable significant impacts on overall marital distress. However, although cognitive interventions by themselves tend to reduce spouses' negative cognitions concerning their marriage, the cognitive restructuring appears to produce limited change in spouses' overt behavioral interactions (Baucom & Epstein, 1990; Baucom, Sayers, & Sher, 1990; Behrens, Sanders, & Halford, 1990). One of the implications of the existing research findings is that cognitive-behavioral marital therapy must indeed be an integration of cognitive and behavioral treatment procedures. The following case study is offered as an example of how such an integrated approach can be applied with a distressed couple.

CASE REPORT

John and Barbara, both in their early 50s and married for 28 years, sought marital therapy at Barbara's insistence, due to her high level of distress concerning their marriage. Barbara initially contacted the therapist by phone and noted that the problems in the relationship were

Norman Epstein • Department of Family and Community Development, University of Maryland, College Park, Maryland 20742.

Comprehensive Casebook of Cognitive Therapy, edited by Arthur Freeman and Frank M. Dattilio. Plenum Press, New York, 1992.

long-standing. She reported that a course of marital therapy with another clinician several years ago had produced only brief improvement. Her description of the marital problems focused on her husband's general detachment from her "unless he wants something from me, or unless we do things on his terms." Barbara suggested that she most likely could motivate her husband to attend at least one therapy session with her by acting very upset, but she was skeptical about the depth of his commitment to changing their relationship.

BACKGROUND INFORMATION

Relationship History

During the first conjoint interview with the couple, the therapist asked them to give an overview of the history of their relationship. John and Barbara reported that they met in their teens, dated few others, and married when they finished college. John owns a thriving business, and Barbara is a successful accountant. For the first 20 years of their marriage, John spent long hours building his business, while Barbara focused on raising their daughter and two sons (now aged 25, 24, and 22) and maintaining their home. Barbara had begun an entry-level accounting job after graduation from college, but she stopped working when their first child was born a year after they were married. Barbara reported that she felt unprepared for parenthood, and as a result she felt anxious and ambivalent about her parenting efforts. She increasingly felt resentment toward John as he spent large amounts of time away from her and their young children. As Barbara described this pattern, John acknowledged that he had focused his attention outside the home, due to both his anxiety about building a successful business and his discomfort with the demands of family relationships.

The couple had a history of chronic tension and periodic verbal arguments, usually elicited by Barbara's "storing up" her resentment and then venting it to John. According to both spouses, John typically would apologize to Barbara for being so preoccupied with his own life and would increase his attention to her for a while. Over time, he would drift back into his detached position, and Barbara's frustration would build again.

Eight years ago, Barbara took additional courses in accounting and became a CPA. She first worked for an accounting firm and then started her own practice, which has grown to include three employees. She reported that with her success came less tolerance for her husband's lack of involvement in their marriage. John works fewer hours than in the past but spends many hours in leisure activities that do not include Barbara (e.g., watching sports on television, playing golf with friends). Recently, Barbara "blew up" (as she described it) and threatened to leave John unless he went to see a marital therapist with her.

In the initial conjoint session, Barbara stated that her husband would be satisfied to let the marriage stay as it is indefinitely, and that she must be the catalyst for change. John agreed with that description overall, saying that he believes that they have a good marriage and often does not notice the problems that his wife notices. He acknowledged that he often drifts into his own world, especially when he experiences stress at work, but he claimed that this pattern is not due to a lack of caring for his wife. His major complaint about Barbara was the aversive manner in which she expressed her displeasure (e.g., yelling, occasionally breaking objects in the house). He also said that he saw her as overlooking positive aspects of their relationship and focusing her attention on any negative events that occurred.

Family Backgrounds

Barbara's parents followed traditional sex roles in their own relationship and apparently applied them in the raising of their children. Barbara remembers little parental support for her career ambitions. She also remembers that throughout her childhood, her mother criticized her frequently for things she said and did. Her father was also critical and periodically was physically abusive to her and her older brother. She reported that she consistently had friends during childhood and adolescence, but that her low self-esteem led her to seek attention by being "outrageous" (e.g., voicing controversial opinions, dressing in unconventional clothing). Barbara stated that her current group of women friends show more interest in her as a person than John does, but she sometimes doubts whether people really like her. She is very pleased with her career success, but she stated that she had to achieve her goals without much emotional support from John.

John grew up in a family that he described as "wonderful." He has a younger brother and sister, and a large extended family. He remembers many large, warm family gatherings. His parents were loving and supportive of their children, but they discouraged expression of personal feelings, especially negative emotions such as anger. Both parents encouraged a high level of achievement. Although they were quite generous with money and gifts, they expected their children to take on summer jobs and work hard. John has always been highly competitive, as evidenced by his strong performance in school, his success in high school sports, and his current intense approach to his work and leisure activities. His business struggled for several years, but he described its ultimate success with considerable pride.

ASSESSMENT AND DIAGNOSIS

The initial one-hour conjoint assessment interview with the couple began with an inquiry about each spouse's definition of the marital problems, as well as their accounts of their relationship history (described above). In addition, each spouse was asked what characteristics attracted them to each other (relevant to an assessment of their expectations of the relationship), how the decision to marry was made, and what life events seemed to have had significant impacts on the relationship. Barbara reported that she had been attracted by John's ambition and sense of direction in his life, his humor, his physical appearance, and the close ties among his family members that were so different from the relationships in her own family of origin. John said that he was attracted by Barbara's unconventional sense of humor, her intelligence, her appearance, and her adventurous spirit. Even in the initial assessment session, the therapist guided the couple in examining how some of the characteristics that they now found distressing were aspects of the qualities that initially attracted them to each other (Abrahms & Spring, 1989).

Barbara identified the birth of their first child as a significant event in the deterioration of their marriage, because she felt abandoned when John participated minimally in the care of the baby. In turn, John remembered Barbara's return to school eight years ago as a time when she paid little attention to him or their children. When the spouses described these events, it was clear that the memories were still vivid for them and were readily triggered by current partner behaviors that each individual interpreted as "selfish."

The conjoint assessment session also identified strategies that the couple used to cope with relationship problems. John and Barbara concurred in their view that Barbara tended to alternate between "sitting on her feelings" and venting her frustration, whereas John avoided communication about problems that surfaced, hoping that Barbara's distress would fade and that further discussion would not be necessary. Barbara tended to ruminate about their conflicts, but John reported that he tended to assume that their marriage was basically a loving one and to focus on positive events. Whenever Barbara had exhibited a high level of anger and had refused to behave affectionately for more than a day or so, John had paid more

attention to her by allotting more time for talking and shared leisure activities.

In addition to relying on the couple's self-reports concerning their interaction patterns, the therapist used the assessment session as an opportunity to observe their communication behavior directly. Consistent with the couple's reports about their coping patterns, Barbara spent more time than John did describing problems, pointing out ways in which John spent time on individual interests rather than on their relationship. Her primary complaint was that John's behavior reflected a lack of interest in her. In turn, John tended to defend himself, discounted some of Barbara's concerns, described the relationship in more positive terms, and expressed little emotion. His primary complaint was that Barbara "searched" in a biased manner for evidence that he did not care, when in fact he was very committed to their marriage. The therapist also observed that neither partner communicated acknowledgment of the other person's views or the subjectivity of their own perceptions and opinions.

Following the conjoint assessment session, each spouse was seen for an individual assessment session focused on personal history (family of origin characteristics and relationships, school performance, quality of friendships, past intimate relationships, work history, health history and status, and any history of psychological problems). The therapist also inquired about each partner's cognitions regarding the marriage's strengths and problems, including the *standards* each held about the qualities their relationship "should" have and the *attributions* each made about the causes of each other's behavior. For example, Barbara expressed the standard that joint activities should nearly always take precedence over the pursuit of individual interests. One of the standards that John held was the belief that members of a couple should focus as much as possible on discussions of pleasant experiences rather than relationship problems. He also held the related standard that in order for a shared activity to be relaxing, it should include no discussion of negative personal feelings, but instead should be a pleasantly distracting diversion.

Concerning attributions, John concluded that Barbara was distressed about his "unwinding" with leisure activities that did not include her because she lacked self-esteem (i.e., he attributed it to a trait within her, rather than to his own behavior). He also attributed her "blow-ups" to fluctuations in the stress she experienced from her work (again, a cause external to him). Barbara reported that she attributed John's involvement in independent activities as a sign that he did not find her interesting (a trait attribution). She also attributed his periodic shifts toward more attentive behavior as insincere attempts to mollify her. Both partners' attributions typically placed the blame for relationship discord on characteristics of the other person.

The assessment of the couple's standards about intimate relationships also included asking them each to fill out a 21-item sentence-completion form* that included stems such as "The roles of work and careers would be . . .," "The way we'd fight would be . . .," "We'd show our appreciation for each other by . . .," and "We would handle any differences in our personal values by . . .". Finally, each spouse's attributions about causes of their marital problems (e.g., attribution to partner's personality, or to partner's malicious intent), as well as his or her expectancies for improvement in the marriage, were assessed with Pretzer, Epstein, and Fleming's (1991) Marital Attitude Survey.

As is typical in cognitive therapy (see Beck, Rush, Shaw, & Emery, 1979), the assessment of cognitive and behavioral factors in the couple's discord extended beyond the formal assessment sessions and included ongoing data collection both within and between treatment sessions. Within sessions, the therapist monitored shifts in each partner's affect and behavior, stopping the interaction and probing for associated cognitions. For example, in one early session, John said that when he gets home after a stressful day, he just wants to "unwind and not think about anything important." As he said this, Barbara's facial expression suggested that she was upset. When the therapist asked her about her reaction, she said that she was angry, and additional open-ended questions by the therapist revealed that Barbara had made the attribution, "He has no interest in being with me and wouldn't care if I disappeared." At that moment, John was able to elaborate on his statement, telling Barbara that he really valued some time to relax when he first walked in the door, but that he would find it enjoyable to spend some leisure time with her. His response still did not satisfy Barbara, who reported her interpretation that John would only like to be with her if they restricted the conversation to pleasant topics. Thus, the ongoing exchange between partners during therapy sessions yielded rich data concerning both the couple's communication style and their cognitions about each other's messages.

Additional information about the spouses' cognitions concerning their interactions was collected by having them complete the Daily Record of Dysfunctional Thoughts (Beck et al., 1979) at home between sessions. The therapist instructed each spouse to record descriptions of upsetting situations between them, as well as the associated automatic thoughts and emotions. When the therapist reviewed the forms with each spouse during conjoint therapy sessions, this afforded Barbara and John the opportunity to examine the validity of their cognitions, provide each other with valuable feedback concerning interpretations of upsetting events, and increase their understanding of each other's subjective experiences.

Based on the interview and questionnaire data, it appeared that John and Barbara had a strong affectional bond and that both were committed to maintaining the marriage. However, the couple's discord seemed to be influenced significantly by several behavioral and cognitive factors. Their problematic communication pattern involved Barbara periodically pursuing and criticizing John, John avoiding conflict and defending himself, and both partners failing to communicate empathy and respect for the other's thoughts and feelings. Furthermore, given their painful history of mutual neglect, they had not developed a constructive way of letting each other know that they wanted to be together *or* that they wanted to be alone. They had developed a balance of individual and shared activities that was much more satisfactory for John than for Barbara, but they were unable to engage in systematic problem-solving discussions to find a more mutually acceptable use of time.

In terms of cognitive factors, each spouse held some unrealistic standards about their relationship and was distressed when the standards were not fulfilled. Furthermore, both partners automatically made a variety of unfavorable attributions about the other's goals and motives, at least some of which appeared to be inaccurate. The therapeutic treatment plan was designed to address all of these processes.

TREATMENT

Therapy consisted of weekly conjoint sessions over six months, with an occasional individual session with one spouse or the other when that person was having considerable difficulty challenging a particular relationship standard. Each session included (a) a brief review of the couple's past week and any homework they completed between sessions, (b) identification of specific conflictual incidents from the week that required processing in the session, (c) active practice in modifying dysfunctional cognitions and behavioral interactions, and (d) design of homework assignments that would extend the couple's application of constructive cognitive and behavioral changes to their daily life.

---

*Copies of the relationship expectations sentence completion form can be obtained from the author.

Behavioral Interventions

Although each session included a mix of cognitive and behavioral interventions, more time was spent on the behavioral components of the couple's interactions during the first few sessions. The initial emphasis on reducing the couple's negative behavioral exchanges is common in cognitive-behavioral marital therapy when it appears that a continuing pattern of aversive interactions is likely to reinforce the spouses' negative appraisals of their marriage (Baucom & Epstein, 1990). In the present case, Barbara and John were more willing to examine the validity of their own negative cognitions when the "atmosphere" of their interactions had become more pleasant.

Communication Training

In the first conjoint treatment session, the therapist presented a summary of the couple's interaction patterns (including some typical cognitions experienced by each partner) that appeared to be related to their chronic discord. After giving the couple an overview of the principles of cognitive-behavioral marital therapy (Baucom & Epstein, 1990), the therapist cited examples from the data that the couple provided during the assessment sessions as illustrations of how negative cognitions and behaviors can contribute to marital distress. Next, it was stressed that the couple needed to alter their negative communication pattern in order to break their long-standing stalemate, a suggestion that made sense to both John and Barbara.

At this point, John and Barbara were introduced to the principles of Guerney's (1977) relationship enhancement approach to communication, whereby each spouse was to be taught both expressive and empathic listening skills. After giving each spouse a written handout outlining Guerney's communication guidelines for the expresser and the listener, the therapist answered their questions about the principles and modeled examples of competent responses. Next, each spouse was asked to select a recent experience that was unrelated to their marriage to discuss with the partner (e.g., John chose a problem that he had with one of his employees). With coaching from the therapist, John practiced telling Barbara about his subjective thoughts and emotions in his situation, and Barbara practiced providing John with empathic feedback that conveyed her understanding of his experiences *and* her acknowledgement that he had a right to those subjective experiences. When John was able to tell Barbara that she had communicated a good level of understanding, they switched communication roles, with John providing empathic listening as Barbara expressed her thoughts and feelings about a disturbing conversation with an old friend.

After each partner had performed competently as expresser and empathic listener, the therapist had them apply the same communication skills to a topic that involved mild conflict in their own relationship. Over the course of the next few sessions, the therapist coached the couple in this form of constructive communication, moving them into discussions of their areas of major marital conflict. The couple reported that they were able to resolve conflicts more quickly at home, with fewer residual hard feelings, and that they were spending more time talking together each week.

Practice in Phrasing Assertive Requests

In order to reduce the couple's aversive behavioral exchanges further, the therapist spent part of two early sessions reviewing each spouse's ways of making and refusing requests. For example, Barbara described how she had wanted to talk to John about a problem with their joint checking account, but she found him watching what she referred to as a "stupid" television program. In the session, she said that she had begun to mention the checkbook problem to John (she reported that her phrasing had been "We've *got* to talk about this before the account is in a real mess!"), but that she quickly backed off when John made a hostile facial expression. John acknowledged that he had felt frustrated by the interruption of his relaxation time and that he probably did make such a face.

At this point, the therapist coached the couple in ways of "replaying" that episode with more empathic *and* assertive responses. For example, Barbara shifted to saying, "John, I know that you are enjoying relaxing now, but there is a problem with the checkbook that is making me nervous. When would be a good time to talk about it?" In return, John shifted to saying, "I can see that it is bothering you and I appreciate your recognition that I need to relax a bit now. I would be willing to discuss the account after the show is over." As was the case with the relationship enhancement communication training, the therapist asked the couple to practice similar shifts toward more assertive communication during subsequent sessions and at home.

Scheduling of Shared Leisure Activities

From the initial assessment, it was clear that one impediment to John and Barbara spending more leisure time together was the difference in their preferred activities. John tended to prefer activities outside the house, whereas Barbara most valued time spent together quietly at home (e.g., talking, playing cards, working on a house project). Each spouse had developed the *expectancy* (prediction) that he or she would not enjoy the other's preferences. On the other hand, when one of them declined to participate in the other's preferred activities, the latter person attributed it to rejection of him or her as a person. Inquiry by the therapist revealed that the spouses both had begun making these arbitrary inferences many years ago, based on a limited number of attempts to share activities.

Consequently, the therapist coached the couple in generating a list of possible joint activities, without evaluating how enjoyable each activity might be. The list of couple activities presented by Baucom and Epstein (1990) was used to supplement the list that the couple compiled from their brainstorming session. Then, the therapist explored both spouses' cognitions about each activity on the list, using Socratic questioning to guide them in challenging any "resistance" they felt toward trying particular options. For example, John expressed reluctance about spending time together arranging a backlog of their family photographs into albums, as suggested by Barbara. His automatic thoughts about the activity included the following:

- "We'll end up talking about upsetting memories that some of the pictures probably will trigger."
- "Barbara gets so obsessed with organizing things that she'll take over and spend all of the time figuring out exactly how to place the pictures in the albums."

John reported that he had a strong degree of belief in these predictions, even though the couple had never worked on photo albums before. The therapist guided him in examining the available evidence regarding his predictions. The following exchange was among those that took place.

THERAPIST: John, have you found that either you or Barbara have tended to get upset and talk about bad memories when you have looked at any of the old pictures in the past?

JOHN: Well, I remember getting into an unpleasant discussion of whether I really cared about Barbara when we looked at the pictures taken at her birthday party last year. When it comes to looking at pictures from our vacations or pictures of the children, we usually end up laughing about something.

THERAPIST: So, what do you think is the probability that something unpleasant will come up? Your original automatic thought predicted that it would happen.

JOHN: It's probably less than 50–50, but it if comes up, it will end up in a mess.

THERAPIST: It seems that you have had another automatic thought, regarding the inevitability that a discussion of unpleasant feelings will get out of control and become really aversive. What do you know about your communication with Barbara, as it is *now*, that supports or contradicts that prediction?

At this point, John was able to discuss how he and Barbara had become much more skilled at expressing empathy for each other's positions, and how they also had experienced success with making requests of each other. He noted that if their conversation became focused on negative memories, he would be able to request that he and Barbara shift away from negativity, especially because their joint goal was to share some pleasant leisure time. He also acknowledged that he could tell Barbara that he understood the importance of dealing with the negative feelings and could make specific plans with her to do so at a future time.

As the therapist and couple examined the list of potential joint leisure activities and explored any reluctance that either spouse had concerning particular options, Barbara and John distilled the list down to several activities that were feasible and interesting to both of them. Over the next few weeks, they began to spend more time together, and they both reported considerable enjoyment from the activities.

Cognitive Interventions

As illustrated by the description above of the intervention designed to increase the couple's shared leisure activities, the efforts to produce behavior changes frequently included some cognitive restructuring. The sessions also increasingly had time devoted to the examination and modification of the couple's cognitions (e.g., standards, attributions, expectancies) that played roles in their day-to-day upsetting interactions.

On a number of occasions, Barbara reported that John had been behaving in a much more attentive and caring manner toward her, which she greatly enjoyed, but that she also had experienced some anxiety and anger toward him. When the therapist inquired about her automatic thoughts associated with the negative emotions (as she recorded them in writing at home or as she experienced them during the session), the following exchange took place.

BARBARA: Why didn't this happen before? Why did it take my acting up to get him to pay attention to me?

THERAPIST: What kinds of answers to those questions have occurred to you?

BARBARA: He doesn't take the *initiative* to think about paying attention to me. He just responds to pressure from me. I'm really not that important to him, and if I don't make his life uncomfortable, he just goes along thinking about the other things that are more important to him. If we stopped coming to therapy, or I stopped making an issue of it, his caring behavior would disappear after a while.

THERAPIST: So, it is hard for you to see John's behavior changes as real or lasting, because you attribute them to your pressure rather than some true caring and motivation on his part. John, what do you make of that? It does seem easy for Barbara to draw a conclusion like that, because you do have a pattern of drifting off until she focuses your attention on it.

JOHN: I can see how she could interpret it that way, and I do tend to take things for granted more than she does. However, Barbara is important to me, and I wouldn't be coming here and putting all of this effort into the relationship if I didn't care about it. I think that this work we are doing is making me aware of ways in which I have tuned out for a lot of my life, and ways in which I can remind myself to keep focused more on what is going on in our daily life. I can't guarantee that I won't drift off when I have a lot on my mind, but I am willing to do whatever I can to remember to pay attention to Barbara. I think that I am doing a good job of it already. I hope that she will let me know if she thinks I'm drifting off, as long as she doesn't attack me. She's been approaching me in a much better way lately.

THERAPIST: Barbara, so let's take a look at your inferences about John's motivation and consider what he just said . . .

This is an example of how the therapist attempts to strike a balance between existing evidence that a spouse's attributions have been based at least partially on accurate perceptions of a problem associated with the partner *and* other evidence that the spouse's attributions may fail to take some more positive data into account. The intervention described above also was designed to focus John on his own responsibility for the problematic pattern and his role in the solution.

The cognitive intervention used most frequently to alter the spouses' unrealistic standards for their relationship (e.g., John's standard that they should focus almost exclusively on discussions of pleasant topics) was an examination of the advantages and disadvantages of trying to live according to a particular standard. The therapist avoided suggesting that a spouse's standard was irrational, but instead collaborated with the individual in listing (usually in writing) its pros and cons. By initially focusing on the "good reasons" why the person has adhered to the belief, the therapist tends to reduce the client's defensiveness about examining its drawbacks. For example, although John's standard about focusing on pleasant topics included a number of advantages (e.g., it resulted in some pleasant times together that might balance some of the couple's memories of former difficult times), it had some significant drawbacks as well (e.g., Barbara's frustration about unresolved issues typically built until she blew up).

In general, as John became aware that the avoidance strategy associated with his belief traded short-term tranquility for long-term discord and stress, he began to look at ways in which he could alter his standard, maintaining basic values that were important to him but removing the components that contributed to chronic marital problems. The therapist guided him in rewriting the above standard to read, "We will make a consistent effort to spend time talking about and doing things that make us both feel good, in order to build intimacy and memories of good times together. However, we also will set aside time to listen to any issues that concern our partner, using the expressive and listening skills we learned in therapy. In this way, frustrations will not fester, and the discussions of more unpleasant issues also can be looked back on as 'a job well done' (and in that sense as satisfying experiences, too)."

Barbara and John's long-standing standards about their relationship also were altered significantly through the repeated use of behavioral interventions that demonstrated their ability to interact in more satisfying ways. In fact, Barbara altered her standard concerning ways in which John should demonstrate caring for her, so that she found it less distressing when he was self-absorbed. Whereas she initially believed that he should not even have the desire or impulse to withdraw into solitary activities, what became more important to her was his nondefensive willingness to experiment with time apart and together. As John discovered that he could influence discussions of problems through active participation rather than avoidance, his belief that leisure time should be restricted to talk about pleasant topics was weakened considerably.

TREATMENT SUMMARY

Treatment of the couple consisted of six months of weekly sessions, mostly conjoint, that initially focused more on the behavioral interactions of the couple but increasingly involved systematic challenging of extreme and distorted cognitions. The behavioral interventions used to alter the couple's pattern of aversive exchanges and withdrawal were communication training (expressive and empathic listening skills), assertiveness training, and problem solving aimed at increasing shared leisure activities. Cognitive interventions focused on increasing the spouses' abilities to identify and challenge their own negative attributions, expectancies, and standards concerning the marriage. The behavioral and cognitive interventions were integrated, such that (a) cognitions eliciting resistance to behavior change were altered, and (b) behavioral experiments demonstrating the ability of the couple to interact more positively were used to change long-standing beliefs that the spouses held regarding their marriage.

During the last month of therapy, the couple was seen every two weeks, and two subsequent monthly follow-up sessions were scheduled. Both spouses reported increased satisfaction with their relationship (including John, who had reported a high level of satisfaction when the couple began therapy but later had revealed considerable frustration with the pursue-withdraw pattern that he and Barbara had developed). The behavioral interventions had facilitated notable change in the couple's ability to talk constructively about areas of conflict, and the focus on identifying mutually enjoyable activities had led to increased time together.

DISCUSSION

Although this case is offered as a realistic representation of changes that can be implemented with distressed marriages, it is important to note that the spouses were both still committed to working toward the maintenance of their relationship, and they were both fairly flexible (i.e., open to examining their own roles in the problems). As any marital therapist will attest, a substantial number of couples who begin therapy have less motivation and openness for collaborating toward change than did Barbara and John. Consequently, it is crucial that the therapist carefully assess each spouse's motivation for therapy and spend as much time as is necessary in exploring cognitive sources of resistance. When an individual spouse is very reluctant to work on the marriage due to hopelessness or strong residual anger over past grievances, it may be necessary for the therapist to schedule a number of sessions alone with that person. Such individual sessions can be devoted to examining evidence relevant to the person's hopelessness about potential change, examining the advantages

and disadvantages of clinging to anger and a desire for retribution, or comparing the pros and cons that the client sees in the options of staying in the marriage versus separating.

There are numerous other clinical issues that can arise in work with couples in which the two parties have different "agendas" for therapy (e.g., the difficult question of whether the therapist should be open to keeping secrets with each spouse) that are beyond the scope of the present discussion. Furthermore, marital therapy appears to have considerable promise for spouses who are both clinically depressed and maritally distressed (Beach, Sandeen, O'Leary, 1990), but it involves a variety of special clinical assessment and intervention issues beyond those described here. Nevertheless, the basic principles outlined in this chapter concerning the implementation of behavioral and cognitive interventions appear to have wide applicability with distressed couples who present with a range of chronic and acute relationship problems.

REFERENCES

Abrahms, J. L., & Spring, M. (1989). The flip-flop factor. *International Cognitive Therapy Newsletter, 5*(1), pp. 1, 7–8.

Baucom, D. H., & Epstein, N. (1990). *Cognitive-behavioral marital therapy.* New York: Brunner/Mazel.

Baucom, D. H., Sayers, S. L., & Sher, T. G. (1990). Supplementing behavioral marital therapy with cognitive restructuring and emotional expressiveness training: An outcome investigation. *Journal of Consulting and Clinical Psychology, 58,* 636–645.

Beach, S. R. H., Sandeen, E. E., & O'Leary, K. D. (1990). *Depression in marriage: A model for etiology and treatment.* New York: Guilford.

Beck, A. T., Rush, A. J., Shaw, B. F., & Emery, G. (1979). *Cognitive therapy of depression.* New York: Guilford.

Behrens, B. C., Sanders, M. R., & Halford, W. K. (1990). Behavioral marital therapy: An evaluation of treatment effects across high and low risk settings. *Behavior Therapy, 21,* 423–433.

Bradbury, T. N., & Fincham, F. D. (1990). Attributions in marriage: Review and critique. *Psychological Bulletin, 107,* 3–33.

Fincham, F. D., Bradbury, T. N., & Scott, C. K. (1990). Cognition in marriage. In F. D. Fincham & T. N. Bradbury (Eds.), *The psychology of marriage: Basic issues and applications* (pp. 118–149). New York: Guilford.

Guerney, B. G., Jr. (1977). *Relationship enhancement.* San Francisco: Jossey-Bass.

Leslie, L. A. (1988). Cognitive-behavioral and systems models of family therapy: How compatible are they? In N. Epstein, S. E. Schlesinger, & W. Dryden (Eds.), *Cognitive-behavioral therapy with families* (pp. 49–83). New York: Brunner/Mazel.

Pretzer, J. L., Epstein, N., & Fleming, B. (1991). The Marital Attitude Survey: A measure of dysfunctional attributions and expectancies. *Journal of Cognitive Psychotherapy: An International Quarterly, 5,* 131–148.

SUGGESTED READINGS

Baucom, D. H., & Epstein, N. (1990). *Cognitive-behavioral marital therapy*. New York: Brunner/Mazel.

Beck, A. T. (1988). *Love is never enough*. New York: Harper & Row.

Dattilio, F. M., & Padesky, C. A. (1990). *Cognitive therapy with couples*. Sarasota, FL: Professional Resource Exchange.

Epstein, N. (1986). Cognitive marital therapy: Multi-level assessment and intervention. *Journal of Rational-Emotive Therapy*, *4*, 68–81.

Epstein, N., & Baucom, D. H. (1989). Cognitive-behavioral marital therapy. In A. Freeman, K. M. Simon, L. E. Beutler, & H. Arkowitz (Eds.), *Comprehensive handbook of cognitive therapy* (pp. 491–513). New York: Plenum.

29

Hypnotherapy

E. Thomas Dowd

INTRODUCTION

Hypnosis is a multifaceted adjunct treatment that is useful in overcoming a wide variety of psychological disorders. However, it should be emphasized that hypnosis is an adjunct procedure only, and is not by itself a therapy (Dowd & Healy, 1986). Thus, hypnosis should always be integrated within a more general psychological treatment plan and should not be used alone. For that reason, I will refer to the psychological procedures described in this chapter as *hypnotherapy*.

Psychological problems can sometimes be alleviated by direct suggestion, that is, by suggesting to the client while in a trance that their symptoms will disappear or be reduced. However, hypnosis in psychological treatment more commonly involves the use of indirect suggestion. In indirect suggestion, the hypnotherapist suggests to the client that they may wish to consider changing a problem behavior, that their symptoms might be reduced, or that they might become more comfortable in the future. The emphasis in indirect suggestion is on the creation of an open-ended, ambiguous hypnotic situation in which the

client is presented with many options for change. The likelihood that the client will resist the hypnotherapist's change attempts is thus significantly reduced, since there is little to resist. The hypnotherapist may also wish to use Erickson, Rossi, and Rossi's (1976) utilization approach, in which any association or mental process that the client brings to therapy is used in service of client change. In this approach, whatever response the client makes may be interpreted as therapeutic change.

Hypnotherapy, especially as used in cognitive-behavioral therapy (Golden, Dowd, & Friedberg, 1987), often involves the treatment of a psychological problem in its present context. Thus, the hypnotherapeutic treatment of anxiety, pain, or depression would focus on its current manifestations rather than on its etiology or past expression. However, there are occasions when the historical background of a particular problem exercises significant control over its current expression. In these cases, problem resolution is accomplished faster and better if the historical and developmental antecedents are dealt with. Hypnotic age regression is ideally suited for this. In age regression, the client is enabled to remember in vivid detail an earlier time in life, often with accompanying cognitive and emotional reactions appropriate to the earlier episode.

The case described in this chapter illustrates all of the above phenomena. In particular, it illustrates the value of a developmental and historical approach to current cognitive restructuring. This cognitive developmental hypnotherapeutic procedure enabled Linda to overcome her fear of the dark.

E. Thomas Dowd • Department of Educational Psychology, Kent State University, Kent, Ohio 44242-0001.

Comprehensive Casebook of Cognitive Therapy, edited by Arthur Freeman and Frank M. Dattilio. Plenum Press, New York, 1992.

Linda came to see me because she had heard that I did hypnotherapy and thought it might be of benefit to her. I should note that it is somewhat common for hypnotherapists to receive (or be referred) clients who essentially prescribe their own treatment. The therapist is then faced with a delicate task: to refuse to use that modality and risk losing the client or to use it and allow the client to prescribe his or her own treatment. This problem is exacerbated by the common belief that hypnosis is a quasi-magical technique that will eliminate entrenched problems with little or no client effort.

Linda was a 35-year-old female with a history of multiple problems, including alcoholism, drug abuse, and low self-esteem. She had spent 1½ years in an alcoholism rehabilitation program and had received additional therapy as well. She felt that she had dealt successfully with a number of her psychological problems, but had recently become aware of how much she was afraid of the dark and how much that had actually affected her life. She stated that she was both afraid of the dark and afraid of things in the dark. When she couldn't see everything, she felt helpless and alone and was afraid that someone might "get her." Previous psychotherapy had resolved several problems, and now she wanted to work on this one.

PROBLEM ASSESSMENT

The client's symptoms followed a repetitive and predictable pattern. She felt quite anxious at night, both at home and away from home, especially if she were alone. She particularly feared walking outside in the dark. When night fell, she made elaborate checks of the locks on her doors and windows at home to ensure that they were securely locked. She repeated this pattern when she went to bed; failure to do so led to extreme anxiety. At first, she preferred to sleep nearest the door (for control). Generally, however, she would wake up during the night, often screaming, and then would want her roommate between her and the door (for protection).

Interview assessment revealed the following family background: Linda's mother and father were both dead, her father having died when she was 4 years old. She had a sister (18 years older) and a brother (10 years older). Her mother had been ill for many years, and Linda had been her primary caregiver. Linda reported that she never really had a childhood and lived in constant fear of her mother becoming sick. She had a warm and close relationship with her mother, although she was never really disciplined. She did not remember her father, but had heard reports that he had been a peacemaker among other family

members. Her relationship with her siblings was described as cordial but distant. In response to my questioning, she expressed the thought that her brother, brother-in-law, nephew, and grandfather were all alcoholics.

Interview assessment also revealed the following personal characteristics: Linda described herself as a "survivor," and stated that it was very important that she remain in control of herself and situations at all times. If not, she said that other people would then be able to control her. She described herself as tense and anxious, with strong perfectionistic tendencies. In her relations with friends, she tended to give more to them than she received, and as a result ended up feeling resentful and used. She was "always there for her friends." Childhood sexual exploration was punished severely by her mother, and she was raped as a teenager by a cousin. She felt until recently that she was to blame for the rape because she did not fight it; now she felt that she did not fight it because she felt worthless and deserving of such treatment. Her relationships with men historically had been poor.

DIAGNOSIS

The client's excessive caregiving activities appeared to result from her strong need for control and from her alcoholic family background (Lawson, Peterson, & Lawson, 1983). As a result, her interpersonal relations were distant and rigid. Perhaps as a result of her early sexual experiences, she appeared to have a strong ambivalence about intimate relationships, viewing them as potentially threatening to her sense of control. There appeared to be a paradoxical reciprocal relationship between intimate relationships and self-esteem. Her poor self-esteem led her to select individuals who treated her badly, thus confirming her self-impression as an unworthy person.

There appeared to be several tacit cognitive assumptions that guided the client's behavior. Her subsequent behavior then confirmed and reinforced the original cognitive assumptions, thus preventing any incorporation of new data into the existing cognitive structure (Carmin & Dowd, 1988; Guidano, 1987). The assumptions were:

- "If I am in control, then I can protect myself."
- "If I am or appear weak, others will take advantage of me."
- "I am helpless relative to other people."
- "Other people cannot be trusted."
- "I am not worthy of being well thought of by others or of having good friends."

TREATMENT

I saw Linda for a total of nine sessions. The first session and much of the second were devoted to problem assessment and diagnosis. Subsequent sessions were devoted to problem exploration and hypnotherapy.

Session 1 (Initial Trance Assessment)

People differ significantly in susceptibility to hypnosis, that is, in their ability to achieve a given level of trance and to experience various hypnotic phenomena (Bowers, 1976; Udolf, 1981). Therefore, it is important to assess each subject for hypnotic susceptibility or, as I prefer, trance capacity. Individuals who possess a greater trance capacity and who are therefore capable of achieving a greater level of trance generally benefit more from hypnotherapy than do those who have less trance capacity. However, motivation to change is also an important factor in the success of hypnotherapy (as, indeed, in all psychotherapy!) and should be assessed as well. Therefore I conducted a simple arm levitation (Udolf, 1981), which she performed satisfactorily. Although she reported that she felt that she was in a trance, she was quite concerned if she had "done it correctly." I told her that everyone experiences trance somewhat differently and that a concern with correct performance would reduce the chances of experiencing trance. I should note that this type of concern is quite common and should be addressed early if the individual is to have a successful trance experience.

Session 2

Part of this session was devoted to exploration of family background. Linda reported that she woke up screaming one night during the last week. She also reported a common dream, that she is running but cannot move. In this dream, she is afraid that someone is after her, but she cannot attach a face or an identity to this person. A topic of exploration during this session was Linda's strong need for control. Because she had proved to be a good hypnotic subject during the first session and because of the apparent centrality of this issue for her, I decided to employ a hypnotherapeutic technique to address this problem.

I used a progressive relaxation induction technique with Linda (Wright & Wright, 1987). Because this technique is quite similar to that employed in systematic desensitization and stress management, it is relatively nonthreatening. In addition, it is difficult to fail at relaxation, so the client is immediately provided with a success experience. In hypnotherapy, it is important to arrange successful trance inductions so that clients will not feel that they have failed, to the detriment of their motivation or the hypnotherapist's credibility. After Linda was in a trance, I conducted a cognitive restructuring hypnotic routine involving the paradoxical situation of increasing control by relinquishing control. Following is a sample of that routine.

> Being in control has been important for you for many years . . . however, you have never really felt in control, isn't that right? (client nods) So, the more you try to be in control, the less you feel in control; the harder you try, the more you fail. Isn't that interesting? (client nods) So, what you have been trying isn't working, right? Perhaps you may be ready to try something new. Being in control is like falling asleep; the harder you try, the less you succeed . . . I would like to suggest to you that the only way you can truly be in control is to allow yourself to give up control. That's right! Only someone who is truly in control can afford to give up control. But remember, you only give up control for a little while, and then you can take it back any time you wish . . . so that you can practice obtaining ultimate control by practicing giving up temporary control . . . and you can feel more in control by practicing being less in control; find increasing comfort in giving up control temporarily . . . feeling more comfortable knowing you can take back control anytime you want.

Since she was a good hypnotic subject, I suggested that Linda would be able to remember only one or two things that I said (partial posthypnotic amnesia). I did this to test the level of trance depth she had achieved (posthypnotic amnesia is characteristic of deeper trance levels), but leaving her the option of remembering one or two things to avoid the possibility of failure. She had no subsequent remembrance of anything I had said, indicating a moderate to deep trance level. I asked her to keep a record the next week of incidences in which she woke up during the night. I also asked her to practice self-hypnosis when she felt fearful, telling herself that her fears were groundless.

Session 3

Linda stated that she had awakened during the night on three different occasions during the week. The first time, she went right back to sleep; the second time, she insisted on changing places with her roommate to be farther from the door. The third time, she woke up and screamed. Otherwise, she reported that she had felt unusually comfortable and relaxed during the week.

We explored Linda's need for control. She stated that if she was in control, she could protect herself. If she was not, she had to trust other people, which was very difficult for her to do. She also stated that she despised weakness in herself and others.

In an attempt to recover her memories of the origin of her fear of the dark, I employed age regression. This technique, useful for good hypnotic subjects, involves a progressive movement back in time, during which the individual may remember previous events with exceptional clarity and detail. There are a variety of age regression techniques; I used calendar imaging. A partial transcript follows.

> I would like you to imagine a calendar in front of you. As I begin to count off the years, I would like you to imagine the pages of the calendar flipping back and yourself going back in time. You will continue going back until you come to a time of special significance for your fear of the dark. When you come to that time, please raise the index finger of your right hand. It is now March 1986. It is now 1985, 1984, 1983, 1982, 1981, 1980 . . . 1960, 1957, 1956 . . . (client raises finger) Good; now I'm going to count backwards by month; raise your finger when I come to the month that has special significance for your problem. December, November, October, September . . . (client raises finger) Good; now tell me what you see.

While in the trance, Linda said that she was 3 years old and was very much afraid of a dark cellar. Further questioning indicated that an older cousin would take her into the cellar, turn off the light, and proceed to terrify her. She would then run up the stairs screaming. When she came out of the trance, she stated that the cellar memory was new to her.

Session 4

Linda reported that she woke up only two nights during the previous week, both times without screaming. She continued to check the doors and locks at night, but did not seem to feel quite as much anxiety. During the week, she had remembered a further incident with the cellar. Her cousin's sister and the sister's boyfriend would take her to the cellar and turn off the light. Linda recalled the anticipatory fear of the light being turned off.

It appeared that Linda's current fear of the dark and related feelings were being influenced by her experiences in the cellar at age 3. Accordingly, I decided to provide a cognitive restructuring of her early memories and fears of being in the dark cellar in an adult context. I used the previously described age regression to bring her once again to 1956. While she was in a trance, I asked her to describe the emotions she experienced regarding the events in the cellar. She reported that she felt panicky, helpless, and out of control. In order to restructure her

childhood thoughts and feelings in an adult context, I used the following hypnotic routine.

> Young people, because they are small and weak, feel helpless and scared because bigger people seem so much more powerful . . . perhaps you feel that way, too . . . As we grow older we become bigger, stronger, and more powerful. Often, however, the old feelings of fear remain; perhaps you feel that way, too. We sometimes don't realize, do we, that we eventually become the person who once seemed so big and so important to us. We still feel like the frightened, helpless child . . . but we need not fear as adults the things we feared as children.

This last sentence was repeated like a refrain as the above hypnotic routine was progressively elaborated and repeated. After leaving the trance, Linda said that she had not realized before how her childhood fears had carried over into her adult life. We discussed how similar the thoughts, feelings, and behavior of her childhood cellar experience were to her adult fears of the dark, particularly regarding her strong need for control as providing a sense of safety and security.

Session 5

A month elapsed between this session and the previous one, since Linda was on vacation. During the vacation, she had visited her family and had become aware for the first time how alone she was. She had become aware that she no longer felt an integral part of her family. She felt she had become more "disorganized," whereas her life was previously very tightly organized and structured. She woke up screaming at night only once during this time, and was only aware of it because her roommate had told her the following morning. She reported that she now felt frightened at night only in her own home.

We discussed at length her emerging understanding that home had never been a secure and safe place for her, either in childhood or now. I reframed her concern over her increasing disorganization and her feelings of separation from her family as steps on the path toward growth and adulthood. Whereas previously she needed excessive control and organization in her life to feel safe, increasingly she was able to tolerate some disorganization and disarray. I suggested that she practice feeling comfortable with periodic disorganization, knowing that she could reestablish control whenever she wished.

Session 6

Linda reported not feeling quite as alone as she did the last week. She woke up screaming only once during the week. She also had been reconsidering her relationship with her roommate, feeling that she really didn't need her as much anymore, and was able to discuss with her the possibility of a breakup. She reported some concern about this detachment from her roommate, as she saw it as similar to her detachment from her family. I reframed this as an increasing independence from others that was part of adulthood.

I reviewed with Linda the gains she had made to this point:

1. She was not "hitting the panic button" nearly as much.
2. She was not waking up at night screaming as much.
3. She was not nearly as afraid of the dark as formerly. When she still had fears of the dark, she was able to tell herself that those fears were groundless and then feel better.
4. She appeared to be reevaluating a number of her relationships with others in terms of what she wanted rather than in terms of what she needed. I interpreted her feelings of aloneness and detachment as moving from needing relationships to wanting them.

Linda agreed that she had a tendency to catastrophize about problems in her life and to want immediate change. I suggested that she view the current changes in her life as indicators of growth.

Linda traced many of her current feelings to the hypnosis induction two sessions earlier. At that time, she reported feeling "like a stone," which was a helpless feeling for her. Since she wanted to understand her past reactions more, I did another age regression, counting backwards (at her suggestion) by age. This was similar to the calendar imagery described earlier, but I counted backwards by year (35 years of age, 34, 33, etc.) until she signaled me to stop at age 20 by raising her finger. At age 20, her mother died and Linda was involved in a relationship with a female teacher, resulting in feelings of love, hate, dirtiness, and anger. She reported, while in the trance, that she felt she needed this female friend to take care of her and protect her. At this time she was raped by her cousin, and her female friend was helpful to her. When Linda came out of the trance, we discussed these past feelings and incidents in light of her current situation.

Session 7

Linda reported that she did not wake up screaming at all during the last week. She realized, after the last session, that she had for a long time experienced a strong need to have someone care for her. During her adolescent years, she became increasingly unsure of her ability to

cope with adult responsibilities. Even mundane tasks began to overwhelm her. She had now begun to realize that this tacit assumption still governed her life.

After she was raped, Linda began to gain weight. She had become dissatisfied with her excessive weight, but was also afraid to lose it. We discussed the function her weight might have served in keeping her unattractive and therefore safe from the attention of men. We also discussed her self-deprecating tendencies and her rather brusque exterior as a coping strategy for keeping people away from her until she felt that she could trust them. She did admit that she was reluctant to allow people to become emotionally close to her and would only do so when she felt such trust; this did not happen often. She reported that it was very frightening for her to think of herself as "attractive."

Session 8

Linda reported that she woke up screaming one night last week, but had almost no panic at all. In addition, her roommate had been gone for several days, and Linda was not afraid of the dark while home alone as she would have been previously. She thought that both of these incidents represented real therapeutic breakthroughs. She had been reevaluating her life goals and orientation and said that other people had commented that she seemed much calmer and apparently was happier. She had a new realization of how much self-deprecation she had engaged in for not being perfect.

In order to elicit and explore more fully Linda's feelings and cognitions regarding important events in her past life, I did another age regression, counting backwards by age as in the previous example. I instructed her to raise her finger when she came to an age that she wanted to explore and understand better; she signaled me to stop at ages 20, 17, 14, 11, and 4. She described the critical incidents at each age, along with associated thoughts and feelings. General themes described included:

- A feeling of desperately needing a significant other, and using her body to meet this need
- Not knowing how to say no to sexual overtures because of the above need
- Feelings of being taken advantage of sexually, but withholding final tacit acquiescence
- Feelings of loss when her father died when she was 4 (she reported feeling much happier and having her emotional needs met much better before her father died)

When Linda came out of the trance, she indicated that her mother had never recovered from her father's death. She therefore had lost not only the emotional support of her father but that of her mother as well, since the latter became very self-absorbed. We discussed Linda's apparent searching throughout her life for the emotional closeness that she had lost with her father's death. This loss had occurred before she was able to verbalize it, thus perhaps leading to a tacit and little-understand search for intimacy and support. At the same time, however, the desperate quality of this search led her to be vulnerable to exploitation by unscrupulous others. Thus, she learned that, while she needed intimacy and closeness, her trust would be betrayed, and therefore she could not trust others to meet her needs. Because of this, her striving toward intimacy was characterized by deep ambivalence.

Session 9

This was Linda's last session and we summarized the gains made in therapy. She reported that she no longer woke up screaming and was rarely afraid of the dark. When she started to become fearful, she was able to reduce it by using self-talk to the effect that her fear was a product of her childhood and was no longer relevant to her adult life. Her friends and colleagues saw her as much less tense, anxious, and driven. She felt happier with her life and was reevaluating her sexual identity. She stated that she had no idea that early events could affect people in the way that they apparently did her.

I encouraged her to contact me again if she felt her problems recurring. She never did and apparently maintained her gains.

SUMMARY

As the reader can see from the above description, a number of different interventions were implemented. First, hypnotherapy was used to elicit the early traumatic incidents in the client's life that underlay her presenting problem, fear of the dark. Second, hypnotherapy was used to assist the client in identifying the tacit assumptions about people underlying the presenting problem. Third, hypnotherapy was also used to enable the client to relive the original emotionality associated with the early traumatic events. Fourth, these hypnotherapeutic sessions were interspersed with discussion sessions designed to help her cognitively and emotionally distance herself from her stated problem (Beck, 1976) by providing a new perspective on it. She was encouraged to view her problem as originating in childhood incidents and having little relevance for her adult life. She was also taught self-talk

coping statements, which she was able to use successfully to reduce her fear of the dark when feeling afraid.

Linda realized several therapeutic gains, not all of which were overtly dealt with in therapy. These outcomes were as follows:

1. Loss of her fear of the dark and disappearance of associated screaming behavior at night
2. Development of self-talk coping strategies
3. New awareness of the power of early events in shaping subsequent behavior, cognition, and emotional responses
4. Better relations with other people
5. Beginning of an exploration of sexuality and sexual identity

DISCUSSION

There are several noteworthy features about this case. First, hypnotherapeutic sessions were alternated with discussion sessions, in which the material elicited in one became the basis for integration in the other. This is quite typical of hypnotherapy. As I mentioned earlier, hypnosis is an adjunct treatment, not a complete treatment. Therefore, it should be integrated into an overall treatment package.

Second, Linda began dealing with life issues that were never the focus of therapy at all—in particular, her sexual identity. I have found that this "ripple effect" is quite common in hypnotherapy, where material elicited under hypnosis is reevaluated and examined not only in succeeding therapy sessions, but in other aspects of the client's life. Milton Erickson, in particular, has described numerous instances of single hypnotherapeutic interventions that have had significant and unexpected effects on the client's life. Of course, this can occur in other forms of psychotherapy as well, but in my experience it is more likely to occur in hypnotherapy.

Third, early experiences were found to have had a significant impact on the client's current functioning. Interventions directed only at current problems can often have a palliative effect, but sometimes fall short of the changes that can result when developmental antecedents of problems are uncovered and understood, and symptoms can then be put into proper perspective. This developmental history is often obtained by verbal exploration, but can sometimes be obtained faster and more completely by hypnotic procedures, which tend to bypass resistance.

I want to caution the reader, however, that hypnotic techniques such as age regression and posthypnotic amnesia are efficacious only with individuals who possess a high level of trance capacity. While most people can be hypnotized to some extent, only certain individuals are capable of "deeper" levels of trance phenomena. Therapists who wish to use hypnosis in their clinical practice are urged to obtain specialized training.

REFERENCES

Beck, A. T. (1976). *Cognitive therapy and the emotional disorders*. New York: International Universities Press.

Bowers, K. S. (1976). *Hypnosis for the seriously curious*. New York: Norton.

Carmin, C. N., & Dowd, E. T. (1988). Paradigms in cognitive psychotherapy. In W. Dryden & P. Trower (Eds.), *Developments in cognitive psychotherapy*. London: Sage.

Dowd, E. T., & Healy, J. M. (1986). *Case studies in hypnotherapy*. New York: Guilford.

Erickson, M. H., Rossi, E. L., & Rossi, S. I. (1976). *Hypnotic realities*. New York: Irvington.

Golden, W. L., Dowd, E. T., & Friedberg, F. (1987). *Hypno therapy: A modern approach*. New York: Pergamon.

Guidano, V. F. (1987). *Complexity of the self: A developmental approach to psychopathology and therapy*. New York: Guilford.

Lawson, G. W., Peterson, J. S., & Lawson, A. (1983). *Alcoholism and the family: A guide to treatment and prevention*. Rockville, MD: Aspen.

Udolf, R. (1981). *Handbook of hypnosis for professionals*. New York: Van Nostrand Reinhold.

Wright, M. E., & Wright, B. A. (1987). *Clinical practice of hypnotherapy*. New York: Guilford.

SUGGESTED READINGS

Crasilneck, H. B., & Hall, J. A. (1985). *Clinical hypnosis: Principles and applications*. New York: Grune & Stratton.

Dowd, E. T., & Healy, J. M. (1986). *Case studies in hypnotherapy*. New York: Guilford.

Golden, W. L., Dowd, E. T., & Friedberg, F. (1987). *Hypnotherapy: A modern approach*. New York: Pergamon.

Wester, W. C., & Smith, A. H. (1984). *Clinical hypnosis: A multidisciplinary approach*. Philadelphia: J. B. Lippincott.

30

Combined Cognitive Therapy and Pharmacotherapy of Depression

Jesse H. Wright

Cognitive therapy and pharmacotherapy have originated from competing etiological theories of mental disorders. However, they are frequently used together in treatment of a wide variety of clinical conditions (Wright, 1987; Wright & Schrodt, 1989). This case report will illustrate how different forms of therapy can complement one another in the treatment of severe depression.

CASE REPORT

Mrs. Keene, a 32-year-old housewife, was brought to the emergency room by her husband after she threatened suicide. She had been depressed for the previous two months. Mrs. Keene had been receiving intensive, psychodynamically oriented therapy; in addition, a tricyclic antidepressant (nortriptyline) had been prescribed by her family doctor. These treatments had failed to reverse the course of a steadily worsening depression. During the

Jesse H. Wright • Department of Psychiatry and Behavioral Sciences, University of Louisville School of Medicine, Louisville, Kentucky 40292 and Norton Psychiatric Clinic, 200 East Chestnut Street, Louisville, Kentucky 40232.

Comprehensive Casebook of Cognitive Therapy, edited by Arthur Freeman and Frank M. Dattilio. Plenum Press, New York, 1992.

initial evaluation, Mrs. Keene reported that "my family would be better off with me dead."

BACKGROUND INFORMATION

Mrs. Keene was the second of two children of an upper-middle-class Kentucky family. Her early childhood was described as "perfect." Mother and father were depicted as loving individuals who "could do no wrong." Her older brother was a star athlete and top student who received a scholarship to a prestigious university. Mrs. Keene's father was a self-made man who extolled the virtues of hard work and moral integrity. Her mother was a quiet person who "sacrificed" herself for the family. They attended the Baptist church regularly.

Although Mrs. Keene's initial recollections of her family were extremely positive, she later identified several problems. Her father had been excessively demanding of himself and others and had been prone to long periods of melancholia. He died of cancer at age 58, four years prior to the onset of Mrs. Keene's depression. Her paternal grandfather also suffered from depression. Other family members remembered her grandfather as having severe mood swings, including periods of hyperactivity and euphoria. He committed suicide shortly after retirement as a college professor. There was no family history of alcohol or drug abuse.

Memories of peer relationships and school experiences indicated that Mrs. Keene suffered from low self-esteem at an early age. When she compared herself to her classmates, she concluded that she was "dumb and ugly." This contrasted with her family members' report that she was a friendly, engaging, and attractive child who was an above-average student. Despite this, she became convinced that she would be unable to make it through college or obtain a good job.

Mrs. Keene's first year at a state university confirmed her worst fears. She couldn't force herself to study, because she thought that it was "no use." For a few weeks she was able to escape into a vigorous social life, but she soon became depressed and stopped attending classes on a regular basis. Halfway through the second semester, she dropped out and returned home. Mrs. Keene had symptoms of major depression at this time; unfortunately, she did not receive treatment.

After about three months, Mrs. Keene was feeling well enough to get a job as a lifeguard. She remembered this period of her life as a "high." All of her academic troubles were forgotten. Her spirits soared. She looked great with a deep tan, and she received much attention from her boyfriends. There was an elevated mood, a quickened pace of activity, and a decreased need for sleep at that time, but the symptoms did not escalate into an overt mania.

Within two years, Mrs. Keene was married and pregnant with her first child. Her husband had recently graduated from college and had returned to Kentucky to help manage a large family business. They were reasonably happy during the first years of their marriage. Mrs. Keene was satisfied with her role as mother of a growing family, while Mr. Keene devoted himself to establishing his career. They had four children within the first eight years of the marriage.

By the time she was 30, Mrs. Keene knew that she was in trouble. Her daughter, Tracy, the oldest child, had been having severe outbursts at school and had even threatened suicide. The second child, Jack, still had enuresis at age 7. Her two preschoolers, Sally and Ted, needed a great deal of attention. Mr. Keene was becoming more absorbed with his work. She wondered if he could be having an affair.

During the year before her hospitalization, Mrs. Keene became preoccupied with her shortcomings as a wife, mother, and woman. She was convinced that Mr. Keene would soon ask for a divorce, even though he had given no signs that he was about to leave. Blame for her children's problems was turned inward because she believed that deficient mothering skills had led to the difficulties. As she looked at herself, all Mrs. Keene could see

was an incompetent, failed housewife who was trapped in an unsolvable situation.

ASSESSMENT AND DIAGNOSIS

The principal method of assessment was a series of intensive diagnostic interviews conducted by the therapist during the first three days of Mrs. Keene's hospitalization. History taking and early cognitive-behavioral interventions were combined in these initial interviews. A family-systems evaluation was completed by the inpatient unit social worker. In addition, records of psychological evaluations of two of the children were obtained, and a conference was held with Tracy Keene's therapist.

The Beck Depression Inventory (Beck, Ward, Mendelson, Mock, & Erbaugh, 1969) and the Hopelessness Scale (Beck, Weissman, Lester, & Trexler, 1974) were given on admission and weekly thereafter. Baseline scores were 37 for the BDI (severe depression) and 19 for the Hopelessness Scale (marked hopelessness). A Medication Attitude Survey developed by the author (Wright, 1989) was used to elicit cognitions about taking medications. Medical history, physical exam, and laboratory studies, including neuroendocrine testing, were also performed. The only significant finding of these examinations was a subtherapeutic plasma level of nortriptyline (15 ng/ml).

TREATMENT

Session 1

The majority of the initial session was spent on the patient's description of her current problems and her background history. Two critical themes emerged that served as entry points for combined cognitive therapy and pharmacotherapy. The first was a profound sense of hopelessness that pervaded virtually all of her perceptions of past, present, and future. The hopelessness was associated with intense suicidal ideation, including having a plan to crash her car into a tree. The second theme was her belief that it was unacceptable to show vulnerability. This was expressed in a number of different ways, such as "I should be able to do this on my own"; "If you have trouble, put on a smile and just keep going"; and "I must be strong." These dysfunctional underlying schemas, identified in the first session, were having several deleterious effects. The schemas accentuated the hopelessness and also were interfering with therapeutic attempts. She had only partially adhered to the medication schedule outlined by her family doctor, and (under pressure from her husband) had gone begrudgingly to outpatient psychotherapy. Now she was talking about being released from the hospital.

Therapeutic work with severely depressed inpatients usually begins at the behavioral level (Thase & Wright, 1991). However, in this case the therapist concluded that changes in fixed depressogenic cognitions would be required in order to forge an effective working relationship with the patient and to reduce her serious risk for suicide. In the first session, the approach was structured and psychoeducational.

After eliciting the patient's history, the therapist observed that Mrs. Keene had a style of thinking that is common in depressed patients and that she also had the physiological changes of depression. A simplified psychobiological model for depression was then described.

THERAPIST: In many ways, the psychological and biological parts of depression seem to play on one another. Nonstop worries take a toll on your body. You're churning all day and most of the night, so your body doesn't get the rest it needs. Being depleted physically also has an effect on your ability to cope with your worries. You just don't have your normal physical resources to use in solving your problems.

MRS. KEENE: Yes. That's me. That's why I've given up. I'm exhausted both mentally and physically. I just can't go on any longer.

THERAPIST: The most important question is what can be done when a person gets into this state. Would you like to hear about some of the possibilities?

MRS. KEENE: Yes, if you think it might help.

THERAPIST: Let's take a look at them together, and then we can decide what to do.

MRS. KEENE: OK.

The therapist then briefly described cognitive and biological interventions as a combined method of treatment. Specific observations were made to relate both cognitive and biological strategies to Mrs. Keene's situation. A comprehensive, integrated approach was emphasized (Wright, 1988; Wright & Beck, 1983; Wright & Schrodt, 1989).

MRS. KEENE: I appreciate hearing about how treatment works. I guess I never got much of an idea of what to expect from my other therapy. But I'm still not sure I want to stay here and go through all of this. Couldn't I just go home and try to manage? I should be able to snap out of this if I really tried.

THERAPIST: What you have just said is a good example of how thinking gets twisted in depression. Would you be willing to look at your thinking to see if it could help you feel better?

MRS. KEENE: I guess so.

THERAPIST: Good. Then let me just read back to you a couple of things you've said today so we can understand how you are thinking. You described yourself this way: "If you have trouble, put on a smile and keep going." Then just a moment ago, you said: "I should be able to snap out of this if I really tried." What are you telling me when you say these things?

MRS. KEENE: I guess I'm saying that I shouldn't have problems, or if I have them, I shouldn't let it show. You know, I should be able to take care of these problems on my own.

At this point, the therapist explained the nature of silent assumptions, or schemas. He then asked Mrs. Keene to consider how these assumptions could be having a destructive effect.

THERAPIST: How does it make you feel when you have problems you can't seem to control, like the ones you described with your children?

MRS. KEENE: Terrible. I feel like a total failure, and I don't see any way out.

THERAPIST: This is an example of how a schema can box you into a corner. You must not have problems at all; if you do have problems, then somehow you must erase them completely on your own. If you can't do this, then what?

MRS. KEENE: I keep trying for a while until it looks impossible, then I give up.

THERAPIST: Is that when you start to think of suicide?

MRS. KEENE: Yes.

THERAPIST: It looks like we've found one situation in which your attitudes have had negative consequences. They even drove you to consider suicide. Do you think there might be others?

MRS. KEENE: I don't know. Do you?

THERAPIST: Well, let's consider how these attitudes might affect treatment for depression. If you think you should be able to do it on your own, how do you view taking medication or receiving psychotherapy?

MRS. KEENE: Yes, I see what you mean now. I never accepted the idea of taking drugs. In fact, I skipped a lot of doses of the antidepressant, and I really never got into the psychotherapy either.

THERAPIST: We don't yet know how you developed these beliefs. We'll try to understand more about this through the course of treatment. But for the time being, the most important thing is to realize that these attitudes or beliefs are only assumptions. They may or may not be completely accurate. How does this sound to you?

MRS. KEENE: Yes, I can see how they have gotten me into deep water. I've shut off people who have tried to help. I guess if I could have done it on my own, I would have already been better.

THERAPIST: No one really wants to be depressed. You have been trying hard, but when depression sets in, medications and therapy are usually needed. The best method is a team approach that combines the efforts of the patient, the therapist, and the medication in the fight against depression. We need to give you tools that you can use in recovery.

MRS. KEENE: That sounds good to me.

The remainder of the initial session was spent on charting a general plan for treatment. It was decided to discuss pharmacotherapy in detail at the next session. Mrs. Keene also was asked to read *Coping with Depression* (Beck & Greenberg, 1974) and to complete several rating scales (Beck Depression Inventory, Hopelessness Scale, Medication Attitude Scale) as a homework assignment.

Session 2

The agenda for the second session included a homework review, further history taking, and a decision on medication. The session began with a review of the ratings on the Beck Depression Inventory (BDI) and Hopelessness Scale; the Medication Attitude Scale rating was reserved for later use. A discussion of *Coping with Depression* helped to socialize the patient to the cognitive therapy method.

The middle section of session 2 was devoted to collecting additional history. The focus was on getting a clear picture of the manifestations of depression experienced by Mrs. Keene and her family members. It was explained that this information would play a significant role in decisions about medication. As noted in the background information section, Mrs. Keene had a mild hypomanic episode after her first depression. She also had a family history of bipolar disorder. As these data surfaced, the therapist used psychoeducational procedures to help Mrs. Keene understand the different forms and treatments of depression.

They then began to explore Mrs. Keene's cognitions about medications. She had completed the Medication Attitude Scale, a 20-item questionnaire that is comprised of 10 negative and 10 positive statements (e.g., "Medications are a crutch"; "I am always the one to get side effects"; "Medication will improve my ability to concentrate") about medication. Although she had endorsed more negative than positive attitudes, her answers were not uniform. For example, she indicated that she might be able to concentrate better if she were on medication. She admitted this attitude had changed since the first therapy

session, in which she learned about the psychobiology of depression.

The ratings on the Medication Attitude Scale were used as a springboard for initiating cognitive-behavioral procedures to enhance the biological component of treatment. The therapist explained the concept of negative automatic thoughts and observed that the prescription of medication might set off a volley of automatic thinking.

THERAPIST: Now imagine that your doctor has suggested that you take an antidepressant and has just handed you the prescription. What are you thinking?

MRS. KEENE: That I don't want this. I don't want anyone to know.

THERAPIST: Any more thoughts?

MRS. KEENE: Yes; I feel weak. I don't want to be dependent. Maybe I'll get hooked.

THERAPIST: Now let's see how accurate these thoughts are.

Guided discovery, a basic cognitive therapy technique, was then used to uncover the arbitrary and dysfunctional nature of Mrs. Keene's automatic thinking about taking medication. This material was used to identify cognitive errors such as absolutistic thinking, selective abstraction, and personalization (Beck, Rush, Shaw, & Emery, 1979). The homework assignment related to this topic was to complete a four-column thought record (event, automatic thoughts, feelings, and rational thoughts) about taking medication. Mrs. Keene became aware that she had been jumping to conclusions about medication and didn't really have full information about the advantages and disadvantages of pharmacotherapy.

The final portion of session 2 was spent discussing side effects, plasma level assays, and use of antidepressants for acute symptom relief and relapse prevention. She was told that her nortriptyline level was below the desired therapeutic range, and that it probably would have been too low even if she had taken her medication as prescribed. A recommendation to increase the nortriptyline dosage was accepted. She also agreed to a homework assignment of reading a pamphlet about tricyclic antidepressants. Collaboration between Mrs. Keene and her therapist increased significantly by the end of session 2. She remained severely depressed, but suicidal thinking was decreased to a moderate level.

Session 3

The third session began with Mrs. Keene's reporting that she had slept much better after receiving an increased dose of nortriptyline. As a result, she had more energy, and she thought that her concentration was improved. The agenda for session 3 included (a) homework review, (b) questions about medication, (c) coping with guilt about her children, and (d) her lack of interest in her environment.

As part of her homework assignment, Mrs. Keene had completed a four-column version of the Daily Record of Dysfunctional Thoughts (Beck, Rush, Shaw, & Emery, 1979) about taking medication. She was able to identify a number of cognitive errors in her automatic thoughts about medication. Two of the columns from the daily record are detailed in the following example:

Automatic thoughts	Rational thoughts
"I should do this on my own."	"This is an absolute statement. My chances of getting better are much higher if I take medication and work hard in therapy."
"I'll be dependent."	"A gross exaggeration. Overgeneralization. You can't get hooked on anti-depressants. I'd rather not take medication, but I won't lose my independence if I do."
"I'm a weakling."	"Personalization. Magnification. Taking medication doesn't make me weak. Depression is a common problem that strikes many people—not just the weak."

This thought record revealed that Mrs. Keene had learned a great deal about her dysfunctional thinking and was able to work toward changing her attributions about taking medication. However, she still had negative thoughts about pharmacotherapy. The therapist saw this as being related to deeply ingrained schemas, but the patient was positive enough about medication at this time to proceed to other areas of the therapy.

Mrs. Keene had intense guilt about her children's problems. She had wanted her children to be "superkids"—bright, attractive, athletic, and sociable. Contrary to expectations, her children had significant problems with behavior control, learning, and peer relationships. The oldest child was particularly troublesome. She had been admitted to the hospital six months ago for a brief period after becoming despondent and threatening suicide. History collected during this session suggested that Mrs. Keene had negatively distorted her role in the chil-

dren's problems, but that there was some validity to her conclusion that the whole family was "sick."

The therapist reasoned that Mrs. Keene would need to examine her perfectionistic standards and learn to make balanced attributions about her family's difficulties. This could help relieve part of the depression; however, specific skills training would probably also be needed. He doubted that medication alone could correct Mrs. Keene's dysfunctional attitudes about herself as a mother and wife, or fully resolve the family-system pathology. This examination process was begun in session 3, as illustrated with the following vignette.

MRS. KEENE: So you can see why I feel like a total failure. My children are turning out to be losers, just like me. It's my fault. I'm so scatterbrained; I never know what to do with them.

THERAPIST: I understand you have real problems with your children. We'll need to work on ways to improve things. But let's first take a look at how this situation has made you view yourself. You mentioned words like "total failure" and "I never know what to do." Could we check the validity of these statements?

MRS. KEENE: OK. Maybe I've exaggerated a bit. I could try to look for cognitive errors.

THERAPIST: That's a good idea. Let's think of a specific example and fill out a thought record on this topic.

They agreed to continue with this theme for homework. The final portion of session 3 concerned Mrs. Keene's low energy and interest. She reported, "I don't want to do anything. How can I try to change the way I act with my children when I feel so tired and unmotivated?" The therapist elected to focus on cognitive-behavioral tools that might relieve depressive symptoms and therefore explained how to use the Daily Activity Record, including mastery and pleasure ratings (Beck, Rush, Shaw, & Emery, 1979). This procedure was added to the homework assignment for the third session.

Sessions 4 and 5

The last two sessions of the first week of hospitalization went more smoothly than the initial segment of treatment. Mrs. Keene was an active participant in the therapy process. She came to each session with a prepared agenda and a therapy notebook; the therapist usually recommends note taking during sessions to enhance learning and remembering (Wright & Salmon, 1990).

Negatively biased cognitions about taking medication appeared to fade quickly by the end of week one. Additional psychoeducational material was presented about the biological effects of antidepressants, side effects were carefully monitored, and the therapist continued to ask for cognitions about medication. Mrs. Keene experienced mild dry mouth; however, advance preparation for this side effect reduced the chances of an adverse response.

MRS. KEENE: Well, I got one of those side effects you mentioned—dry mouth. It's really not too bad. I just drink a little extra water and try to forget about it. You told me that mild side effects indicate I'm probably getting enough medication to do the job. It helps to think about it that way.

THERAPIST: Are you having any other problems with the medication?

MRS. KEENE: No, but I'm still pretty depressed. It hasn't seemed to help a whole lot so far.

THERAPIST: What do you make of that?

MRS. KEENE: I don't know. Part of me says, "That's what you should expect; nothing will help." But another part of me remembers what you told me about how long it takes the drug to act. It's still too early to tell.

THERAPIST: That's right, it's still too early; and even if the nortriptyline doesn't do all we want, there are other options that we can consider.

Sessions 4 and 5 included further work on Mrs. Keene's low self-esteem and her difficulties coping with family problems. Standard cognitive therapy procedures were employed. Also, the Daily Activity Scale was used to obtain baseline behavioral data and to identify activities that could help build her sense of confidence and increase her ability to experience pleasure. Specific behavioral assignments were made on a daily basis.

Although Mrs. Keene made significant gains in utilizing cognitive therapy techniques in the first week of treatment, she remained severely depressed. The BDI after the first five sessions was 30; the Hopelessness Scale score improved more dramatically (from 19 to 11). Classic vegetative symptoms of depression continued, including low energy and interest, poor appetite, and insomnia.

Sessions 6 Through 10

A plasma level assay for nortriptyline obtained in the middle of week two was within the therapeutic range for this drug, and there had only been a modest improvement in symptoms of depression. This led the therapist to suggest that a trial of lithium carbonate augmentation therapy be considered. He explained that lithium can enhance the effectiveness of tricyclic antidepressants. Mrs. Keene's history of possible bipolar symptoms added further weight to the argument for lithium therapy. It was also suggested that lithium carbonate might be the best long-term treatment for her condition because of the risk for rapid mood-cycling induction by tricyclic antidepressants. Mrs. Keene had an interesting response to this discussion.

MRS. KEENE: So you think I'm a manic-depressive. You know, I always wondered about that. It scared me a lot—I don't want to be like my father and grandfather.

THERAPIST: We're not sure yet whether you have bipolar disorder, but there is enough of a suggestion to tell us that lithium might be a real help. Talking about this seems to have stirred up some strong memories.

MRS. KEENE: That's for sure. My father always said that we should be strong, to "never give in." I think grandfather's suicide really got to him. They were both so proud and fought so hard. I guess they had a fatal flaw—and so do I.

THERAPIST: I can see that this is hard for you.

MRS. KEENE: (begins to cry) Yes, I'm so sad for all of us. I can see why grandfather killed himself.

THERAPIST: Yes, it is sad that you have had to face this condition. I wonder, though, if you are viewing it as accurately as you can. It sounds like your father and grandfather tried to fight depression by themselves and didn't have too much success.

They then explored her belief that depression is a "fatal flaw." Considerable evidence was found that depression can be successfully treated. Also, Mrs. Keene was able to see that she was a unique person with her own blend of strengths and weaknesses. There were more differences than similarities between Mrs. Keene and her father and grandfather.

A number of other therapeutic interventions were utilized during the second week of hospitalization. These included behavioral procedures (daily activity recordings and graded task assignments), psychoeducational interventions (eliciting and explaining side effects, lithium pamphlets, reading materials about depression), and modification of automatic thoughts and schemas. One of the sessions during the second week was devoted to family therapy.

Cognitive-behavioral techniques used during week two will be illustrated with a vignette from session 10. One of the agenda items concerned follow-up from the family session held the day before.

MRS. KEENE: My husband doesn't realize how bad it is. He's at work all day and doesn't see what it's really like.

THERAPIST: How bad is it?

MRS. KEENE: It's chaos! Nobody listens to what I say. They just scream and do what they want to do. I can't stand the screaming, so I let them get away with everything.

THERAPIST: Let's see what part of the problem is due to how you perceive the situation, and also what you can do to start to cope with it more effectively.

The therapist then asked Mrs. Keene to identify cognitive errors in her description of the home scene and to articulate some of her positive attributes as a homemaker. They were able to establish that she had considerable abilities, but that she was being inconsistent and needed to learn ways of encouraging appropriate behavior from her children. Several strategies were outlined to help Mrs. Keene manage problems in her home situation. These included role-playing exercises, family therapy sessions, reading assignments, and discussions with a psychiatric nurse who had raised a large family.

By the end of the second week of therapy, Mrs. Keene's depression was reduced to a moderate level (her BDI was 21). Suicidal thinking was minimal, and she was hopeful for further recovery. The medication regimen included nortriptyline and lithium carbonate.

Subsequent Sessions

Mrs. Keene continued to improve and was discharged in the middle of her third week of hospitalization. Sessions 11 and 12 focused on low self-esteem (including examination of maladaptive schemas) and relapse prevention. The predominant technique used to prepare for discharge was cognitive-behavioral rehearsal (Beck, Rush, Shaw, & Emery, 1979). Adherence to pharmacotherapy recommendations was also stressed.

The Medication Attitude Scale was readministered, and a marked change in cognitions about medications was recognized. However, the patient still had a somewhat dysfunctional perspective on the long-term use of medications. She hoped that eventually she would be able to "do it on my own"; however, she agreed to at least a six-month trial of lithium carbonate, and she accepted the therapist's suggestions for behavioral procedures to enhance treatment adherence (Rush, 1988). The treatment plan also included short-term use of nortriptyline, weekly follow-up cognitive therapy sessions, and family therapy with a social worker. The BDI at discharge was 15; the Hopelessness Scale score was 6.

Mrs. Keene continued to take lithium and nortriptyline as an outpatient. Cognitive therapy sessions were beneficial in helping her to take a problem-solving approach to her difficult home situation. Mrs. Keene also began to focus on her personal growth and development after she recognized that she had fallen into the trap of

"sacrificing" herself for her family—just as her mother had done. Within three months, Mrs. Keene was enrolled in courses at a local college in order to help her prepare to open a small business.

Her BDI was 7 after the first 12 weeks of therapy (12 inpatient and 9 outpatient sessions). By this time, Mrs. Keene was fully committed to ongoing pharmacotherapy and was utilizing self-help cognitive therapy exercises on a daily basis. The frequency of sessions was tapered to once a month for an additional three months. After six months of therapy, Mrs. Keene had no significant symptoms of depression or mania. Nortriptyline had been stopped after three months of treatment. The long-term therapy plan was to continue lithium carbonate and to have therapy visits once every three months.

SUMMARY

A 32-year old depressed woman with a history suggestive of bipolar disorder was treated with cognitive therapy combined with pharmacotherapy. The patient had marked hopelessness, intense suicidal ideation, and severe depressive symptoms early in treatment. Dysfunctional schemas had undermined previous treatment efforts.

Cognitive therapy helped the patient understand and adhere to pharmacotherapy recommendations, while pharmacotherapy improved sleep and other vegetative functions. The treatments were presented as an integrated package of effective interventions for depression. The patient recovered fully and continued with a maintenance program of lithium carbonate and cognitive therapy.

DISCUSSION

The combined treatment approach, as illustrated here, seeks to promote a two-way facilitation between therapies. In the treatment of Mrs. Keene, cognitive therapy was used to uncover and modify negatively distorted thinking and maladaptive behavior. This effort was targeted at Mrs. Keene's hopelessness, poor self-esteem, and low level of self-efficacy. Cognitive therapy was also utilized to identify dysfunctional attitudes about being ill and taking medication. If pharmacotherapy would have been used alone, this dimension would have been missing.

Pharmacotherapy with nortriptyline and lithium carbonate helped to relieve the acute symptoms of depression, including insomnia, loss of appetite, low energy, and decreased ability to concentrate. Disturbance of these functions may interfere with a patient's ability to participate effectively in the psychotherapeutic process (Wright & Schrodt, 1989). There is also good evidence that antidepressants can play a role in reversal of negatively distorted thinking (Simons, Garfield, & Murphy, 1984).

This case illustrates how cognitive therapy may be particularly beneficial in the treatment of a suicidal patient. Antidepressants may take 10 to 14 days or more before they exert a significant effect. However, cognitive therapy can rapidly address hopelessness, and thereby reduce suicidal risk, prior to the onset of action of medications. Mrs. Keene's suicidal ideation diminished significantly in the first few days of treatment.

There also is a role for combined treatment in relapse prevention. Lithium carbonate is the accepted maintenance therapy for patients with bipolar disorder, but cognitive therapy can help arm the patient with problem-solving techniques that can maximize the chances of good psychosocial functioning. In addition, cognitive therapy procedures can reduce the risk of nonadherence to a long-term pharmacotherapy regimen (Cochran, 1982).

Cognitive therapy with this severely depressed inpatient was somewhat unusual because work was done on underlying schemas early in treatment. The more common approach is to start with behavioral techniques and relatively superficial cognitive interventions (Thase & Wright, 1991). Patients with marked depression may have significant problems with learning and memory that make it difficult for them to grasp complex or abstract therapeutic procedures (Wright & Salmon, 1990). Thus, there is some risk that moving too fast with therapy will overload the patient and have a paradoxical effect of increasing hopelessness.

The therapist thought that Mrs. Keene had the capacity to work on schemas during the first week of therapy, but he was prepared to change topics if this initiative was not successful. Fortunately, she was able to benefit from schema modification in the early phase of treatment. This had an important influence on her acceptance of an aggressive pharmacotherapy program and appeared to contribute significantly to her recovery.

REFERENCES

Beck, A. T., & Greenberg, R. L. (1974). *Coping with depression*. New York: Institute for Rational Living.

Beck, A. T., Rush, A. J., Shaw, B. F., & Emery, G. (1979). *Cognitive therapy of depression*. New York: Guilford.

Beck, A. T., Ward, C. H., Mendelson, M., Mock, J., & Erbaugh, J. (1969). An inventory for measuring depression. *Archives of General Psychiatry, 9*, 295–302.

Beck, A. T., Weissman, A., Lester, D., & Trexler, L. (1974). The measurement of pessimism: The hopelessness scale. *Journal of Consulting and Clinical Psychology, 42*, 861–865.

Cochran, S. D. (1982). *Effectiveness of cognitive therapy in preventing non-compliance with lithium regimens*. Paper presented at the annual meeting of the American Psychological Association, Washington, DC.

Rush, A. J. (1988). Cognitive approaches to adherence. In A. J. Frances & R. E. Hales (Eds.), *The American Psychiatric Press review of psychiatry* (vol. 7). Washington, DC: American Psychiatric Press.

Simons, A. D., Garfield, S. L., & Murphy, G. E. (1984). The process of change in cognitive therapy and pharmacotherapy for depression. *Archives of General Psychiatry, 41*(1), 45–51.

Thase, M. E., & Wright, J. H. (1991) Cognitive behavior therapy with depressed inpatients: an abridged treatment manual. *Behavior Therapy, 22*, 579–595.

Wright, J. H. (1987). Cognitive therapy and medication as combined treatment. In A. Freeman & V. Greenwood (Eds.), *Cognitive therapy: Applications in psychiatric and medical settings*. New York: Human Sciences Press.

Wright, J. H. (1988). Cognitive therapy of depression. In A. J. Frances & R. E. Hales (Eds.), *The American Psychiatric Press review of psychiatry* (vol 7). Washington, DC: American Psychiatric Press.

Wright, J. H. (1989). *Medication attitudes and treatment compliance*. Paper presented at the International Congress of Psychosomatic Medicine, Madrid, Spain.

Wright, J. H., & Beck, A. T. (1983). Cognitive therapy of depression: Theory and practice. *Hospital and Community Psychiatry, 34*(12), 1119–1127.

Wright, J. H., & Salmon, P. (1990). Learning and memory in depression. In D. McCann & N. S. Endler (Eds.), *Depression: New directions in research, theory and practice*. Toronto: Wall and Thompson.

Wright, J. H., & Schrodt, G. R. Jr. (1989). Combined cognitive therapy and pharmacotherapy. In A. Freeman, M. D. Simon, H. Arkowitz, & L. Beutler (Eds.), *Handbook of cognitive therapy*. New York: Plenum.

SUGGESTED READINGS

Rush, A. J. (1988). Cognitive approaches to adherence. In A. J. Frances & R. E. Hales (Eds.), *The American Psychiatric Press review of psychiatry* (vol. 7). Washington, DC: American Psychiatric Press.

Wright, J. H. (1987). Cognitive therapy and medication as combined treatment. In A. Freeman & V. Greenwood (Eds.), *Cognitive therapy: Applications in psychiatric and medical settings*. New York: Human Sciences Press.

Wright, J. H., & Beck, A. T. (1983). Cognitive therapy of depression: Theory and practice. *Hospital and Community Psychiatry, 34*(12), 1119–1127.

Wright, J. H., & Schrodt, G. R. Jr. (1989). Combined cognitive therapy and pharmacotherapy. In A. Freeman, M. D. Simon, H. Arkowitz, & L. Beutler (Eds.), *Handbook of cognitive therapy*. New York: Plenum.

31

Inpatient Treatment

Mary Helen Davis and G. Randolph Schrodt, Jr.

INTRODUCTION

The practice of cognitive-behavioral therapy (CBT) in an inpatient setting involves the expansion of the traditional individual psychotherapy format to a multidisciplinary team (Bowers, 1989, Davis & Casey, 1990; Shaw, 1981). Inpatients frequently present with severe, complex conditions that may require family, group, and pharmacologic interventions in addition to individual cognitive behavior therapy. An integrated cognitive-behavioral milieu can provide expanded opportunities for a patient to incorporate the principles of change that are learned in individual therapy sessions. The CBT emphasis on collaborative problem solving can also provide a cohesive organizing philosophy for the treatment staff (Schrodt & Wright, 1987).

The purpose of this chapter will be to demonstrate the techniques of cognitive-behavioral therapy in an inpatient unit. Examples of individual therapy sessions, the community meeting, group therapy, family therapy, and treatment planning are illustrated.

Mary Helen Davis and G. Randolph Schrodt, Jr. • Department of Psychiatry and Behavioral Sciences, University of Louisville School of Medicine, Louisville, Kentucky 40292 and Norton Psychiatric Clinic, 200 East Chestnut Street, Louisville, Kentucky 40232.

Comprehensive Casebook of Cognitive Therapy, edited by Arthur Freeman and Frank M. Dattilio. Plenum Press, New York, 1992.

BACKGROUND INFORMATION

Ann was a 24-year-old white female referred to the inpatient psychiatric unit because of escalation of suicidal ideation, expressions of hopelessness, and persistent vegetative signs of depression that included insomnia, decreased appetite with weight loss, pronounced fatigue, impaired concentration, and inability to function at home or in her job.

Ann presented after a breakup with her boyfriend of two years. She provided a history of depressive episodes since adolescence and had sought outpatient therapy on two previous occasions. Ann had attempted trials of "some medication," but discontinued treatment after three to four visits. Although Ann acknowledged frequent thoughts of suicide, she denied any past attempts except for "a small aspirin overdose when I was 15 that I never told anyone about." She admitted to problems with impulse control on occasions, and had injured herself by hitting a brick wall with her fist while angry. A history of marijuana and alcohol use in college was reported, but she denied any use over the past two years. The patient was employed in the accounting department of a bank, but recently had work difficulties secondary to problems concentrating and being irritable with her coworkers. There was an absence of close relationships or support, and the patient perceived her family as distant and uncaring. In addition, the patient responded affirmatively to a history of sexual abuse, but would not elaborate in the initial assessment.

ASSESSMENT AND DIAGNOSIS

The initial assessment included a one-hour clinical interview followed by a nursing assessment. Background information was obtained, including social and family histories. At admission, her score on the Beck Depression Inventory (Beck, Ward, Mendelson, Mock, & Erbaugh, 1969) was 38, which is indicative of severe depression.

In addition to obtaining background information, the initial session was devoted to establishing a therapeutic relationship. It was assumed that this would be a potentially problematic task because of the patient's level of hopelessness, skepticism about treatment, historically poor relationships, and history of sexual abuse, as well as previous disappointments with the medical profession.

A patient handbook that described the unit, treatment team members, rules, regulations, and activity schedule was given as part of the orientation to the unit. The patient also received a "Cognitive Behavior Program" folder that included introductory reading material, an overview of cognitive therapy as it is used in the inpatient unit, and a homework notebook. The material was designed to convey the expectation that the patient would play an active role in her treatment and recovery.

THE COMMUNITY MEETING

The community meeting has been an integral part of the therapeutic milieu of many inpatient units (Arons, 1982; Oldham & Russakoff, 1982). This large group gathering of patients and staff can play a vital role in the cognitively oriented inpatient psychiatric unit. The meeting is task oriented, making it suitable for utilization in short-term units in general hospitals. Similar to individual sessions, the cognitive community meeting is structured, and a formal agenda is set. A typical agenda might include the following: (a) introduction of new patient members; (b) orientation to rules and unit policies; (c) discussion of changes in privilege status; (d) conflicts with other patients or staff; and (e) termination with patients being discharged.

In Ann's first community meeting, the group leader asked new patients to introduce themselves and explain why there were in the hospital.

ANN: I'm not comfortable talking about myself in front of a group of people I don't know.
BETH: I felt the same when I first came to the hospital. It gets easier when you learn that the staff and groups really can help you.

GROUP LEADER: We understand that groups can, at first, seem intimidating; perhaps you'll be able to share more tomorrow.

Turning to Cathy (also recently admitted), the group leader then asked the same question.

CATHY: I'm here because I've been so depressed I can't seem to function anymore; I've been like this ever since my husband asked for a divorce. I can't seem to care about anything.
DON;: I went through a divorce last year. I blamed myself for the longest time. I've only recently learned to begin to put some of that experience into a perspective. I can see it hurts you a lot, but believe it or not, things do get better. The staff and program here have helped me a lot.

After taking care of other community meeting agenda items, the group leader reminded the group, "For those of you who find group therapy on your daily activities schedule, we ask you to be prepared by thinking of your agenda item or specific issue that you want to discuss."

The community meeting serves as an introduction to the cognitive milieu. Encouraging individuals to disclose their reasons for hospitalization helps them formulate their problem list and reinforces that the process of treatment will be a collaborative experience, with shared responsibility. In addition, the sense of hopelessness and demoralization that often accompanies admission to an inpatient unit is often diminished as new patients interact with others in various phases of their recovery.

INDIVIDUAL SESSION 2

Ann started her second therapy session with a request for discharge, stating, "I want to go home; I told you this wouldn't work." Upon questioning Ann about what had precipitated such an abrupt change from the previous day, the following thoughts were elicited:

- "It's hopeless; I won't get better."
- "Nobody understands me."
- "I'm too different from those other people out there."
- "If I talk about the things that are bothering me, I'll go crazy."

Ann's difficulty in trusting others had become apparent in the large group meeting. Her automatic thoughts about the situation were laden with distortions. Guided discovery revealed several schemas, including "I can never talk to anyone because they don't believe me"; "I'm a failure, I always have been"; and "Good things happen to other people, not to me."

Rather than immediately confronting the patient on her apparent distorted beliefs (which may have reinforced the schema that she was never understood or believed), the therapist attempted to engage her in exploring the validity of the statements she was making by gathering additional data or evidence. Her schema about "not being believed" appeared to be related to the failure of important adults to accept her disclosure of sexual abuse as a child. With the help of her therapist, Ann was able to design an experiment in the inpatient unit to check out the validity of her overgeneralized assumption: (a) Attend the groups on her activity schedule for one day; (b) record information on how well she was "believed and understood"; and (c) attempt to identify any similar or shared issues with other patients and staff she came into contact with during the day.

GROUP THERAPY

Group therapy with a cognitive focus was held twice a week for 90 minutes. Ann attended her first cognitive-behavioral group session later that afternoon with her roommate and six other patients. One of the cotherapists began the group by writing each member's agenda on the blackboard. Several group members had their agendas ready to report and included topics such as homework assignments, follow-up of family conferences or out-of-unit passes, and new issues from individual therapy sessions. When Ann was asked if she had an agenda she responded, "I don't know."

COTHERAPIST: Since this is your first group, it might be useful to have someone explain how our group works and the purpose of establishing an agenda. Anyone want to give it a try?
DON: The agenda lets us make the best use of our time and gives everybody a chance to talk about what's on their mind.
CATHY: Group gives me a chance to get other people's ideas about dealing with my problems.
BETH: When we set our agenda, we might not get to every issue, but we can deal with the important ones. I'd like to talk about my conference with my husband this afternoon.
COTHERAPIST: Let me write that down. Ann, can you think of anything you'd like to put on the agenda?
ANN: My boyfriend.

The completed agenda was as follows:

- Don—Dealing with boredom from retirement
- Cathy—Yesterday's conference with daughter
- Beth—"I'm so sad, I can't stand it"; anniversary of son's death
- Michelle—Worried about bills; threatened loss of job
- Jean—Review of homework; Daily Record of Dysfunctional Thoughts (DRDT)
- Tracy—Conference with husband; probably a divorce
- Ann—My boyfriend

One of the cotherapists assisted the group members in prioritizing the agenda and commented that coping with loss appeared to be a recurrent issue among the group members. Ann listened quietly as the other group members discussed life events they experienced: the loss of personal meaning that was triggered by retirement; fear and apprehension in response to threatened divorce; guilt and emptiness from a child's death in a car accident; sense of personal inadequacy from loss of a job and inability to support one's family.

Ann became involved as the group progressed, and she offered supportive and constructive suggestions. Another group member—her roommate—commented, "While we are talking about loss, why don't you tell the rest of the group the story about your boyfriend?" Encouraged by the quiet attention of the group, Ann consented.

ANN: Tom and I met during our senior year in college. I had some other relationships that had gone poorly, but when I met him my whole life changed. I was happier than I had ever been in my entire life. We moved in together, talked about getting married when we were settled in our jobs. I don't really know what went wrong. He lost his job. I guess I bitched too much, I don't know. Two weeks ago, I caught him with another woman. I drove him to it. Sometimes I think I'll never be able to have a good relationship.
JEAN: Honey, you're lucky to be rid of the creep.
DON: You're so young to say you'll never have a good relationship. You're attractive, smart, got a good job. There's a thousand guys who would be wild about you and treat you right.
COTHERAPIST: You seem to believe that you somehow caused the breakup and take full responsibility. (writes on the board "I drove him to it" and "I'll never have a good relationship") You also have concluded that you'll never have another satisfying relationship. These seem to be very emotionally powerful statements that cause you a lot of sadness.
ANN: (tearful) I just feel so bad.
JEAN: You sound just like me, always blaming yourself

for things that go wrong, jumping to conclusions. In the last couple of weeks, I have come to think about things differently. I catch myself when I start to think in negative twisted kinds of ways. These thought records help a lot.

COTHERAPIST: Maybe it would help Ann to see what you mean by thought record. Perhaps you could share your homework with the group?

As Jean reviewed the DRDT, the therapist provided some didactic explanation of specific techniques of cognitive modification, including reattribution and "thinking in shades of gray" (Burns, 1989). Before the group ended, the therapist and group members focused on Ann to check out how she was and offered the suggestion that she write down the reasons she would "never have a good relationship" for the next group session.

THE TREATMENT PLANNING MEETING

The treatment planning meeting includes attending physicians, residents, medical students, nursing staff, psychologists, occupational and recreational therapists, social workers, and others involved in the care of a given patient. The agenda of this weekly meeting includes (a) problem identification with delineation of specific symptoms and stressors; (b) setting of short-term goals that are defined in operational terms so that progress can be monitored by both patient and staff; (c) clarifying specific assignments of responsibility for therapeutic roles; and (d) long-term goals and aftercare planning (Figure 31-1).

Other issues may need further exploration, especially when dealing with difficult patients. At times, the staff's attitudes and attributions about the meaning of a patient's behavior need to be identified and discussed. Taking the time to understand the caregiver's beliefs and assumptions about patient care can promote consistency and decrease opportunities for countertherapeutic splitting and acting out of patients and staff in the inpatient setting (Schrodt & Wright, 1987).

Once completed, the treatment plan is reviewed with the patient. This review reinforces the collaborative nature of treatment and establishes the objectives of multidisciplinary interventions. In conjunction with the treatment plan, a clinical monitoring approach is used to assess progress and the attainment of specific goals.

Ann was surprised to see her treatment plan. The thought that so many professionals had come together to discuss her problems was interpreted positively. When the clinical monitoring program was explained by her assigned nurse, Ann reported that she felt "more in con-

trol." As her reading assignments were reviewed, Ann felt encouraged to have received *Feeling Good* (Burns, 1980) on day 2 instead of day 3 (interpreting this as rapid advancement through the program).

INDIVIDUAL SESSION 5

Ann had begun to engage in treatment, attend groups, and complete homework assignments in her individual therapy when she experienced a sudden downturn in mood, with increased expression of hostility. Her fifth therapy session began with the following exchange.

ANN::   I don't want to set any damn agenda.

THERAPIST: How would you like to approach our time together, then?

ANN: You're the one who is supposed to have all the answers. I'm the patient, remember?

THERAPIST: One answer that I don't have right now is what happened between our meeting yesterday and now. There's been a clear shift in your mood.

ANN: Bingo, Sherlock! Go ahead and put that on your stupid agenda.

THERAPIST: All right, I'll add that to the list. I'd suggest we also review your homework assignment, and I had hoped to introduce you to a new technique. Is there anything else you want to talk about?

ANN: No.

THERAPIST: Can we be curious about what this sudden downturn in your mood is all about?

ANN: You can be as curious as you want.

THERAPIST: It's obvious that you are angry. I'd like us to be able to understand that better.

ANN: I'm sorry, I don't mean to give you such a hard time; I'm upset. I don't know what's wrong, but I've been feeling this way since last night.

THERAPIST: What happened last night?

ANN: I don't know. I got an unexpected call from my mother last night, and as the evening wore on I got more and more upset.

THERAPIST: Were you having thoughts related to the conversation with your mother?

ANN: You have to know my mother. She never listens to anything I say. She doesn't care very much about me. She just called to get me upset. (becomes tearful)

THERAPIST: I can see this is really upsetting to you. Have you ever discussed this with her?

ANN: No! Are you kidding?

THERAPIST: Seriously, you have a family meeting scheduled for later this week. It might be a good opportunity.

ANN: No way; discharge me.

NORTON PSYCHIATRIC CLINIC
INITIAL-MULTIDISCIPLINARY TREATMENT PLAN

Name: _____

Date: _____

Therapist: _____

Staff present: Attending MD, resident MD, RN, Occupational therapist, Recreational therapist, M.S.S.W.

Discussed with
patient by: _____

Diagnosis:	Patient strengths/resources:
I. Major depression Substance abuse (in remission) R/O PTSD (Hx. of sexual abuse) II. R/O borderline personality disorder	Verbal Educated Employed

Long-term goals: Improved coping ability; reduction of depressive symptoms; medication compliance

Estimated length of stay: 14 days

Problem list:

1. Major depression
   (+) suicidal ideation
   ↓ sleep, ↓ energy, ↓ concentration
   ↓ appetite with weight loss
   ↓ functioning
   ↑ hopelessness
   ↑ medication non-compliance

2. Past history of alcohol abuse, marijuana

3. Psychosocial stressors
   - breakup with boyfriend
   - isolation from family
   - history of sexual abuse (recurrent memories)
   - job stress/dissatisfaction

Short-term goals/patient outcomes
State behaviorally:*

1. Absence of suicidal ideation
   ↓ BDI score from 38 to 20
   ↑ sleep 6-8 hours
   ↑ appetite stabilize weight
   ↑ baseline level of functioning
   Improve medication compliance

2. Obtain history of use patterns
   Maintain sobriety under stress

3. Improve coping with relationship loss
   Identify sources for support in life
   Decrease impact of past trauma on current life
   Explore employment options

Treatment/interventions
Indicate responsible person and discipline:

1. Initiate Prozac trial (MD)
   Explore attitudes and attributions regarding meds (MD, RN)
   CBT 5x/week, group 3x/week
   Occupational therapy
   Dietary consult (RD), psych. testing

2. Tox screen, review labs, collateral history, addictive dis. consult, re: relapse prevention under times of stress. Attend chemical dependency awareness group.

3. Collateral family and social work history, educational material on sexual abuse, determine attributions of experience to current perceptions of self. (MD, RN, Voc. Rehab referral)

* Or as measured by clinical rating scales.

Figure 31-1. Norton Psychiatric Clinic Initial-Multidisciplinary Treatment Plan.

THERAPIST: Look, the decision about the meeting will ultimately be yours. You have some time to think about the pros and cons of such a meeting. I'm just suggesting that we look at this situation a little closer. Look at how angry you've felt since that phone call, how it's affected your mood—

ANN: (interrupting) OK, OK, maybe I'll think about it. What else was on your agenda?

THERAPIST: As I mentioned earlier, I had a new technique I was hoping to introduce to you. I'm not sure how far you've gotten in the book, *Feeling Good*, but this is described in some detail there.

ANN: I just read through Chapter 3, about all the ways my thinking can get messed up.

THERAPIST: That's fine. I'd like to explain an additional concept to you, then you can read about it further in the book. This is called the Daily Record of Dysfunctional Thoughts, or DRDTs. You may have discussed this technique in group therapy this week. It's a technique to help better understand how an event like that telephone call from your mother can make you feel so upset. (hands patient a blank DRDT form) Let's take a look at the first two columns. These can be used for monitoring the connection between an event like a phone call and how that affects the way you are feeling.

ANN: Like last night when I was so angry and didn't know why. OK, so I connect it to that phone call. A lot of good that does me.

THERAPIST: Well, it can help you see what triggers your anger or depressed mood. That might help others, like me or the staff, to understand your anger isn't really intended for them.

ANN: (laughing) OK, how many times do I have to apologize? Really, though, I get your point. I do that a lot at work, too—get upset about one thing and let everybody around have it. That was in Chapter 3, overgeneralization or something.

THERAPIST: You're learning. That brings us to this sheet. If I remember correctly, your thoughts about that phone call were, one, "My mother never listens to me"; two, "She doesn't care about me"; and three, "She called to get me upset." (writes these in columns)

ANN: But that's all 100% true! Oh, no—that's all-or-nothing thinking. I take it back; it's mostly true. Let me have that paper. I'm going to add proof to my beliefs. [See DRDT in Table 31-1.]

THERAPIST: Obviously, not knowing your mother, I'm not in a position to accept or challenge the validity of those thoughts; nevertheless, I understand your strong belief in them.

ANN: You better.

THERAPIST: Indulge me a few more moments. Let's change the heading of the next column. We'll strike "rational" and replace it with "alternative" thoughts. What might be some other ways of thinking about that phone call?

TABLE 31-1 Daily Record of Dysfunctional Thoughts

Event	Emotion	Automatic Thoughts	Rational Thoughts
Phone call from home. Mother talking about neighbor's vacation.	Anger–100% Sad–90%	"She didn't even ask about my treatment. She's going on and on about their stupid vacation; she never listens to me. She deliberately wants to make me more upset. She wishes she didn't have to be bothered by me anymore; she wishes I were dead."	"Nobody in the family can talk about problems. Why should I expect anything to be different now? If I really wanted her to know what was going on, I could have told her." 50% "She called me because she cares about me." 10% "If she didn't want to be bothered, she wouldn't have called." 20% "It would be too big an embarrassment for her if I committed suicide." 90% "Even if she doesn't care about me, it doesn't mean other people don't care. I can live."

ANN: That means I can come up with some other options without having to believe they are true. (therapist nods; Ann takes the DRDT form and writes in column)

THERAPIST: (reviewing completed DRDT) You're getting the idea. Suppose you took one of those alternative thoughts and could change the percentage of belief you placed in it, how do you imagine that might impact on the way you feel?

ANN: You mean like what I rated 10%, if I could change that one to, say, 50%—it would make all the difference in the world to me.

THERAPIST: So you can see some value of examining those initial thoughts a little closer.

ANN: On paper, yeah, but what does that prove? I already know I'd feel better if I had a different life.

THERAPIST: Perhaps it could be useful to explore some of those alternative thoughts a little deeper, maybe even put them to a test.

ANN: Like what?

THERAPIST: If I dare bring up that family meeting again, you seem to have different ideas regarding the effect of telling your mother what is going on and what your treatment involves.

ANN: I already know what it would be; she wouldn't listen.

THERAPIST: (suggesting what Ann is doing) Fortune-telling?

ANN: (replying in kind) Manipulating me into a family meeting? I'll do it just to prove you wrong.

THERAPIST: I don't know who is right or wrong. All I'm saying is we need more evidence. Maybe we can collect that kind of data from a family meeting.

This vignette illustrates a problem commonly encountered in inpatient cognitive-behavioral therapy. In addition to acute psychiatric disturbances such as major depressive disorder, many inpatients present clinical evidence of a chronic personality disorder. Beck, Freeman, and Associates (1990) have described how the structured, directive, problem-oriented approach of cognitive-behavioral therapy can provide a framework for understanding and dealing with these interpersonal problems.

FAMILY SESSION

The participants in the family session included the social worker, Ann, and her mother, Mrs. J. Mr. J. was not present, although he was invited to attend. The session began with Mrs. J. apologizing for Mr. J.'s absence.

MRS. J.: Your father couldn't make it. He sends his apologies, but a business meeting came up.

ANN: He's always too busy for me.

SOCIAL WORKER: Before we get too far, it might help if we establish the agenda, just like in our individual sessions. (stops to explain briefly to patient's mother the task of agenda setting)

Continuing, the social worker suggested that Mr. J.'s absence be placed on the agenda. Mrs. J. requested information about Ann's illness and treatment, as well as ways the family could be supportive. Ann declined additions to the agenda. The social worker asked Ann what she thought about her father's absence.

ANN: He doesn't care. He doesn't want to be here; he's always too busy for me.

MRS. J.: He cares very much for you. You just never understand about his professional obligations.

ANN: There you go blaming me again. You wanted to know ways you could be supportive, and when I try to tell you, then it's my fault because I don't understand this or that.

MRS. J.: Wait; I'm not going to make excuses for your father. I'm disappointed that he couldn't come to this meeting, too. He leaves me to make all the decisions about the children. Talk about blame; I blame myself for your difficulties. I never seem to know the right thing to say or do, so sometimes I just end up avoiding talking about things to you. Like the other night, I wanted to call to be supportive and I didn't want to make you more upset, so I just started chatting about neutral topics—and before you knew it, we were into one of our blowups, and I guess we both hung up the phone upset.

SOCIAL WORKER: What do you think about what your mother just said?

ANN: I can't believe I heard what she just said; that's the first time I've ever heard you say you were disappointed in Dad or that you blame yourself for my problems. I've always felt like I've disappointed the whole family, always letting everybody down.

MRS. J.: No, I've thought about a lot of things since you've been admitted to the hospital. I know this isn't your fault. We just aren't very good about facing problems. Your father uses his work to escape family problems and I try to avoid them, hoping they'll resolve themselves. I should have known or should have done something when you took that aspirin overdose in the 10th grade, but I couldn't; I didn't know what to do. I've blamed myself for all these years—I couldn't even ask you why. I'm so ashamed of myself.

ANN: How did you know about that? You never said a word to me. You mean you're blaming yourself for something that happened nearly 10 years ago?

SOCIAL WORKER: There seems to have been a fair amount of misunderstanding and problems communicating within the family. Perhaps substituting curiosity for blame will make it easier for everyone to begin to fill in the blanks and work through some of these problems, so they won't continue to have such an impact on your life and relationships.

MRS. J.: How do we start?

SOCIAL WORKER: Well, if you both agree, we could continue to have further family sessions. You and your husband could participate in our family night programs that include sessions on cognitive therapy and communications skills.

Surprised by her mother's unexpected display of understanding and support, Ann experienced an almost immediate improvement in mood, energy, and enthusiasm. Although Ann had doubts about seeing major changes in the relationship with her father, she began to talk more frequently with her mother and later had an out-of-unit pass to eat lunch with her.

Cognitive-behavioral approaches to a number of family and couples problems have recently been described, many of which are applicable in inpatient settings (Epstein, Schlesinger, & Dryden, 1988). Communication skills, assertiveness, and methods of conflict resolution can be taught in psychoeducational groups, and additional reading material may be suggested (Beck, 1988).

DISCHARGE PLANNING

By the end of her second week of hospitalization, Ann reported that she was feeling better, with renewed hope and no suicidal thoughts. Although she still had residual depressive symptoms, including occasional-onset insomnia and fatigue, she felt that she could now function on an outpatient basis. Her BDI score had dropped to 16, and she began to formulate plans for discharge and return to work.

Considerable anxiety can be generated at the thought of leaving the hospital, connecting to a new outpatient therapist, returning to the work or home environment, and dealing with the questions and reactions of family and friends. A transition group can often help to bridge the gap between inpatient and outpatient levels of care. Transition groups include recently discharged patients and provide both support and reinforcement of the concepts and skills learned in the hospital. Ann attended such a group for eight sessions after her discharge.

Prior to discharge, Ann agreed to take responsibility for contacting the nurse each morning when she was

scheduled to take her antidepressant. Outpatient adherence to her medication regimen was further reinforced in psychoeducational groups on the psychobiology of depression. Her cognitively oriented psychiatrist carefully explained the side effects and expected benefits of the medication, and attempted to identify any maladaptive attitudes and beliefs about pharmacotherapy of her depressive disorder (Wright & Schrodt, 1989).

Seventeen days after admission, Ann was discharged. She was seen by her psychiatrist for 30 sessions over the next year, and continued medication for six months. One year after her discharge, she was clinically asymptomatic, with a BDI of 5.

SUMMARY

This 24-year-old depressed woman with multiple psychosocial stressors and poor interpersonal relationships was successfully treated in an inpatient unit via a cognitive-behavioral treatment approach. The inpatient setting provided an active, coherent, problem-oriented environment, which fostered a collaborative therapeutic alliance. This patient, although initially resistant to engaging in treatment, was able to benefit from psychopharmacological interventions and cognitively oriented individual, group, and family therapies. The positive experience of hospitalization promoted compliance with outpatient follow-up that focused on the modification of maladaptive schemas that were identified in the hospital.

This patient's outpatient therapy was extended beyond the usual 12 to 15 sessions typical for cognitive therapy of depression. However, many patients hospitalized for the treatment of depression present with greater symptom severity and other problems such as substance abuse or character pathology. These complicated cases may require extended treatment to accomplish therapeutic goals and assure optimal outcome.

DISCUSSION

Most patients with nonpsychotic depressive disorders can be effectively treated on an outpatient basis. However, serious risk of suicidal behavior, incapacitating symptoms such as profound hopelessness and helplessness, and/or failure of outpatient therapy may necessitate hospitalization. In an inpatient setting, cognitive-behavioral therapy has been studied as an adjunctive treatment with evidence of enhanced clinical response and reduced relapse rates (Bowers, 1990; Miller, Norman, & Keitner, 1989).

Other inpatient units—such as the one described in this case history—use cognitive-behavioral theory as an organizing treatment philosophy. CBT is a short-term, active, problem-oriented treatment approach that can be adapted for use in large and small groups, family therapy, and treatment planning. Cognitive-behavioral strategies may enhance compliance and response to biological therapies, which remain a primary treatment modality on inpatient units.

The case described illustrated several important phases of inpatient treatment, including (a) establishment of a collaborative therapeutic alliance; (b) identification of target symptoms and goals; (c) use of cognitive-behavioral techniques to modify dysfunctional beliefs that led to a client's sense of isolation, helplessness, hopelessness, and suicidal thoughts; and (d) the consolidation of therapeutic gains and relapse prevention.

REFERENCES

Arons, B. S. (1982). Effective use of community meetings on psychiatric treatment units. *Hospital and Community Psychiatry*, *33*, 480–483.

Beck, A. T. (1988). *Love is never enough*. New York: Harper & Row.

Beck, A. T., Ward, C. H., Mendelson, M., Mock, J., & Erbaugh, J. (1969). An inventory for measuring depression. *Archives of General Psychiatry*, *9*, 295–302.

Beck, A. T., Freeman, A., & Associates. (1990). *Cognitive therapy of personality disorders*. New York: Guilford.

Bowers, W. A. (1989). Cognitive therapy with inpatients. In A. Freeman, K. M. Simon, H. Arkowitz, & L. Beutler (Eds.), *Comprehensive handbook of cognitive therapy* (pp. 583–596). New York: Plenum.

Bowers, W. A. (1990). Treatment of depressed inpatients: Cognitive therapy plus medication, relaxation plus medication, and medication alone. *British Journal of Psychiatry*, *156*, 73–78.

Burns, D. D. (1980). *Feeling good: The new mood therapy*. New York: William Morrow.

Burns, D. D. (1989). *The feeling good handbook*. New York: William Morrow.

Davis, M. H., & Casey, D. A. (1990). Utilizing cognitive therapy on the short-term psychiatric inpatient unit. *General Hospital Psychiatry*, *12*, 170–176.

Epstein, N., Schlesinger, S. E., & Dryden, W. (Eds.). (1988). *Cognitive-behavioral therapy with families*. New York: Brunner/Mazel.

Miller, I. W., Norman, W. H., & Keitner, G. I. (1989). Cognitive-behavioral treatment of depressed inpatients: Six- and twelve-month follow-up. *American Journal of Psychiatry*, *146*, 1274–1279.

Oldham, J. M., & Russakoff, L. M. (1987). *Dynamic therapy in brief hospitalization*. Northvale, NJ: Jason Aronson.

Schrodt, G. R., Jr., & Wright, J. H. (1987). Inpatient treatment of adolescents. In A. Freeman & V. B. Greenwood (Eds.), *Cognitive therapy: Applications in psychiatric and medical settings* (pp. 69–82). New York: Human Sciences Press.

Shaw, B. F. (1981). Cognitive therapy with an inpatient population. In G. Emery, S. D. Hollon, & R. C. Bedrosian (Eds.), *New directions in cognitive therapy* (pp. 29–49). New York: Guilford.

Wright, J. H., & Schrodt, G. R. Jr. (1989). Combined cognitive therapy and pharmacotherapy. In A. Freeman, K. M. Simon, H. Arkowitz, & L. Beutler (Eds.), *Comprehensive handbook of cognitive therapy* (pp. 267–282). New York: Plenum.

SUGGESTED READINGS

Beck, A. T., & Freeman, A. (1990). *Cognitive therapy of personality disorders*. New York: Guilford.

Freeman, A., Simon, K. M., Beutler, L. E., & Arkowitz, H. (1989). *Comprehensive handbook of cognitive therapy* (chap. 29). New York: Plenum.

Davis, M. H., & Casey, D. A. (1990). Utilizing cognitive therapy on the short-term psychiatric inpatient unit. *General Hospital Psychiatry*, *12*, 170–176.

32

Poststroke Depression

Mary R. Hibbard, Susan E. Grober, Paula N. Stein,
and Wayne A. Gordon

INTRODUCTION

As medical technology advances, survival rates from stroke are steadily improving. There are over 1 million stroke survivors in this country (National Center for Health Statistics, 1977). Combining this statistic with the rapid "graying" of the American society, the rehabilitation community has begun to focus attention on providing a broader range of interventions for stroke survivors. Despite the fact that the majority of stroke patients are depressed (Gordon, Hibbard, Egelko, et al., 1990; Robinson et al., 1983; Ruckdeschel-Hibbard, Gordon, & Diller, 1986), traditional rehabilitation efforts have focused largely on the physical and language losses following stroke. Thus, poststroke depression (PSD) presents as a major impediment to maximizing the quality of life for stroke survivors.

Treatment for PSD has typically involved the use of

antidepressant medication (e.g., Lipsey, Robinson, Pearlson, Rao, & Price, 1984). Although antidepressants can be effective, these drugs are often contraindicated because of preexisting medical conditions (cardiac arrhythmias, seizures, glaucoma, etc.), drug interactions, or patient refusals. Therefore, psychotherapy emerges as the treatment of choice for the majority of stroke patients. For psychotherapy to be effective, modifications of existing techniques and practice are required to deal with this often cognitively impaired population. This chapter will highlight these modifications through a case presentation.

Before treatment is initiated, an accurate assessment of a patient's mood is essential. This evaluation must address issues that can impact both the patient and the observer's reports of PSD. More specifically, poststroke cognitive deficits in abstraction, memory, perception, and language can radically alter a patient's understanding and view of the world, and may impact the patient's ability to evaluate his or her emotional state accurately, while neurological sequelae (e.g., hypoarousal, lability, and aprosodias) can impact the observer's ability to diagnose PSD accurately. Thus, assessment must be expanded to include (a) an examination of the patient's cognitive and functional changes, as well as the patient's awareness of these changes; (b) independent evaluations of a patient's mood from people familiar with the patient (the family, the nurses/attendants, etc.); and (c) a clinical interview. This broad-based approach to PSD diagnosis enables the clini-

Mary R. Hibbard, Wayne A. Gordon, and Paula N. Stein • Department of Rehabilitation Medicine, The Mount Sinai Medical Center, New York, New York 10029-6574. Susan E. Grober • Section of Physical Medicine and Rehabilitation, Norwalk Hospital, Norwalk, Connecticut 06880.

Comprehensive Casebook of Cognitive Therapy, edited by Arthur Freeman and Frank M. Dattilio. Plenum Press, New York, 1992.

cian to diagnose the patient's mood accurately and to determine where and in what direction to focus psychotherapy.

BACKGROUND INFORMATION

Mr. M., a 60-year-old, high-school-educated actor, lived with his wife in an apartment in a large city at the time of treatment. Until the time of his stroke, Mr. & Mrs. M. had enjoyed a common interest in acting. They socialized with a small network of friends and had a wide circle of acquaintances. Their active professional lives obscured preexisting problems that the couple had in effectively communicating with each other. Prior to his stroke, Mr. M. had assertive difficulties and was never an "introspective" individual. Because of these long-standing dynamics, Mr. M.'s illness precipitated friction within the couple surrounding these issues. Mr. M.'s interests and hobbies were minimal; his major focus was his acting career.

MULTIMODAL ASSESSMENT OF MOOD

The clinician assessed the patient's functional status, cognitive abilities, and awareness of stroke-related changes. In addition, independent data about the patient's mood was obtained from three sources—the patient himself, his wife, and the clinician. This multimodal approach allowed the clinician to incorporate several evaluations of Mr. M.'s mood and to use the most accurate data sources when making a diagnosis (for a detailed description of this process, see Hibbard, Gordon, Stein, et al., in press).

Functional Status

Mr. M. suffered a left cerebrovascular accident three months prior to evaluation. Physical sequelae included a mild loss of right leg strength and a significant loss of right arm movement. Mr. M. was clearly distressed over the loss of his right arm functioning. While initially expressively aphasic, Mr. M. had experienced significant recovery of his language skills by the time of evaluation; however, he continued to experience moderate word-finding difficulties during the interview. Although he was aware of these deficits, his expectations were unrealistic, as he believed he would have a "complete" recovery of his physical functioning and his language abilities. His expectations were supported by positive feedback he received from his participation in outpatient rehabilitation speech, occupational, and physical therapies.

Cognitive Status

On formal assessment, the patient had a moderate expressive and mild receptive aphasia. In addition, Mr. M. was concrete in his thinking and exhibited significant language comprehension and memory deficits. Mr. M. had no awareness of his concreteness, memory deficits, or comprehension impairments. Furthermore, he minimized his actual language difficulties, considering them to be limited to a "mildly annoying" word-finding problem.

Mood State

Clinical interviews were completed separately with the patient and his wife. In addition, the patient rated his mood on the Beck Depression Inventory (BDI), while the clinician and his wife rated the patient's mood on a modified Hamilton Rating Scale for Depression (HRSD). These data (see Table 32-1) suggest that Mr. M. had limited awareness of the extent of his physical and cognitive losses, as well as his dysphoric mood. However, behavioral manifestations of dysphoria were noted by both the clinician and his wife, i.e., irritability, sleep and appetite changes, feelings of hopelessness, loss of energy, etc. Given Mr. M.'s limited awareness and concrete thinking, the clinician and wife's reports were utilized for diagnosis, since they were the more accurate reports of the patient's mood. While Mr. M. was diagnosed as being clinically "not depressed" due to the low magnitude of his symptoms, the clinician suggested a follow-up re-evaluation in six weeks.

On re-evaluation, Mr. M. appeared significantly more depressed to both his wife and the clinician. Yet Mr. M. continued to minimize his emotional distress, as well as his cognitive and physical losses (see Table 32-1). The discrepancies regarding the level of Mr. M.'s depression, as reported by the patient and independent observers, are a common poststroke pattern that reflects a patient's overall lack of awareness. This case highlights the need for a broad-based approach to data collection when attempting to diagnose PSD. At this point, Mr. M. was diagnosed as depressed and referred for cognitive-behavioral psychotherapy.

In the present chapter, a modified cognitive-behavioral psychotherapy approach for the treatment of Mr. M.'s depression is highlighted (for a more detailed approach to treatment, see Hibbard, Grober, Gordon, & Aletta, 1990a). Due to the extent of his stroke-related cognitive losses, a combination of behavioral and educational interventions was emphasized in the initial phase of his treatment (phase 1). Cognitive techniques were embedded within the latter phase of Mr. M.'s treatment

TABLE 32-1 Longitudinal Mood Assessment (Mr. M.)

	Initial evaluation	Re-evaluation	Mid-therapy evaluation	Post-therapy evaluation	One-year follow-up
Patient					
BDI	7 (3, 4)[a]	8 (4, 4)	12 (6, 6)	6 (2, 4)	3 (0, 3)
Level of awareness of poststroke sequelae[b]	4	4	0	0	0
Clinician					
HRSD	11 (3, 8)	19 (8, 11)	21 (8, 13)	7 (1, 6)	3 (1, 2)
Wife					
HRSD	12 (4, 8)	17 (7, 10)	26 (8, 18)	14 (6, 8)	8 (4, 4)
Diagnosis	Not depressed; follow-up evaluation indicated	Major depression	Major depression	Not depressed	Not depressed

[a]Numbers in brackets represent subtotals of somatic and nonsomatic complaints.
[b]Higher scores are indication of greater unawareness; maximum score = 8.

(phase 2) in proportion to the level of his awareness of poststroke changes. Fourteen principles of cognitive psychotherapy utilized in PSD treatment are summarized in Table 32-2, and are referenced as they apply in this case report. Serial reassessments of Mr. M.'s mood are presented that reflect the effectiveness of these therapeutic endeavors.

PHASE 1: INCREASING AWARENESS, EDUCATION, AND MOURNING

Mr. M. began therapy with minimal awareness of the extent and severity of his losses and unrealistic expectations about his potential recovery. These factors were taken into account when deciding upon the initial approach and goals of treatment. Phase 1 goals were to increase the patient's awareness of his stroke sequelae (including his depression); to educate the patient and his wife about his stroke losses; and to help the patient initiate the process of mourning. To accomplish these goals, a predominantly behavioral and educational approach was utilized (principle 1).

During initial sessions, Mr. and Mrs. M. were seen jointly in an attempt to increase the patient's awareness of, and provide realistic information about, Mr. M.'s stroke sequelae (principles 1, 4, 12). To decrease the patient's minimization of his depression, focused interventions were used. For example, both Mr. and Mrs. M. independently completed a BDI as it related to Mr. M.'s mood. A comparison of the differences in scoring of the BDI gave the therapist an opportunity to explore differences in the couple's perceptions about Mr. M.'s mood, as well as to identify areas of distress for the patient. Within this con-

text, the patient discussed a major source of discomfort (difficulty sleeping) and related that he had difficulty falling asleep because of recurring anxious thoughts about his paralyzed arm. He referred to his thoughts as a "tape that plays automatically at night" centering around a theme of recovery: "When is my arm going to get better? I just keep thinking . . . when, when, when? I just know it will get *all* better; I have to be patient, that's all." The therapist avoided directly challenging Mr. M.'s beliefs about achieving a complete recovery and refocused the discussion on Mr. M.'s understanding of stroke recovery in general, as well as his knowledge about other stroke patients. This nonconfrontational strategy was employed to avoid decreasing the patient's motivation prematurely in his outpatient rehabilitation. It became clear that neither the patient nor Mrs. M. had a clear understanding of what a realistic recovery from stroke might be. Nor did they know others who had experienced strokes with whom they could compare Mr. M.'s progress. Mr. M. also avoided discussion of his disability or his potential recovery with his doctor, his therapists, or other patients.

Highly structured assignments were designed that facilitated Mr. M.'s gathering realistic data about his own stroke recovery (principle 3). These fact-finding tasks included helping the patient make a list of questions to ask his doctors, his physical therapist, and other rehabilitation patients he encountered while in therapy. When exploring the patient's feelings about meeting other stroke patients, Mr. M. related that he was always a shy person who had difficulty meeting new people. He readily admitted that most people saw him as being whatever personality he had played in his most recent movie. While normally, Mr. M. loved this attention from others, he now avoided being in the limelight and felt uncomfortable receiving any atten-

TABLE 32-2 Principles of Cognitive Therapy in the Treatment of Poststroke Depression

1. Cognitive functioning moderates the treatment strategies used.
2. Cognitive remediation enhances the patient's ability to profit from therapy.
3. New learning and generalization are difficult for stroke patients.
4. Patient awareness of depressive symptomatology moderates therapeutic strategy.
5. Mourning is an important component of treatment.
6. Premorbid life-style and interests provide a context for understanding current behavior.
7. Understanding the discrepancy between actual and perceived losses is essential to treatment.
8. Reinforcing even small therapeutic gains improves mood.
9. Emphasis on the collaborative nature of the therapeutic relationship facilitates a working alliance.
10. To ensure continuity of treatment, session flexibility is essential.
11. Fluctuations in medical status impact the course of treatment.
12. The distortions of family members must be addressed in therapy.
13. Family members' mourning must be addressed.
14. Family members are important therapeutic helpers.

tion from strangers since he was unable to assume the role of a competent actor. This avoidance, combined with his language losses, served to isolate him further from the support often given by fellow patients. To help Mr. M. seek out other stroke patients from whom he could get support and information, social skills training and role-playing were utilized, which the "actor" in Mr. M. really enjoyed. Together with the therapist, Mr. M. rehearsed his new role as a person who had suffered a stroke and wanted to reach out to other people.

During the fourth session, Mr. and Mrs. M. reported increasing tension and arguments at home. These disagreements were focused on what the wife perceived as Mr. M.'s lack of compliance with tasks at home and in his rehabilitation program. One such disagreement went something like this:

MRS. M.: He's more forgetful now. I'm out in the kitchen, and I ask him to do a few simple things for me. I go back a few hours later and nothing's done! He doesn't have much to do now—I don't understand why he doesn't help me!

MR. M.: I think I'm as helpful as before the stroke. (angry) But I don't even remember this event she's talking about!

MRS. M.: See, he can't even remember it as a problem! That makes me even more angry and frustrated. He's getting lazy—that's no way to treat me!

While such lack of follow-through after a stroke can be mistakenly attributed to noncompliance, it more frequently represents an underlying cognitive failure on the part of the patient. However, these cognitive deficits can manifest themselves as communication difficulties that place additional stress on a marriage. To decrease tension between Mr. and Mrs. M., the therapist described how cognitive deficits impact poststroke communication skills (principle I). Since the therapist felt Mr. M.'s cognitive deficits were underlying many of the couple's current miscommunications, Mr. M.'s specific deficits in abstract thinking, memory, and comprehension were then discussed in detail. By reframing Mr. M.'s "faulty" behaviors as cognitively based, the therapist educated both Mr. M. and his wife as to the nature of these altered communication patterns. In response to this intervention, Mrs. M. stated, "I'm less angry at him; I guess I didn't realize his problems would also be mine as well." Thus, the immediate results of this approach were to (a) defuse Mrs. M.'s anger, (b) increase the wife's awareness that changes in Mr. M. would also impact her, and (c) validate Mr. M.'s perception that his wife was punishing him when he felt he had not intentionally done anything to upset her (principles 3, 12).

This vignette highlights how poststroke changes become dynamic problems affecting not only the patient but also significant others in the patient's life. Thus, it is often necessary to work within couple/family systems when treating PSD (principles 12,13). The therapist also worked with Mrs. M. to modify her overly verbal and abstract communication style in order to maximize Mr. M.'s compromised abilities. The therapist initially modeled brief, less verbally complex responses. Specific suggestions about Mrs. M.'s need to speak in simple brief sentences, and to clarify her requests with Mr. M. to assure that he had adequately understood them, were stressed. The couple's misperceptions of Mr. M.'s "noncompliant" behavior were also used to highlight how each individual had cognitively distorted the communication problem in a manner reflective of their premorbid personalities—Mr. M. tending to minimize difficulties, while Mrs. M. would exaggerate them (principle 6).

Understanding the discrepancy between Mr. M.'s actual and perceived losses was another essential focus of therapy (principle 7). Mr. M's initial complaints focused solely on the loss of his right arm function. He appeared to ignore issues related to his speech and cognitive limitations that were equally important to his career as a professional actor. As a result of his fact-finding homework assignments (talking to his MD, his therapist, and other patients about stroke/recovery), Mr. M. began to acknowledge that total recovery of his right arm might be unrealistic. In addition, he became aware that his speech and memory deficits, though amenable to therapy, would remain a problem for him. In sharing this information with the therapist, Mr. M. began the belated process of mourning (principle 5). The patient became more verbal about his disability and its impact on his profession. He stated in an angry voice, "I can't accept my arm not getting better; right now, it looks like a dead chicken wing . . . I feel like a cripple! Who wants a tongue-tied actor with a crippled arm?" Further exploration revealed that Mr. M. was worried not only about his career, but about issues of body integrity and the social stigma that surrounded his losses. As the patient stated, "I didn't tell the world I've had a stroke—but with this stupid arm and my lousy speech, everyone will know!"

Concerns about body image, stigma, and mourning became the major foci of subsequent sessions. These themes are common in the treatment of all stroke survivors. Within this context, distortions about Mr. M.'s losses were labeled by the therapist (principle 7). For example, Mr. M. described himself as being "*totally crippled,*" when in fact he could walk independently, had full use of his left arm, and had gross movement of his right arm. This information was used to dispute his distortion. As is typical with many stroke patients, Mr. M.'s realization that full recovery might not be possible resulted in increased resistance to continued participation in his rehabilitation program. This self-defeating attitude was challenged to prevent Mr. M. from prematurely discontinuing a program that could maximize his functioning and/or teach him compensatory skills. Since the patient's compliance with home exercise had already decreased dramatically, a behavioral contract was drawn up that allowed Mr. M. flexibility in the times he would perform home exercises (thus working with his resistance), but simultaneously required that he attend all of his outpatient rehabilitation program.

The behavioral contract was reviewed within sessions to ensure compliance and enhance carryover from session to session. The patient's progress in his classes was reinforced to help Mr. M. focus on small areas of functional gain that he made in therapy (principle 8). Like many stroke patients, Mr. M. employed what the therapist labeled as "black/white thinking" in his own evaluation of his progress. For example, Mr. M. would state, "So what if I can lift a five-pound weight with my hand? I still can't use my hand for anything purposeful." The therapist highlighted his distortions and helped the patient begin to challenge his own rigid self-statements. Over the next several sessions, Mr. M. became sensitized to the frequency with which he minimized his abilities and began to relate his depressed mood to many of his critical self-statements. Thus, a more traditional cognitive psychotherapeutic approach to treatment was now possible given the patient's increased awareness of his depression and his deficits.

To summarize, the initial phase of treatment was focused on increasing Mr. M.'s awareness of his cognitive, physical, and emotional losses secondary to his stroke. To accomplish this goal, treatment included patient education and had a behavioral emphasis. As Mr. M.'s awareness increased, cognitive principles were slowly embedded within therapy. The patient's spouse was included in many sessions to increase her own understanding of Mr. M.'s situation. This approach allowed both Mr. and Mrs. M. the opportunity to begin a necessary, but delayed, mourning process and decreased the mounting marital discord that so typically follows the onset of a major disability.

MOOD REASSESSMENT

Three months after initiation of treatment, Mr. M.'s mood was re-evaluated (see Table 32-1). Mr. M. was fully aware of his cognitive/physical losses, but continued to minimize his depression. As in his earlier assessment, the clinician and his wife reported Mr. M. to be more depressed; however, at this evaluation, Mrs. M noted greater depressive symptoms in her husband than did the clinician. Mrs. M.'s report of her husband's mood actually reflected her own increased level of depression as she began to realize that her husband's losses had permanently impacted her as well. This is a common finding in spouses of stroke patients, one that clinicians need to be careful of in an evaluation process (Stein, Gordon, Hibbard, & Sliwinski, 1992). At six months poststroke onset, the patient's speech and physical therapies had been terminated, since the rehabilitation team felt that Mr. M. had achieved his "maximal rehabilitation gains." Mr. M. continued to be seen for twice-weekly psychotherapy.

PHASE 2: RESTRUCTURING

During this second phase of treatment, the clinician shifted to modified cognitively based interventions. Treatment issues included: (a) mourning of cognitive and language losses, (b) correction of depressinogenic distortions about current abilities, (c) remediation of cognitive deficits, and (d) improving the quality of poststroke life. Because Mr. M. was now fully aware that his speech and cognitive losses were permanent, a marked increase in his depression was noted both at home and within the therapy. For example, Mrs. M. reported, "Over the last month, [Mr. M.] has really changed. He jumps all over me whenever I try to be supportive to him." In response, Mr. M. angrily replied, "I am sick and tired of people thinking they know what is best for me. I hate it when you try to placate me. I'm not sick . . . I'm permanently changed." This pattern of increased depression following an increased awareness of the permanence of poststroke losses is commonly observed in PSD and often necessitates mourning at different phases of treatment as different losses are recognized. Mrs. M. also became increasingly depressed as she realized that Mr. M. would not recover to be the exact person he was before his stroke. Mrs. M.'s mourning focused around the loss of her previously successful and charming partner, as well as the impact of his loss on her own social functioning. As a result, joint sessions were interspersed with individual therapy to facilitate the continued process of mourning for both Mr. and Mrs. M. (principles 4, 5, 13).

While exploring issues surrounding his increasing depression, Mr. M. admitted that he was becoming increasingly insecure about his cognitive skills. As Mr. M. stated, "I'm totally unsure of myself now . . . I never know when I'll forget something or hear something the wrong way . . . I never know when I'll make a fool of myself." Cognitive interventions used during this phase initially focused on exploring situations in which the patient experienced a perceived cognitive failure (principle 7). To facilitate this goal, the patient was instructed to keep a diary of his memory and speech problems. Since the patient was unable to write with his dominant hand, his wife recorded these events in his diary for him (principle 14). While time was allowed for the patient to grieve these losses, exaggerated or distorted self-statements stemming from his compromised abilities were actively challenged. For example, Mr. M. had noted in his diary that he had received a call from a local actor's workshop to attend a session. While these workshops were formerly a weekly activity on the patient's social calendar, Mr. M. had not attended them since his stroke. He used the following reasoning for his continued refusal: "Why go? I might be asked a question, and won't be able to answer quickly enough. No one wants a silent, crippled actor to help them act." On reviewing this statement, Mr. M. identified the words *silent* and *crippled* as being exaggerated, and replaced these distortions with "some problems finding words quickly" and "a right arm that's partially paralyzed." After monitoring his negative statements, Mr. M.

began to explore other areas of intact expertise that he could still bring to this group. As an outcome of this exploration, Mr. M. was able to state in a humorous fashion, "I guess I do have other skills to offer—how to make facial gestures, use postures, and ways to cover up when you forget a line . . . if the young actors don't like it, the hell with them!" Thus, simple cognitive exercises enabled Mr. M. to entertain the resumption of a formerly valued social activity.

Graduated task assignments were utilized to help bolster the patient's confidence so he could again participate in the workshops (principle 3). A series of social events with friends and family members were planned that involved both Mr. and Mrs. M. participating in increasingly larger social groups. Mr. M. was asked to evaluate his interpersonal abilities and have his wife record both his and his wife's opinions about the events in his diary. This technique was used to facilitate Mr. M.'s memory for the event as well as to enhance his self-evaluation skills. It also provided Mrs. M. an opportunity to give feedback about her perceptions of the event and Mr. M.'s behaviors. These notes were discussed and reviewed jointly in session in an attempt to enhance communication between Mr. and Mrs. M. (principles 7, 12, 14). As Mr. M. experienced gradual success in these preplanned activities, his amount of social dialogue slowly increased. As his final task, Mr. M. was asked to attend the actor's workshop, first as an observer and then as a participant. With repeat visits to the workshop, Mr. M. slowly increased his spontaneous exchanges with fellow actors and began to attend these sessions on a regular basis. These exercises served the dual purpose of structuring a re-entry of Mr. and Mrs. M. into their former social network as well as the workshop. Thus, both Mr. and Mrs. M. slowly began to resume important aspects of their former life-style.

As Mr. M.'s mourning gradually resolved, he began to discuss his annoyance at his continued dependency on his wife for many daily activities. For example, he complained of "being tired of having my wife sign all my checks. I feel powerless. I want to be able to do this for myself." While Mr. M. had been resistant to the idea of learning compensatory left-hand writing earlier in therapy, he now appeared ready to learn these skills. A series of writing exercises were designed that Mr. M. could practice as homework assignments. He faithfully completed these assignments, and within three weeks he had learned to sign his name legibly with his left hand. Mr. M. discounted this accomplishment as he stated, "So what? I can write my name, but it took me five minutes to do it—before it took seconds—and it looks like a child wrote it!" The patient was encouraged to challenge his prestroke-to-now comparisons, and to provide alternative statements which reflected his realistic poststroke gains (principles 7, 8). By creating alternative ways of viewing his newly learned writing skills, Mr. M. finally stated, "Even if my signature looks different, I can now control my own finances again." Thus, use of such compensatory strategies served to maximize Mr. M.'s functioning and enhanced his sense of independence (principle 2). (For a list of select cognitive remediation techniques appropriate for therapy use, see Hibbard, Grober, Gordon, Aletta, & Freeman, 1990b).

As Mr. M.'s writing skills improved, he was taught to record information he wanted to remember (e.g., appointments, things to do) in his diary as a compensatory tool to augment his frequent memory losses. The patient took notes during sessions on issues discussed and wrote down preplanned assignments to be completed between sessions. The therapist asked Mr. M. to review these notes during the week to "refresh his memory." In addition, Mr. M. recorded distressing events or issues that arose during the week that he wanted to discuss with the therapist. These issues became the agenda for subsequent sessions and allowed Mr. M. a more active, collegial role in determining the focus of the therapy sessions (principle 9). Thus, cognitive remediation strategies served to enhance both the patient's cognitive functioning and session continuity for this memory-impaired individual.

The last phase of treatment focused on helping the patient approximate his previous life-style as closely as possible given his realistic poststroke limitations (principle 6). While Mr. M. had successfully resumed many of his social involvements (e.g, visits with select friends, going to the actor's workshop), he continued to turn down acting positions, claiming he was "not ready for public scrutiny". Exploration of his assessment of his current versus previous acting abilities, as well as his perceived and real limitations, were discussed in a series of sessions. This resulted in Mr. M.'s reformulating what roles he could comfortably assume. On his own, Mr. M. decided to resume speech therapy in an attempt to maximize his acting opportunities. He insisted that the focus of these sessions would be his practice of oratory skills by using new scripts he had been given to review as his practice materials. He was also taught how to use cue cards to remember better the lines he was to say. Slowly, Mr. M. began to consider potential acting offers, but he remained very cautious in his selection process. However, by the end of therapy, Mr. M. had accepted his first acting position— a small role in which he had one line to say. He was eager to resume a modified acting career and appeared to have come to grips with his limitations, which altered but did not eliminate, his previous aptitudes and life-style.

To summarize, phase 2 treatment focused on allowing Mr. M. to mourn his speech and memory losses, providing him with compensatory strategies to enhance his cognitive functioning, and rebuilding Mr. M.'s prestroke life-style within the limitations of his poststroke abilities. The therapist, while continuing to utilize behavioral techniques, integrated cognitive strategies. Active challenging of exaggerations and distortions, particularly surrounding Mr. M.'s current (as contrasted with prestroke) abilities, became the major focus of therapy sessions. Mr. M. assumed a more active role in therapy as the emphasis of treatment became more collaborative in nature. Mrs. M.'s role during phase 2 was initially one of a therapeutic helper; she listed both her and her husband's impressions of his social interactions, as well as issues Mr. M. wanted to discuss in ensuing sessions, within his memory diary. As Mr. M. became more active his reliance on his wife decreased, and he began to function more independently. Structured social interactions involving both Mr. and Mrs. M. were used to help the couple overcome the social isolation they had experienced since Mr. M.'s stroke.

MOOD REASSESSMENT: COMPLETION OF THERAPY

Re-evaluation was completed after six months of treatment. As noted in Table 32-1, Mr. M. was now fully aware of his stroke-related losses and their impact on his personal and professional functioning. He denied feelings of depression at this evaluation. As a result of cognitive remediation and speech therapy, modest improvements were noted in the patient's speech and memory skills. The clinician also rated the patient as not depressed. Mrs. M. continued to see her husband as mildly depressed; her appraisal of her husband's mood again appeared to reflect her own reactive depression. As is typical of many PSD spouses, Mrs. M. was seen individually for several sessions to deal with her own losses surrounding the permanent changes in her partner and her life-style.

MOOD REASSESSMENT: ONE-YEAR FOLLOW-UP

As noted in Table 32-1, Mr. M.'s mood at this assessment remained stable. While he admitted to occasional bouts of sadness, he continued to challenge any self-critical statements, which served to limit his dysphoria and to give him some control over his mood and self-esteem. He had taken on several acting jobs, and all had gone well. In general, he was pleased with his progress. At this point, his spouse was no longer depressed. The couple's relationship was stable, with both partners accepting that "while life has changed, it's basically OK."

CONCLUSIONS

Cognitive therapy with depressed stroke patients places a series of unique demands on the therapist. Clinicians must not only be familiar with the principles and practice of cognitive therapy, but also be aware of the impact of the physical, cognitive, and social sequelae of stroke on this process. As discussed in this chapter, the therapist who works with this population must be flexible, creative, and patient. He or she must also, at times, function as a family therapist, marriage counselor, and cognitive remediator. If the clinician is able to understand the unique psychosocial, medical, and cognitive needs of these individuals, the rewards are immense. Patients who have often given up on themselves—and may have been given up on by their families and friends—frequently make great gains toward leading revised but rewarding lives.

REFERENCES

Gordon, W. A., Hibbard, M. R., Egelko, S., Riley, F., Simon, D., Diller, L., Ross, E. D., & Lieberman, A. N. (1990). Issues in the diagnosis of post-stroke depression. *Rehabilitation Psychology*, *36*(2), 71–87.

Hibbard, M. R., Gordon, W. A., Stein, P. S., Grober, S., & Sliwinski, M. (in press). A multimodal approach to the diagnosis of post-stroke depression. In W. A. Gordon (Ed.), *Advances in stroke rehabilitation*. Andover, MA: Andover Publishers, Inc.

Hibbard, M. R., Grober, S. E., Gordon, W. A., & Aletta, E. G. (1990a). Modifications of cognitive psychotherapy for the treatment of post-stroke depression. *Behavioral Therapist*, *13*, 15–17.

Hibbard, M.R., Grober, S. E., Gordon, W. A., Aletta, E. G., & Freeman, A. (1990b). Cognitive therapy and the treatment of post-stroke depression. *Topics in Geriatrics*, *5*, 43–55.

Lipsey, J. R., Robinson, R. G., Pearlson, G. D., Rao, L., & Price, T. R. (1984). Nortriptyline treatment of post-stroke depression: A double-blind study. *Lancet*, *1*, 297–300.

National Center for Health Statistics. (1977). *Profile of chronic illness in nursing homes, United States, August 1973–April 1974* (Vital Health Statistics, Series 13, No. 29). Hyattsville, MD: U.S. Department of Health, Education and Welfare.

Robinson, R. G., Starr, L. B., Kubos, K. L., & Price, T. R. (1983). A two-year longitudinal study of post-stroke mood disorders: Findings during the initial evaluation. *Stroke*, *14*, 736–741.

Ruckdeschel-Hibbard, M., Gordon, W. A., & Diller, L. (1986). Affective disturbances associated with brain damage. In S. Filskovs & T. Boll (Eds.), *Handbook of clinical neuropsychology, vol. 2* (pp. 457–472). New York: John Wiley.

Stein, P. N., Gordon, W. A., Hibbard, M. R. & Sliwinski, M. (1992). An examination of depression in the spouses of stroke patients. *Rehabilitation Psychology*, *37*(2), 121–130.

SUGGESTED READINGS

Beck, A., Rush, A. J., Shaw, B., & Emery, G. (1979). *Cognitive therapy of depression*. New York: Guilford.

Gordon, W. A., Hibbard, M. R., Egelko, S., Riley, F., Simon, D., Diller, L., Ross, E. D., & Lieberman, A. N. (1990). Issues in the diagnosis of post-stroke depression. *Rehabilitation Psychology*, *36*(2), 71–87.

Hibbard, M. R., Gordon, W. A., Egelko, S., & Langer, K. (1986). Issues in the diagnosis and cognitive therapy of depression in brain damaged individuals. In A. Freeman & V. Greenwood (Eds.), *Cognitive therapy applications in psychiatric and medical settings* (pp. 183–198). New York: Human Sciences Press.

Hibbard, M. R., Grober, S. E., Gordon, W. A., & Aletta, E. G. (1990). Modifications of cognitive psychotherapy for the treatment of post-stroke depression. *Behavioral Therapist*, *13*, 15–17.

Hibbard, M. R., Grober, S. E., Gordon, W. A., Aletta, E. G., & Freeman, A. (1990). Cognitive therapy and the treatment of post-stroke depression. *Topics in Geriatric Rehabilitation*, *5*, 43–55.

Hibbard, M. R., Gordon, W. A., Stein, P. S., Grober, S., & Sliwinski, M. (in press). A multimodal approach to the diagnosis of post-stroke depression. In W. A. Gordon (Ed.), *Advances in stroke rehabilitation*. Andover, MA: Andover Publishers, Inc.

Stein, P. N., Gordon, W. A., Hibbard, M. R., & Sliwinski, M. (1992). An examination of depression in the spouses of stroke patients. *Rehabilitation Psychology*, *37*(2), 121–130.

III

Extended Case Studies

33

Schizophrenic Disorders

Carlo Perris, Gullan Nordström, and Louise Troeng

INTRODUCTION

Cognitive-behavioral therapy has been applied to a broad range of patient problems, mostly of the neurotic type, including depression, anxiety, phobia, and panic. The application of cognitive therapy to the more chronic and serious schizophrenic disorders has been a far more recent development (Perris, 1988, 1989). Because of the genetic and neurochemical elements of schizophrenia, "talking therapy" has not been seen as a prime component of therapy for this large and quite diverse group. It can, however, be a central part of a comprehensive treatment program including hospitalization during acute phases, aftercare living arrangements, outpatient medication, individual and group therapy, and vocational counseling.

The importance of the therapist–patient relationship, based on the concepts of building a secure base and collaborative empiricism, is emphasized. We will illustrate how cognitive psychotherapy can be implemented with severely disturbed patients. The treatment has been

Carlo Perris • Department of Psychiatry, Umeå University Hospital, S-901 85 Umeå, Sweden and WHO Collaboration Center for Research and Training in Mental Health, Umeå University, S-901 85 Umeå, Sweden.   Gullan Nordström and Louise Troeng • Ersboda Cognitive Treatment Center, Stävgränd 73, S-902 63 Umeå, Sweden.

Comprehensive Casebook of Cognitive Therapy, edited by Arthur Freeman and Frank M. Dattilio. Plenum Press, New York, 1992.

carried out following the principle of dealing first with less problematic issues in the life of the patient, and later on working with core problems that manifest themselves in delusional experiences.

The importance of guiding the patient in carrying out a review of early experiences that might have contributed in promoting the development of dysfunctional self-schemas is stressed in the therapy. At the conclusion of treatment, the patient in this case was coached to obtain and maintain regular employment.

This case history deals with the long-term cognitive-behavioral treatment of a 34-year-old female whom we will name Eva. She has been suffering from a schizophrenic syndrome since age 19; prior to the beginning of this treatment, the patient had been in continuous contact with the adult psychiatric services for approximately eight years.

Since the treatment lasted for about three years, the scope of the report will be limited to emphasize significant areas of intervention in order to illustrate how cognitive psychotherapy can be applied with severely disturbed patients. During treatment, Gullan Nordström and Louise Troeng were the patient's main therapists, whereas Carlo Perris served as the supervisor and only met with Eva at irregular intervals.

SETTING

Eva was treated at one of the small community-based treatment centers for young patients with severe mental disorders that have been developed at Umeå in northern Sweden since 1986. Eva was a stable guest for a first period between August 1986 and July 1987, and later on for a second period between August 1988 and July 1989. In the nonresident time, she was seen as an outpatient on a weekly basis.

A detailed description of the treatment centers mentioned in this report has been made available elsewhere (Perris, 1988, 1989). hence, only their main characteristics and a general outline of the treatment program will be reported. It must be emphasized, however, that access to a special-purpose treatment center is not an indispensable prerequisite for conducting cognitive-behavioral therapy with severely disturbed patients. On the other hand, it is generally acknowledged (Perris, 1989) that the possibility of establishing a long-term psychotherapy treatment on an inpatient basis greatly facilitates the development of a purposeful working alliance between the therapist(s) and severely disturbed patients.

TREATMENT CHARACTERISTICS

The treatment program is based on cognitive-behavioral principles and is comprised of various elements (milieu, group, and individual therapy) that are related to each other and are assumed to interact in promoting the progress of the patient toward a higher level of personality integration. In particular, observations made during the life at the center, or at the group therapy sessions, can be used as a basis for discussion in the individual therapy. Conversely, topics discussed in the individual therapy sessions may lead to homework assignments to be carried out in the ordinary daily life at the center, or in a subsequent group therapy session. Two therapists are assigned to each patient. They work as staff personnel at the center and supervise the daily activities and participation turns in the group therapy sessions. Each patient staying at the center participates in two group therapy sessions and two individual therapy sessions each week.

ASSESSMENT

Besides a continuous clinical monitoring of the patient's condition, a battery of test instruments are administered at fixed intervals throughout the treatment. This battery is comprised of:

- the Automatic Thoughts Questionnaire (ATQ) (Hollon & Kendall, 1980).
- the Dysfunctional Attitude Scale (DAS) (Weissman & Beck, 1978).
- the Cognitive Style Test (CST) (Wilkinson & Blackburn, 1981).
- the Social Function Scale (SFS). This fourth instrument has been constructed at our department and is aimed at mapping the level of social functioning of the patient. It is available in two parallel versions: the SFS-Pat (to be used as a self-rating instrument completed by the patient) and the SFS-St (used for ratings made by the staff). Each version of the SFS is comprised of 20 sentence-completion items rated on a graded scale ranging from "very easy" (1) to "very difficult" (10). Examples of the items included in SFS-Pat include "to be able to assert my opinion without being overtly aggressive is for me . . ." and "To be able to establish reasonable priorities whenever I have to do several things is for me . . ."; examples of the questions included in SFS-St include "To start a conversation when people unknown to him/her are present is for him/her . . ." and "To be able to verbalize feelings experienced in various situations is for him/her . . .". Unpublished preliminary evaluations suggest that both instruments are satisfactorily reliable (inter-rates rho coefficient = 0.75 to 0.87).
- a Locus of Control Scale (LOC) (Eisemann, Perris, Palm, Palm, & Perris, 1988).
- a highly reliable (inter-raters rho = 0.97) scale for the staff rating of inpatient behavior (RASIB) developed at our department.

Other instruments include (a) a self-rating scale for the rating of personal parent child-rearing attitudes (EMBU) (Perris, Jacobsson, Lindström, von Knorring, & Perris, 1980); (b) a special-purpose scale constructed for mapping the subjective experience of interpersonal relationships; (c) a subscale of the Comprehensive Psychopathological Rating Scale (CPRS) (Perris, Schalling, & Sedvall, Åsberg, 1978), (d) the Beck Depression Inventory (BDI) (Beck, Ward, Mendelsohn, Mock, & Erbaugh, 1961); and (e) the subscales dealing with attentional processes of the Test of Attentional and Interpersonal Style (TAIS) (Nideffer, 1976). Videotapes of individual therapeutic sessions, patient diaries, and drawings made by the patient are also used.

Access to an item analysis of the test instruments used in the overall evaluation program allows therapists, at a very early stage of treatment, to pinpoint dysfunctional cognitions by less communicative patients. It also facilitates developing a clinical conceptualization of the patient's difficulties.

PAST HISTORY

Eva was born as the second child to lower-class parents in a small village outside Umeå. She grew up in a crowded, small farmhouse that lacked even the most elementary hygienic facilities (e.g., there was no toilet in the house). Occupants of the house included Eva's parents, a sister (who was 10 years older), two maternal uncles, and the maternal grandparents (who lived downstairs and were cared for by Eva's mother). The grandmother had been hospitalized in a mental hospital on a few occasions; her hospital diagnosis was that of a recurrent psychotic unipolar depression. She was described by Eva's parents as "strange" most of the time, and as occasionally manifesting acts of violence against her relatives. She eventually died when Eva was 6 years old.

Eva completed her primary schooling without any problems. Afterward she attempted, on several occasions, to achieve some professional training but was never able to complete any of the training courses she began. She had several occasional employments, but none lasted for very long. At age 29, she was able to complete a sheltered vocational training as a kitchen aide. She was unable, however, to keep an appointment she had been given later on as a part of her vocational rehabilitation. Thus, Eva was economically dependent on the social insurance system when she started her treatment.

At the time of her referral to the center, Eva had lived in her own apartment for several years. She had a stable relationship with a man of her age whom she had known for several years, though they did not live together. She had no children.

When Eva was first referred to the cognitive treatment center in 1986, her history of manifest mental illness had lasted for about 15 years. She had been in contact with psychiatric care almost without interruption for the last 8 years, mostly as an outpatient, but also as an inpatient for two periods of about two months each in 1979 and 1981. Her manifest problems began at the age of 16, when a pronounced change in her behavior was first observed. Apparently, she had been friendly, outgoing,and cheerful as a child and a young teenager. Afterwards, and apparently without any reason, she became shy, experienced difficulties in interacting with other people, and complained of feelings of estrangement and unreality. She felt as if she was living in a kind of fog and described experiences of depersonalization. She remembered that she felt as if she were "two different persons at the same time," but was unable to expand on this idea. She was at that time in the care of a child psychologist, but the symptomatology remained practically unchanged.

At age 22, she first came in contact with the adult psychiatric services complaining of the same symptoms as before (depersonalization, derealization, withdrawal, and anhedonia), which had now lasted for almost six years. She had also begun to express delusional ideas of reference and was convinced that others were negatively influenced by her. These symptoms had made it difficult for her to complete her studies, or to keep any of the few jobs she had attempted.

Between 1978 and 1980, Eva participated in individual supportive dynamic psychotherapy on an outpatient basis at the same time as she was treated with a neuroleptic medication at a low dosage (flupenthixol, 4 mg daily). At the end of the therapy, on whose termination both she and her therapist had agreed, she showed a brief improvement of a few months' duration. Very soon, however, the improvement was followed by a new and more pronounced exacerbation of her symptomatology, which prompted her second hospital admission in 1981. At that time, Eva was afraid to be alone in her apartment, since she was convinced that her neighbors were persecuting her and had menaced her with a knife. Before being admitted to the hospital, she had also refused to drink any water, since she was convinced that "they" had managed to poison it. She avoided going out of her apartment for fear of being assaulted. When panic-stricken, she would contact her sister by telephone in the middle of the night and visit her, and her sister would feed her. At admission, she refused to speak for a few days, since she was convinced that her speech and even her thoughts could negatively influence the personnel in the ward.

An increase in the dosage of the neuroleptic medication led to a symptomatological improvement and to her discharge from the hospital after 40 days of treatment. Since that time she had been in contact with the outpatient unit and had participated, on a somewhat irregular basis, in a series of community-based supportive group meetings. Her symptomatology had been less pronounced than before, but she had never been completely free from symptoms. She complained of tiredness, passivity, feelings of unreality, and vague ideas of reference. She continued her neuroleptics at a low dosage rather irregularly, along with a benzodiazepine derivative (lorazepam) because of insomnia and the rather diffuse somatic complaints, which were seen by the staff as a manifestation of anxiety.

ESTABLISHING A THERAPEUTIC WORKING RELATIONSHIP

The development of a therapeutic working relationship is a necessary prerequisite for any treatment, and especially so in the case of severely disturbed patients; its unfolding occurs over a long period of time. The principles upon which the relationship with these patients must be built are based on the conception of a "secure base" (Bowlby, 1979). It is from this base that the patient is expected and encouraged to explore his or her environment and to build up a self-reliant self-schema. For this process to be successful, it is necessary that the therapist(s) formulate a conceptualization of the patient's views of self, the world, and the future (what Beck, 1976, has defined as the "cognitive triad") as early as possible. In the case of patients with a severe psychotic disorder (perhaps even more so than with other types of patients), it is imperative that such a conceptualization is successively revised when new information is obtained in the unfolding of the treatment.

A preliminary conceptualization of Eva's interpersonal schema (Safran & Segal, 1990) focused on her experience of the environment as hostile and on her poor self-esteem. Later on, when data concerning Eva's current experiences could be related to experiences during her upbringing, other dysfunctional basic assumptions became evident. (e.g., "It doesn't matter what I do—nobody cares"; "One had to be nice at any price not to be rejected").

BEGINNING OF TREATMENT

Eva was withdrawn, shy, suspicious, and ambivalent when she first came to the center in August 1986. She had been favorably impressed by the familylike atmosphere of the setting and wanted to stay. On the other hand, she was uncertain whether she would be able to share the life at the center with the other patients and with the members of the staff whom she had not met before. She complained of somatic symptoms (mostly undefinable disturbing sensations in her head) and was moderately to severely depressed, with a BDI score of 22.

To overcome her initial difficulty, she was allowed a few days' trial during which she was expected to spend only a few hours each day at the center and to sleep at home until she felt that she wanted to stay as a resident. This decision was in keeping with an awareness of Eva's negative feelings toward any kind of external pressure concerning what she had to do. After a few days, Eva decided to stay at the center at night, but her social

interaction with the other guests and the personnel remained very guarded for quite a while. She would sit in a corner with some handwork, or whenever possible, remain isolated in her room, where she wrote in her daybook or completed the forms that were part of the assessment program.

SOCIALIZATION AND FORMULATION OF THERAPY GOALS

After a few days at the center, Eva was able to formulate some main goals for her treatment. Such a formulation is one part of the standard procedure in our program and is reached in connection with one or more interviews aimed at an inventory of the problems with which the patient wants to work. It also represents the beginning of the socialization to the principles of cognitive therapy and with the video recording of the sessions. The emphasis of the interview(s) is put on problems, rather than on symptoms. The following segment of one such interview with Eva illustrates the procedure. It also shows how the two therapists alternate in conducting the interview without interfering with each other.

THERAPIST 1:: Well, Eva, you have now been at the center for a few days. Do you think that you will be able to stay with us for a period as agreed?

EVA: It is nice . . . Yes, I feel that I will be able to stay here and to get some help.

THERAPIST 1: What makes you think that it will be easy for you to stay with us?

EVA: Well . . . people are kind to me . . . nobody pushes me to do things I don't want to do.

THERAPIST 2: Do you often think that other want you to do things when you don't want to?

EVA: Yes . . . everyone wants me to do what they want, without taking into account my wishes.

THERAPIST 2: How come?

EVA: Hmm . . . It is because I am unable to say no when I would like to do just that.

THERAPIST 1: What would happen if you said no?

EVA: I don't know . . . it is so difficult. I am unable to say no.

The first therapist explained at this point the relationship between thoughts, feelings, and behavior, and emphasized the importance of finding out what Eva thought when she felt compelled to act against her will. In particular, the therapist pointed out that Eva frequently used the expression "I feel" instead of the more appropriate "I think" or "I believe." She explained the concept of collaborative empiricism and the importance of working on the basis of specific everyday situations before probing further.

THERAPIST 1: It would be helpful if you could give us some example of a situation in which you felt pushed to do things that you did not want to do. It will make it easier to try to find out what kind of thoughts you may have had at that time that made you feel upset. Let's write down an example.

EVA: Well, a few days before coming to the center I wanted to buy some nice black shoes, which I had my eye on for some time. I went to the shop with a friend of mine to buy them, but she said that they would not suit me. She would not let me buy them.

THERAPIST 1: And what happened?

EVA: I felt both sad and angry. I did not buy them. We went away . . . I was disappointed with myself.

THERAPIST 1: (writes down on a sheet of paper) Well, we have this situation when you wanted to buy the shoes and your friend discouraged you. Then you said that you felt sad and angry. Is that correct?

EVA: Yes.

THERAPIST 1: Now, try to imagine once again the moment when your friend told you not to buy the shoes you wanted. What kind of thoughts occurred to you at that moment?

EVA: I don't know. I thought that I am never able to decide what to do; others can decide better . . . I am a grownup now, but I still am a complete failure. Everyone tells me what to do as if I did not have any right to decide for myself.

THERAPIST 1: (after writing down the automatic thoughts and Eva's consequent behavior) What would have happened if you had decided to buy the shoes?

EVA: My friend would have been disappointed. She would have decided to not go out shopping with me anymore.

THERAPIST 2: How do you know that?

EVA: It always happens that way. When I don't do what others want me to do they get angry at me.

THERAPIST 1: Have you ever tried to refuse to do things that others wanted you to do?

EVA: Not for a long time.

THERAPIST 2: Is this a problem for you to not be able to refuse to do what others want you to do?

EVA: Yes.

THERAPIST 2: Would this be one of the issues that you would like to work on during your stay here at the center?

EVA: Yes.

THERAPIST 1: OK. We will do that using the same method as we did now. We will explore together which other solutions could have been possible, and what you would have felt if you had behaved in some other way. But now let's go back to something you said before. You mentioned that you feel unable to decide by yourself despite the fact that you are a grownup. Is that always the case?

EVA: Well, I think that I can decide when I am on my own, but whenever I am with someone else, especially my relatives, then . . . I don't know . . . It is impossible for me to contradict people.

THERAPIST 1: What do you think would happen?

EVA: They would not agree. They would say that I am troublesome; they could decide to not want to meet me anymore.

THERAPIST 1: Has it happened to you that people have refused to associated with you because you contradicted them on some occasion?

EVA: I never did that, but I'm sure it would happen.

THERAPIST 1: Do you think that this would be another important issue to explore during your treatment?

EVA: I don't know; maybe.

Eva's fear of asserting herself, coupled with very poor self-esteem, had been a major issue in her life. Other goals that she was eventually able to formulate in successive interviews included a desire to overcome difficulties in establishing contact with others (thus avoiding being isolated), a wish to improve her ability to concentrate, and a desire to learn to be able to express feelings in an appropriate way. Much later during her treatment, Eva was able to add an additional goal that was obviously related to her delusional experiences—the wish to learn how to avoid being influenced by, and negatively influencing, other people.

Eva's negative thoughts of unworthiness appeared to stand out in her answers to the Automatic Thoughts Questionnaire (ATQ) that she completed at several occasions during her treatment (see Figure 33-1). The completion of the SFS scales aimed at assessing social functioning also revealed a profound disturbance in Eva's ability to interact socially. Examples of questions in the two scales on which both Eva and her therapists agreed were:

- Difficulty in starting a conversation when together with others
- Inability to show disappointment or anger
- Inability to appropriately respond to expressions of disappointment or anger by others

On the basis of those ratings, a series of exercises was planned for Eva to try a different behavior in agreed-upon situations in order to test what would happen in reality. In addition, she was encouraged to keep a record of the

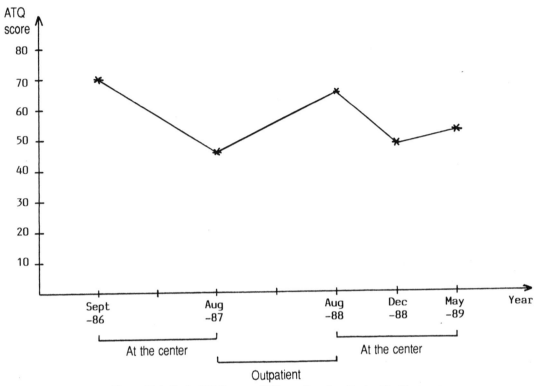

Figure 33-1. Eva's ATQ Scores at Different Occasions During Her Treatment.

fellow patients' behavior toward her when she had refused to do something that she did not want to do, or in connection with other social interactions when she had tried to manifest disappointment or anger. The following segments of interviews illustrate this part of the treatment.

THERAPIST 1:   What would you like to speak about today?

EVA: I am angry . . . It's the same old thing here at the center. It is the same as it has always been.

THERAPIST 1:   What do you mean?

EVA: The other patients want to decide all the time. They never listen to what I would like. They're all hostile.

THERAPIST 1:   Could you tell us about some specific situation that happened?

EVA: This morning, for example. We had worked together at the house chores and I wanted to have a coffee break, but they just laughed. I was angry because it was late and we should already have had our coffee break.

THERAPIST 1:   Well, what did you do?

EVA: I went up to my room to write in my daybook.

THERAPIST 1:   What did you write?

EVA: That I was angry . . . that everyone seems to be able to decide what to do without any respect for others' wishes.

THERAPIST 2:   Were you satisfied?

EVA: (with emphasis) No! I was angry.

THERAPIST 2:   What would you have preferred to do?

EVA: To tell them that when people live together in a place like this, everyone has the right to say what they want. I wanted my coffee break.

THERAPIST 2:   Was there any special reason why you could not say what you wanted or get your coffee by yourself?

EVA: One can't quarrel all the time.

THERAPIST 2:   Is it necessary to quarrel? Could you just tell them that you would prepare for the coffee break for everyone?

EVA: They were ignoring me. If I had tried to prepare the coffee break, they would have ignored me even more.

THERAPIST 1:   Would it be of any help to you if or when a similar situation again occurs, to do what you would prefer to do and to notice whether the other patients actually become angry, or ignore you? In that way you could test whether your expectations are correct.

Eva: What if they get angry?

Therapist 1: Let's try at least once. We would work out together afterwards how to cope if the others should react by becoming angry—is that OK?

Eva: Well, I will try, but how?

At this point, the therapists helped Eva to identify a possible situation when she could try to assert her wish. They agreed that such an occasion could easily occur when the patients were watching TV, if Eva decided to change the channel. Eva was coached and helped to rehearse how she could express her wishes and to imagine what kind of interaction would follow. She was also instructed to notice any change in the other patients' behavior toward her after such a critical incident. The following is a segment of an interview that took place a few days later.

Therapist 1: Did you have any occasion to put in practice what we rehearsed last time?

Eva: Well, yes, I tried . . . two days ago.

Therapist 1: Good! Tell us what happened.

Eva: Actually, it had nothing to do with watching the TV. Two days ago, all of the patients decided to go out to spend some time in a bar and to get something to eat. They all wanted to have some pizza, and I preferred a hot dog. Afterwards they all wanted to go to the movies, but I said that it was late and that we had to go back to the center, and it was OK. All the others followed me to the center.

Therapist 2: That was great! You have been able to apply what you had learned in a completely different situation. Was it difficult?

Eva: A little . . . I was uncertain about what would have happened. I thought that if they had tried to influence me, I would have answered using what we had rehearsed together, even if it did not concern watching another TV channel.

Therapist 1: Did you notice any particular reaction from the other patients?

Eva: Not in particular. I have written down what they said and how they have behaved toward me since that occasion. (shows her daybook, in which she had made notes of the other patients' behavior) They have not changed their behavior.

Therapist 2: Well, this seems to be a meaningful way to test whether your expectations are correct. Your writing down of your observations can be helpful in exploring both your experience of various situations and the way you have coped with them.

Eva continued to keep records of various situations in which her wishes happened to be in contrast with those of other people. Successively, she was able to test a variety of responses appropriate to various situations. She was able to generalize her appropriate behavior to situations that were different from those for which she had been prepared by cognitive rehearsal. Decisive for her progress was the fact that no assignment was ever imposed on Eva. On the contrary, she was coached to suggest which behavior she wanted to try and to rehearse how she would like to behave before any attempt was made to guide her toward any homework. Positive feedback was given to her at the completion of each task. Her attempts to test out her ideas in the early phase of treatment were planned by the therapists to occur in situations that were relatively uncharged emotionally.

In the course of these exercises, which continued with increasing complexity for the whole duration of treatment, it became apparent that Eva (as is the case with many other patients in her situation) was unable to grade her expressed feelings appropriately and was unable to interpret correctly feelings expressed by others. Hence, she was invited to participate in group sessions in which the patients learned through modeling and feedback to recognize and to distinguish different feelings, to appreciate their intensity, and to express them appropriately.

CHALLENGING DELUSIONAL EXPERIENCES

Eva's contact difficulties, however, were not only due to her inability to assert herself. They also had a delusional base that became more and more evident as Eva experienced the center as a safe place where she could trustfully express her inner feelings. The following excerpt of an individual session—which occurred at a time when Eva spent most of her time in her room, appeared particularly suspicious, and refused to go out of the center—illustrates some of her experiences.

Therapist 1: You have mostly stayed in your room for the last few days. Is there any special reason why you prefer not to go out?

Eva: Hmm. . . I don't care to go out.

Therapist 1: All the other patients go out for some time every day, and so far you haven't joined them. Do you have any special reason for not joining them for a walk?

Eva: I don't want to go out because I don't want to get angry.

Therapist 1: I must confess that I am unable to follow what you mean; would it make you angry to go out?

EVA: Well, every time I go out there is something upsetting me. I don't like to feel bad afterwards.

THERAPIST 1: Do you mind telling us what it is that makes you feeling bad?

EVA: It is what other people think.

THERAPIST 1: I am afraid I still don't understand what you are referring to.

EVA: (with some irritation) I told you. It is what other people think that make some upset.

THERAPIST 2: Could you tell us in detail about one such upsetting situation you have recently had?

EVA: Well a few days ago, for example, when I went out there were some workers working close to the street . . .

THERAPIST 2: And? Tell us what happened.

EVA: Nothing. I had to turn back.

THERAPIST 2: What caused you to turn back?

EVA: I don't know. I just had to.

THERAPIST 1: Let's look a little closer at this situation. You were going for a walk when you saw some people working. You say that nothing happened; nevertheless, you had to turn back. Is that correct?

EVA: Yes.

THERAPIST 1: Do you remember any thoughts you had when you saw the workers?

EVA: Well, I thought that they were looking at me as if I were an odd person, a crazy woman. It was menacing. I felt that I had to defend myself from them . . . I had to turn back.

THERAPIST 1: Did they say anything to you?

EVA: No . . . they were working.

THERAPIST 1: In which way were they menacing you?

EVA: I don't know . . . it is as if the whole world is against me. I am helpless. You can never understand what it feels to be constantly menaced . . .

THERAPIST 1: In which way did they show that they thought that you were an odd person?

EVA: I could see it in their faces . . .

THERAPIST 2: What did it look like when they had those thoughts?

EVA: I don't know . . . you can see it. You're trying to confuse me . . .

THERAPIST 2: Well, let's assume that you interpreted the expression of those workers correctly,. Could you have acted in some other way besides turning back?

EVA: No. The only possibility was for me to turn back. You don't understand.

At this point, Eva was unable to produce any alternative explanation for her interpretation of the situation. She was also unable to think of any alternate behavior but turning back. Even the therapists' probing of how one is

able to recognize that someone thinks that another person is "odd" or "crazy" was unsuccessful. Despite her well-cared-for appearance, Eva was convinced that everyone could "see" that she was "odd." Hence, the therapists decided not to pursue the challenging of the experience. Instead, they probed further to obtain additional information about the pervasiveness of the delusional experiences and about the degree of conviction in Eva's beliefs.

THERAPIST 1: Does it often occur that you have the experience of people looking upon you as if you were an odd person?

EVA: Well, everyone is able to see that I am a strange person.

THERAPIST 1: In which way do you think that you are different from other women?

EVA: I know that I am.. People can see it on my face . . . I am able to understand it when I see how they look at me. Otherwise, why should people be looking at me when I go to some place?

THERAPIST 2: It seems to me that this is a major issue for you. Would you like to work on this problem with us to see if we can reach any solution?

EVA: I don't think that there is any solution . . .

The process of helping Eva to challenge her delusional experiences had proved to be very hard and had lasted for a long time (see below). She had, on several occasions in the early stage in treatment, given the impression of having some understanding of the pathological nature of her referential experiences. Her conviction of the correctness of her delusional interpretation of other's behaviors and reactions was very strong indeed.

The following excerpt from her diary shows the extent of her delusional experiences:

> I wish that they [Eva's closest relatives, although this did not become clear until much later in treatment] would leave me alone, but I don't know what to do . . . It's terrible . . . Everyone believes me to be much better than I am. I should be able to give the impression that I don't care, but it is meaningless. They are capable of reading my thoughts. Do you have any suggestion about what I should do? I cannot succeed any further [in my therapy] because they push me down. It is as if they were able of thinking my thoughts . . . They want me to be a robot in their hands.

Eva actively avoided in subsequent sessions any discussion of her misinterpretations. She insisted, instead, that all efforts should concentrate on helping her to prepare herself for some suitable part-time job. An accentuation became evident with her experience of strange sensations in her head that did not respond to the analgesics she occasionally used, and were coupled with irritability and restlessness. She claimed that her disturbances had to be related to some vague organic cause and insisted on wanting a referral for a "somatic investigation of her head." Since at that time we had in progress a CAT scan study of patients suffering from a schizophrenic disorders, such an investigation was proposed to her. When the CAT scan was to be performed, however, she refused to participate because of feelings of "claustrophobia" after looking at the apparatus.

Eva was offered a part-time job as part of a vocational rehabilitation program administered by the social insurance system toward the end of the first year that she spent at the center as a resident. She decided to leave the center, against the advice of her therapists. Eva maintained stubbornly that she was satisfied with the degree of improvement that she had reached, and that she wanted to test whether she had really become able to stay on her own. Whenever the therapists attempted to bring up the topic of her delusional experiences, suggesting that she should remain at the center for an additional period to solve this problem, her response was that those experiences were not a problem that disturbed her anymore, and thus, there was nothing that needed to be solved.

A THERAPEUTIC INTERLUDE

Between July 1987 and August 1988, progress in Eva's treatment occurred very slowly, with several ups and downs. She met regularly with her therapists once a week on an outpatient basis, but the contents of the therapy sessions were shallow and the sessions were judged by the therapists to be not particularly productive. Mostly, Eva wanted to discuss how to solve small practical difficulties at her working place, or other everyday trivia. Occasionally she brought up hints about difficulties with her parents, but she consistently refused to discuss her relatives—and in particular, her relationship with her mother—in any depth.

At her working place, Eva was appreciated by her immediate superior and, apparently, had no major problems with her coworkers. She met her boyfriend regularly and planned to spend her summer vacation with him in 1988.

LATER PHASE OF TREATMENT

The part-time employment that Eva had obtained as part of the vocational rehabilitation came to an end toward the end of June 1988, when Eva began her planned vacation. There would have been an opportunity of finding some alternative suitable employment if Eva had wanted it. Instead, at the end of her apparently uneventful vacation, Eva expressed a wish to spend a new period at the treatment center. She reported that she had realized that her therapeutic gain had only been partial. She said she was aware that she had not taken full advantage of the opportunity she had been offered at the center "to once and for all get rid of all her problems," because she had lacked the necessary motivation to deal with issues that could have been stressful. The therapists noticed a slight general impairment in her condition: She was more suspicious, more guarded in her contacts, and less talkative than she had been at the end of her first period at the center and during the early phase of her treatment as an outpatient. On almost all ratings carried out at that occasion, she also showed slightly higher scores than those obtained at the end of the first treatment period (see Figures 33-1, 33-2, 33-3, and 33-4).

A Renewed Attempt to Deal with Eva's Delusional Experiences

It was during the second period of staying at the center that Eva was able to face the broad scope of her psychotic experiences, and that she was willing to work actively at dealing with them. Crucial in this respect was an occasion, a few weeks after she had been at the center, when the patients and the staff had agreed on going to the theater. Eva was ambivalent as to whether she wanted to join the others or remain alone at the center for the evening. The following interview segment illustrates the breakthrough that occurred at that time.

THERAPIST 1: Is there anything in particular that you want to discuss?

EVA: Well . . . there is this problem with going to the theater.

THERAPIST 2: What is the problem?

EVA: I don't know. I am not sure that I want to go. On the other hand, I have always very much liked the artist [a well-renowned comedian who occasionally performed in town] who will perform. I have only seen him on TV, and I like him very much. It would be nice to see him in a live show.

THERAPIST 1: Then it's simple. You will see him if you go to the theater. Why would you not want to go?

EVA: It is because of the same problem we have spoken about on previous occasions. It is very difficult for me to go to the theater.

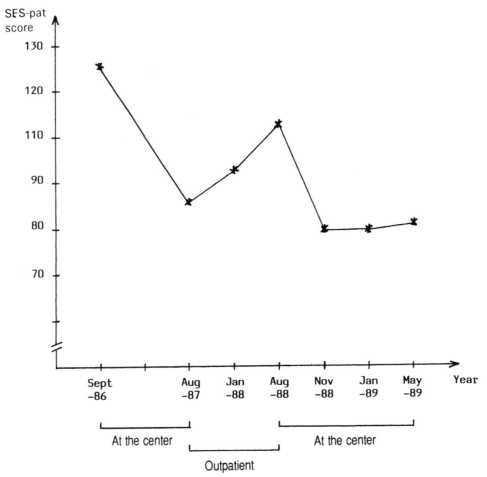

Figure 33-2. SFS Scores (Self-Rating) at Various Intervals During Treatment.

THERAPIST 1: Could you be a little more specific about this difficulty of yours?

EVA: (long pause) It is because of the spotlights . . .

THERAPIST 2: What about them?

EVA: (pause) I am sure that when I enter the theater, the spotlights will be on me . . . Everyone will see that I am a strange person.

THERAPIST 2: Have you been at the theater before?

EVA: No, I have not. I have always been afraid of the spotlights. And besides . . . I am not sure that I would be able to laugh or to applaud appropriately. People would see and understand that I am sick. On the other hand, what would I do if I remained alone at the center for the whole evening?

At this point, the second therapist led Eva to reflect that she very likely would feel unsatisfied with herself if she decided to remain alone at home. The therapists also helped Eva, by using a Socratic interview technique, to realize that the spotlights are usually first turned on only when the actors are on stage, and that they are always directed toward the stage and not toward the audience. There would hardly be any risk that the spotlights would be focused on her. Eventually, Eva accepted the validity of this way of looking at the problem.

THERAPIST 1: Let us now turn to your other problem. What could you do to be sure that you will laugh or applaud at the right time?

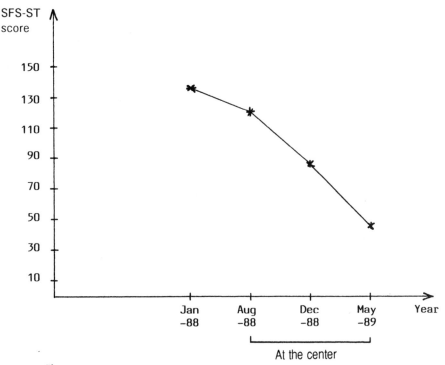

Figure 33-3. SFS Scores (Therapists' Rating) at Various Intervals During Treatment.

EVA: I don't know.

THERAPIST 1: Who is going to the theater, besides you?

EVA: Well . . . all of the people here at the center are going.

THERAPIST 1: OK. You are supposed, then, to go together with all of the others. Where do you expect that you will sit when at the theater?

EVA: Near to the other patients or to some of the staff, I guess.

THERAPIST 1: Right. Now think, do you believe that the other patients and the staff are able to applaud appropriately?

EVA: Yes . . . I think so.

THERAPIST 1: What could you do, then, so that also you applaud at the right time?

EVA: (pause): When you say that . . . maybe, I could wait and watch what the others will do.

THERAPIST 1: Right. You see, one possible solution—if you should feel uncertain about how to behave, you could be attentive to what the other patients and the members of the staff will do. Is that OK?

EVA: You are right.

THERAPIST 1: Do you think that you will feel more comfortable now when you know some clue you can use to adjust your behavior?

EVA: Yes.

THERAPIST 2: Well, what is your decision?

EVA: I think that I will come with you. Will I have an opportunity of sitting close to you?

THERAPIST 2: Of course, if you want to.

At this point, the therapists should have dealt more closely with the very nature of Eva's fears. However, they judged that the available time before the end of the session was too short to deal in a meaningful way with such an important topic. They expected that Eva's experience of the visit to the theater would prove to be a positive one, thereby serving as a base for further experience and discussion. If so, it was expected that it would have been easier at a later occasion to address the irrationality of her fears. They also assumed that if, at that time, Eva had become upset by a discussion of her referential ideas, she could have decided not to go to the theater, which she probably would have experienced as a major failure for her.

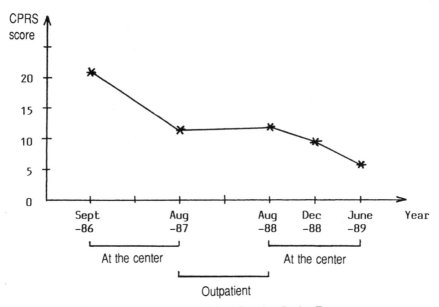

Figure 33-4. DAS Scores at Various Occasions During Treatment.

Eventually, Eva went to the theater and enjoyed the performance. In particular, she was proud of having been able to laugh and to applaud appropriately without waiting for any cue from the others. She was surprised by having completely forgotten about her fear of the spotlights. Two days later, at the session from which the following segment has been abstracted, she was in good spirits.

THERAPIST 1: How do you feel today?

EVA: Much better than I have in a long time.

THERAPIST 1: Is there any special reason why you feel better?

EVA: Well, I am glad to have overcome my fear of going to the theater. I enjoyed the performance so much . . . I believe that it will be easier for me in the future to go again to some show if I want to.

THERAPIST 1: That will be nice for you. Now, when you think back, what do you think had been helpful for you in this occasion?

EVA: I think that having been able to prepare myself in advance had been most helpful.

THERAPIST 2: Is there any conclusion you can draw from this experience?

EVA: Well . . . I could do the same in the future—that

is, prepare myself in advance when I am going to be exposed to new situations.

THERAPIST 2: Right. Now, is there anything in particular you want to discuss today?

EVA: No . . . not in particular. You might suggest . . .

THERAPIST 1: What about looking a little closer at the fears you mentioned before going to the theater, now that you have had an opportunity of testing them in practice?

EVA: Is that necessary?

THERAPIST 1: I think so. You have admitted that fears of that kind are an obstacle to your participation in various activities.

EVA: Yes, I think they are.

THERAPIST 2: Do you remember what your real fears were before going to the theater?

EVA: Oh, yes! It was my knowledge that people look at me because I am a strange person. I feel watched all the time. That makes it impossible for me to think clearly.

THERAPIST 2: Hmm, that says a whole lot. How do you judge what you say to be true?

EVA: That's the way it has been that way for a very long time . . . I know that it is so.

THERAPIST 2: Well, let's examine each of your statements one by one. Which of your expectations proved to be true?

EVA: Well . . . actually, none of them.

From this point on, the therapists begin to probe about Eva's referential experiences in general. She admitted that she felt "watched," and complained that "the others" were hostile toward her. She said that she believed that everyone was able to see that she was a strange person, and that for this reason they behaved with hostility toward her. This was the main reason, Eva said why she preferred to keep to herself, avoiding as far as possible any interaction with other people.

By using the technique of pinpointing and analyzing various specific situations in detail and by having access to her diary, the therapists succeeded in making Eva aware of her own expectations when meeting new people. Eventually, she was able to realize that it was almost exclusively when she herself felt stressed and uncertain about her own behavior that she expected others to be particularly critical of her and to look at her as if she were a strange person. She believed that others were capable of reading her thoughts, thereby making her even more uncomfortable. With the therapists' guidance, Eva became aware that whenever she felt unsure of how to behave in unfamiliar situations involving other people, she put herself in a "referential attitude" (Arieti, 1962). Eventually, she also proved able to understand the negative impact that an interpersonal schema comprising a conception of the environment as hostile had on her behavior and, thus, on the reactions shown by others. Graded homework assignments allowed her to test in vivo the tenability of alternative ways of looking at the environment and to discuss them in the therapy sessions.

This process of successively increasing insight, easy to summarize in a few lines, in reality unfolded during several months. Eva could, during that time, easily shift between periods when she worked productively both in the therapy sessions and as a part of her homework assignments, showing a progressive acceptance of the irrationality of her thoughts and periods when she was irritable and uncooperative and tried to stay away from the center with the same rationalization as before—that is, that she had to train herself to live in her own flat. On the whole, however, it became easier and easier to help her in identifying stressful situations that promoted delusional experiences and to discuss how she could functionally cope with them.

Encouraged to pay particular attention to automatic thoughts in various situations, Eva became able to identify their frequent self-defeating characteristics. Also, she became interested in attempting to train more functional self-instructions, as it is illustrated by the following segment of an interview. Prior to this excerpt, the first therapist had inquired about Eva's homework and asked her what she would like to talk about.

EVA: I have tried to identify those situations when I feel particularly uncomfortable. I mean those occasions when I feel as I were paralyzed and would like to just disappear.

THERAPIST 1: Would you like to talk about any such occasion?

EVA: (shows her notebook, in which she had written down various situations and the related feelings, thoughts, and alternative thoughts according to the five-column technique) Well, the situation which I have written down here was that I had to do the shopping for the meal at the center and went into a shop. There was a lot of people doing their shopping and waiting for their turn at the counter. I felt disturbed and wanted to run away . . .

THERAPIST 2: Could you be more precise about the kind of feeling you experienced?

EVA: I don't know . . . maybe I was anxious. It was unpleasant; I wanted to run away.

THERAPIST 1: OK. let's see . . . which were the thoughts that you recalled?

EVA: I thought, "I am behaving strangely. I am behaving in a deviant way. Now everyone will stop and look at me. Everyone will laugh at me." I wanted to leave without waiting for my turn.

THERAPIST 2: And what, in fact, did you do?

EVA: Well, I remembered what we are talking about in our sessions. I remained in the shop and I started telling myself, "Eva, do you know that these are your irrational fears? If you look around, you will realize that nobody is particularly interested in you. Nobody looks at you more than you yourself look at others. Also, if they did, that does not necessarily imply that they are hostile."

THERAPIST 1: Did it help?

EVA: Yes. I repeated those sentences a few times and was able to relax. I remained in the store to do my shopping.

THERAPIST 1: How did you feel when you were able to challenge your self-defeating thoughts?

EVA: I was satisfied with myself. I wasn't tense any longer.

THERAPIST 1: Right. Have you tried this procedure on other occasions as well?

EVA: I am learning to do that. Do you think that it will be useful?

THERAPIST 1:   Judging from what you have just told us, I would think so.

THERAPIST 2:   Would you lose anything if you tried?

EVA: Well . . . no. I don't think so.

Dealing with Recollection of Past Experiences and with a Possible Reconstruction of the Development of Dysfunctional Cognitions

In time, with her progressive openness in dealing with topics that she for a long time had refused to touch upon, Eva began to ask about possible explanations of her beliefs. Early in treatment, especially at the time when her somatic complaints were in the foreground, she had repeatedly maintained that her disturbances must have had a somatic origin. Later on, she became more and more aware that one important component of her distress could be found in the fact that she lived under the pressure of harsh "personal rules" (Wessler & Hankin-Wessler, 1986), and she wondered how those could have come about. On one of these occasions, Eva's therapists gave her a short lecture on what is known about the possible development of basic dysfunctional schemas and encouraged her to write down memories of her upbringing, which she felt had been particularly important for her.

The therapists had access to Eva's family history and to the data concerning Eva's memories of her upbringing collected by means of the EMBU. From the scoring of the EMBU questionnaire, in fact, what emerged was the picture of an intruding mother, harsh and punishing in her attitudes, who had made use of rearing practices based on the engendering of shame. Her father, in contrast, had been experienced as more understanding and warm, but weak. Eva had experienced her parents' child-rearing practice as not having any sense of consequence. The lack of a close, sharing relationship between Eva and her mother was even more evident in her answers to a questionnaire (developed at our centers) aimed at investigating to which people in their environment a patient felt that he or she could turn to discuss different topics and confide when in trouble. Particularly significant was the fact that Eva did not include her mother as among the people to whom she could confide.

Eva's mother never visited at the center, and Eva did not consent for the therapists to visit her parents at their home. On the other hand, the therapists were able on some very few occasions to get in touch with Eva's mother by telephone. On those occasions, she did not convey the impression of any warmth or concern for her daughter's

treatment. Eva's father, on the other hand, visited her a few times and showed an empathic interest in Eva's progress. When asked about his view of his family, he described his wife as a woman always strained by the burden of a big household, almost obsessively concerned with duties, and unable to show any warm feelings.

Encouraged by the therapists, Eva wrote down in her notebooks those memories that she felt had been the most impressive and important to her. Those notes—amounting to four thick books—were analyzed in the individual therapy sessions. On those sessions, Eva was encouraged to rehearse some of her most negative experiences (to try to elicit the feelings experienced at that time) and which thoughts those experiences could have provoked (in order to explore alternative interpretations of the various situations). Thus, during a few months, the content of the therapy sessions shifted back and forth between revision of Eva's childhood memories and Eva's everyday life experiences at the center. While it is impossible for us to deal with the specific contents of those early memories, out of consideration for Eva's integrity, the report of a few short abstracts of her reflections at the center at that time can give a flavor of the turmoil that she experienced:

- "I am experiencing a positive feeling that I have never had before. I don't dare to hope that it will last . . . I will live these days one by one and see what happens."
- "I feel more trustful of other people than I have ever been for a long while . . . What will happen if I will feel bad again?"
- "I feel so sad . . . I have had to take some tablets [lorazepam] to stand out my distress. It is a failure to have to take tablets to feel relaxed. It feels as if I were cheating myself."
- "I cannot stand when the other patients are laughing . . . Even though I feel happier, still I am unable to laugh with the others."
- "Everything stands still in my head today. I would like to go downstairs and just scream . . . scream at everyone . . . On the other hand, I could take some tablets and feel better . . . but I would lose my positive feelings as well . . . The choice is mine."
- "I have been able to avoid taking tablets for a few days. It's been hard work, but I feel so much more satisfied with myself. I believe that I am slowly moving forward . . . I think that the other patients have realized that I feel better. I'm able to talk with them in a more relaxed way and to participate in their jokes. On the other hand, I feel that there still is something wrong with me . . . However, I feel

that I am coming closer and closer an alternative way of being and thinking [*sic*]."

- "I was able to feel sadness, anger, joy, disappointment, etc. Are there particularly emotional persons? Sometimes I think that I'm such a person. Is this one of the reasons why I became ill? Because I feel so easily hurt?"
- "I have gotten back a feeling I have had before. I cannot describe what kind of feeling it is. It is not pleasant . . . I am almost afraid of being together with the other patients, and at the same time I don't know what my fear consists of."
- "It is several weeks since I took any medication. It had been very difficult, but I've succeeded. Is there any hope that I can be cured once and for all?"

Eva became aware that most of her dysfunctional personal rules of living could have had their origin in her inability to establish a relationship of basic trust with her mother. She became able to see her mother's behavior less critically, though not without a certain degree of sadness. However, no real rapprochement occurred.

Issues of Transference and Countertransference

The life at the center and the consistent use of two therapists contributed to diluting the transference that develops in any prolonged treatment. However, transferential behavior became especially manifest when Eva felt pushed by the therapists to deal with topics that she felt were particularly stressful. On those occasions, Eva was stubborn, irritable, and sad at the same time. In particular, she revealed her identification of her current environment with her parents, and especially with her mother, in several transparent notes in her notebooks:

- "I am really angry with G. and L. They try to influence me to do things which I don't want . . . They believe that I'm a little girl that can be bullied as they wish . . ."
- "I would like it if L. were better able to understand what I want."
- "Everything looks as if it were artificial. Nobody at this place is able to show his or her real feelings."
- "I don't dare to react according to my feelings, because I don't know whether my feelings are healthy. Is there anyone I can trust?"
- "I feel more easily hurt than ever. I would like to work actively with G. and L., but at the same time I want to be left alone to avoid being hurt."

The therapists made a consistent use of positive transference throughout the treatment in order to convey to Eva the feeling of having found a secure base. Especially on those occasions in which Eva was afraid of being rejected or ignored, they behaved in such a way to actively disconfirm her negative expectations with their affectionate behavior, and to enhance her sense of trust.

TERMINATION OF TREATMENT: COACHING EVA BACK TO WORK

Termination of treatment is seldom a difficult issue at our centers. This is mainly due to the fact that our conceptualization of the therapeutic relationship is theoretically based on Bowlby's concept of attachment (Bowlby, 1969–1980) rather than being focused on theories of dependence or resolution of transference. Hence, it is expected that even when the active treatment has come to an end, the patient will still feel attached to the therapists who for such a long time have become his or her substitute family. In the same way that teenagers who leave their parental home to live on their own, however independent, can still rely on the emotional bond to their parents, so can our patients rely on their therapists when therapy is finished and they no longer meet on a regular basis. We believe that such an attitude is a necessary prerequisite for treating patients who suffer from severe mental disorders. In addition, in follow-up planning, booster sessions greatly contribute to mitigating the immediate impact of separation at the end of the active treatment.

The last few months that Eva spent at the center were devoted to guiding her in finding a suitable job. This was made possible by the cooperative efforts of the members of the vocational rehabilitation system that operates everywhere in Sweden. Eventually, a position was found at a nursing home run by the town's social service, which fit with Eva's vocational training and her previous working experiences.

To minimize the risk of failure, the therapists accompanied Eva to her new working place and, in turn, stayed there as participant observers during her first week at work. At the end of each working day, a short session was scheduled in which Eva was given the opportunity of summing up her impressions of the day. On those occasions, Eva's feelings and thoughts in relation to the new people she had met and the various situations to which she had been exposed during the day were analyzed in detail and worked through utilizing the cognitive-behavioral techniques that she had been taught throughout her time at the center.

Initially, Eva reported the occurrence of dysfunctional thoughts—mostly related to her fear that her performance would appear as poor to her coworkers, thus leading to rejection. She was afraid of prejudicial attitudes by her coworkers because of her mental illness. As a consequence, her performance was below her real capacity for a few days. The rehearsal of the experiences of each day at the following therapy sessions, however, helped Eva in a very short time to develop a more adaptive internal monologue that proved to be effective. During the second week, when Eva went alone to her work, she was able to identify self-defeating cognitions easily and to both challenge and correct them. For example, she told her therapists:

> When I get the thought that my coworkers may be critical of what I am doing because I'm a failure, I have learned to stop the old train of thoughts by telling myself, "Stop it Eva! Don't give in to your crazy thoughts." I have found that it works . . . I'm able to analyze the situation from other angles and to counteract my old proneness to misinterpret.

Presently, Eva has moved back to her apartment and has been able to work for a little longer than six months without any problem. She visits her parents from time to time and dates her boyfriend with whom she had spent a nice and quiet vacation. She feels safer in her new role and behaves more confidently and openly when she meets other people. Her contact with the center is presently limited to occasional telephone calls to her therapists just to tell them that everything is OK.

Medication

Throughout her treatment, both at the center and on an outpatient basis, Eva had been on medication with haloperidol (2 mg/day). She felt comfortable with such a dosage and does not suffer from apparent side effects. For some time, Eva had also had lorazepam, which she had mostly used as a hypnotic at a dosage of 1 mg at bedtime. Occasionally, however, she had increased the dosage up to

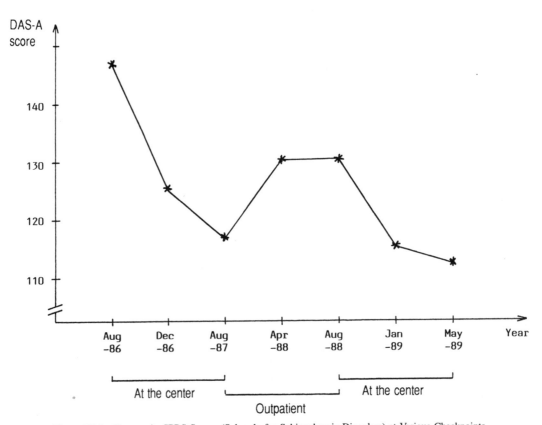

Figure 33-5. Changes in CPRS Scores (Subscale for Schizophrenic Disorders) at Various Checkpoints.

1 mg two or three times a day when, as mentioned earlier, she felt more stressed. She had always been concerned with the risk of becoming dependent on benzodiazepines, and therefore she had kept careful notes in her notebooks of the amount of medication she had used so as to avoid any abuse.

ISSUE OF ASSESSMENT

Some results of the ratings carried out throughout the treatment have been given above. At this juncture, we wish to add that a decrease in rating scores occurred also in the DAS-A (which was consistently used) and on the CPRS (see Figures 33-4 and 33-5). In contrast, results obtained with the CST remained practically unchanged (see Figure 33-6).

One reason why no more pronounced changes were obvious on the various tests used in our assessment, despite Eva's clear clinical improvement, could be that those tests were originally conceived to be used with depressed patients; therefore, they may not include items that would be pertinent for mapping more specific dysfunctional cog-

nitions in patients suffering from a more severe disorder of a schizophrenic type. Until more suitable instruments are developed, access to videotapes of therapy sessions and (whenever possible) to diaries and notebooks in which the patient reports the progress of therapy are a necessary complement to the continuous clinical monitoring and notes made by therapists to be able to describe in detail the therapeutic process.

CONCLUDING REMARKS

Throughout this chapter, we have reported on a three-year-long treatment of a young woman suffering from a schizophrenic syndrome in order to show how cognitive psychotherapy can be implemented with patients suffering from a severe disorder. Considerations of space have imposed limits on the scope of our presentation. Another constraint has been the obligation not to report in detail several issues discussed in therapy, especially those concerning Eva's childhood and her relation to her mother, because they could lead to an identification of the patient. These limitations are important because they

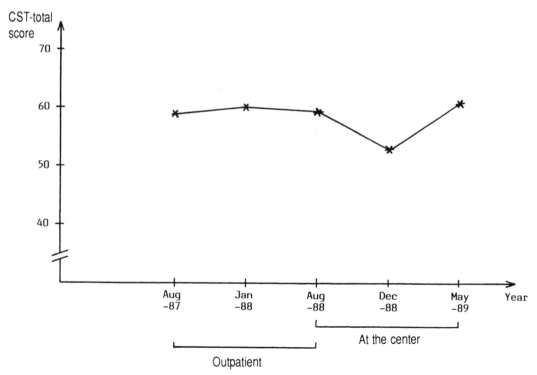

Figure 33-6. CST Total Scores During Outpatient Treatment and Second Stay at the Center.

thwart the possibility of giving a full picture of the therapeutic process that went on. We believe, however, that
even with such limitations the reader will be able to get a
general picture of the conduct of therapy with a severely
disturbed patient and of the various steps that were taken
in its implementation.

Finally, we do not claim to have "cured" Eva from
her mental illness. What we believe to have achieved,
instead, is an enhancement of her competence, which
includes both a modification of several dysfunctional basic assumptions that had ruled her life so far and an
increase in her adaptive ability in dealing with problematic interpersonal situations in her everyday life. She has
developed a more confident view of herself and a more
hopeful view of her future. In particular, we believe that
she has been able to incorporate and construct her own
cognitive tools that will help her to cope successfully with
situations that she previously would have experienced as
hopelessly straining.

REFERENCES

Arieti, S. (1962). Hallucinations, delusions, and ideas of reference treated with psychotherapy. *American Journal of Psychotherapy, 16,* 56–60.
Asberg, M., Perris, C., Schalling, D., & Sedvall, G. (1978). The
CPRS—Development and applications of a psychiatric rating
scale. *Acta Psychiatrica Scandinavica,* suppl. 271.
Beck, A. T. (1976). *Cognitive therapy and the emotional disorders.* New York: International Universities Press.
Beck, A. T., Ward, C. H., Mendelsohn, M., Mock, J., & Er-
baugh, J. (1961). An inventory for measuring depression. *Archives of General Psychiatry, 4,* 561–571.
Bowlby, J. (1969–1980). *Attachment and loss* (vols. 1–3). Pen-
guin Books.
Bowlby, J. (1979). *A secure base.* London: Routledge.
Eisemann, M., Perris, C., Palm, A., Palm, U., & Perris, H.
(1988). LOC—presentation of a Swedish instrument for as-
sessing locus of control. In C. Perris & M. Eisemann (Eds.),
Cognitive psychotherapy: An update (pp. 45–49). Umeå,
Sweden: DOPUU Press.
Hollon, S. D., & Kendall, P. C. (1980). Cognitive self-statements
in depression: Development of an automatic thoughts ques-
tionnaire. *Cognitive Therapy & Research, 4,* 383–395.
Nideffer, R. M. (1976). Test of attentional and interpersonal style.
Journal of Personality and Social Psychology, 34, 394–404.

Perris, C. (1988). Intensive cognitive-behavioral psychotherapy
with patients suffering from schizophrenic psychotic or post-
psychotic syndromes: Theoretical and practical aspects. In C.
Perris, I. M. Blackburn, & H. Perris (Eds.), *Cognitive psycho-
therapy: Theory and practice* (pp. 324–375). New York:
Springer-Verlag.
Perris, C. (1989). *Cognitive therapy with schizophrenic patients.*
New York: Guilford.
Perris, C., Jacobsson, L., Lindström, H., von Knorring, L., &
Perris, H. (1980). Development of a new inventory for assess-
ing memories of parental rearing behavior. *Acta Psychiatrica
Scandinavica, 61,* 265–274.
Safran, J. D., & Segal, Z. V. (1990). *Interpersonal process in
cognitive therapy.* New York: Basic Books.
Weissman, A. N., & Beck, A. T. (1978). *Development and
validation of the Dysfunctional Attitude Scale.* Paper presented
at the annual meeting of the Association for the Advancement
of Behavior Therapy, Chicago.
Wessler, R. L., & Hankin-Wessler, S. W. R. (1986). Cognitive
appraisal therapy (CAT). In W. Dryden & W. Golden (Eds.),
Cognitive behavioral approaches to psychotherapy (pp. 196–
223). London: Harper & Row.
Wilkinson, I. M., & Blackburn, I. M. (1981). Cognitive style in
depressed and recovered depressed patients. *British Journal of
Clinical Psychology, 20,* 283–292.

SUGGESTED READINGS

Arieti, S. (1962). Hallucination, delusions, and ideas of reference
treated with psychotherapy. *American Journal of Psychotherapy, 16,* 56–60.
Bowlby, J. (1988). *A secure base.* London: Routledge.
Brenner, H. D., Hodel, B., Kube, G., & Roder, V. (1987).
Kognitive Therapie bei Schizophrenen: Problemanalyse und
empirische Ergebnisse. *Nervenarzt, 58,* 72–83.
Greenwood, V. B. (1983). Cognitive therapy with the young adult
chronic patient. In A. Freeman (Ed.), *Cognitive therapy with
couples and groups* (pp. 183–198). New York: Plenum.
Hole, R. W., Rush, A. J., & Beck, A. T. (1979). A cognitive
investigation of schizophrenic delusions. *Psychiatry, 42,* 312–
319.
Perris, C. (1988). Intensive cognitive-behavioral psychotherapy
with patients suffering from schizophrenic psychotic or post-
psychotic syndromes: Theoretical and practical aspects. In C.
Perris, I. M. Blackburn, & H. Perris (Eds.), *Cognitive psychotherapy: Theory and practice* (pp. 324–375). New York:
Springer-Verlag.
Perris, C. (1989). *Cognitive therapy and the schizophrenic disorders.* New York: Guilford.

34

Family Treatment with an Acting-Out Adolescent

Yona Teichman

"Disguise fair nature with hard-favour'd rage."

—Henry V, William Shakespeare

Cognitive therapy was conceptualized and developed as an individual modality of therapy for treating depression (Beck, Rush, Shaw, & Emery, 1979). Despite the fact that Beck et al. (1979) attributed great importance to the interpersonal context, they perceived the patient as an "individual thinker." According to their definition, the model they presented was an "autonomous cognitive model" that was "divorced from the current environment" (p. 22). In the decade that followed, cognitive therapy was applied to a wide variety of symptoms and psychopathologies, and expanded from solely individual to group and family intervention.

The expansion of cognitive therapy to an interpersonal treatment modality requires a theoretical adaptation. Such an adaptation was offered by Teichman (1986) and Teichman and Teichman (1990) in their "reciprocal model of depression." Originally, the model was devel-

oped to point out the interpersonal aspects of depression, but actually it is a general model that applies to a wide range of problems. The reciprocal model is based on integration of system theory (Bertalanffy, 1964), Bandura's (1978) concept of "reciprocal determinism," and the basic rationale of cognitive therapy. The Beck et al. (1979) model and Bandura's (1978) model can be seen as complementing each other; Beck et al. neglected the interpersonal aspects, and Bandura neglected the intrapersonal processes—particularly the role of affect. The reciprocal model represents both. It contends that a model of human experience, functional or dysfunctional, has to include four elements: cognition, affect, behavior and environmental context. Following systems theory, it is suggested that any experience involves a dynamic reciprocal interrelationship among these four elements, which constantly influence each other. The outcome of these reciprocities is reflected in all of them and initiates endless cycles of mutual influence on the intrapsychic and interpersonal levels.

Each of the four elements may be further classified. For example, emotions may be negative or positive; behaviors may be overt or covert; environmental feedback may be direct or indirect, and cognitions may be primarily related to self, experience, and future (the cognitive triad

Yona Teichman • Department of Psychology, Tel-Aviv University, Ramat-Aviv, Tel-Aviv 69978, Israel.

Comprehensive Casebook of Cognitive Therapy, edited by Arthur Freeman and Frank M. Dattilio. Plenum Press, New York, 1992.

of Beck et al., 1979, which applies mainly to an individual perspective) or to self, others, and relationships (Teichman, 1986; Teichman & Teichman, 1990, which are more relevant to an interpersonal perspective). The basic unit of the reciprocal model that applies to an interaction between two individuals is presented in Figure 34-1.

The underlying assumption of the reciprocal model is that cognitions, feelings, behaviors, and environmental feedbacks are in constant reciprocal process among themselves. The reciprocities occur on intrapersonal and interpersonal levels. Symptoms develop as a result of distortions that produce dysfunctional reciprocities and relationships. In cases of long-lasting pathology, the distortions are reflected in the cognitions, feelings, and behaviors of all individuals who are involved in a significant relationship, and in the transactions among them. Families with members who suffer from pathology or adjustment problems are caught in repetitive cognitive, emotional, and interactional reciprocities that maintain the problem. These ideas lead us to consider the patient and his or her family and to apply diagnostic procedures and therapeutic interventions within the family context. This line of thinking is especially valid when the identified patients are adolescents or children.

A therapist who views cognitions, emotions, behaviors, and interactions as interrelated will wish to discover the reciprocities that maintain the dysfunctionality and to intervene in such a way that the relevant reciprocities will change. The reciprocal model provides a conceptual paradigm for tracing the intrapersonal and interpersonal components involved in maintaining dysfunctionality. This paradigm may serve as a frame of reference for evaluating, defining, and demonstrating to the patients and their family members the underlying reciprocities that guide their personal and interpersonal functioning and elucidate the consequences of these reciprocities. Broadening the insight of each participant regarding his or her part in maintaining the dysfunctionality may be used to encourage and motivate reevaluations and a search for alternative patterns of interpersonal relationships. The task of the therapist is to lead and facilitate this process.

Since the model emphasizes reciprocity, it is possible to assume that change occurring in any of its components will cause change in all the other components. Indeed this model, unlike the original cognitive model, does not advocate any preferred target for intervention or sequence of change. In every family, it is the therapist's task to evaluate the full reciprocal pattern (which includes cognitions, emotions, behaviors, and feedback loops) and to lead the patients and their family members to recognize them and explore alternatives that will lead to better adjustment. It may be suggested that significant therapeutic results will be achieved when the intrapsychic and interpersonal reciprocities change.

Working with families according to the reciprocal model leads to a reconsideration of some of the traditional cognitive intervention techniques. The mere fact that more than one patient participates in the therapeutic process produces a different situation and different needs. First of all, especially in the onset of therapy, it is not recommended to concentrate on one participant and explore in depth his or her cognitions or intrapsychic recip-

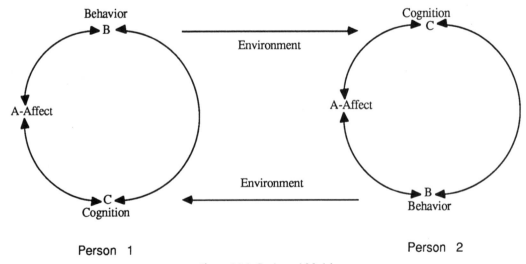

Figure 34-1. Reciprocal Model

rocities. Such procedure may alienate other participants, but most importantly may convey that the participant in the hot seat is assigned the patient's role. This contradicts one of the main rationales of interventions with families, which aim to convey that the whole family maintains the problem and needs to change in order to advance adjustment, and that the main targets of intervention are the interpersonal reciprocities. In one of the first applications of cognitive techniques to couples (Rush, Shaw, & Khatami, 1980), the therapists tried to solve this problem by concentrating on homework material obtained from the Daily Records of Dysfunctional Thoughts (DRDTs) that were filled out separately by the spouses. In a later application (Dattilio, 1989; Dattilio & Padesky, 1990), the therapist first met each spouse individually and socialized them to the cognitive orientation, language, and techniques. Then he started to see them as a couple, and soon encountered the problem of how to engage both spouses while focusing on the thoughts of only one of them. Dattilio's (1989) solution to the problem was to ask the passive spouse to write down her thoughts in order to work on them in a latter stage.

In working with families of three or more, or when intervening in crisis situations, it is difficult to prolong the process by investing time in a preliminary socialization of the patients to cognitive techniques. A way has to be found in which it will be possible to explore both intrapsychic and interpersonal reciprocities of thoughts, feelings, and behaviors efficiently and in the presence of other family members. Such a technique will be presented in this chapter. The technique is based on using verbal, behavioral, or affective expressions or interactions that occur in the session as a source from which underlying cognitions about the self, others, and relationships may be inferred. The interactions may occur spontaneously or may be elicited by the therapist. They may take place between or among any family members, or between the therapist and individual or several participants.

The therapeutic process involves a focused examination of the interactions in a way that expands awareness regarding intrapsychic and interpersonal reciprocities of cognitions, emotions, and behaviors. It aims toward a gradual understanding, reevaluation, and change of dysfunctional repetitive patterns in which the family members are involved and that maintain symptoms or adjustment problems. The cognitive techniques are conveyed in a less didactic way, but they are mastered by all the participants simultaneously. When the family members have enough familiarity with relating to underlying cognitions and to sequences of cognitions, affects, and behaviors, it is possible to introduce the use of DRDTs, to assign homework, or to use family members as co-therapists.

Based on their own experience and witnessing the work being done with others, family members can be very helpful in pointing out to each other dysfunctional beliefs and identifying dysfunctional reciprocities. This process, however, has to be guided and supervised by the therapist.

This last topic brings up another point regarding the slightly different role of the cognitive therapist in a couple or family situation as compared to the classical approach. In the traditional approach, Beck et al. (1979) stress very much the subtle leadership of the therapist, and the importance of Socratic questioning and collaboration in setting agendas and in building the session. In couple or family therapy, the leadership of the therapist has to be more obvious. It is very difficult to accomplish a structured intervention with a couple or family without assuming leadership and guiding the process in a designated direction. This may be performed in a delicate manner, but the participants have to be aware of this aspect of the therapist's role. A nice example of such leadership can be found in an application of cognitive marital therapy with a couple described by Dattilio (1989). In Dattilio's (1989) work, we see a therapist who leads the couple to focus on conflicts that he has chosen to point out, or who instructs them to adhere to rules that were suggested by him.

The case that will be described in this chapter, will illustrate the application of the principles derived from the reciprocal model to the treatment of a family with an acting-out adolescent. The material will be organized according to groups of sessions. In each group of sessions, typical dialogues will be presented, and theoretical or practical issues will be pointed out. The main focus of interest will be the analysis of beliefs about the self, others, and relationships, and their intrapsychic and interpersonal consequences. Work on cognitive distortions like all-or-nothing thinking, overgeneralization, or arbitrary inferences and attributions will be highlighted as well.

CASE REPORT:
BACKGROUND INFORMATION

The Y. family came to therapy because of problems with their oldest son Ron, aged 15 years and 6 months. He was tall, handsome, intelligent, and very well mannered in the interviews. Ron was under police investigation because of his harassing teachers by telephone (calling at 3 a.m., ordering cabs and ambulances for them, ordering delivered food, and threatening them or their family members; the most violent call was to a teacher with cancer, telling her and her son that she would soon die). He was also accused of teasing children, especially unpopular girls, and threatening them if they complained about what he had done. The last incident of this sort occurred on a school bus: He and two other boys dragged a girl to the rear end of the bus, touched intimate parts of her body, and insulted her. An older boy who came to her rescue was physically attacked by the three.

Following these events, Ron was expelled from school. During the semester he spent in school he hardly attended classes, and when he was in class, he was a discipline problem. He took few tests, mainly in science subjects; his achievements on the tests were high. An additional problem in school was his refusal to wear the required school uniform.

At home, Ron was violent toward his two younger sisters (13 and 8) and toward his parents. He refused to participate in any family activities, to do any house chores, or to comply with any standards regarding behavior at home. He did not eat with the family, and went and came as he pleased. His room was a mess, and no one entered it. His mother summed the problem up by stating that they all lived in terror of him.

Ron had many friends. Most of his buddies were dropouts, or close to that, from well-to-do families. Their favorite pastime was to hang around discotheques; at times, they got involved in petty criminal activities. Neither Ron nor any of his friends were involved with alcohol or drugs. Ron also had many girlfriends—the girls were from well-to-do families, and most were good students. They tried to help him at school, mainly by giving him homework to copy.

Ron's parents were in their 40s. The father (Mike) was a successful businessman and a scholar. He had a Ph.D., had written several highly regarded books in his field, and taught a course at a university. The mother (Ziva) was an English teacher. She studied for many years in different universities, but never completed a degree. Economically they were very well off and lived in an exclusive neighborhood.

Ron's physical and mental development were normal. He was slightly taller than his peers, and looked older than his stated age. He liked different sports and excelled in athletics and swimming. His verbal ability was high, and he liked to express himself verbally and enjoyed arguments. Since kindergarten, Ron had experienced discipline problems. According to him, he had started cutting classes as early as the first grade; his mother explained that it was difficult for him to sit on the small chair and to concentrate. His grades were reasonable, but if he did not like a teacher, he would not study the subject. As he grew older, both learning and discipline problems increased. When Ron was 7 years old, he was referred for psychological treatment. He saw a psychologist several times but refused to continue with treatment. At this stage he be-

came more and more difficult at home, and physically violent toward his younger sister.

When Ron was 10 years old, the family moved to England while his father worked on his Ph.D. and wrote a book. They hoped that the change in atmosphere and stricter discipline in the English school would have a positive effect on Ron. Indeed, Ron did much better in the English school: Being a foreigner, he was given an academic moratorium, and he gradually adjusted to the school. Nevertheless, his behavior at home became increasingly more difficult. During the time the family stayed in England, Ron did not make any friends. He felt rejected because he "did not belong." Toward the end of the stay in England, he befriended one boy and was very happy about it.

After spending three years in England, the family moved for almost a year to France. Ron had to adjust to a new culture, a new language, and a new school. Again, academic achievements became secondary, and the main effort was directed at mastering the language. In France, Ron was once more friendless and unhappy, but did not have discipline problems.

Upon the family's return to Israel, Ron went to a regular high school and was placed in the 10th grade. He started with good intentions, but very soon encountered difficulties. Although he could communicate in Hebrew, he could not use the language at a 10th-grade level and soon found himself behind his class in most subjects. When the fact that he was failing became clear, he started to cut classes, to misbehave, to act out violently toward teachers and students, and to make a point of not wearing the school uniform. Despite this behavior, he became extremely popular socially. He made many friends in his neighborhood and at school. Boys and girls liked him. He was witty, smart, always well dressed, and when he chose, very well mannered and polite. Gradually, boys who were good students started to avoid him, but still Ron had many friends. He considered this to be the "most important thing in life" and "the best thing that has happened to me since I came back to Israel." Friends became the only thing he cared about.

INITIAL ASSESSMENT

All five family members were invited to participate in the first session. After a short introduction, the mother described an argument that she had that day with Ron regarding her calling one of his friends in order to find him. Ron, using very rude language and a threatening voice and expression, informed her that it was none of her business and that she was not allowed to call his friends.

The father did not react to Ron's way of talking to his mother. He started to clarify with the mother which friend did she call, what time it was, and so forth. I addressed both parents and asked them what their reaction was to Ron's way of communicating with them. The mother made a sign of resignation, and the father expressed a vague disappointment. When asked about this subject, Ron became even angrier and announced that he "cannot speak with them" and that the conversation "will be the same as usual." After being in the room less than 10 minutes, he got up and left the office, slamming the door behind him. The session continued without his physical presence, though his "aura" persisted in the room. The parents and sisters described their difficulties with Ron and gave most of the background information. The helplessness and hopelessness of the parents were very clear.

Both parents were nervous. The father was very tense and monopolized the conversation. He often raised his voice, bit his lips, opened his eyes wide, and generally created an uneasy atmosphere. The mother had a nervous tic, cried easily, and spoke seldom and in a low voice. She appeared depressed. The girls were cooperative and polite, but also very passive. Whenever any of the participants talked, the father would interrupt either to present things his way or to make "clarifications" that proved the speaker wrong. The resemblance between the father's and son's styles was unmistakable—only the father was more sophisticated, and his domination was accepted by the others.

Based on previous experience of treating noncooperative adolescents and their families (Teichman, 1981), it was suggested that at the beginning Ron and his parents would meet with the therapist separately, but that the ultimate goal would be to enable the family to meet together and discuss their problems. Counting on Ron's fear of the police and his confusion because of being out of school, he was invited by a letter from the therapist "to present his point of view with no interference, and to discuss in what way he can deal with his situation." He was asked to call in order "to find a convenient time for both of us." Ron called, and the meeting was arranged. In order to acquaint the reader with the psychological atmosphere in which Ron developed, the sessions with the parents will be presented first, followed by the sessions with Ron and, finally, the conjoint sessions.

SESSIONS WITH PARENTS

The parents were seen 12 times. The first session with them was a combination of continued assessment, introduction of the therapeutic orientation, and a start of the therapeutic interventions. The parents' attitudes toward therapy differed. The mother had a previous therapeutic experience and was able to see that Ron's problems were related to the family constellation; she was interested in exploring "the entire background." The father was far more reluctant to explore problems. He claimed that Ron had problems since he was very young, and criticized what his wife was saying. He commented that although she had been in therapy, "she was never serious about it, and it did not accomplish anything." He accused her of being unable to stand up to Ron and of not maintaining any consequences for Ron: "With her, a rule is never a rule in our house." He was extremely critical of the way she expressed herself—finding inaccuracies in her words, pointing them out, or defining them as lies. When this happened she would try to correct herself, to explain or clarify, but she did not have much chance. Such incidents would usually divert the conversation and lead to a different subject.

Using the unbalancing technique (Minuchin & Fishman, 1981), the therapist indicated she also believed that a significant part of Ron's problems was related to the family context, that the whole system contributed to the development and maintenance of the problems. The recommended therapy was cognitive family therapy. It was described as a process that provided insight about the reciprocity among cognitions, emotions, and behaviors of each of the family members, as well as how the personal reciprocities affected the ways in which they perceived each other, felt toward each other, and related to each other. The mother's willingness to cooperate was expected, but the father agreed only because "this seems logical and I hope I learn a lot." A typical example of an assessment intervention is described below. The assessment stage is represented in questions directed to both participants, which enabled them to enact their characteristic way of dealing with problems and of relating to each other.

THERAPIST: (addressing both parents) I understand that you are concerned about Ron's behavior at home.
MOTHER: We don't approve of his friends, and we think that at this time he should be less involved with them.
THERAPIST: (still to both parents) What do you do about it?
MOTHER: I try to explain, and to talk with him.
FATHER: When was the last time you spoke with him?
MOTHER: I think it was yesterday, you were there.
FATHER: What exactly did you tell him?
MOTHER: I told him to stay home because we promised the police that he will stay at home.

FATHER: I hate when you don't tell the whole truth. What else did you tell him?

MOTHER: I don't know what you mean.

FATHER: Think clearly, don't confuse things—what else did you tell him?

MOTHER: It was a conversation. Do you want me to repeat the whole conversation?

FATHER: Only the important things.

This exchange between the parents provides sufficient material to explore their underlying cognitions about themselves and others, but the therapist decided to probe how rigid the system was and whether it would be possible to shift the blame from the mother to the father.

THERAPIST: (to father) I understand you were there; what do you consider important? What did you do about it?

FATHER: I want her to understand what is important, and to show how she confuses things.

MOTHER: Do you mean that I told him he could invite friends to stay with him at home?

FATHER: Yes, yes, this is very important. We don't want him to associate with these friends, so why do you invite them? You know that they close themselves in his room for hours.

MOTHER: You were the one who told me to invite his friends instead of his going out.

FATHER: Again, you didn't understand. I meant when there is *no choice*.

MOTHER: I thought there was no choice.

FATHER: You didn't try hard enough.

The therapist's attempt to include the father as a responsible partner was skillfully avoided by him, but it is important to note that both partners participated in this maneuver. The father continued to blame, and the mother actually invited the blame. Her attempt to share responsibility was ineffective. Even at this very early stage in treatment, it seemed clear that this was an ongoing pattern of interaction. In the very beginning of the conversation, when the therapist addressed both parents, the mother started to lead the conversation, exposing herself to the obvious consequence of her husband's criticism. Although both of them were present at home in the incident they reported, she was active in dealing with Ron, and the father was an observer. In the assessment session when she started to report the incident with the telephone, the father assumed the role of a clarifier. Despite the importance of this pattern, the therapist decided to continue the assessment and examined both parents' ability to relate to their cognitions and feelings. The initial focus was on the

father. His task was relatively easy; he was asked to focus on this thoughts regarding his wife.

THERAPIST: I suggest we explore the conversation you just had. (to father) How do you feel right now?

FATHER: Shall I tell you how I feel? I am very angry and disappointed.

THERAPIST: Can you share with us what makes you angry and disappointed?

FATHER: My wife! She will never learn to deal with Ron, and she will never learn to analyze a situation correctly.

THERAPIST: It seems to me that you give up too soon. Instead of losing hope, let us better understand what is going on between the two of you. When you see things the way you just described, what do you think about your wife?

FATHER: I don't want to insult her.

MOTHER: I know what he thinks, at home he does not spare me, he uses a different language.

THERAPIST: (to mother) Would you allow him to use the language here that he uses at home, so that we shall be able to explore the process as close to the "normal" as possible?

MOTHER: Yes. I am interested in your knowing the actual situation.

THERAPIST: Let us learn together what is going on. (to father) What would you say at home? What do you think about your wife?

FATHER: Well, if you want the truth, I think she is stupid!

MOTHER: (shrugging her shoulders) This is what I hear all the time.

This segment of the interaction clearly points out the father's cognitions about the mother, as well as the fact that both of them are aware of these cognitions. In the next segment, we shall see the mother's cognitions about herself and about her husband, as well as their affective and behavioral consequences.

THERAPIST: Let us return to the conversation we just had about Ron's friends. I would like to look at it from Ziva's point of view. (to mother) Can you remember that part and relate to it? For instance, besides the issue that was discussed, did you have any thoughts about yourself?

MOTHER: Sure. I thought that I am falling into the usual trap, of being accused and blamed.

THERAPIST: And what do you think about yourself in such situations?

MOTHER: As he says, I think I am very stupid, I should have known better than that. I have stopped believing in myself. I have never had self-confidence, but now whatever small amount I had, I have lost completely. I doubt if I can trust myself to decide what kind of bread to buy.

THERAPIST: What do you think about Mike?

MOTHER: I think that he is very strong, that his thinking is clearer than mine, and that I don't have a chance in arguments with him. He will always have the last word.

THERAPIST: (to father) Did you know that this is what Ziva thinks about you?

FATHER: Well . . . I guess I do.

THERAPIST: (to mother) How do you feel in these situations?

MOTHER: Miserable.

THERAPIST: Did you ever think what these thoughts and feelings lead you to do?

MOTHER: I give up, feel ashamed, and am disgusted with myself.

In the rest of this session and in the next one, the therapist continued to explore the spouses' cognitions about themselves, each other, and the way these cognitions were represented in their behavior toward each other. The following picture emerged: Mike considered himself very competent, strong, clear minded, and efficient. He saw Ziva as completely incompetent, weak, confused, indecisive, and unable to confront problems. He believed that his responsibility was to point out her mistakes and to protect her from doing harm. Ziva was in full agreement with Mike's definition of both of them. She tried to avoid mistakes and to please him. The fact that she continuously failed made her miserable. Mike felt disappointed with Ziva, but satisfied with himself and with the way she perceived him. The messages he received from her enhanced his self-worth; the messages she received from Mike frustrated her and decreased her self-worth.

In the third and fourth sessions, an attempt was made to examine how these attitudes were reflected in the wider family context and to probe the reaction to confrontation. Referring to Mike's tendency to criticize Ziva and correct her, the therapist initiated the following dialogue.

THERAPIST: Do the children hear it, does Ron hear it?

FATHER: I don't see the point of this. I don't want to waste time and money; if this is how you want to continue, I'll leave.

THERAPIST: This reminds me of Ron. When he did not like the things that came up here, he left us. Even though it makes you angry, I would very much like you to stay. This can be very helpful and productive. Don't take much time to think about the right answer, just tell us the first thing that comes to your mind. What did you think of at the moment you became so angry?

FATHER: I heard an accusation!

MOTHER: I did not accuse.

THERAPIST: (to mother) Let's stay for a moment with Mike. (to father) What do you think when you believe that you are being accused?

FATHER: I think it should not occur. It is not appropriate.

MOTHER: (to father) But you accuse all the time!

FATHER: I try to—to show you your mis—to help you out of the mess you get yourself into.

THERAPIST: It seems that both of you feel accused. Mike, we heard what Ziva thinks and feels in this situation. Based on what you experienced just now, can you tell us about yourself?

FATHER: It is an unpleasant feeling.

THERAPIST: Yes, I know, but if you want to understand why you feel so bad, try to identify what you thought before you felt this way.

FATHER: I thought that when she implies I do wrong things in front of the children, that it means that I am not a good father, and that I caused Ron to be the way that he is.

This dialogue demonstrates the therapist's control of the situation, and the focus on the "hot cognitions" experienced in the session. It is evident that Mike had difficulty seeing his faults or admitting mistakes. When doubt was expressed about his behavior, he became hostile and wanted to avoid the confrontation by leaving. The stress caused him to generalize, concluding that one particular mistake made him responsible for all that happened to Ron, and that this meant he was a bad father. This way of thinking may explain why he avoided an active approach in dealing with problems, and preferred to tell others (mainly his wife) what to do and then criticize what they had attempted. Despite his own sensitivity to criticism, when he criticized, he defined his behavior as "help." Another aspect of the problem is highlighted below.

THERAPIST: When you thought that you are a failure in such an important thing, in being a good father to your son, how did you feel?

FATHER: I became very emotional.

THERAPIST: It seems to me that when you feel the way you felt right now, you don't want others to know about it, and you show them a different feeling. Can you recognize that feeling? We saw it here in this room.

FATHER: You mean anger?

THERAPIST: Yes, that is what I saw. I think that anger helps you out of a situation you consider difficult.

FATHER: I hate to be emotional . . . to show my feelings.

THERAPIST: Which feeling or feelings do you need to cover up?

FATHER: (hesitates) Fear, guilt . . . sadness.

THERAPIST: Why? What do these feelings mean to you?
MIKE: I don't know, I only know this is the way it is.

At this point, the therapist had a choice of concentrating either on the issue of the meaning of threatening feelings or on the reactions to perceived accusations. Since both would eventually lead to the same basic assumptions, and accusation was of relevance to both spouses, the decision was to focus on the perceived accusation.

THERAPIST: (to father) This is a very important issue, and we shall try to understand it later on. Now, I would like you to explore something else that is related to feeling accused, something that is relevant to how you define your relationship with your wife, and perhaps with other people as well. When you feel accused by her, or in her presence, what do you think she thinks about you?
FATHER: She must think the same things I think about myself, that I am a failure as a father.
THERAPIST: And suppose she thinks this way; what does that mean to you in terms of the two of you? (Ziva indicates a desire to join the conversation) Ziva, I appreciate your patience very much, but let him just complete this trend of thoughts. You will be able to express yourself in just a moment.
FATHER: If she thinks about me this way, it is very sad.
THERAPIST: Can you take this idea one step further? Why is it so sad?
FATHER: Because, this means that I am a failure in her eyes.
THERAPIST: (to mother) What did you want to say?
MOTHER: I wanted to say that I did not mean anything about his fatherhood. I only wanted to point out that he is capable of mistakes, too.

Here we see even more clearly Mike's inability to differentiate between making a mistake and being a failure. Unfortunately, he attributed his way of thinking to his wife; the tendency to attribute his extreme attitude to others made blame intolerable. Ziva, on the other hand, was interested in a relatively small-scale achievement. She wanted to limit his feeling of omnipotence and to gain some small measure of self-esteem. This problem was highlighted in the following way.

THERAPIST: (to father) Did you hear her response? Does that make you think in a different way?
FATHER: I don't know.
THERAPIST: I hear a discrepancy between what the two of you are saying.
FATHER: I think I went too far again.
THERAPIST: In what way did you go too far this time?

FATHER: She said what she meant, but I heard her saying a different thing which is much beyond it.
THERAPIST: Can the two of you think about how such situations can be avoided?

At this point, a constructive, future-oriented attitude was introduced. The therapist challenged both spouses to work together on a problem they had discovered. The main idea was that the more they trusted themselves and respected each other, the more they would be able to check out things with each other and help each other to clarify and challenge arbitrary generalizations or attributions. This brought some positive experiences into the relationship, but in order to achieve a more meaningful change and maintain it, a deeper understanding of their basic assumptions about the relationship was necessary. They needed to understand why they were involved in a relationship that repeatedly produced interactions which enhanced his self-esteem and reduced hers. In other words, why did Mike need constant reassurance about himself, and why did Ziva "help" him to achieve it, despite the price she paid? Answering these questions was the most difficult part of the therapy. In the next four sessions, these questions were addressed in different ways and from different angles. Some examples are provided below.

THERAPIST: (to both parents) I understand that there was a problem with finding a school for Ron for the next year. What did you do?
MOTHER: We started to discuss this problem and to look into the matter. Then the pattern repeated itself: I ran around, spoke with different people, and made appointments with others. Ron came to some of the places with me. When Mike heard about it, he found fault with everything I did. I admit that I did make mistakes, but *some* of my decisions were correct.
FATHER: First of all, I think it is too early to deal with this problem! At this point, we have to invest in Ron's adjustment to this school. I don't understand why you took him with you, and why you went to schools during the rush hour. You had to travel a full hour.
THERAPIST: (ignoring the school issue, addressing both parents) We have been interested in and discussed patterns that repeat themselves. Can you identify what keeps this pattern going?
MOTHER: I have no idea.
FATHER: Do you mean to say that I like it this way? That I do it on purpose? That in this way I make her think I know everything?
MOTHER: You have to admit that you like this feeling, that you can never be wrong or guilty of anything, and putting me down most probably makes you think that you are always right.

THERAPIST: This is an important contribution, but what about your part, Ziva? How do you maintain the pattern from which you suffer?

MOTHER: I don't know.

THERAPIST: Let's learn from what just happened here. Can you think back to the beginning of the conversation and what happened?

MOTHER: You asked us about the new school, and I told you that we worry about this problem, then we told you what happened.

THERAPIST: Ziva, who told me about your mutual worries, who dealt with the problem?

MOTHER: If I remember correctly, I did . . . do you think that this is what I do wrong?

THERAPIST: What do you mean by "this"?

FATHER: See how it goes? She can't define things clearly. You will never know what she means.

At this point the conversation started to drift to the question whether Ziva was or was not clear, but this was interrupted by the therapist.

THERAPIST: Here you go again. I assume that when this will be over, Mike will think that he is very articulate, and will feel good about it, and you, Ziva, will think that you are stupid and feel miserable about it. I suggest that instead we try to understand in what way you, Ziva, bring blame and criticism on yourself. Before the topic was changed to how Ziva expresses herself, we saw that Ziva took the lead in trying to solve the problem regarding the school issue. She also started the discussion here in the session.

Both parents looked puzzled at this definition. Neither partner considered Ziva a leader in this relationship, and the therapist reflected their perceived surprise.

THERAPIST: Both of you look puzzled. Is there a problem in seeing Ziva as a leader?

FATHER: (hesitating) I would not say she is a leader.

MOTHER: I am not a leader, but I try to deal with problems.

THERAPIST: Did you ever think about why you rush in to solve everything?

MOTHER: The only reason I can think of is that I am trying to prove again and again that I am capable of dealing with problems. I want to prove myself, and I always fail.

THERAPIST: You mean you want to be able to think that you are competent. That's a good goal, but what goes wrong? Why is it that despite the fact that you work so hard, you fail?

MOTHER: I see what you mean. You mean that I do too much, and that is why I fail.

THERAPIST: This is certainly worth a deeper exploration, and a good opportunity for homework for both of you. I would suggest that you examine this pattern at home. Try to find out, Ziva, how you succeed in drawing Mike's fire at you—and why your reaction, Mike, is so predictable. What goes on in your mind when you react to Ziva? Observe yourselves and get acquainted with your thoughts and feelings when this occurs, and write them up on the thought records you have.

Both spouses recorded several incidents in which Ziva offered to take responsibility and Mike criticized her for doing a wrong thing, choosing a wrong alternative, or not differentiating between important and unimportant aspects of a problem. In addition to the already-familiar themes of Ziva's need to prove herself and Mike's need to interfere with that, a new theme emerged. Ziva wrote, "I have to try my best to solve this problem; I have to protect him." The therapist pointed this out in the next session, asking what she had in mind.

MOTHER: (after a long deliberation) I think I protect Mike by not letting him deal with the difficult issues. I don't think he can live with the experience of failure, or with the idea that he did not solve a problem in a perfect way.

THERAPIST: This means that you also attribute thoughts to Mike, and the kind of thoughts you attribute to him make you think that you are actually stronger than Mike.

MOTHER: Yes, I assume this is what it means.

THERAPIST: (addressing Mike) Did it ever occur to you that Ziva may think that she has to protect you? Is there something that she knows about you that could cause her to think this way?

FATHER: She is right. I cannot stand failure, and everything I do has to be perfect.

THERAPIST: Would you agree that it makes her actually the stronger between the two of you?

FATHER: (cynically) That's an interesting idea. I have never thought about it in this way. This means that she does not want me to feel bad, so she acts stupid, and I can feel better about myself?

THERAPIST: Could you think about it again? Does she really act stupid in order to help you?

MOTHER: I act. This gives you, Mike, the opportunity not to act, and to define whatever I do as stupid.

FATHER: I think that this is very stupid. How can you say that you are the active one? I make all of the important decisions, and then act upon them.

MOTHER: Yes, but after I do all the background work and the steps to be taken are obvious. I am sure that when we shall have all the information about the school, and there is an agreement to accept Ron, you will go and shake hands with the principal.

THERAPIST: It means that you have a very elaborate system to protect your husband. We know that you want to spare him failure, but I wonder whether you have another reason that leads you to believe that it is so important to protect him.

MOTHER: Because it was the only way to keep this relationship.

THERAPIST: You want this relationship very much, and you think that it can be maintained only if Mike feels that he is the dominant partner. In order to give him this feeling, you disguise your strength and help him to maintain an image of a strong man. Why? What do you gain?

MOTHER: Yes, this was never as clear to me as it is now. I guess that I need a strong man. I never thought much of myself. I am dependent and weak. I have never believed in myself. Mike gives a feeling of confidence, he knows so much, he is a good provider, and I like the good life. It is strange to look at things differently, to see that I can trust my judgment, that I can deal with problems, and that Mike is not so powerful, that he needs me.

THERAPIST: (addressing Mike) How does this strike you? Do you also think that this relationship can last only if you are the dominant partner, and that you need constant reassurance that indeed you are?

FATHER: (looking away) I shall have to think about it. This is very loaded; I need time to digest it.

Using positive definitions like "helping" and "protecting," the therapist led Mike and Ziva to reveal their expectations of each other that determined their basic assumptions about their relationship. Her assumption was that the relationship was vital for her self-confidence; she could not deal with life on her own, and therefore she had to maintain the relationship on Mike's terms (i.e., to contribute to his self-esteem by making sure that he was spared from experiencing failure). On the other hand, she also wanted to enhance her self-worth by gaining approval from a person who seemed incapable of giving her that approval. He could not approve, because this would mean that she deserved respect as well. This was a no-win situation for Ziva and for Mike. These basic assumptions influenced the way in which they interacted and felt, and their feelings and behaviors were interpreted in a way that strengthened their initial cognitions about themselves and each other, and the cycle perpetuated itself. Using the scheme of the reciprocal model, the complete picture may be summarized as shown in Table 34-1.

The reversal of roles that was accomplished by uncovering Ziva's strong side and Mike's weaknesses (needs) necessitated a reevaluation of the whole scheme of cognitions about themselves, others, and the relationship. It also changed the transactions between the spouses. Mike was encouraged to become actively involved in dealing with most of the problems they faced regarding Ron, and to experiment with failures, doubts, and imperfection. Ziva was encouraged to get some distance, to be less involved, and to give up looking for small accomplishments that would enhance her self-esteem. After 12 sessions, they reached a point where neither expected the protection of the other. They realized that they enjoyed each other's support but did not depend on it, and that it was possible to criticize and at the same time to respect the other. One could reject destructive criticism without destroying the other or the relationship.

At this stage, Ron also made significant accomplishments in his therapy. It is interesting to look at his initial steps and to note the correspondence between his cognitions and those of his parents. It is also interesting to examine how the interplay of the cognitions of the three of them influenced the reciprocities in the family. First, we shall look at the work with Ron in the 20 individual sessions he had, and then at the reunion between Ron and his parents in the conjoint sessions.

SESSIONS 1 THROUGH 5 WITH RON

When Ron was alone, he was very polite and very much a gentleman. At the beginning, he was somewhat reserved, but communicative; later he became at times provocative, but overall maintained a cooperative stance. He tried to minimize his part in the phoning and bus incidents and to present himself favorably. Ron was seen twice a week. Most of the first five sessions were devoted to establishing trust, rapport, and a collaborative relationship. This was achieved by dealing with the realities of the police investigation and decisions that had to be made regarding a new school. In the beginning, Ron was seen individually, and it was possible to socialize him to cognitive therapy in the traditional way (Beck et al., 1979). This was accomplished by gradual expansion of his attention to his thoughts, as well as to the relationship among cognitions, feelings, and behaviors. Whenever possible, the interpersonal context was preferred: The focus in the five first sessions was on the social context (friends), and in the sessions that followed on the family context. This sequence was based on the assumption that the family context was more threatening to him.

The dialogue that follows is from the second session. It revealed an intrapsychic loop that represented one of Ron's central sequences of cognitions, feelings, and be

TABLE 34-1 Intrapsychic and Interpersonal Reciprocities of Mike and Ziva

Mike	Ziva
Cognitions about himself	*Cognitions about herself*
I have to be sure I am strong, competent, intelligent, efficient; I cannot stand failure; everything I do must be perfect. Any failure or mistake means that I am worthless and a complete failure.	I am stupid, dependent, incompetent, unable to think clearly, confused; I have to prove that I am also capable to deal with reality.
Cognitions about Ziva	*Cognitions about Mike*
She is stupid, weak, and confused; she cannot solve problems. She needs protection.	He is intelligent, clear minded, competent, successful, but also needs reassurance that he is perfect. He cannot experience failure, and needs protection.
(Interpretation of Ziva's cognitions about himself: She is afraid of me; she respects me.)	(Interpretation of Mike's cognitions about herself: He does not respect me.)
Cognitions about the relationship	*Cognitions about the relationship*
The relationship should prove my strength, power, importance, and intelligence.	This relationship gives me confidence, and the kind of life that gives confidence. I can stay in it on his terms by making him feel strong and faultless.
Feelings	*Feelings*
When expectations fulfilled: content and satisfied. When experiencing criticism or failure: fear, guilt, shame. Since the meaning of these feelings is devastating, they are disguised and expressed as anger. Anger restores positive self-regard.	Miserable, nervous, sad, depressed. These feelings lead to repeated attempts to please or to a giving-up attitude.
(Feelings toward Ziva: mainly irritation, anger, disapproval.)	
(Interpretation of Ziva's feelings: she feels bad about herself and good about me.)	(Feelings toward Mike: threat, fear, but also pity.)
	(Interpretation of Mike's feelings: he feels good about himself and bad about me.)
Behavior	*Behavior*
Avoidance of active involvement but very active in verbal aggression, for which Ziva provides ample opportunities. Aggression is interpreted as strength and competence, and thus reinforces initial cognitions and feelings about self and Ziva.	Overactivity that accumulates experiences, defined by Mike and herself as failures. These repeated experiences are interpreted as stupidity, bad judgment, incompetence, and thus reinforce initial cognition and feelings about self and Mike.
(Interpretation of Ziva's behavior also reinforced cognitions about him and herself.)	(Interpretation of Mike's behavior also reinforced cognitions about her and himself.)

haviors. This loop organized many aspects of his life. Like his father, Ron could not acknowledge any weakness or experience of fear. Even when the fear was legitimate, it was unacceptable; such experiences were a threat to self-esteem, and they had to be concealed. Ron also adopted his father's way of dealing with what he defined as weakness—when threatened, he expressed anger or hostility. This usually helped him to have his way with others and gave him a feeling of restored strength.

THERAPIST: What did you think when you found out that, in the investigation, your best friends put all the blame on you?

RON: At the beginning I did not believe it, but they showed me the signed statements. Also, my friends stopped calling or visiting. It was very frightening.

THERAPIST: What did you think at that time?

RON: I became really nervous; one night I could not sleep. I did not know what to do.

THERAPIST: Tell me, what went through your mind when you had these fears?

RON: I thought that they will arrest me, and that I shall have to be with criminals. I was afraid that they will rape me.

THERAPIST: This is really frightening. Do you remember any other thoughts you had?

RON: I thought they all should go to hell!

THERAPIST: When you think this way, what do you feel?

RON: I don't care.

THERAPIST: This is a helpful answer. (Ron looks surprised) Can you tell me what you felt right now, when I asked you about your feelings?

RON: (puzzled) I felt angry.

THERAPIST: Can you pinpoint what made you angry?

RON: I believe it was because I did not know what to tell you.

THERAPIST: You mean you felt lost?

RON: I think I did.

THERAPIST: And what did you think about yourself?

RON: I did not like myself.

THERAPIST: Can we assume that when you feel lost, you get angry at yourself and at those who make you feel this way?

RON: Yeah . . .

THERAPIST: What makes it so difficult for you?

RON: To be afraid is to be a baby, to be weak, to let others think they can boss you around.

THERAPIST: In what way does anger help?

RON: (hesitates) I guess it makes me feel strong again.

It is interesting to note that with Ron, as well as with his parents, basic patterns that occurred in daily life repeated themselves in the interactions with the therapist. Fear and feeling lost were unacceptable when he was under investigation, or when he did not know how to deal with the therapist. In both instances, he defined these feelings as weakness; this triggered an anger response, which was interpreted by him as strength. The therapist chose to focus on the interaction in the session and defined Ron's negativism in positive terms ("This is a helpful answer"). Such a definition interfered with the usual sequence: Ron remained the weak one in the relationship, but it was difficult to be aggressive. He continued to cooperate, and with the therapist's guidance, explored what happened to him in the session. This understanding was later generalized to other experiences in therapy and in other situations.

In the following sessions in this sequence, Ron came to understand that many of his behaviors were related to the way he conceptualized weakness and related to it. Thus, he was able to relate his aggression in school to his feeling incompetent because he could not cope with the academic demands. He also understood that his demonstrative objection to the school uniform was a way of proving to himself (and others) his strength, and to compensate for lack of achievements with "good looks." His tremendous investment in friends was also related to the same issues. The belief that guided his overinvolvement

with friends was that "people who are popular are strong."

SESSIONS 6 THROUGH 12 WITH RON

After many rejections and disappointments, Ron was accepted into a good school in the same area where he studied before. However, he and his parents had to sign a document that the acceptance was conditional, and that the first discipline problem would cause an expulsion from the school. They also had to agree that Ron would stay in this school only until the end of the academic year; in the following year, he would have to transfer to another school. In this part of therapy, there were also many realities that had to be attended to, most of which had to do with adjustment to the new school. When Ron started to go to school, it became evident that he lacked basic study skills. Due to his frequent transfers from country to country and school to school, Ron was often granted a status of "a foreigner." This status was willingly accepted by Ron and was used as an excuse to avoid difficulties at school.

In order to prevent another failure in the new school, one of the first priorities in this sequence of sessions was to improve Ron's study skills. Attention was devoted to topics like planning his time, deciding setting priorities, doing homework, studying for tests, and so forth. A very helpful technique for dealing with these problems was the use of a weekly activity schedule and ratings of mastery and pleasure of the different activities that were assigned to him (Beck et al., 1979). When Ron started to experience mastery, he started to enjoy studying and began to devote long hours to schoolwork. This led to a drastic cut in the time he spent with friends. Soon he received positive feedback from teachers, and despite the fact that he failed the first test, on some of the tests that followed he received excellent grades.

SESSIONS 13 THROUGH 20 WITH RON

After establishing a basis for adjustment at school, the interest was devoted again to cognitive interventions aimed at expanding Ron's awareness of his thoughts, feelings, and relationships within the family context. As can be expected, the most prevalent theme in this context was also related to the weakness–strength continuum.

THERAPIST: I would like to come back to the first time we met, to the meeting with your parents. I am curious what made you leave the session. What did you think about when you got up and left?

RON: I thought that it would be the same as usual, that my father will put me down, and accuse me.

THERAPIST: When father puts you down, what do you think about yourself?

RON: I have to fight back.

THERAPIST: I understand, but I would like to know what thoughts about yourself make you fight back.

RON: Thoughts that I am stronger.

THERAPIST: Think carefully, Ron. Is this the first thought that comes to your mind, or can you find one that comes even before thinking that you are stronger?

RON: I don't know.

THERAPIST: Would you like to find out? I am sure that there are previous thoughts. Since you say that this is the usual situation, I would suggest that at home you use the Daily Record of Dysfunctional Thoughts, which you have learned to use before. When it happens in real life, when you have an argument with your parents, try to recognize the very first thoughts that come to your mind and write them down. Also, pay attention to the feelings that accompany these thoughts and write them down, too.

Ron came to the next session with the descriptions of two incidents. Once he wanted to go out with friends and his parents opposed it, claiming that it was too late in the day. Nevertheless, Ron left the house without permission. The second time, Ron demanded that his sister stop using the VCR, because he wanted to watch a different movie. His parents interfered and took his sister's side. After the first incident, in the dysfunctional-thoughts column Ron wrote, "They don't understand. They will not make me do what they want. I am not a silly baby; I will not let them." After the second incident, he wrote, "They always help her. I am older, but they make me weak and her strong." In both incidents, in the feelings column, he wrote in bold letters, "very angry."

THERAPIST: This is a very good work. Can you see the answer to our question from the previous session?

RON: (reads the material again) You mean that I am afraid to be weak?

THERAPIST: I see that there is an order. First you think about weakness, and then about strength. What do you make out of this sequence?

RON: It is possible that when I think that I am weak, I become angry and try to prove that I am strong.

THERAPIST: And what happens then?

RON: I get into a fight.

THERAPIST: It seems to me that we speak about a rule that very often guides you. Do you recognize the rule?

RON: About weakness? I hate weak people.

THERAPIST: That is why you react so strongly when you suspect that you may appear weak.

RON: It has to be clear.

THERAPIST: In order to be sure, I think that sometimes you test your strength.

RON: What do you mean?

THERAPIST: Read the two incidents you reported again. Do you see a difference?

RON: You mean that in the incident with my sister I was testing?

THERAPIST: What do you think?

RON: (laughs) It's possible.

At this point Ron was able to acknowledge his preoccupation with the weakness–strength issue at home as well. More important, however—as will be demonstrated in the next segment—was his ability to draw the first ties between these issues and the family situation.

THERAPIST: When you think about your family, who would you say is strong, and who is weak?

RON: Father is strong; all the others are weak.

THERAPIST: And what about yourself, where do you belong?

RON: I am even stronger than my father, because he cannot do anything to me.

THERAPIST: Could it be that you became so strong in your family in order not to feel weak?

RON: I assume that it is the same rule everywhere.

THERAPIST: Who could make you feel weak at home?

RON: Only father. Mother does not have a backbone. Everyone tells her what to do. She doesn't know what she wants. No matter what she says, I can make her do whatever I want. She said she will not drive me to school. Who do you think drove me to school today?

THERAPIST: What would you think about yourself if you would listen to your mother?

RON: It's impossible.

THERAPIST: Would it make you think you are weaker than she is?

RON: Sure.

THERAPIST: And what do you think about yourself when you make her do whatever you want?

RON: That I am the boss.

THERAPIST: What about your father?

RON: He thinks he is always right. He argues all the time and tells all of them what they should do.

THERAPIST: What does the fact that he cannot tell you what to do mean to you about yourself?

RON: As I told you before, this means that I am stronger than him.

THERAPIST: This must be very difficult. You have maneuvered yourself into a very difficult position. All the time you are on guard, protecting your superiority in the family. I assume that you need to protect it because you are not sure about it. What makes you unsure?

RON: I don't understand what you mean.

The examination of Ron's cognitions about himself, others, and relationships, as well as their intra- and interpersonal reciprocities, indicates that they are very similar to those of his father. However, Ron had the ambition to be superior to his father. This ambition caused constant rivalry and struggles at home, and was generalized to other settings as well. At this point, Ron could not understand this notion. In putting himself above his parents, he was actually fighting his dependency on them (weakness). Gradually, after repeated explorations of the related beliefs, Ron started to admit his dependency on his parents for everyday needs, for the luxuries he liked, and particularly because of his problems with the police and at school. At the beginning, his attitude was, "I deserve it; they are my parents." Later he was able to say, "It may be OK to need parents' help and to admit it," and finally he realized that "one cannot cheat all the people all the time." When Ron reached this stage, the question was whether his parents would be able to unite as a parental subsystem and stop Ron's confusion about his power by setting limits on him and by providing an example that allowed expression of weakness and strength by both of them.

THE CONJOINT SESSIONS

The idea to meet again with his parents was suggested to Ron after 10 weeks of therapy (20 sessions). In the beginning he was reluctant, but after further consideration, he agreed to give it a trial "in order to test out whether now we shall be able to stay in the same room for a full hour." This agenda was appreciated, but when the family met, the therapist defined an additional goal: "to see if we can get a better understanding into what ways you cause each other to maintain frustrating relationships, and to reevaluate whether there is a choice." This task was accomplished within eight sessions, from which the following excerpts reveal representative themes.

Three main topics were encountered in the conjoint sessions: first, Ron's attempt to impersonate his father and to compete with him; second, the change in the parents' relationship; and third, the parents' ability to control Ron and set limits. The best opportunity to encounter the first topic came up in a metaphorical way. Ziva said in one session that the other day Ron had "borrowed" his father's shoes and gone to school in them. The father said he thought this behavior may have a symbolical meaning.

THERAPIST: What meaning do you attribute to this behavior?

FATHER: To me, it means that he wants to follow in my footsteps.

THERAPIST: It is a nice feeling for a father when his son wants to follow his example.

FATHER: Not always.

THERAPIST: (to Ron) Did you ever think about this? Did you ever see that you try to resemble your father?

RON: Only in the fact that both of us think that we are always right.

THERAPIST: You mean that both of you think you are not allowed to make mistakes, or to be in a situation where someone knows something more or better than you do?

Later in the session, there was further development in dealing with the resemblance between father and son, and a gradual transition to the second topic (the change in the parent's relationship). The way all three participants expressed themselves and interacted demonstrated the change that was achieved in underlying cognitions and in relating to each other. Occasionally a regression occurred, but insight followed very quickly.

FATHER: I think that my starting point was that as a man, I should have presence, be assertive and dominant. That I am not allowed any sign of weakness, indecision or hesitation. (to Ron) Apparently I have taken it too far, and that is what you learned from me.

THERAPIST: In what way did you take it too far? Ron could not know what you think, he could infer it from what he heard you say, or what he saw you do.

FATHER: I guess he heard and saw my roughness with people. It is true that I am very critical of others.

THERAPIST: Was there any particular person that he saw you criticize?

FATHER: I see what you mean. I am sorry to say that it was mainly his mother.

THERAPIST: Could you ask Ron's reaction to what you said? What does he think right now?

FATHER: Ron, did you ever hear me speak like this?

RON: No.

MOTHER: I didn't either.

THERAPIST: Do you think that your father was stronger before, or is he stronger now?

MOTHER: To me, it is obvious; I respect him much more now.

RON: I still think that it is better not to let others know when you make a mistake.

As can be seen, the father reached remarkable awareness regarding his beliefs about himself and the influence they had on his son. He also spoke about his wife in an entirely different way. On the other hand, although in the individual sessions Ron reached significant achievements as well, in the conjoint session he regressed to old patterns of relating to his parents. Nevertheless, he allowed himself to be involved and even to contribute to the sessions. As will be seen in the next segment, he was not the only one who regressed.

THERAPIST: (to Ron) What is your reaction to your mother's statement? Why do you think she respects your father more now?

RON: It doesn't matter; in a minute she will say something different.

FATHER: He is right. This can really happen.

THERAPIST: I was afraid of this. I hear your old way of thinking about yourself and Ziva; can you also hear it?

FATHER: Yes, it still comes out automatically.

THERAPIST: Suppose you could turn the tape back, and react to what Ron said differently. What would you say?

FATHER: This is difficult.

THERAPIST: Yes, I know; maybe you could ask Ziva to help you.

Here, in Ron's presence, the therapist introduced a complete change in the family's structure. She agreed with the definition that the task was difficult and suggested that the ever-competent father had difficulties and could ask for help from the "incompetent" mother.

FATHER: (looks at his wife) What could I have said differently?

MOTHER: You did not have to say anything, or if you wanted, you could tell Ron that you care whether I respect you or not. When he hears it, he will most probably think that something is wrong with you.

THERAPIST: (to father) Do you care?

FATHER: Yes, I do. (to Ron) I respect your mother, and I want her to respect me.

THERAPIST: You need her respect, and you always needed it, but you thought that in order to gain it, you have to put her down. Now you have tried a simpler way. Do you realize what you did?

FATHER: I gave her respect, and I said I care for her respect.

THERAPIST: Ron, I wonder what you think now. Is your mother right? Do you think that there is something wrong with your parents?

RON: It does not sound like them.

In the next segment, we can see the change in the mother as well.

THERAPIST: Where do you stand now regarding the decision about a school for next year?

MOTHER: I have learned my lesson. I am not going to open this issue up.

THERAPIST: I see; you decided to leave the floor to the men. That is a good idea.

FATHER: I would like to tell you that she has really changed. It is not difficult to respect her.

MOTHER: It is true that I stand up much more for things that I believe in, and I don't get involved in silly arguments with any of you. Nevertheless, the one who really changed is Mike. I can also tell you that what has happened to us has an effect on Ron. The music in our home is entirely different.

The new strength that each of the parents experienced and their new loyalty allowed them to ally with each other and to act together on issues they considered important vis-à-vis Ron. When Ron realized that his parents supported each other, and that he could not manipulate one against the other, he also realized that antagonism and hostility could not prove his strength and that he had to look for alternative ways to gain respect. This enabled the parents to regulate the amount of time Ron spent with his friends, the way he talked to them, and the way he behaved toward his sisters; the three of them were even able to plan a summer vacation together. Initially, Ron objected to spending the vacation with his family, and his parents' reaction was a good example of their new authority.

RON: I told you at home that I don't want to go with you. It is not going to be fun, and I am not interested to visit all this old castles. I want to go with my friends to Eilat [a seaside resort in Israel].

FATHER: This year, you cannot go with your friends. If you prove yourself responsible during the next year, you will be able to make your summer plans as you please for the following year.

MOTHER: Instead of making it difficult, I suggest that you join us in the planning stage. We shall be happy to include places that are of interest to you. In this way, you have a chance to enjoy the vacation much more.

The change in Ron was first manifested in school. He was able to complete the school year without any discipline problems and with relatively good academic accomplishments. Both students and teachers respected him for the way he dealt with the problems he encountered. As a student who was away for years and joined a class during the middle of the year, his achievements were indeed remarkable. In the last week of school, Ron was invited to participate with his class in all of their social activities; after receiving his report card, he was invited by the principal to stay in the school for the next two years until his graduation.

It took Ron several more months to be able to act upon his new understanding of himself and his parents at home. The fact that both the relationship between the parents and the atmosphere at home changed made him change as well. At the beginning, there was a lot of testing on his part; then he found out that the change in his parents was fundamental and permanent. The realization that his parents had stopped nourishing his self-image by negativistic interactions led him to look for ways to gain respect through positive participation and belonging.

SUMMARY

A therapeutic intervention with an acting-out adolescent and his parents was described. The therapy process was guided by a theoretical model that expands cognitive therapy from an individual orientation to a family orientation. The main assumption of this approach is that cognitions, feelings, and behaviors are in constant reciprocity among themselves and with those of significant others. The full scope of these reciprocities was the focus of the treatment.

Due to the fact that therapy was conducted with three very intelligent people who were highly motivated because of the crisis they experienced, the process was quick, intensive, and produced meaningful changes. The changes were manifested in the behavior of the partici-

pants in therapy and inferred from their coping with everyday tasks.

REFERENCES

Bandura, A. (1978). The self system in reciprocal determinism. *American Psychologist, 33*, 244–258.

Beck, A. T., Rush, A. J., Shaw, B. L., & Emery, G. (1979). *Cognitive therapy of depression.* New York: Guilford.

Bertalanffy, L. A. (1968). *General systems theory: Foundation, developments, applications.* New York: George Braziller.

Dattilio, F. M. (1989). Cognitive marital therapy: A case report. *Journal of Family Psychotherapy.*

Minuchin, S., & Fishman, H. C. (1981). *Family therapy techniques.* Cambridge: Harvard University Press.

Rush, A. J., Shaw, B., & Khatami, M. (1980). Cognitive therapy of depression: Utilizing the couple system. *Cognitive Therapy and Research, 4*, 103–113.

Teichman, Y. (1981). Family therapy with adolescents. *Journal of Adolescence, 4*, 87–92.

Teichman, Y. (1986). Family therapy of depression. *Journal of Psychotherapy and the Family, 2*, 9–39.

Teichman, Y., & Teichman, M. (1990). Interpersonal view of depression: Review and integration. *Journal of Family Psychology, 3*, 349–367.

SUGGESTED READINGS

Epstein, S., Schlesinger, S., & Dryden, W. (1988). *Cognitive-behavioral therapy with families.* New York: Brunner/Mazel.

Dattilio, F. M., & Padesky, C. A. (1990). *Cognitive therapy with couples.* Sarasota, FL: Professional Resource Exchange.

35

Multiple Personality Disorder

Catherine G. Fine

INTRODUCTION

Long believed to be a rare and apocryphal psychiatric condition (Klutf, 1987), multiple personality disorder (MPD) is presently understood as a relatively common but often misdiagnosed syndrome. Putnam, Guroff, Silberman, Barban, and Post (1986), in a study of 100 MPD patients, found that the average MPD patient is correctly diagnosed only about seven years after initial mental health assessment for symptoms referable to MPD. During that time frame, he or she can expect to receive an average of 3.6 erroneous diagnoses. These misdiagnoses have as much to do with graduate training programs, Hollywoodian perceptions, and overt skepticism about a disorder (Dell, 1988) that carries with it supposed flamboyant and attention-seeking behaviors (though this type of presentation occurs in only 6% of the cases; Kluft, 1985) as it does with MPD patients' decided attempts to dissimulate or deny their condition (Kluft 1985, 1987) to their therapists and to themselves. MPD is a condition of secrecy; if the presentation were truly overt, delay in diagnosis would be the exception rather than the rule (Kluft & Fine, 1989).

Catherine G. Fine • The Institute of Pennsylvania Hospital, Philadelphia, Pennsylvania 19139.

Comprehensive Casebook of Cognitive Therapy, edited by Arthur Freeman and Frank M. Dattilio. Plenum Press, New York, 1992.

DEFINITION, PHENOMENOLOGY, AND ETIOLOGY OF MPD

MPD is increasingly understood as a dissociative adaptation to traumatic childhood events (Braun & Sachs, 1985; Coons & Milstein, 1986; Fagan & McMahon, 1984; Kluft, 1984a,b, 1987); it is considered a childhood-onset post-traumatic chronic stress disorder (Putnam et al., 1986; Spiegel, 1984). In two large series of 100 and 355 MPD patients, respectively, 97% of the patients reported histories of physical and/or sexual abuse (Putnam et al., 1986; Schultz, Braun, & Kluft, 1989). It is believed that the child victim of severe abuse rapidly exhausts his or her nondissociative ego defenses and begins to rely on more effective dissociative ones. Initially, the child uses dissociation in response to severe trauma, but eventually, he or she will mobilize these defenses in order to deal with any stressful experience.

MPD is characterized by recurrent disturbances in identity and memory (Nemiah, 1980). Watkins and Watkins (1982) propose that anyone's mental apparatus can be thought of as a series of ego-states (patterns of behavior and experience bound together by a common principle, yet separated from one another by differentially permeable boundaries) with slight perceptions of subjective differentness. However, there is no sense of loss of personal identity nor true discontinuity across ego-states; there is no denial of ownership of these states. For example, we are the same person (and know we are the same person) whether we are working with our patients, cleaning the house, or making love, even though there may be desired alterations in consciousness and perceptions. In contrast, the MPD ego-states (or personalities or personality states) have more rigid and impermeable self-boundaries, little ongoing sense of self, and characteristically inconsistent patterns of behaviors and feelings in response to a given stimulus. The memory disturbances may be as distinct as individual personalities' unawareness of one another, with consequent global amnesia for the periods of time that others are in control of the body. But MPD may also involve various permutations of partial, intermittent, and/or one-way amnesia that can include a sense of historical recollection of the events without a sense of participation in them (Kluft & Fine, 1989). To confuse the picture further, the memory problems may be manifested as a subjective sense of no memory problems because all gaps have been obscured by confabulations and "amnesia for amnesia" (Kluft, 1985).

GOALS OF TREATMENT

There are two ways of understanding the goals of treatment for MPD: (a) achievement of congruence of purpose and motivation across the different parts of the mind (Kluft, 1985), or (b) experiencing completeness of events and continuity of history over time, using Braun's model of dissociation as a referent (Fine, 1989b).

The Kluft Model: A Psychodynamic Model

The severe deficits and lacunae in the observing and synthesizing functions of the ego in the MPD patient make efforts to relieve distress and improve functioning tenuous at best. The different personalities in the MPD patient have mental functions and contents that are neither unified nor uniformly accessible. In addition, the parts of the mind (i.e., personalities) that can be in treatment do not always choose to be or to remain in treatment. The basic impairments to treatment arise secondary to the impact of dissociation on the mind and because of the individual personalities' narcissistic investment in their perceived self-representation. It should be clearly understood at treatment onset that, regardless of what the patient says, the MPD patient is committed to treatment across certain personalities only some of the time—and often resistant to treatment across many more personalities most of the time.

The different personalities often have different perceptions, different attitudes, different memories, different problems, and therefore different priorities, one of which may not be therapy. For treatment to succeed, the various personalities must make themselves accessible both to the therapist and to one another. Congruence of purpose and motivation must be established between the different personalities in order to facilitate their integration into one stream of consciousness and to begin to alleviate the patient's distress and dysfunctions. Satisfactory erosion of the amnestic barriers between the personalities proceeds as unification of the different streams of consciousness progresses.

The Fine Model: A Cognitive Model

Braun's (1988) BASK model of dissociation has considerable descriptive and explanatory power. It states that people, when in a nondissociated state, experience events almost simultaneously across four dimensions: they have *knowledge* of the events, they can associate *behaviors* to those events, they have *sensations* (physical and/or proprioceptive) during them, and they feel *affects* as well. For people in a dissociated state, any or all these interconnections can be severed and recombined. Each dissociated ego-state carries with it a cognitive experience, which shapes that part's affect. Uncovering this cognitive mode is very much like listening for Luborsky's (1984) "red thread" within a symptom-context approach in his work on patients' core conflictual relationships. Discovering the red thread of the patient's cognitive reality will protect the therapy from disruptions from the patient's resistances and the therapist's countertransferential withdrawal, as both struggle against inner obstacles to face the patient's genuinely painful material (Fine, 1990). The treatment goal for the MPD patient therefore becomes the reconnection of an event across all four BASK dimensions, that is, to recontextualize all aspects within an event and then to reassociate the event within contiguous events in the patient's life (i.e., to help recontextualize for meaning).

THE COGNITIVE-AFFECTIVE REALITIES OF THE MPD PATIENT

The Impact of Dissociation on the Cognitive Reality of the MPD Patient

In their seminal work with abused children, Fish-Murray, Koby, and van der Kolk (1987) have found that molested children think differently than nonabused children. People with multiple personality disorder (MPD) are reported to have a mean age of abuse onset at 4.5 years (Schultz et al., 1989). It would follow that the cognitive development of MPD patients must have been interfered with, and normal development impeded, by the abuse they sustained. Clinical experience supports this contention; sometimes, clinicians feel as if they are struggling with not merely an affectively overwhelmed patient, but rather a patient who is *seemingly* delusional, learning disabled, and/or perceptually handicapped. In reality, both patient and clinician alike are in the grips of tackling cognitive lacunae and distortions that have arisen secondary to the effects of dissociation on the cognitive development of the child.

Age of onset of abuse, its intensity, and its duration will differentially affect the child's cognitive development. Problems in the Piagetian accommodative and assimilative functions (Piaget, 1971) will impart to the child a distorted view of the world. In the same way that depressed individuals often look at the world through dark-colored glasses, the victim of severe child abuse will understand, interpret, and respond to his or her environment as if abuse were either ongoing or imminent. Fish-Murray et al. (1987) report that abuse affects the organism's capacity to accommodate, rendering self-correction difficult. The cognitive structures are more fixed than variable and lack optimal flexibility. An abusive environment will predispose to "abuse schemas" that reflect the traumatic history of the individual and will render adjustment to a nonabusive environment difficult.

Abuse may also interfere with assimilation. The assimilative function is relatively all-or-none; you either assimilate or you don't. If no assimilation takes place, the cognitive schemas may remain fixated at a previous developmental level and never aid in the formation of schemas that reflect the current history of the individual. The schemas thus remain meaningless and unintegrated or reflect the semantics of a previous ontogenic level. Is it not uncommon to encounter personalities within one MPD patient who have no knowledge, memory, understanding, or mastery over some cognitive domains, whereas other personalities excel in the identical arenas. The clinical evidence points to two ongoing and non–mutually exclusive mechanisms to explain these findings: cognitive regression and/or cognitive substitution/replication (Fine, 1990). It is heuristically plausible that abuse not only severs the knowledge dimension from the other three dimensions (as described by Braun, 1988), but may force the knowledge dimension to shatter into smaller units of information (i.e., into fragments of knowledge). Thus, knowledge may be broken into its schematic elements. The actual consequences of a reduction of cognitive structures to their elemental parts by random dissociative intrusions may be different when it occurs in children than when it occurs in adolescents or adults. In children, dissociation interrupts the normal cognitive-associative functions, as well as pulls apart the already-established schemas. Adults who have been severely abused in child-

hood (such as MPD patients) have to deal with an impaired cognitive foundation that will be reworked in therapy with initially faulty cognitive tools.

The therapist's task is challenging, because many MPD patients have relinquished the cognitive flexibility needed to learn from experience; they choose instead to maintain a pathological cognitive homeostasis. If the faulty beliefs remain untouched, the consequent distorted cognitive schemas will condemn the patients to a position of continued helplessness in adulthood rather than facilitating their recovery.

The Affective Realities of the MPD Patient

Few MPD patients enter treatment saying, "I can't think straight; that's why I feel so bad." The identifying complaints for which MPD patients typically present for help are vague and often lead the therapist to consider a number of affective disorders. Depression and anxiety are by far the more frequent emotions reported by MPD patients, but panic attacks, multiple phobias, and hypomania are also common (Bliss, 1985; Putnam et al., 1986). A plethora of affective symptoms coexist to render this pleiomorphic syndrome difficult to diagnose. Acute emotional reactions are the norm and are often elicited by situations (i.e., people/places) that, through stimulus generalization, have become associated with their abuser(s) or abuse(s). The more generalized the stimulus trigger has become, the more disabled the patient will be (Fine, 1990).

Feelings in the MPD patient run a similar spectrum to those in non-MPD patients; however, they appear either more transient and elusive or more established and unchanging. An essential part of the therapy becomes uncovering these affects and making sense of them. Patient and therapist alike need to know what the feelings mean in the context of the patient's history and how they impinge on his or her life today. This fundamental understanding requires abreactive work.

In working an abreaction, it is essential that the affective component be retrieved, released, and accepted in order for the information that could not originally be assimilated be integrated now. The content and meaning of the experience cannot be clear without the affective component. Reattaching feelings to an incident that may have seemed irrelevant to both therapist and patient could reveal that that one experience formed the affective foundation on which dozens of predictions and beliefs were scaffolded (Fine & Comstock, 1989).

If it is understood that neither the therapist nor the patient truly and completely know what the hierarchy of cognitive- affective building blocks are until the end of therapy, then all cognitions and all affects need to be approached with the same purpose—that is, to realign them in some way to make sense of the world. This reorganization is possible because, whether the MPD patient is aware of it or not, his or her overdetermined affective responses are subtended by multilayered and often intertwined cognitive distortions that need to be discovered and rectified before the abreactions can be helpful. Therefore, the next section of this chapter will examine cognitive distortions that the therapist is likely to encounter in MPD patients.

Cognitive Distortions and Pseudodelusions: The Cognitive Substrate of the MPD Patient

Many MPD patients share the same distorted cognitions present in their nonmultiple depressive cohorts; indeed, depressive symptomatology is present in over 80% of MPD patients (Putnam et al., 1986). Though depressogenic thoughts (Beck, Rush, Shaw, & Emery, 1979) are the unfortunate plight of the MPD patient, the quality of the distortion is quite distinct from that of non-MPD patients. The cognitive distortions of MPD patients are more established and have the quality of deep-rooted perceptual deficits. A surface consideration of the MPD patient's thought determinants would lead therapists who are naive to the diagnosis and treatment of MPD to interpret the stated cognitions as delusions, rather than psuedodelusional artifacts that reflect the impact of dissociation on the mind (Fine, 1990).

These distortions form the bases of the MPD patient's cognitive realities; they stem from faulty information processing of the varieties described by Beck et al. (1979). They lead to the following determinants of thought: (a) dichotomous thinking; (b) selective abstraction; (c) arbitrary inference; (d) overgeneralization; (e) catastrophizing; (f) time distortion; (g) distortion of self-perception; (h) excessive responsibility; (i) circular thinking; (j) misassuming causality.

One prototypical case (which is a clinical composite) will be presented throughout this chapter. The patient is a 35-year-old, single, female Caucasian who has been in treatment for MPD for two years. Her presenting complaint was anxiety compounded by bouts of depression still not relieved after a number of therapy trials, the last one having lasted more than three years. Her abuse started in infancy at the hands of her mother, who sexualized her at an early age (a few months old) while changing her diaper, and eventually included her father, who was an alcoholic. In childhood, she and her siblings were introduced to group abuse at the hands of her parents' friends.

At treatment onset, no history of abuse was known to the personality functioning in the world.

Dichotomous thinking is a response set in which there is a tendency to classify experiences into one of two extreme categories. This manner of thinking affects all personalities in the MPD patient to some degree and is a cognitive expression of dissociation. The person who develops MPD cannot tolerate the coexistence of two pieces of affectively charged, inconsistent data at the same time—for instance, "the father who loves me" cannot also be "the father who rapes me." MPD patients may develop personalities who maintain the love for the father, others who hate the father, and still others who have no idea who their father is.

For example, one of the distortions experienced by a child alter ego is that somehow she will never fit into this world. This child personality sees herself as damaged and unworthy of being here: "I stick out like a sore thumb. I will never be like everybody else." This distorted belief is reinforced by the fact that the child personality remembers her parents degrading her using the identical words. Another personality is "a survivor"; she will do whatever she needs to do to get by, lie by omission or commission, or manipulate to get people around her mobilized to her benefit ("I can handle *anything* and *anybody*—just watch me"). The drawback for her is twofold: (a) people around her start avoiding her to not get hurt by her (which of course feeds into her fears of isolation and not belonging); and (b) she leaves little room for learning new coping strategies.

Selective abstraction represents a stimulus set in which certain elements or characteristics of an event are taken out of context. Some salient features do not seem to be integrated into the event's perception; therefore, the meaning of the event is derived from an incomplete/constricted data base that often leads not only to ambiguous semantics, but to blatantly incorrect conclusions. For example, an angry alter personality would refuse to talk with a "weakling" passive alter personality because she remembered the passive one submitting to the abuse ("I ain't seen no gun held to her head; I don't gotta speak to no pushovers"). As part of the exploration into her past, the angry alter personality saw the abuser hurting the passive one and the passive one just laying there. The angry alter personalty felt that the passive one could have stopped, overpowered, kicked, or bitten. The angry one, as she reviewed in her mind the abuse scene, genuinely did not see the scalpel in the abuser's hand. A slow and meticulous reexploration opened up the communication between these two alter personalities.

Arbitrary inference is a response set that involves drawing specific conclusions without the evidence in support of them. The overlap between this and the first two categories is self-evident. For example, an adolescent personality felt that she did not fit in this world. Rather than facing her fears forthright, she chose to discount it as "just as bad, just as evil, just as sick, just as dangerous as the abusive world in which I grew up"; therefore, there was no point in examining memories further. When asked where she got her data, she brought a newspaper into therapy sessions and starting pointing to the numerous crimes and murders that our metropolis bears. The patient was asked to check a variety of media sources (magazines of all kinds, newsletters for survivors of abuse, help-oriented groups, etc.) to include more balanced data in her final decision.

Overgeneralization/undergeneralization is a response set in which incorrect conclusions are drawn from a restricted sample or from nonexistent data. It often corresponds to the stimulus set of selective abstraction and, of course, is parallel to dichotomous thinking. Many of the patient's personalities adhere to the syllogism, "My father is bad; he is a man; all men are bad." In an attempt of find a remedy to her belief about men, one of her personalities chose to eliminate men from her interactional sphere. She chose to become a lesbian and has been involved in a long series of unsuccessful homosexual relationships.

Catastrophizing/decatastrophizing is a response set that, when first mobilized in the abuse child, was not a distortion, but an acknowledgement of reality. The child's circumstances *were* truly catastrophic. Unfortunately, the persistence of cognitions that tend to catastrophize "normal" events act as conditioned stimuli that maintain dysfunctional conditioned emotional responses.

For example, a teenage personality who maintained the memory of her father making her ingest drugs (minor tranquilizers) before raping her was on a date at a local restaurant that had an outdoor elevated terrace. A woman at a nearby table took out a pillbox. A series of connected thoughts raced through the personality's mind: pillbox—pills—drowsy—rape. She panicked, screamed at the woman, and climbed out the window to escape. Fortunately for the patient, she was on the ground floor. She later described her panic to be so great that she didn't even remember being on the ground floor, and had she been on the third floor, she would have jumped anyway.

On the other hand, the *la belle indifference* stance that can prevail when some alters decatastrophize any event (regardless of its seriousness) can be equally destructive to the patient. For example, the patient was overwhelmed by the discovery of new child personalities. When such a new layer appears, it is best to anticipate that an abuser alter personality (an internal introject of the external abuser) may also be near discovery. An initial sign of this latter presence is a tendency in the patient toward reenactment and/or acting out. The therapist's recommendation to explore inwardly for the possible existence of this abuser was initially met with denial, as were the signs of impeding, uncontrolled abreactions. Waking up one morning smeared in her own blood after some self-mutilative gestures (of which she was amnestic), however, was a confrontation she could no longer ignore. She had decatastrophized a serious discovery and taken away from herself the possibility of crisis prevention.

Disorientation/distortions of time, place, or person are response sets in which the MPD patient thinks that he or she is in a different year/month/day/season or city/state/country and feels and acts accordingly. The MPD patient in this circumstance seems to live in multiple realities (Loewenstein, 1990, personal communication). For example, a new personality in the patient's system consistently refused to speak with me and was actually keeping others in check as well. I came to understand that she felt we were still in the 1950s and that I might be a friend of her mother's. She had tried at one time to tell a grown-up about what was going on at home; being her mother's acquaintance, the adult questioned the mother—who, of course denied any abuse. The patient was then raped more violently by her mother until the pain was so severe that the patient reported losing consciousness. Her resulting distrust in confiding in me was understandable and was redressed by helping her reorient to the present.

Distortion of self-perception is a response set typical of abused individuals and probably reaches its epitome in MPD patients, where different personalities actually perceive themselves as being separate people—rather than one person with several personalities—because of their autohypnotic hallucinogenic capacity. They think differently and, as a consequence, feel and act differently. It is understood that challenging a hypnogogically created image is fairly fruitless and is usually as productive as challenging the delusions of a schizophrenic; in fact, such efforts are usually counterproductive. For example, a child personality in this patient felt that it would be all right to walk around with a blanket (part of her self-image) so that she could feel safe. In my office, she would sometimes suck her thumb and act regressed. Rather than challenging her on "who are you really," repeated comments on the importance of putting behaviors into words rather than action seemed to enable the child personality to "grow up" by facing the memories (nodules of unresolved conflicts) that seem to maintain her cognitive functioning at the preoperational level.

Excessive responsibility or irresponsibility is a response set that typically leads to excessive reactions to opportunities for self-flagellation/self-blame and guilt.

Young personalities tend to be overwhelmed by taking excessive responsibility for events over which in reality they had little control. In addition, some adult alternate personalties who have trouble understanding that they cannot change that for which they were amnestic also struggle with this distortion. Excessive irresponsibility is the reverse of excessive responsibility; it leads adolescent alter personalities and/or angry ones into reenacting abuse scenarios and therefore setting themselves up for revictimization as adults (Kluft, 1990). A depressed and depleted child alter personality maintained that she must have been a "bad girl," even though she did not know what she did wrong, because "daddies don't do things like this to little girls unless they are bad—real bad."

Circular thinking is a response set where the premise for the conclusion becomes the conclusion, and the conclusion becomes a premise, and so on. It is a fairly common style in adult alter personalities, but can be challenged fairly easily in them. It is more problematic in child alter personalities who are cognitively arrested and have not yet negotiated the necessary Piagetian stages to achieve resolution and closure. The developmental level of personality puts a ceiling on the ability to analyze and dispel circular thinking. An example (already discussed in the section on excessive responsibility) is where the child feels that she deserved to be hurt: "I am bad, therefore I deserve to be hurt. I am hurt because I am bad."

Misassuming causality is a response set that is often connected to taking excessive responsibility and to circular reasoning. This style clearly maintains personalities and eventually the whole individual in fixed styles of thinking, constricted affect, and predetermined behaviors. When ingrained in this style, the person or personality does not learn from experience because there are difficulties in predicting events from precursor incidents, as well as difficulties stemming from unfortunate connections drawn between unrelated events.

For example, a child personality believes that something she does or does not do will either elicit the abuse or stop it. Her father would tell her that she was a bad girl because she made a spelling mistake recopying her homework (in grade 2 or 3), and therefore she brought on the abuse herself; had she not made spelling mistakes, he never would have raped her. According to the father, it was all her fault, and she deserved what she got. As this patient progressed in the therapy, she became increasingly aware of how the locus of control for the abuse was within her father and not within her (i.e., she became able to recontextualize).

As the therapist reviews with the patient the cognitive distortions, it becomes increasingly clear to both parties not only that the patient is locked into dysfunctional beliefs, but also how interconnected the presently unrealistic beliefs are. It feels as if the MPD patient is always warring with some aspect of a double-bind paradigm.

The Double Bind Revisited: The Double-Double Bind

Gregory Bateson (1972) speaks of the following ingredients as necessary for a double-bind situation:

1. Two or more persons (in the MPD patient, there is the victim of abuse and the abuser/perpetrator).
2. Repeated experience (in the MPD patient, the abuse often occurs over a protracted period of time, often years).
3. A primary negative injunction (the MPD patient learns to avoid punishment rather than to seek reward or positive reinforcement; for example, the patient as a child would be told that if she did not allow the father to have sex with her, then he would burn her, cut her, etc.).
4. A secondary negative injunction conflicting with the first at a more abstract level and, like the first, enforced by punishment or signals that threaten survival (the MPD patient will pick up this information, which is communicated at a nonverbal level or even a verbal level, but which conflicts with what is physically occurring—for example, the father rapes his young daughter as he tells her that he is doing this because he loves her).
5. A tertiary negative injunction prohibiting the victim from escaping the field. The average age of abuse onset in the MPD population has been determined to be around 4.5 years of age (Schultz et al., 1989). More recent clinical observations, though still anecdotal, suggest that severe abuse often occurs when the child is still negotiating the sensorimotor stage, that is, before the age of 18 months. Therefore, no actual physical escape is possible.
6. Finally, the double bind is firmly established when the complete set of initial ingredients is no longer necessary and therefore the victim has learned (or been conditioned) to perceive her universe in double bind patterns. The MPD patient often speaks in terms of feeling hopeless, helpless and overwhelmed at relatively minor daily incidents and that really nothing has changed since her childhood. Without the help of the therapist, the MPD patient's reality is an ongoing flashback where many behaviors are re-enactments of past set ups.

The MPD patient's use of dissociation seems connected to this double-bind module where the patient has "incorporated within her mind the paradox in its totality by making co-consciousness impossible" (Spiegel, 1986). The MPD patient's beliefs and assumptive world are crystallized and fixed within this double-bind paradigm. The seeming impermeability of his or her cognitive distortions, as well as the steadfast and predictable affective storm that often follows confrontation about the distorted beliefs, clearly follow Bateson's (1972) prediction; Bateson believes that panic or rage will be precipitated when any part of the double-bind sequence is entered. The MPD patient is conditioned to expect external violence when any disruption is made to the pathological equilibrium established via the personalities.

A obvious solution to the double-bind situation would be to follow a recommendation made popular in the movie *War Games*. The solution to the dilemma posed by the no-win situation strategized in the movie led the computer responsible for national security to use logic and decide that "the only winning move is not to play." For the MPD patient more than any other patient, this recommendation is hard to follow. In the same way that MPD patients' cognitive distortions involve polarized perspectives, they seem equally invested in polarized double binds. MPD patients tend to lock themselves into mutually exclusive double-double binds; this means that if they do not choose to conceptualize or respond to a problem in one constricted fashion, they have an unfortunate tendency to consider an equally rigid, stigmatized alternate double-bind.

For example, a child personality of the patient believed that "I am hurt by Daddy because I am bad, and I am bad because Daddy hurts me." When the double bind was challenged and the patient was told that daddies are not supposed to hurt their little girls, they are supposed to love their little girls, the patient's cognitions flipped into a new set of explanations consonant with the affect of the initial series of cognitions: "If daddies are supposed to love their little girls and not hurt them, and my daddy hurt me, then I must be unlovable." The patient was unable at the time to make the appropriate attribution of responsibility (to the father rather than to herself) and therefore reequilibrated her cognitions to a familiar, yet defeated affect.

Consequently, the therapist cannot challenge only one double bind at a time when working with the MPD patient. The therapist must gently question *all* the concurrently active double binds surrounding a theme and leave the patient unsettled and puzzled, but not imbalanced for fear of precipitating all-too-familiar polarized response sets. In summary, the therapist establishes in the patient

gentle cognitive dissonances as an introduction to a cognitive therapy treatment model.

COGNITIVE STRATEGIES IN THE TREATMENT OF MPD

The Cognitive Therapy Model in the Treatment of MPD

Cognitive therapy has been blessed and cursed with the reputation of being an easily learned, technique-oriented treatment modality that achieves symptom relief rapidly. Given that the treatment of MPD is neither quick nor geared to symptom relief, the roles of the various techniques need to be understood in terms of the reconnecting, uniting, and processing of dissociated experiences in the patient's life. To achieve this goal, a variety of cognitive techniques are mobilized to bring the patient to a point of remembering and assimilating through abreaction the once-dissociated feelings. Behavioral changes are brought about by affect changes and through the support of adjunctive behavioral strategies. These interventions occur in a structured therapy and in an environment of consistency, predictability, and safety where the cognitive therapist engages the MPD patient to use an experimental model to test via hypotheses the validity in her present life of his or her long-held beliefs (Fine, 1988c).

Cognitive Restructuring with MPD Patients

Using an experimental model will help the patient challenge the distorted beliefs of the past or of today, formulate alternative solutions, and start applying them. For the patient, it is finally getting down to the business of reality testing. Two fairly traditional cognitive restructuring approaches are relevant to the treatment of MPD. These involve (a) looking at the evidence to support a belief once it is elicited, and (b) looking for interpretations other than the ones initially stated by that personality (as well as considering the reasons for the initial interpretation). Regardless of the therapist's ongoing strategies, the first step involves collecting the patient's automatic thoughts.

What Automatic Thoughts Go Through Each Personality's Mind?

Asking MPD patients to attend to the thoughts that spontaneously occur to them serves several purposes: (a) It helps patients focus by forcing them to slow down their thinking and to examine the content of their cognitions;

(b) it helps them to be less vague and to acknowledge a certain responsibility and connection between what takes place in their heads and what occurs external to them—consequently, it serves in decreasing the denial surrounding the diagnosis; (c) it helps differentiate the thoughts that the patient is willing to acknowledge as his or hers from those thoughts of other personalities; and most importantly, (d) it helps establish the data base on which reality testing can occur. These thoughts are to be understood as hypotheses that need to be tested within an experimental model.

What Alternative Explanations Are There for These Thoughts?

To help the patient in hypothesis testing, patient and therapist together try to elicit alternative explanations to inflexibly held beliefs. Initially, the therapist models these strategies for the patient; then, the patient is expected to do this independently (of course, the therapist may need to go through this process a number of times, working with each personality independently). The therapist–patient dyad may ask the following questions.

What would an outside observer conclude? Asking personalities to imagine the opinion of an objective outside observer gets them to decenter for their perspective of the problem rather than understanding the thinking error from their own enmeshed, masochistic or possibly narcissistic way (Kluft, 1987). Difficulty with decentering is common among MPD patients who, either through developmental lag or regression, struggle with egocentric thinking. This "observer" strategy works well with adult alter egos when dealing with issues of shame, responsibility, self-blame, and guilt. It proves less successful with young personalities, who consider as "objective" the views of the abusing parents or of the abusing introject if they can decenter at all. Adult and adolescent personalities come to learn in this way that a thought can mean different things to different people; they learn that meanings cannot be assumed and often require contextual reframing.

What is really going on with this event (reattribution work)? For reattribution work to occur, the MPD patient must already be quite fluent at generating alternative explanations for the thought/belief (see previous section). Reattribution training involves helping the personality to modify maladaptive causal attributions to more realistic and appropriate ones. For instance, MPD patients typically understand life according to Seligman's (1979) learned helplessness model. They tend to attribute aversive events to internal, unstable, and global causes, and positive ones

to external, unstable, and specific causes. The challenging of distorted cognitions and their replacement with appropriate attributions of responsibility slowly but effectively redress negative self-attributions. These cognitive techniques, which are a precursor of the MPD patient's correct recontextualization, require careful planning and sensitivity in jarring the false assumptions. Fully understanding how cognitive dissonance should be established in MPD patients is an essential ingredient for successful treatment.

Establishing cognitive dissonance. Festinger (1957) postulates that dissonance is a state of psychological tension that motivates the organism to reduce tension by reducing the dissonance. The amount of pressure to reduce dissonance, according to Himmelfarb and Eagly (1974), is a function of the magnitude of the dissonance aroused; the implication being that the more dissonance is aroused, the more likely the organism/patient will want to reduce the tension. This is hardly a novel concept to the cognitive therapist; however, the therapist working with the MPD patient must guide his or her interventions and challenges (as stated previously) based on the overall personality characteristics of the MPD patient and on possible existence of the double-double binds established between and within personalities.

Dissonance in the MPD patient can be established across a number of dimensions. At treatment onset, the steps to instill dissonance are successive; as treatment proceeds, they become concurrent. The previously described BASK model of dissociation (Braun, 1988) tells the therapist exactly where and how to question the patient on his or her rigidly formed understanding of the world. The BASK model speaks of the coexisting four levels that, when integrated in childhood, form a person's experience of external reality—that which is outside the self and which dictates internal reality and perceptions. Therefore, faulty information processing would be detected and challenged at the cognitive, affective, and behavioral levels and at the level of the patient's physical sensations.

Cognitive-cognitive dissonance involves considering cognitive differences either within one personality or between several personalities and focusing on some of the inconsistencies in the cognitive processes. For example, one piece of knowledge is incongruent or just cannot exist with another belief: a personality observing another personalty being abused by the patient's father deprecated the latter for her seeming compliance, only to find on closer observation that the father was armed. The second personality's belief, "If I move, I die," is initially inconsistent with the first personality's belief, "Don't be a pushover; fight him, kick him, bite him." The two personalities meeting and "talking over" their different perspectives led the second personality to feel stronger and less helpless (yes, she could fight back) and the first personality to think before she acted and to consider all aspects of a situation.

Cognitive-affective dissonance or incongruence is to be expected in MPD patients, where patients often say they don't know how to feel. At other times, how they feel seems unrelated—or the polar opposite—to what they describe. This incongruence becomes their cognitive-affective status quo. In MPD, it is not uncommon to discover personalities who have knowledge of some of the abuse, but seem to relay it in a detached or telegraphic manner; it is best described by a *la belle indifference* style of relating tragic life events. It is almost as if the history that these personalities are giving or the event that they are relating refers to someone else's life, not theirs. Regardless of what they say, they seem to disown the experience altogether.

For example, the personality who identified with the "enabling" part of the mother agreed quite readily that the father's behavior was "tragic"; it was only later in the therapy, when I asked this personality to embrace of the child alters and feel this child's feelings that a true connection with the actual abuse occurred. This example is one of a "nonfeeling" alter personality. Another example would be when a personality who is identified with the abusing part of the mother hears the child personalities talk about their distress and actually laughs gleefully because "children are meant to be hurt." Part of the cognitive affective connection for that personality revolves around the belief, "When I can hurt a child, I am happy."

Cognitive-sensation dissonance occurs when a flawed connection develops in how an MPD patient interprets some of his or her body experiences. MPD patients commonly have personalities that are anesthetic to pain, and consequently, the patient can become unable to evaluate situations in the present that can be harmful. For instance, a serious infection resulted when an anesthetic personality stepped in to take the pain of a wound. It became important for the therapist to work with the anesthetic personality and help her learn not to emerge necessarily as soon as the body experienced pain. This personality needed to unlearn the connection, "The body is in pain—I will make the pain go away."

Another problem emerges when normal adult life choices had, in childhood, been connected by some personalities to pain. At one point, the patient's sexual life had become seriously impaired when personalities who equated sex with pain surfaced in her current life circumstances. These personalities needed to unlearn the connection between sexual intercourse and the experience of pain.

Cognitive-behavioral dissonance can often be elicited in the patient in light of the frequent passive-influence phenomena that MPD patients experience. For example, a violent personality started emerging as a more soft-spoken, mild-mannered one was trying to normalize a horrendous family event. As the latter personality was saying, "How difficult it must have been for Dad to keep me under control; I feel sorry for him . . . but I could never strike a child—I never get that angry," she found herself pounding the couch with white knuckles. Her noticing the incongruence between what she was saying and what she was doing allowed her to become aware of an alter that contained her anger.

Pacing the Recovery of the Memories: Tactical Integration as a Cognitive Model for Crisis Prevention

The present chapter describes a tactical integrationist's perspective of working with MPD (Fine, 1991). This philosophy takes into account the needs of both the patient and the therapist. MPD patients traditionally struggle with feeling out of control and vulnerable. The tactical integrationist's perspective focuses on establishing a strong cognitive foundation geared to the development of mastery and control for the patient (Fine, 1991). The therapist, too, would in many cases prefer a more structured, less chaotic therapy, rather than a Nantucket sleigh ride (Kluft, 1989). Therapists who maintain an outpatient practice and who are reluctant to hospitalize MPD patients (for the patient's lack of financial resources, or the psychiatric community's lack of trained psychiatrists in this field, or not to lose the continuity of care that is essential for the patient's recovery, or not to disrupt unduly the patient's professional and/ or personal life) need to devise a concrete strategy for the patients to contain the often overwhelming affects. The tactical integration model helps the patient develop mastery over not only the content of the therapy but also its process.

The therapy is a collaborative one between a consistent, predictable, and empathic therapist who has clearly delineated boundaries that he or she is able to enforce and an easily overwhelmed MPD patient who will understandably be long in trusting the therapist. For purposes of clarity, the therapy itself can be divided into two general phases: preunification and postunification. The preunification phase of the therapy involves the returning to the main stream of consciousness of all the dissociated parts/personalities; it is probably the aspect of MPD therapy that is most unlike any other traditional therapy. The postunification phase of treatment begins after the last final integration of the last personality and continues until termination, and will not be discussed in this chapter.

The preunification phase of treatment for the tactical integrationist carries with it two contiguous steps: an initial suppression of affect phase, followed by a dilution of affect phase.

Preunification Phase Therapy: Suppression Phase

This phase of treatment involves getting to know the MPD patient through his or her defensive vehicle of choice: the personalities. Indeed, it is not helpful to the MPD patient to immediately start remembering the original or even later traumas of his or her life. Patient and therapist must first establish a working relationship as the patient becomes familiar with the ground rules of therapy (Fine, 1989a). The beginning of the therapy is designed to build the foundation on which the arduous processing and powerful abreactive events will unfold; this basis involves extensive cognitive groundwork.

Mapping of the personalities. In the first few sessions, I will often ask the MPD patient to take a large sheet of paper, to place his or her name (i.e., the name of the host personality) in the center of it and to either fill in or have other personalities fill in their respective names. I ask the personalities to place their names on the paper in a way that would describe how similar or dissimilar they feel toward or about one another. Depending upon either the total number of personalities or the number of personalities in conscious awareness, the page may look quasi-blank or like a scattergram. This mapping will become a baseline against which all subsequent mappings can be compared. It is fairly common to observe groups of personalities clustered together for reasons foreign to them; continued exploration often reveals common core conflictual relationships (CCRT; Luborsky, 1984) among the members of the cluster. This mapping, along with the therapist's actual clinical interview, constitutes a first unifying step in the MPD patient's treatment.

Uncovering the cognitive distortions. Once some of the personalities have been delineated, they one by one need to tell their story—to talk about themselves, what they know, and what they remember, without at this point going into the details. It is important for the therapist to keep in mind that personalities are originally created through autohypnosis and therefore continue to respond nicely to "distancing" suggestions such as, "All that you need to do at this time is talk about what happened as if you were watching it on a TV screen, way, far away from

you." It is important to attend to each personality's stated problem (Braun, 1986), as all other parts of the mind listen in. The different parts of the mind need to recognize one another and one another's needs; they need to compare histories respectfully and learn to agree to disagree.

Uncovering the "story lines" within the various personalities serves as a distraction from the affect (at a time where it would be unmanageable), as well as a road map to the life events that need to be faced by all personalities. It also allows the therapist time to challenge carefully the cognitive distortions present in all personalities, so that the abreactive work that will follow allows for a corrective emotional experience rather than a retraumatization. In other words, when the time will come to "feel the feelings," the therapist and the patient alike will know (in part) the content of the abreactive material. This contrasts with following the thread of the person's affective reality, which is tied to victimization in childhood and very much linked to childlike thinking and perceiving.

Preunification Phase Therapy: Dilution Phase

Diluting the affect clearly starts when the therapist asks the various personalities to tell what they remember of their lives "as if" it happened on the TV. The personalities need to adjust to the sheer horror of what happened to the other parts of the mind before they start dealing with the fact that it happened to them, too. It is helpful at this point for patient and therapist to review yet one more time the mapping of the personalities. The groups/clusters of personalities start making more sense in that there may be a cluster of personalities who remember experiencing oral rapes, another group that knows about vaginal rapes, and a third group that knows about anal rapes. The affect surrounding these events is best initially shared within the same cluster of personalities rather than across clusters or with the host. It is less traumatizing to all personalities concerned and reduces the feelings of revictimization by the therapist; therefore, the affect gets initially contained, retained, and processed within clusters and among like personalities. Consequently, by the time it the affect seeps to other personalities or the host, it will be more diluted and less 'raw.'

A second precaution to dilute affect and decrease the negative impact of abreactive work is to do fractionated (rather than full) abreactions. Abreactions are necessary in the treatment of the MPD patient to help the different parts of the mind reconnect their perceptions of reality to the present reality. The purpose of the abreaction is therefore to inform, to educate, or to reeducate in order to release the repressed affect, to complete content, and to reformulate cognitive schemas and beliefs, as well as to release somatically encapsulated trauma (Comstock, 1986). Abreactions are necessary to reconnect all four dimensions of the previously described BASK model (Braun, 1988), to ward off further amnesia, and to achieve continuity of life experiences (Fine, 1989b). The detailed course of abreactions in the treatment of MPD is best described elsewhere (Comstock, 1986), but what is essential is that these abreactions be done systematically and completely.

The fractionated abreaction involves achieving this goal in small increments. Rather than doing one complete abreaction in one (extended) or several therapy sessions, the feelings are slowly reconnected to discrete aspects of the history, with cognitive restructuring throughout. This process parallels using systematic desensitization to achieve mastery over a phobic stimulus, rather than flooding procedures. With the patients, I liken the fractionated abreaction to climbing a mountain; they do not have to climb all of the mountain in one day, but they do have to know where the major ledges and the safe and protected resting places are. These natural halts are possible for the patient because of the a priori cognitive work. The patients feel more in control because they can actually tell me, or themselves, how far up the (affective) mountain they have gone (e.g., 60%) and how far they have yet to go (40%). The abreaction to follow may put them at 80%, allowing them to note their progress as they continue the arduous "climb." Therefore, these fractionated abreactions allow the patient to pace the necessary therapeutic work by diluting the affect.

A final common method to dilute affect is through the "blending" of personalities. Personalities can be temporarily joined for any number of purposes, as described in detail elsewhere (Fine & Comstock, 1989). Blending must be done for the growth of the patient and not for any reason that would benefit the therapist either alone or primarily; consequently, countertransferential needs must be carefully monitored. It also ought to be emphasized that time-limited blending is not to be confused with fusion or integration of personalities.

To dilute the affect, the therapist may propose to blend personalities to learn from abreactions. Abreactions are necessary, but painful, treatment components. Time-limited blending can be helpful to facilitate some abreactions. Blending can make abreactions less scary; for example, a small frightened child alter personality needed to do her abreaction, but a protective personality had great difficulty allowing the abreaction to proceed as she did not want the small child alter personality to suffer. The protective personality agreed to blend in with the frightened child and "help" her through the abreaction by staying with her. As a result, the child was much better able to

navigate through her abreaction and to see what had happened. At the end of the time, the personalities split apart again as agreed, but several times during the next few days, they reblended to comfort the child.

Blending of personalities can help different personalities experience an alternative point of view from their traditional all-or-none stance, which is often backed up by a strong affective component. They can learn in a powerful way that other alternatives are also possible and even plausible for them. This experiencing of a different way of thinking and feeling through blending teaches them the worth of hypothesis testing, because they learn that indeed there are other options and that they need not respond in their traditional knee-jerk way. For example, a personality who went to the same dentist for years always performed oral sex for him without a thought as to a possible option. Talking in therapy about "just saying no or changing dentists" did not increase her sense of choice; when he would unzip his pants, she would simply do as she knew to do. Blending another personality in with her before the next dental appointment gave her (and the dentist) a very different experience.

Attempts to dilute affect through blending are noteworthy; however, a few caveats are necessary. First of all, it is ill-advised to force a blending. The personality needs to erode the amnestic barriers slowly and be ready to merge with another alter personality. If the blending is forced, the consequences may be paradoxical and leave the alter personality more fearful, devastated, and decided in his or her attempt to avoid or reduce communication with other personalities.

In addition, certain personalities would do better *not* to merge or blend, because the intensity of the potentially destructive emotion might culminate in action. Abusive alter personalities ought not to be blended together until the intensity of their desire to hurt someone has abated and suicidal alter personalities ought not to be blended together until the suicidality is ameliorated.

Examples of Cognitive Interventions with Different Kinds of Personalities

Working with Depressed Personalities

A depleted, forlorn personality who had very little contact with the outside world had as a central theme "not being part of the world" and a belief that she "would never fit in."

PATIENT: I don't fit in anywhere.
THERAPIST: Nowhere?
PATIENT: I can't connect; I don't belong anywhere.

THERAPIST: How do you know this? (i.e., what was the data to support her self-deprecatory statements?]

PATIENT: No one talks to me!

THERAPIST: I am speaking with you.

PATIENT: (long pause) Yeah.

THERAPIST: Is it hard to speak with me? [starting the Socratic process]

PATIENT: No.

THERAPIST: Do you feel that I listen?

PATIENT: Yes.

THERAPIST: Do you feel that you connect with me?

PATIENT: Yeah.

THERAPIST: So it is really not accurate that you cannot connect, nor that people don't listen to you or even that no one talks to you. We have been doing those things together (emphasis on the collaboration] for a long time now.

PATIENT: Well . . . that's true.

THERAPIST: I think that you now have to look and see who else you may have forgotten about, others with whom you also spend time with and connect.

(Patient starts naming people, places, and things that were shared among them.)

THERAPIST: So, even though sometimes you may feel as if you don't fit in and as if you cannot connect . . . that just isn't true . . . Your feelings do not reflect today's reality, but the reality of the past . . . you need to learn to bring your feelings into the here and now.

Working with Angry/Violent Personalities

One of the angry adolescent alter personalities of this patient stated that she was angry at the world. As the exchange continued, she acknowledged that she was really angry at herself for not having been a better "protector" personality; regardless of her best efforts, the child personalities got reabused.

PATIENT: (screams) Everybody's an AH [asshole]! (therapist is silent) Don't you think? You probably think I'm an AH, too.

THERAPIST: No, as a matter of fact, I don't [therapist being truthful; otherwise, silence or a confrontation would have been advised].

PATIENT: (grunts, shrugs her shoulders) I can't do anything right.

THERAPIST: OK, let's look at exactly that. You are going to give me a list of things you do well to protect the body and things you do poorly. And you are going to write them down as we talk . . . I want to see this, and you have to see it. (hands over a piece of paper; patient fills out pretty balanced list) So, looks like you can protect

yourself and the other personalities well in some circumstances, and not so well in others. Are you saying that making one mistake makes you an AH?

PATIENT: No.

THERAPIST: Oh, so it's making two mistakes? Maybe it's three strikes and you're out? Maybe after three mistakes, you're an AH?

PATIENT: (very annoyed) Why do you want to know this—why, why, why?

THERAPIST: I figure it may be helpful in my work—so that my next patient, when she comes in, I can say, "Lady, this is your third mistake; you are officially an AH."

PATIENT: (smiles and calms down) No, she wouldn't be an AH after three mistakes . . .

THERAPIST: Oh, really? Why not?

PATIENT: She is only human . . .

THERAPIST: And you, are you human or above that?

PATIENT: No, I'm human . . . my problem is I feel below that most of the time.

The patient was able to calm down with a combination of tactics that challenged her all-or-none thinking with humor and started addressing the feelings that underlie her anger (i.e., her feelings of helplessness).

Working with Childlike Personalities

A child personality was struggling with flashbacks surrounding sexual abuse in her room at night. She was having difficulty, because she thought she was still there and that her father was going to walk through the door any minute.

PATIENT: I can't stay, I can't stay. I've got to go, now . . . now. He will find me . . . hide . . . hide . . .

THERAPIST: (calls personality by name) Do you remember me?

PATIENT: Yes, yes, but he is going to get me, and he will get you, too . . . run . . . run . . .

THERAPIST: No, he won't get me, and he won't get you.

PATIENT: Yes, he will—please, please, don't make me stay . . .

THERAPIST: Do you feel safe in my office?

PATIENT: Yes, yes, yes.

THERAPIST: What does my office look like?

PATIENT: (starts describing, listing objects, colors, etc.; runs into trouble) The pink pillow, the purple pillow . . . the . . .

THERAPIST: (hands over red pillow)— Here, look, what color is this?

PATIENT: Red; it's red.

THERAPIST: What color was your room as a child?

PATIENT: Blue . . . it was blue. (starts calming down)

The therapist continued to use evocative imagery and a split-screen technique, wherein the patient was asked to describe in detail each of the rooms—the childhood bedroom and the therapist's office—in excruciating detail to learn the difference between the here and now and the past.

SUMMARY

Working with adults who have been severely abused in childhood (such as MPD patients) is accessible to most cognitive therapists who are willing to do long-term therapy rather than short-term therapy geared to symptom relief. The cognitive therapist is particularly well suited to work with MPD patients, because the tenets of the cognitive model are also the necessary prerequisites to a stable and effective therapy that strives to unify the mind of the dissociated patient. The cognitive therapist can challenge the numerous and intertwined cognitive distortions as the affective dimension gets slowly reconnected to the MPD patient's unfolding history. The straightforward collaborative directedness of the cognitive model allows patients to learn that some environments, like the therapist's office, can be predictable and safe—and from that point on, by calculated risk taking, they can come to learn about the world in which they have been living without a sense of participation and make it their world, too.

REFERENCES

Bateson, G. (1972). *Steps to an ecology of mind*. New York: Ballantine.

Beck, A. T. (1976). *Cognitive therapy and the emotional disorders*. New York: International Universities Press.

Beck, A. T., Rush, A., Shaw, B. F., & Emery, G. (1979). *Cognitive therapy of depression*. New York: Guilford.

Bliss, E. L. (1984). A symptom profile of patients with multiple personalities, including MMPI results. *Journal of Nervous and Mental Diseases, 172*, 197–202.

Braun, B. G. (Ed.). (1986). *Treatment of multiple personality disorder*. Washington, DC: American Psychiatric Press.

Braun, B. G. (1988). The BASK model of dissociation. *Dissociation, 1*(1), 4–24.

Braun, B. G., & Sachs, R. G. (1985). The development of multiple personality disorder: Predisposing, precipitating and perpetuating factors. In R. P. Kluft (Ed.), *Childhood antecedents of multiple personality*. Washington, DC: American Psychiatric Press.

Comstock, C. M. (1986). The therapeutic utilization of abreactive experiences in the treatment of multiple personality disorder. In Braun, B. G., *Dissociative disorders: 1986*. Chicago: Rush University.

Coons, P. M., & Milstein, V. (1986). Psychosexual disturbances in multiple personality: Characteristics, etiology and treatment. *Journal of Clinical Psychiatry, 47*, 106–110.

Dell, P. F. (1988). Professional skepticism about multiple personality. *Journal of Nervous and Mental Diseases, 176*, 528–531.

Fagan, J., & McMahon, P. (1984). Incipient multiple personality in children: four cases. *Journal of Nervous and Mental Diseases, 172*, 26–36.

Festinger, L. (1957). *A theory of cognitive dissonance*. Stanford, CA: Stanford University Press.

Fine, C. G. (1988a). The work of Antoine Despine: Diagnosis and treatment of a child with multiple personality disorder. *American Journal of Clinical Hypnosis, 31*, 32–39.

Fine, C. G. (1988b). Thoughts on the cognitive-perceptual substrates of multiple personality disorder. *Dissociation, 1*, 5–10.

Fine, C. G. (1988c). *Mood cognition and multiplicity*. Paper presented at the World Congress of Cognitive Therapy, Oxford, England.

Fine, C. G. (1989a). Treatment errors and iatrogenesis across therapeutic modalities in MPD and allied dissociative disorders. *Dissociation, 2*, 77–82.

Fine, C. G. (1989b). *Cognitive aspects of hypnotherapeutic interventions with dissociative disorders patients*. Paper presented at the 32nd annual meeting of the American Society of Clinical Hypnosis, Orlando, FL.

Fine, C. G. (1990). The cognitive sequelae of incest. In R. P. Kluft (Ed.), *Incest-related syndromes of adult psychopathology*. Washington, DC: American Psychiatric Press.

Fine, C. G. (1991). Treatment stabilization and crisis prevention in the treatment of MPD. In R. J. Loewenstein (Ed.), *Psychiatric clinics of North America*. Philadelphia: Saunders.

Fine, C. G., & Comstock, C. M. (1989). Completion of cognitive schemata and affective realms through the temporary blending of personalities in the treatment of MPD. In Braun, B. G., *Dissociative disorders: 1989*. Chicago: Rush University.

Fish-Murray, C. C., Koby, E. V., & van der Kolk, B. (1987). Evolving ideas: The effect of abuse on children's thoughts. In B. van der Kolk (Ed.), *Psychological trauma* (pp. 89–110). Washington, DC: American Psychiatric Press.

Himmelfarb, S., & Eagly, A. H. (1974). *Readings in attitude change*. New York: John Wiley.

Kluft, R. P. (1984a). Multiple personality in childhood. *Psychiatric Clinics of North America, 7*, 121–134.

Kluft, R. P. (1984b). Treatment of multiple personality disorder: A study of 33 cases. *Psychiatric Clinics of North America, 7*, 9–29.

Kluft, R. P. (1987). Childhood multiple personality. In R. P. Kluft (Ed.), *Childhood antecedents of multiple personality*. Washington, DC: American Psychiatric Press.

Kluft, R. P. (1987). Making the diagnosis of multiple personality disorder. In F. Flach (Ed.), *Diagnostics and psychopathology* (Directions in Psychiatry Monograph Series). New York: Norton.

Kluft, R. P. (1989). Today's therapeutic pluralism [Editorial]. *Dissociation, 1*, 4.

Kluft, R. P. (1990). Incest and subsequent revictimization: The case of therapist–patient sexual exploitation, with a description of the sitting duck syndrome. In R. P. Kluft (Ed.), *Incest-related syndromes of adult psychopathology* (pp. 263–286). Washington, DC: American Psychiatric Press.

Kluft, R. P., & Fine, C. G. (1989). Multiple personality disorder. In J. G. Howells (Ed.), *Modern perspectives in the psychiatry of the neuroses*. New York: Brunner/Mazel.

Luborsky, L. (1984). *Principles of psychoanalytic psychotherapy: A manual for supportive-expressive treatment*. New York: Basic Books.

Nemiah, J. C. (1980). Dissociative disorders. In H. Kaplan, A. Freedman, & B. Sadock (Eds.), *Comprehensive textbook of psychiatry* (3rd ed.). Baltimore: Williams and Wilkins.

Piaget, J. (1971). *Biology and knowledge: An essay on the relations between organic regulations and cognitive processes*. Chicago: University of Chicago Press.

Putnam, F. W., Guroff, J. J., Silberman, E. K., Barban, L., & Post, R. M. (1986). The clinical phenomenology of multiple personality disorder: A review of 100 recent cases. *Journal of Clinical Psychiatry, 45*, 172–175.

Seligman, M. (1975). *Helplessness: On depression, development and death*. San Francisco: Freeman.

Schultz, R., Braun, B. G., & Kluft, R. P. (1989). Multiple personality disorder: Phenomenology of selected variables in comparison to major depression. *Dissociation, 2*, 45–51.

Spiegel, D. (1984). Multiple personality disorder as a posttraumatic stress disorder. *Psychiatric Clinics of North America, 7*, 101–110.

Spiegel, D. (1986). Dissociation, double-binds and post-traumatic stress in multiple personality disorder. In B. G. Braun (Ed.), *Treatment of multiple personality disorder*. Washington, DC: American Psychiatric Press.

Watkins, J. G., & Watkins, H. H. (1982). Ego-state therapy. In L. E. Abt & I. R. Stuart (Eds.), *The newer therapies: A source book*. New York: Van Nostrand Reinhold.

SUGGESTED READINGS

Braun, B. G. (Ed.). (1986). *Treatment of multiple personality disorder*. Washington, DC: American Psychiatric Press.

Kluft, R. P. (1985). *Childhood Antecedents of Multiple Personality*. Washington, DC: American Psychiatric Press.

Kluft, R. P. (1990). *Incest related syndromes of adult psychopathology*. Washington, DC: American Psychiatric Press.

Putnam, F. W. (1989). *Diagnosis and treatment of multiple personality disorder*. New York: Guilford.

36

The Treatment of Chronic Pain

Bruce N. Eimer

As articulated in the cognitive-behavioral literature, the chief agenda for psychotherapy with the chronic pain patient is twofold. The first aspect is to teach the patient pain-coping and pain-reduction strategies. The second aspect is to teach the patient how to employ cognitive techniques for disputing beliefs that would undermine his or her acceptance of responsibility for employing coping and self-management techniques.

The cognitive-behavioral literature has not adequately addressed a third important aspect of the problem of chronic pain: the problem of cognitions and behaviors that trigger as well as maintain pain. These would include self-defeating cognitive habits, anticipatory anxiety, avoidant behaviors, behavioral excesses, and dysfunctional posturing and movement patterns.

The enigma of chronic benign pain is that it is a noxious signal from the body that is disproportionate to any identifiable physical threat. As with anxiety, it usually leads to preoccupation with noxious stimuli. Paradoxically, activities that could reduce such preoccupation are often avoided as the person in pain may not feel up to such engagement.

Bruce N. Eimer • The Behavior Therapy Center, Jenkintown, Pennsylvania 19046.

Comprehensive Casebook of Cognitive Therapy, edited by Arthur Freeman and Frank M. Dattilio. Plenum Press, New York, 1992.

Relatedly, many patients with chronic muscle-derived pain develop a fear that excessive movement will trigger an exacerbation. Thus, they limit their range of movement for fear of reinjury. Also, as in anxiety and phobic states, hyperviligance toward cues associated with threatening situations is common. These factors contribute toward the evolution of a chronic state of psychophysiologic hyperarousal with bracing and protective guarding of the musculature.

The behavioral avoidance of situations associated with pain and restrictions in activity level limit the patient's access to reinforcers. Dysfunctional musculoskeletal posturing and chronic hypervigilance create undue physical stress in the body by increasing muscle tension and spasm, triggering muscle ischemia and exhausting the sympathetic nervous system. Excessive cognitive preoccupation with pain, disability, and personal limitations lead to depression. All of the above maintains the pain cycle.

This case report was developed to demonstrate some strategies and techniques for assessing and modifying cognitions and behaviors that can maintain and exacerbate chronic pain. The presentation describes the clinical implementation of a protocol integrating cognitive techniques and biofeedback training in conjunction with the use of behavioral methods (termed *biobehavioral*). The importance of setting clear goals based on the initial assessment of the patient and of limiting interventions to treatable and manageable problems is emphasized in this case report.

CASE REPORT

Emily was a 67-year-old married woman who presented with a 15-year history of chronic pain. Her list of symptoms included an irritable bowel; frequent diarrhea; abdominal pain; weakness, malaise and fatigue; disturbed sleep; anxiety; depression; concentration difficulties; occasional light-headedness and dizziness; frequent headaches; facial and jaw pain; neck, shoulder, and back pain; and sciatica. She was referred to the author by her gastroenterologist, who had been helping Emily manage her irritable bowel condition with medication. Emily stated that the referring physician had suggested that I might be able to teach her relaxation strategies for reducing stress, and that this in turn might help her achieve a reduction in her various symptoms.

Emily dated the onset of her condition to a bad case of the flu that she had developed 11 years ago and from which she felt that she had never fully recovered. Emily had made the rounds of numerous medical specialists in her attempts at finding the etiology of her unabating flulike condition and relief from her symptoms. All medical tests had yielded negative results from the standpoint of finding an identifiable medical cause.

BACKGROUND INFORMATION

Emily was currently unemployed and lived with her husband, Herbert. This was Emily's first marriage and her husband's second. Herbert had three children from his first marriage and had been a widower before meeting Emily. The couple had been married for 25 years and did not have any children from their marriage.

Emily characterized her relationship with her husband as devoid of intimate communication. The couple had never consummated their marital relationship, as Herbert suffered from "impotency" for as long as Emily had known him. Emily jokingly reported that they got along well, since she had her days to herself to do as she pleased while Herbert was at work. Herbert was a public school teacher who had recently retired; Emily readily admitted that she resented Herbert's retirement.

Emily reported that she was very close with her mother and that she had lived with her until she married Herbert at the age of 42. Emily's parents had divorced when she was 30, and after her father moved away, she permanently lost track of him. Emily also had a 58-year-old brother whom she saw infrequently. Another brother died at birth when she was a young child.

Emily's educational background included a high school diploma and about 45 college credits. Her work history reportedly had been stable until she developed a problem with anxiety and panic attacks the year that she was married. As a consequence of her anxieties, she left her full-time position as a financial analyst with a firm in which she had worked her way "up the ranks." She was treated with medication and "talk therapy" by a number of psychiatrists over the years, with poor results. She remained unemployed for a few years and then took a part-time job as a bookkeeper. She held onto this job until her anxiety problem worsened again, and she had not worked since.

Emily also had been involved in a motor vehicle accident approximately eight years earlier in which she had sustained some neck and back injuries. She reported that subsequent to the accident, she had developed anxieties about driving.

She admitted to the occasional use of alcohol in the past for self-medication of her anxieties, but denied drinking at the current time. She denied using illegal drugs or narcotic analgesics. She stated that her father had a drinking problem.

INITIAL ASSESSMENT (SESSION 1)

The first session consisted of a two-hour initial assessment in which a complete history was taken of Emily's presenting symptomatic complaints. Information was also obtained about associated symptoms and behaviors, significant life events, childhood, family and marital history, medical and psychiatric treatment history, personal and family substance abuse history, and educational and vocational history. These clinical data have been summarized above.

A thorough analysis of Emily's presenting problem of chronic pain entailed assessing the discrete *types* of pain she suffered and the circumstances associated with the *initial onset* of each pain complaint. The *bodily location* of each type of pain was determined, and information was obtained on identifiable *pain triggers*. Data was gathered on *pattern and frequency of occurrence*, *duration*, and *severity* for each type of pain. Information was also obtained about *coping strategies*, *previous treatments*, and *medication usage*.

Emily denied current usage of narcotic analgesic medication. She reported taking the following medications on an as needed basis: buffered aspirin for her pain, Imodium for her diarrhea, Bentyl for her irritable bowel, and simethicone for flatulence and gastric bloating.

In addition to the clinical interview, data was obtained through the administration of a number of paper-and-pencil questionnaires. Emily was presented with a shortened version of the McGill Pain Questionnaire (MPQ) and with the Multidimensional Pain Inventory (MPI; Rudy, 1989). The MPI is a 61-item questionnaire that provides a multiaxial assessment of the medical-physical, psychosocial, and behavioral-functional dimensions of chronic pain. This inventory yields a statistically derived multidimensional coping profile, as well as a summary classification of the chronic pain patient's coping abilities.

Emily was asked to complete these questionnaires at home and to mail them back before the next session. It was explained that in this way they could be scored, interpreted, and then reviewed with her in the second sessions. She was also asked to complete a Beck Depression Inventory (BDI) and Burns Anxiety Inventory (BAI).

SESSION 2

Feedback on the results of the initial assessment was delivered to Emily in the second one-hour session. Also, a preliminary problem list was written, goals were formulated, and recommendations were offered.

Emily's responses to the MPQ allowed her pain to be categorized into above the waist and below the waist pain. Her headaches were described as intermittent and as being dull, occasionally throbbing, pulling, and tight with the pain distributed as in a tight band around her head. The jaw pain was described as tight and aching. The neck, shoulder, and back pain was characterized as heavy, tender, exhausting, gruelling, radiating, nagging, and occasionally numbing. The abdominal pain was described as gnawing, sometimes shooting, boring, penetrating, burning, nauseating, grueling, and wretched. The leg or sciatica pain was characterized as pulsing, shooting, boring, sharp, and radiating.

Emily complained of feeling limited in her ability to find relief from her pain. However, for the above-the-waist pain, heat applications, rest, careful movement, and working were thought to provide relief some of the time. The occasional use of a cervical collar was also reported. For the abdominal and below-the-waist pain, the as-needed ingestion of her antispasmodic medication and lying down were reported to be the remedies.

Many factors were associated with pain exacerbations. Emily perceived her pain as having a "life and mind of its own." She felt that there were times when even the slightest activity or movement triggered pain. She did express the awareness that staying in any position, especially sitting, for more than a few minutes was likely to produce or worsen pain. She was keenly aware of driving as being a pain trigger.

Not surprisingly, Emily's responses on the MPI revealed perceptions of high pain severity, high life interference, and diminished control over her pain as well as life events. Her MPI pain profile classification was that of a "dysfunctional" coper. Affective distress was rated as being high. Although support from her spouse was rated as being fairly high, other indicators pointed to a significant degree of social alienation. General activity levels were reported as being low.

Emily scored in the moderately to severely depressed range on the BDI, earning a total score of 32. On the BAI, she revealed numerous indicators of anxiety, with a salient component of anxious thoughts and physical symptoms.

Based on the initial assessment, a problem list was compiled, treatment goals were discussed, methods were proposed for achieving these goals, and an ordering of priorities was suggested. A multimodal list of each identified problem and potential goals is presented in Table 36-1.

The therapist clarified at the outset that it was not advisable to expect to address very problem on the list. It was explained that the problems were interactive and that the successful alleviation of any targeted problem would have positive effects on the others. It was suggested initially that sessions be scheduled on a weekly basis. After confirming Emily's agreement with the treatment plan formulation, the therapist offered some suggestions about the order in which the problems might best be addressed.

THERAPIST: Well, Dr. P. has suggested that relaxation training is in order to teach you how to handle stress in a more healthy manner. I think this is a good place to start because most pain persons whom I have treated have found that, once they begin to really use relaxation techniques regularly, they experience less pain.

EMILY: I'm all for that!

THERAPIST: So, let's begin to teach you how to relax in our next session. In the meantime, I'd like to give you some more homework.

EMILY: This is just like school!

THERAPIST: Yes, in some ways, just think of part of what we might do here as an individualized pain-management school, and of me as kind of like a teacher or a coach.

EMILY: Are you going to grade me? If you are, I'll probably fail.

THERAPIST: Your grades will be delivered in the form of hurting less as long as you do your homework!

EMILY: (laughs) OK, go ahead. Tell me what I have to do.

THERAPIST: I'd like you to keep a sort of pain diary.

EMILY: (interrupting) You mean you want me to pay more attention to my pain that I already do?

TABLE 36-1   Emily's Multimodal Problem List and Suggested Treatment Goals

Modality	Problem	Goal
Behavior	1. Avoidance behaviors	To engage in feared activites
	2. Passivity/timidity	To express opinions and negative feelings appropriately
	3. Pain behaviors	To display fewer pain behaviors (e.g., grimacing, complaints
Affect	1. Anxiety/tension	To manage anxiety
	2. Irrational fears	To express less discomfort and increased tolerance when exposed to feared stimuli (e.g., driving)
	3. Depression	To experience less dysphoria
		To express more satisfaction with self and events
		To accept own imperfections
		To develop more interests
		To develop increased energy
Sensory	1. Preoccupation with physical symptoms	To learn distraction techniques
		To make fewer references to symptoms in conversation
	2. Muscular bracing and guarding	To learn how posture affects pain levels
		To learn muscle relaxation
		To reduce dyspoenesis
	3. Lack of control over severe pain	To learn pain-control strategies
		To learn relaxation strategies
		To learn what triggers and relieves pain
		To learn how activity, mastery, pleasure, and cognitions relate to mood, pain, and energy level
Imagery	1. Destructive images of body processes	To become aware of pain images and develop antidote images
Cognition	1. Self-critical thoughts	To recognize thoughts
		To respond rationally
		To recognize strengths
		To accept failures without self-putdowns
		To take safe risks
Interpersonal	1. Lack of honest communication with spouse	To express positive as well as negative feelings directly and appropriately
	2. Social alienation and trust issues	To make attempts to engage in more intimate communication
	3. Unresolved grief	To talk about feelings about past losses and to determine how related thoughts affect current relationships
Drugs/Biological	1. Sleep disruption	To learn sleep-hygiene behaviors
		To explore indications for use of tricyclic antidepressants to restore deep sleep
	2. Use of pain medications	To understand the iatrogenic outcomes of long-term use
	3. Medical diagnosis	To understand medical care options
		To resolve need to have an etiologic diagnosis
	4. General fatigue and fatigue on awakening	To reduce overall fatigue
		To develop expectations of increased energy levels

THERAPIST: Well, that's not exactly the end I have in mind. You see, I want you to learn a technique called self-monitoring, which is a specific method of rating the amount of pain you feel at different times of the day. It will enable us to discover pain triggers and pain patterns.

EMILY: So what's the point?

THERAPIST: The point is that you have to understand a problem and properly diagnose it before you can fix it. So, just as an automotive mechanic needs to learn where the noise is in your car, what it sounds like, and when you hear the noise so that he can accurately diagnose and then repair the problem, so, too, we need to learn about the factors that affect the changes in your pain.

EMILY: That makes sense. So, how do we start?

The therapist then handed Emily a daily self-monitoring record and proceeded to explain how to use it. For the remainder of the session, the therapist discussed with Emily the way to do self-monitoring. It was suggested that Emily make entries on the daily self-monitoring record every two hours. It was also explained that self-monitoring would establish a pretreatment baseline and would enable them both to chart her progress and improvement over the course of treatment. A follow-up appointment was scheduled for the next week.

SESSION 3

The third session began by reviewing the daily self-monitoring records that Emily had filled out over the course of the past week. A sample of one of Emily's daily self-monitoring records is presented in Figure 36-1. As can be seen from the sample, the record allows the patient to keep track simultaneously each day of activities, subjective ratings of mastery (M) and pleasure (P), energy levels, mood, accompanying thoughts, pain levels, and medication usage.

Examination of Emily's self-monitoring records revealed that her levels of pain fluctuated quite markedly over the course of the day. This was pointed out to her. Seeing this on paper led Emily to comment that the self-monitoring was teaching her that maybe there was some "lawfulness" to the fluctuations in her pain. The therapist then reminded Emily of her earlier comment that her pain had "a life and mind of its own," and she responded that maybe the two of them could discover what it would take to persuade her pain to change its mind and "leave me the [expletive deleted] alone!"

Examination of Emily's self-monitoring records for the week also revealed a number of patterns that were discussed. First, Emily discovered that she engaged in few activities that gave her a sense of either mastery or pleasure. Second, she expressed the realization that her life was quite boring, and that she had an inordinate amount of time to think about little else besides her pain. Third, the negativity of her recorded thoughts was pointed out. It was then suggested that perhaps there was a connection between the nature of her automatic thoughts and her mood. No attempt was made at this time to suggest any connection between Emily's thoughts and her pain levels; this idea would have been premature, and most likely would have been met with strong resistance.

The next item on the agenda was to begin relaxation training. First, the therapist delivered the following rationale for conducting biofeedback-assisted relaxation training:

> You are here because you have not been able to control your pain and your other symptoms. How is it that you can control many things in your body—for example, you can wiggle your toes, wrinkle your nose, raise your arms, and so on—but yet you cannot control the acid in your stomach, the motility of your bowels, the muscles in your head, neck, and back, your blood pressure, and so on? Well, the answer is that every single bodily function you've learned to control gives you natural feedback, like you know where your left foot is, but you don't know what's going on in your back or gut right now unless you have pain there. Biofeedback instruments make you as aware of what's going on inside your body as you are aware of the location of your left foot. Thus, they remove the blindfold of learning, and you can learn to control the physical reactions in your body that cause your pain or make it worse.

After delivering the rationale for biofeedback, the therapist explained the biofeedback instrumentation, assured Emily that there were no risks involved, and then demonstrated how the instruments work. Emily was then connected to the computerized instruments.

Next, the therapist conducted a computerized baseline psychophysiological stress profile assessment. It was explained that the purpose of this assessment was to determine in which physiologic modalities Emily was most reactive. The procedure involved simultaneously monitoring frontalis muscle activity (EMG), skin perspiration changes (termed *electrodermal response* or EDR), skin temperature (TEMP), and heart rate (HR) while Emily was sequentially presented with different task demands and relaxation conditions. Essentially, this procedure was equivalent to computerized psychophysiologically monitored mental status examination.

The task demands or stressors employed were (a) asked Emily to recall and talk about when her pain was at its worst; (b) asking her to perform various arithmetic computations in her head; (c) asking her to recall and talk about her motor vehicle accident; asking her to talk about

Pain Rating Scale
0 1 2 3 4 5 6 7 8 9 10

no   worst pain
pain   imaginable

Mastery Rating Scale (M)
0 1 2 3 4 5 6 7 8 9 10

none   maximum
                             mastery

Pleasure Rating Scale (P)
0 1 2 3 4 5 6 7 8 9 10

none   extremely
                             pleasurable

Energy Rating Scale
0 1 2 3 4 5 6 7 8 9 10

no   extremely
energy   energetic

Mood: (Categories)
A-anxious   G-tense
B-bored   H-happy
C-tired   I-irritated
D-depressed R-relaxed
E-angry   O-other
F-afraid   (specify)

Date: __4/88__

Time	Place & Activity	M(0-10) P(0-10)	Energy Level (0-10)	Mood	Accompanying Thoughts	Pain (0-10) abdomen	Pain (0-10) head & neck	Pain (0-10) shoulder & arm	Pain (0-10) back & leg	Meds
7 AM	In bed	M=0,P=0	1	A,C, D,G	What a bad night. I just can't sleep anymore. It's going to be a rough day, I'm so stiff.	5	5	5	7	2-A 1-S 1-I 1-B
9 AM	Kitchen-making tea	M=1,P=4	3	B,C	I have to go shopping. I don't feel up to it.	3	6	4	8	
11 AM	Driving to market	M=3,P=2	5	A,E	I hate this traffic. My head feels like it's going to explode.	6	9	7	5	
1 PM	Kitchen-making lunch	M=0,P=2	3	O	I'm so hungry. I hope I don't get the runs after eating. I want to be comfortable.	4	5	3	4	2-A 1-B
3 PM	Lying in bedroom	M=0,P=8	1	C,R	I can't keep my eyes open. I feel so much better lying down. I don't want to think.	1	2	2	2	
5 PM	Cleaning living room	M=0,P=3	2	E	I took a 2 hr. nap and I'm still so tired.	1	8	4	5	2-A
7 PM	Eating dinner with husband	M=1,P=3	4	I,E	Herbert had no right to retire. I've lost my personal space.	5	7	6	3	1-I
9 PM	Watching TV in den	M=1,P=6	2	B,R	Nothing	1	5	3	3	
11 PM	Watching TV in den	M=1,P=4	1	B,C	Should I go to bed now or stay up another hr.? I probably won't fall to sleep anyhow.	1	6	3	6	2-A

COMMENTS: A=Ascriptin   I am so angry at Herbert. He had no right to retire. We have so little in
           S=Simethicone   common. I settled in this marriage. I have no control over this. I do care
           I=Imodium   for him though. He has been supportive of me as much of a basket case as I
           B=Bentyl   have been.

Figure 36-1. Emily's Self-Monitoring Record.

her husband's retirement; and (d) asking Emily to listen to loud and stressful prerecorded sounds. Each task was presented for a few minutes and then followed by a "recovery period" during which she was instructed to relax as best she could.

The computerized printout of the stress profile was reviewed with Emily. It revealed severely elevated muscle activity in the upper body that was highly reactive to stress (EMG readings averaged 11 microvolts), moderately cold extremities (hand temperature averaged 78 degrees Fahrenheit), highly reactive skin perspiration response with elevated skin conductance baseline levels (EDR readings ranging from 20 to 62 micromhos), and moderately reactive—but within normal limits—heart rate (HR readings ranging from 72 to 96 beats per minutes).

The connections between breathing, the stress response, anxiety, and pain was then briefly explained, and the importance of learning to breathe properly was emphasized. Emily was then introduced to diaphragmatic breathing and asked to self-monitor her breathing over the course of the week. She was also reminded to continue to record daily on her self-monitoring records.

SESSION 4

Emily's daily self-monitoring records were reviewed at the beginning of the session. She was then asked if she had learned anything about her breathing that week. Emily reported that she had observed herself frequently holding her breath, especially when she felt tense and was in pain. The therapist then modeled the proper way to breath diaphragmatically and demonstrated how Emily could use her hands as a natural form of biofeedback for shaping her skills in diaphragmatic breathing. She was connected to the computerized biofeedback instrumentation, and after recording baseline physiologic data, she was taught a biobehavioral variation of Benson's "relaxation response."

> Just get comfortable. Sit up straight with your back well supported. Feet flat on the floor and well grounded. You may close your eyes or you may keep them open. Place your left hand on your abdomen and your right hand on your chest. Begin to breath slowly and evenly, fully from your abdomen. Feel your abdomen rise as you slowly inhale and fall as you slowly exhale.

In order to facilitate and shape Emily's use of her diaphragm, imagery was suggested of a beach ball in her belly inflating and deflating through an "air valve" in her navel as she inhaled and exhaled. It was suggested that Emily mentally repeat the cue word "breathe" each time she exhaled.

This procedure was tape recorded as it was conducted. It was followed by the recording of instructions for progressive muscle relaxation and suggestions for warming of the extremities, slowing heart rate, developing mental calmness, and increasing feelings of comfort and well-being. The tape was then stopped, and Emily was asked to think of some adjectives to describe how she was feeling at that moment. She responded that she was feeling "relaxed, comfortable, light, and limp." After checking with her to make sure that these represented good feelings, the same adjectives were repeated back to her in the form of suggestions on the tape.

Emily was given the tape and a written sheet of step-by-step instructions summarizing the entire relaxation procedure. It was suggested that she listen to the 20-minute tape twice daily over the next week. Emily was also reminded to continue her daily self-monitoring at two-hour intervals. However, in addition, she was asked to record an entry each time that she listened to her relaxation tape. It was suggested that she enter her mastery and pleasure ratings after listening to the tape, and her ratings of energy level, mood, and pain both before and after she listened to the tape.

SESSION 5

The session was initiated by inquiring about Emily's use of the relaxation tape. She responded that she had listened to the tape an average of once a day. Review of her relaxation entries in her daily self-monitoring records revealed slight reductions in pain levels after listening to the tape. Emily's pleasure ratings of the exercise averaged at around 5; her mastery ratings of her ability to relax evidenced a slight increase over the course of the week.

After reviewing her homework, Emily was connected to the biofeedback instrumentation. A three-minute psychophysiologic baseline was taken, and then Emily was asked to relax to the best of her ability, using the procedures that were on the tape. Twenty minutes were spent coaching Emily to lower her upper-body EMG levels and to increase her skin temperature with suggestions of hand warming and increased blood flow to the extremities. Beginning from baseline averages of 8.2 microvolts for frontalis EMG and 82 degrees Fahrenheit for hand temperature, Emily demonstrated the ability to lower her EMG to around 4.0 microvolts and to raise her hand temperature to 88 degrees Fahrenheit.

During the remainder of the session, Emily ventilated her frustrations with the medical establishment's failure to pinpoint a specific etiology for her overall condition. At this point, the therapist (after qualifying that he did not have a medical license or the medical training to make medical diagnoses) suggested that Emily's symptomatic presentation and history had many similarities to patients he had seen with the medical diagnosis of fibromyositis. The clinical features of fibromyositis were discussed in the remaining few minutes of the session.

SESSIONS 6 THROUGH 8

At the outset of the sixth session two weeks later, Emily reported that she had obtained a referral to a rheumatologist who had diagnosed her as having fibromyositis. He had prescribed Desyrel, a tricyclic antidepressant, to be taken at bedtime. Tricyclics are generally the pharmacologic treatment of choice for patients with fibromyositis who suffer from disturbed sleep patterns. The therapist made sure Emily understood that the rationale for use of the Desyrel was to help in restoring normal deep-sleep patterns. It was explained that sleep restoration could be expected to result in a reduction of her pain, malaise, and fatigue.

Emily continued to self-monitor, and her daily records were reviewed at the outset of each session. She continued to complain that her pain had "a mind of its own," as evidenced by recorded pain exacerbations even when she felt she had been "doing all the right things." To these statements, the therapist responded that it was impossible to control all stressors, that stress was cumulative and insidious, but that it was her responsibility to identify her stressors and to practice strategies for minimizing their ill effects.

As she had become discouraged with practicing relaxation at home and yet reported pain relief after biofeedback-assisted relaxation sessions in the office, the therapist explored with Emily her underlying thoughts about using relaxation. This guided inquiry revealed that she believed that she was not accomplishing anything when she sat and listened to the tape or practiced relaxation without the tape. This belief was disputed with the argument that if she felt better after doing relaxation, then she would be capable of greater productivity when she resumed her activities. Thus, it was suggested that doing "relaxation work" could be thought of as a quiet time to reconstitute her body's resources and restore her energy levels, comfort, and pleasant mood.

Biofeedback-assisted coaching of relaxation and physiologic self-regulation skills was consistently provided for part of each session. Emily's relaxation work was always reinforced by end-of-session reviews of computer printouts that revealed her progress both within and be-

tween biofeedback sessions in developing self-regulation skills.

SESSIONS 9 THROUGH 11

The agenda for these sessions involved teaching Emily the cognitive model of mood disturbances and illustrating the connection between thoughts, feelings, and physiology through biofeedback. Emily had already experienced in previous sessions how her thoughts were associated with measurable physiological changes in her body. She had also associated biofeedback self-regulation skills with noticeable reductions in her pain levels. Therefore, it was hypothesized that she was ready to accept the idea that the replacement of stress-producing thoughts with alternative stress-reducing thoughts would allow her to achieve a greater measure of pain control, and consequently hurt less.

In line with current biobehavioral work, the concept of identifying stress-producing thoughts was termed cognitive stress profiling. Relatedly, the idea of learning "cognitive judo" was presented as a way of conceptualizing an effective means of defense against the unthinking acceptance of stress-producing automatic thoughts that made pain hurt more.

Next, Emily was introduced to the Daily Record of Dysfunctional Thoughts (DRDT). She had already been recording her thoughts on her daily self-monitoring records, so this was familiar. Emily also was provided with a written sheet cataloging the major classes of cognitive distortions and those most typically used by pain patients. She was asked to identify the categories that seemed typical of her thinking and to recall situations when she had employed those types of thinking.

THERAPIST: Do any of these categories or ways of thinking seem vaguely familiar to you?

EMILY: No, none of this describes me! (laughs)

THERAPIST: Are you sure you never let one drop of black ink color your whole beaker of clear water?

EMILY: What are you implying, that I have let pain take over my whole life?

THERAPIST: That really is a leading question, you know, and I take the Fifth on that one!

EMILY: Come on now, don't run scared, tell me what you really think now!

THERAPIST: OK. I think that if you would be willing to be as direct and forthright in confronting some of the thoughts that we've already examined on your daily self-monitoring records as you just have been in confronting me, then you could make great progress in recovering from the rut you have been in.

EMILY: That's a good answer!

THERAPIST: What is this, a test?

EMILY: Yes, your grades will be delivered in the form of helping me to get rid of my pain!

THERAPIST: Well, I'm glad that we're still together on this.

EMILY: Yes, we definitely are!

The therapist gave Emily a stack of DRDTs and suggested that, as homework, she record her automatic thoughts and catalogue the types of distorted thinking she was employing whenever she felt especially low, angry, anxious, tired, or in pain.

Emily was also taught a form of self-hypnosis during these sessions. Hypnosis was defined to Emily as a beneficial altered state of consciousness that was self-attained and self-controlled. It was suggested that self-hypnosis would be an excellent tool for replacing negative thoughts and images with helpful ones and creating positive feelings and experiences. It was explained that one could develop skill in attaining such an altered state through the practiced application of the subskills of self-suggestion, physical relaxation, and the vivid use of imagination. It was further explained that with practice, Emily could learn how to apply these skills to attain a pleasant state of effortless absorption in a positive experience when it was appropriate to do so.

One hypnotic induction that the author has found to be quite effective with many pain patients is called the "candle technique." This induction works well in hetero-hypnosis and is easily adapted to self-hypnosis. A hypnotic state was induced in Emily with the candle technique using an elaboration of the following abbreviated verbalization.

First, Emily was asked to rest back comfortably and to begin by taking a few slow, deep breaths. Then, standard suggestions for muscle awareness and rapid relaxation were delivered. The therapist then asked Emily to stare at a lit candle that was placed slightly above eye level directly in front of her.

> Keep staring at the flame, and as you continue to do so, I would like you to be aware of three other things that you see in your peripheral vision, without moving your head . . . Continue to allow your breathing to be slow and restful as you remain aware of these three things . . . Now, I would like you to become aware of three sounds that you hear as you continue to stare at the flame . . . And while you remain aware of these, I would like you to also become aware of three sensations in your body that you can feel right now as you continue to be aware of those three things that you can see and those three things that you can hear.

The therapist then proceeded to ask Emily to become aware of two things that she saw out of her peripheral vision that were different from the first three, as she continued to stare at the candle. The same progression was followed for two other things heard and two other sensations felt. Then the sequence then progressed to one additional thing seen, one additional thing heard, and one additional sensation felt. All the while, suggestions for eye fatigue, slowing down, and relaxation were interspersed. Emily attained a very deep level of relaxed inner absorption, and while she was in this state, a number of direct suggestions for diminution of pain and for positive coping were delivered. Then, instructions for the use of the candle technique (including and excluding the availability of an in vivo candle) were delivered in the form of post-hypnotic suggestions. These suggestions were reinforced when Emily was fully awake and alert, and a written sheet was given to her summarizing the steps.

SESSIONS 12 THROUGH 14

Hypnotic skills training was conducted over the course of the next three sessions. Emily was taught a number of other hypnotic-induction techniques so that she might have a menu of options from which to choose. She was also taught how to construct her own self-suggestions.

Various techniques for cognitive disputation of dysfunctional thoughts were modeled and rehearsed in the office, using material derived from her DRDTs as well as material brought up in the sessions. These techniques included (among others) labeling cognitive distortions, questioning the evidence, reattribution, scaling down all-or-nothing thinking, estimating probabilities of feared consequences, considering alternate interpretations, listing options and alternatives, and imagining coping with her worst fears.

Emily was given the homework assignment of completing all columns of the Daily Record of Dysfunctional Thoughts. As she became proficient at rationally responding to her automatic thoughts, the therapist began selectively to incorporate her rational responses into hypnotic suggestions.

Emily was also taught about the uses and the abuses of imagery. Emily's images of her different pain symptoms were elicited, and "antidote" images were constructed. Emily was taught to remind herself to think of these antidote images spontaneously as well as in response to her pathogenic pain images. The antidote images were also incorporated into hypnotic suggestions, and it was suggested that Emily utilize them in delivering her self-suggestions during self-hypnosis.

In addition, Emily was taught how to run mental rehearsals. Essentially, this involved inducing a relaxed state and then imagining herself accomplishing things she wanted to accomplish. She reported that this technique helped her to "get psyched" to get things done that she in the past would have put off. She specifically reported that running mental rehearsals helped somewhat in coping with her fatigue in the morning. She regularly used relaxation and self-hypnosis at bedtime and now incorporated suggestions and images of peaceful, restful sleep and of awakening in the morning refreshed, alert, rested, energetic, and motivated.

SESSIONS 15 THROUGH 17

Having developed various cognitive and biobehavioral self-regulation skills, Emily was now quite resourceful at distracting herself from her pain symptoms. Sessions 15 through 17 were largely devoted to reinforcing all that she had learned and generalizing her skills to different situations. She also became aware of how anxiety in various situations (e.g., driving a car) caused her to tense and brace the muscles of her upper body and clench her jaw. She learned how this led to the onset of tension headaches, jaw pain, neck pain, shoulder pain, and pain radiating down her left arm. Her driving anxieties were targeted for future desensitization.

SESSIONS 18 THROUGH 20

A biofeedback-assisted desensitization protocol was implemented incorporating videotaped depictions of 11 driving themes presented from the "associated" perspective of a driver or passenger. The protocol, termed *video-assisted desensitization* (VAD; Brick & Eimer, 1990), involved first determining which of the 11 driving themes needed to be included in the desensitization procedure and their order of presentation. This determination was made by exposing Emily to each driving theme while simultaneously monitoring her physiologic responses (i.e., heart rate, skin perspiration, and frontalis muscle activity) and subjective ratings of distress recorded on a 0-to-10 scale of subjective units of discomfort (SUDs). Each driving theme was automatically repeated in 10 consecutive frames. This preedited video feature provided Emily with sufficient exposure to each theme before she indicated her subjective units of distress to the stimulus presentation.

The videotaped themes selected for the desensitization procedure were those that resulted in any one or more of the following responses: (a) notable bracing of the body

and/or reactive gesturing; (b) verbalizations of discomfort and/or SUDs ratings of 3 or more; or (c) notable reactivity in one or more of the physiologic modalities monitored. The selected themes were then arranged in a psychophysiologic anxiety hierarchy so that exposure to the themes could proceed from the least to the most anxiety-arousing themes.

The actual procedure involved first employing biofeedback-assisted coaching to help Emily attain a baseline level of relaxation. Then, the initial videotaped depiction in the hierarchy was presented while Emily was coached to maintain her baseline levels of relaxation in each physiologic modality. If she evidenced a marked rise in arousal, the videotape was stopped, and Emily was coached back to baseline relaxation. Once this was achieved, the videotape theme segment was rerun. A given theme was presented for as many exposures as was needed until Emily was able to maintain baseline relaxation levels—in other words, until "psychophysiologic habituation" was achieved.

This procedure was followed for each videotaped theme in the hierarchy. In addition, Emily was coached to employ coping self-talk during exposure to the stimuli. She was also given positive suggestions that reframed driving as an opportunity to enjoy pleasures and conveniences of which she had been deprived.

Emily reported very positive responses to the VAD procedure. She reported that she had begun to see driving as another opportunity for practicing self-regulation training and that she was driving more often and feeling more comfortable. This was borne out by her entries in her daily self-monitoring record.

SUBSEQUENT SESSIONS

Subsequent sessions focused on some of the other problems on Emily's multimodal problem list. These included her bouts of dysphoria, her anger, her self-critical thoughts, her dearth of honest and intimate communication with her husband, her feelings of social alienation, her unresolved grief about past losses, her sleep disruptions, and medication issues.

As Emily developed more control over her reactions to her pain and fatigue, she began to develop interests that distracted her from her symptoms. She reported that she still had "bad days" painwise, but that she was better able to respond to irrational automatic thoughts about *having* to do more than she was capable of doing. A number of sessions were partly devoted to teaching Emily how to perform activities to schedule (instead of to tolerance) so that activity levels were not contingent on pain. This was introduced through the concept of pacing; she was taught how to determine baseline activity levels that did not exacerbate preexisting pain, and how to shape increased activity levels without experiencing significant increases in pain.

Cognitive disputation work continued to be done to reinforce her ability to respond to her depressogenic self-talk when she felt excessively fatigued or uncomfortable. She also was encouraged to continue to use self-hypnotic techniques with pain-antidote imagery and rational self-suggestion.

Sessions also focused on identifying and disputing self-critical thinking. She practiced controlled risk taking, as discussed by Ellis (1988), and was guided in learning how to accept failures without "self putdowns." Emily kept daily lists of her strengths, and she became familiar with an American Chronic Pain Association (ACPA) publication listing the "basic rights of the chronic pain person." Eventually she joined a chronic pain support group that was organized through the ACPA.

Emily identified with many of the ACPA's descriptions of the chronic pain person's issues. She found that her new ACPA support network, her ongoing therapy, and the use of cognitive and biobehavioral self-help skills helped her to cope with the fears of reinjury that in the past had limited her range of motion and levels of activity.

Emily understood the iatrogenic effects of the long-term use of narcotic analgesics. This was reviewed, and also the concept of minimizing the as-needed (termed PRN) ingestion of any of her medicines was discussed. She was encouraged to work with her physicians to limit the use of medications to those that were deemed medically necessary and to take those medications according to schedule, as opposed to PRN.

It should be noted that Emily did not find any tricyclic antidepressants that worked for her as she and her physician tried out several according to proper medical protocol. She was unable to tolerate the side effects, the worst of which for her was excessive drowsiness throughout the morning. Nevertheless, Emily found that self-hypnosis, listening to relaxation tapes before bed, diet modification (especially eliminating caffeine), and following various behavioral sleep-hygiene principles helped to improve her sleep patterns to some degree.

Several subsequent sessions were devoted to discussions about past personal losses, Emily's thoughts and feelings about her husband's retirement, and her marital communication problems. The advantages and disadvantages of involving her spouse in therapy to work on these issues was addressed at this point, and Emily chose to defer this approach. Emily was seen for five more "booster" sessions, which were spaced at biweekly to monthly intervals.

The total duration of treatment was 15 months, with a total number of 33 sessions. Periodic follow-ups over the course of a year revealed a maintenance of treatment gains as Emily continued to practice her self-management skills, to learn about chronic pain and fibromyositis, and to remain active in her chronic pain support organization.

ACKNOWLEDGMENTS. The author wishes to thank his patient for participating as a collaborator in this case presentation. Robert H. Brick is gratefully acknowledged for sharing generously his ideas and expertise in the area of behavioral desensitization strategies. He has provided abundant collegial support over the years and offered many helpful editorial comments on this chapter. Also, the author wishes gratefully to acknowledge Jack Hartje, who provided a solid conceptual foundation for implementing systematic biofeedback training protocols with chronic pain patients, and Pamela Ladds for her seasoned input on the implementation of biobehavioral interventions.

In addition, the author wishes to thank the many others whose research and writings on chronic pain have contributed to the development of his clinical approaches with pain patients. They include, among others, David Corey, Penney Cowan, Richard Hanson, Barbara Headley, Kenneth Gerber, Thomas Rudy, and Dennis Turk.

REFERENCES

Brick, R. H., & Eimer, B. N. (1990). *Video-assisted desensitization: A user's manual*. Philadelphia: The Behavior Therapy Center.

Ellis, A. (1988). *How to stubbornly refuse to make yourself miserable about anything—yes, anything!* Secaucus, NJ: Lyle Stuart.

Rudy, T. E. (1989). *Multiaxial assessment of pain: Multidimensional pain inventory, user's manual*. Pittsburgh, PA: Pain Evaluation and Treatment Institute, University of Pittsburgh School of Medicine.

SUGGESTED READINGS

Burns, D. D. (1980). *Feeling good: The new mood therapy*. New York: New American Library.

Corey, D. (1989). *Pain: Free yourself for life*. New York: New American Library.

Cowan, P. (1990). *American Chronic Pain Association: Leaders manual*. Monroeville, PA: American Chronic Pain Association.

Eimer, B. N. (1988). The chronic pain patient: Multimodal assessment and psychotherapy. *Medical Psychotherapy, 1*, 23–40.

Eimer, B. N. (1989). Psychotherapy for chronic pain: A cognitive approach. In A. Freeman, K. M. Simon, L. E. Beutler, & H.

Arkowitz (Eds.), *Comprehensive handbook of cognitive therapy* (pp. 449–465). New York: Plenum.

Golden, W. L., Dowd, E. T., & Friedberg, F. (1987). *Hypnotherapy: A modern approach*. New York: Pergamon.

Hanson, R. W., & Gerber, K. E. (1990). *Coping with chronic pain: A guide to patient self-management*. New York; Guilford.

Headley, B. J. (1988). *Back in balance: A chronic pain workbook*. Stillwater, MN: Pain Resources.

Turk, D. C., & Rudy, T. E. (1990). Chronic pain: Behavioral approaches to assessment and management. In A. Bellack, M. Hersen, & A. Kazdin (Eds.), *International handbook of behavior modification*. New York: Pergamon.

IV

Epilogue

37

Cognitive Therapy in the Year 2000

Arthur Freeman and Frank M. Dattilio

As this casebook comes to a close, two important aspects of the present volume have, we hope, become obvious. The first is the diversity of theoretical and technical positions represented by the contributors. It is interesting that there are differences of opinion, and a wide range of techniques that have come together under the broad banner of cognitive therapy. The second is the clear and active debunking of several of what Freeman (1986) and Freeman, Pretzer, Fleming, and Simon (1990) have called "the myths of cognitive therapy."

In the last few years, the cognitive revolution has, like so many other revolutions, matured and changed. We no longer take the defensive and reactive stance that was characteristic of the early years of the cognitive-behavioral movement. In those early days (a mere 15 years ago), many individuals representing particular domains within the cognitive-behavioral camp were hunting for their own territory. As each piece of turf was identified, many arbitrary lines were drawn. One was often asked to which school of therapy one subscribed: Were you an RETer, a Beckian, a Meichenbaumian, or a multimodal therapist?

Arthur Freeman • Department of Psychiatry, Cooper Hospital/University Medical Center and Robert Wood Johnson Medical School at Camden, Camden, New Jersey 08103. • Frank M. Dattilio • Center for Cognitive Therapy, Department of Psychiatry, University of Pennsylvania School of Medicine, Philadelphia, Pennsylvania 19104.

Comprehensive Casebook of Cognitive Therapy, edited by Arthur Freeman and Frank M. Dattilio. Plenum Press, New York, 1992.

Having delineated the general allegiance, the next step was to make sure of the party loyalty. For example, it was verboten to refer to any dynamic constructs (e.g., the unconscious, countertransference). To do so would label one as a backslider and a reactionary.

When Mahoney and Freeman (1985) edited a volume on the role of cognition in psychotherapy, one of the published reviews of the volume was bellicose at best and shrieked its condemnation of the inclusion into that volume of what the reviewer saw as the same old, worn theories. What prompted this response were the editor's attempts to integrate into contemporary cognitive therapy the work of such "old" figures as Albert Bandura, John Bowlby, Silvano Arieti, Harry Stack Sullivan, Viktor Frankl, Alfred Adler, and Karen Horney. Some old stuff! This early attempt to offer an integration to the cognitive approach was denounced because it suggested somehow giving into the old guard against whom some real or imagined battle was being waged. It was, for some, a need to reinvent the wheel. Historically, it is of interest that the active, directive, here-and-now approach that so characterizes the cognitive therapy model of the 1990s was well established in the work of Horney, Sullivan, and Adler. It would probably have been unthinkable in those early days for a cognitive therapist to publish a volume that emphasized the importance of interpersonal process in cognitive therapy; an excellent volume with that title was recently published (Safran & Segal, 1990).

The increase in professional interest in cognitive-behavioral work since 1972 has been phenomenal; Norcross, Prochaska, and Gallagher (1989) have noted a

600% increase. The increased interest has led to increased demands for training workshops, for better and more sophisticated assessment tools, and for information—eventuating in the publication of many recent volumes in cognitive therapy (including, of course, the present volume).

COMMON DENOMINATORS IN COGNITIVE THERAPY

Despite the theoretical differences that may exist among the authors in this volume, several commonalities emerge. The common denominators include the data base of the model, expectation for activity of the patient within the therapy, the directive stance of the therapist, the collaborative nature of the therapeutic relationship, the goal/problem orientation of the therapy, the focus and structure of the therapy, the time-limited nature of the therapy, the psychoeducational nature of the therapy, and the concern for relapse prevention (Freeman & Davis, 1990).

Data base. The cognitive therapist works from a base of information that involves extensive assessment of many aspects of the patient's thoughts, beliefs, affect, and behavior. It is from this data base that the conceptual framework is developed, rather than starting from a theoretical base and assuming that the patient's problems must be drawn from the theory rather than from the available data. For example, if a patient says something with great emphasis, we as cognitive therapists would likely pay greater attention to it, rather than dismissing it as reaction formation. Of course, if the patient forgets to mention something, it may be unimportant rather than a focus of therapy as repressed material.

Activity. The patients discussed in these cases all were encouraged to be an active part of their therapy. Rather than coming to therapy to be "therapized" or worked on once or twice a week, the patient in cognitive therapy is an active part of his or her own change process. The reader saw this in many of the cases, most often in the homework that therapists and patients generated as part of the therapy session. By adding homework to the in-session therapy work as independent work outside the session, the therapy can proceed much more quickly. In addition, the homework (and the higher general activity of the patient in the therapy) makes the changes and insights far more subjective. Patients can own what they learn, rather than depending on the therapist either telling them what they think or feel, or interpreting to the patient what the patients's internal processes are.

Directive. It might be said that if there are two persons in the consulting room for therapy, one of them should have an idea of a direction for that therapy. Ideally (it is hoped), it should be the therapist. Rather than the therapist taking the role of simply restating, reframing, reformulating, or interpreting, the therapeutic work described herein demonstrates rather dramatically the directive nature of cognitive therapy work. While mainly using a guided approach, there are many times that the patient can be helped by the therapist suggesting, advising, clarifying, and directing the therapy. For some patients, the therapist can lead the therapy by using multiple-choice formats where the therapist offers several choices for the patient to choose between. For the most part, however, the use of Socratic questioning and guided discovery is well demonstrated.

Collaborative. While being directive and active, the therapists describing their work have clearly demonstrated the importance of the therapeutic relationship. If there is not a strong working alliance or relationship between the patient and therapist, the patient may be less likely to comply with the therapeutic regimen. This process, often called *resistance*, needs to be viewed in the broad context of the therapeutic relationship. The lack of compliance may be divided into two areas: those problems due to patient issues, and those due to therapist issues. Patient issues include the lack of skill to comply, negative expectations of the success of therapy based on previous failures, concerns about the results or consequences of the therapeutic outcome, or questions about the results of changes on significant others. Therapist issues include the lack of skill with a particular patient or clinical problem, belief in the hopelessness of the patient's plight, or difficulty in establishing a collaborative set.

Structure. The focus and problem orientation of cognitive therapy is probably one of the most significant elements of the therapy. The need for targeting specific problems is in direst opposition to vague, amorphous psychotherapy treatment that drifts unguided hither and yon. (We call this the "Hansel and Gretel" approach to therapy. The patient goes through the session, dropping crumbs behind him or her labeled "When I was younger . . . ", "I remember . . . ", or "My mother . . . "; the aimless therapist runs along behind the patient, scooping up the crumbs and hoping that the patient will get to where he or she is supposed to be going. When time has run out, the therapist ends the session and the patient, like Hansel and Gretel, is lost in the forest.) By identifying specific targets for therapy, the treatment has a direction that can be seen and agreed to by therapist and patient. In point of fact, not developing a focused and strategic goal in therapy might even constitute a lack of informed consent from the patient for the therapy work. The cases in this volume have all demonstrated the value of focusing the therapy overall, and the individual session specifically.

Time limited. The typical outcome studies of the efficacy of cognitive therapy (e.g., Rush, Beck, Kovacs, & Hollon, 1977; Blackburn, Bishop, Glen, Whalley, & Christie, 1981; Murphy, Simons, Wetzel, & Lustman, 1984) have used a cutoff point of ending the therapy and evaluating the result. While this has generally been 12 to 20 sessions, it does not mean that cognitive therapy must be done within 20 sessions. The therapy descriptions in this volume demonstrate that with the focus of the therapy comes with an attempt to limit the therapy so that it does not become interminable. At times, this time limit may be externally imposed by third-party payers who provide the funding for therapy. In any case, trying to limit the therapy to an particular number of sessions has the effect of keeping the therapist honest. The therapist must be actively involved in moving the therapy apace, rather than sitting back and allowing the therapy to unfold in some vague direction.

Psychoeducational. The problems that contribute to the patient's problems are not always intrapsychic (i.e., totally within the patient). For many patients, their problems are in part or more fully a product of major interpersonal deficits on the part of the patient, or of problematic interactions (Bandura, 1977; Sullivan, 1953). The cognitive therapy model includes large components of skill building, education, and practice.

Relapse prevention. When does therapy end? The cognitive therapist, having taken a time-limited view, sees the therapy as having a beginning (problem definition, building collaboration and rapport), a middle (problem focus, schematic identification and modification, problem resolution), and an end (achieving closure on the therapeutic relationship, relapse prevention). The last phase of therapy, relapse prevention, works to help the patient to identify clearly and have mastery of the cognitive and behavioral skills of the therapy, to review through role-playing and homework the problem-solving skills, and to have proficiency in maintaining and using the impulse control strategies learned in the therapy.

DEBUNKING COGNITIVE THERAPY MYTHS

Having defined what cognitive therapy is, we can examine several of the commonly held myths of cognitive therapy so that they can finally be put to rest (Freeman, 1986; Freeman et al., 1990).

Myth #1: The cognitive therapist does not use information and material from the patient's past. As the reader can see, the therapists in this volume do not focus on the past, or expend large amounts of therapy time in exploring issues and problems of the past. It is, however, clear that the behaviors of the patient were acquired through direct observation and modeling from significant others. This learning took place in the early to middle childhood years. The schemas that are the focus for the therapy are obviously a product of early life experience and not simply an occurrence and product of the moment.

Myth #2: The cognitive therapist eschews the use of medication as a part of the therapy. In treating many patients, medication is a part of the therapeutic regimen. While the outcome studies of the cognitive therapy for depression have tested cognitive therapy versus antidepressant medication versus a combination of the cognitive therapy and medication, this in no way means that cognitive therapy and appropriate pharmacotherapy are mutually exclusive. As demonstrated in several of the cases, therapy and medication are complementary.

Myth #3: The cognitive therapist does not use the therapeutic relationship. Good therapy is good therapy is good therapy. The development, building, and maintenance of the therapeutic relationship is well demonstrated herein. Therapeutic collaboration is a vital component in the therapy. The relationship does not become the focus of the therapy (transference), but rather is used as a microcosm of the patient's style of relating.

Myth #4: Cognitive therapy is the power of positive thinking. The power of positive thinking is the work of Dr. Norman Vincent Peale (1954). While positive thinking is neither bad nor discouraged for the patient, the therapy is more focused on helping the patient to make manifest the internal dialogue that maintains the depressive or anxiogenic state. The cognitive therapist does not try to argue the patient out of his or her negative thoughts by pointing to positive thoughts or the fact that others have even greater life difficulty. The use of positive affirmations or aphorisms (e.g., "I'm good," "I'm OK, you're OK," or "Good things come to those who wait") is similarly not the focus of the therapy; rather, it is acquiring the ability to challenge negative and dysfunctional thoughts.

Myth #5: Cognitive therapy is too simple. While the therapy possibly lacks the elegance and complexity of some other models, *straightforward* is too often confused with *simplistic*. The cognitive therapist tries to follow the law of parsimony, that is, looking for simple rather than complex solutions. This may well mean that the cognitive therapist may not borrow descriptions of problems or titles for syndromes from Greek drama, but rather tries to deal with problems directly. It takes as long to train a cognitive therapist as it does to train any therapist to practice any model of treatment effectively.

Myth #6: The cognitive therapist works only on symptom relief and not on underlying issues. While many of the cases focus on the presenting problems as the centerpiece of the therapy, whenever the therapist works at schematic change, the underlying dynamics are addressed. While these dynamics are not the same as the hydraulic dynamics of the analyst, the construct of "underlying issues" is a theoretical one. If one does not accept the idea that problems are the result of underlying conflict, then focusing on any so-called underlying issues may be of little value. The work of schematic change is dynamic and important.

Myth #7: The goal of therapy is clear thinking, but insight or clear thinking is not the only goal of cognitive therapy. We would question the goal of being a clear-thinking depressive or a straight-thinking panic patient. For the patient who presents for therapy with depression, anxiety, panic, or any other disorder, the goal is affective change. In fact, with many of the most difficult patient disorders (such as the personality disorders), not only is the affect change a goal of therapy, but affect is the major tool in helping to change dysfunctional behavior and beliefs.

RESISTANCES TO COGNITIVE THERAPY

As a result of the growth, maturation, sophistication, popularity, and broad international dissemination of cognitive therapy, some of the resistances to the expansion of cognitive therapy treatment and education will, it is hoped, fall by the wayside. Goisman (1988) has identified several of the most common resistances, which are listed below.

Therapist role conflict. There are three major issues involved in setting up a role conflict for many therapists. Most therapists have been trained to maintain a relatively inactive verbal stance. The structured model described and advocated in all of the cases here is also at variance with the nondirective and unstructured treatment model generally taught as appropriate. The guided discovery approach (Beck, Rush, Shaw, & Emery, 1979) is also at variance with the free-associative model advocated by the psychodynamic therapies.

Role modeling. For many years, younger therapists seeking role models were put into conflict by the older, more senior faculty being more psychodynamically oriented; it was the younger, more junior faculty that were behavioral or cognitive-behavioral. This has changed as the generation of behavioral and cognitive-behavioral faculty has been promoted to senior faculty status. A second role conflict was that the senior role models were primarily medical faculty and biologically oriented, while the cognitive and behavioral faculty were psychologists. In the unfortunate pecking order that prevails in our profession, the medical/psychiatric faculty are usually in the positions of power and administration. The impact of the more behavioral-psychologically oriented therapies has, however, made great impact on the medical community—due in large part to the training and leadership of several influential physicians and psychiatrists, several of whom are represented in this volume.

Treatment model conflict. It is in this area that much of the difficulty and professional resistance has occurred. A question that we have frequently heard in the course of our teaching has been, "What about the underlying or real problems?" The implication is that the cognitive model, taking a symptom relief approach, discomforts those who have been trained to believe the symptom is merely a symbol of some deep, core conflict, and that symptom relief will only lead to symptom substitution. Further, by focusing on the overt behavior rather than the unconscious spurs to the behavior, cognitive therapy is quite different from the more traditional therapies. One of the common complaints or criticisms of the cognitive model is that it appears mundane and functional, rather than having the grand, philosophical view of the psychoanalytic model.

The theoretical and philosophical differences between the traditional insight orientation and the cognitive model have also led to direct disparagement. A commonly voiced view is that psychoanalysis may be likened to the gold standard, and other therapies are seen as useful, but made of "baser metals." This disparagement has been also likened to psychoanalysts viewing the analytic/dynamic therapies as the "Rolls-Royce of therapies" and the others as simply quick-fix therapies (Goisman, 1988). The position of the dynamicists is that if given the choice of therapies with bright and motivated patients, psychodynamic work would be the treatment of choice. This last idea—that is, that there are certain patients who are good candidates for cognitive therapy—is, we hope, put to rest as the result of the case material presented in this volume. We have tried to present the broadest selection of cases to demonstrate the efficacy, utility, breadth, and depth of the model.

As always, any ending is also a beginning. Our hope and expectation is that the readers of this volume will be able to utilize the case treatment protocols directly with their patients. In other cases, there will be a need to adapt and modify the material presented. In any case, our goal has been to present material that can be used in the practice and research into the further applications and development of cognitive therapy well into the 21st century. We wish you well.

REFERENCES

Bandura, A. (1977). *Social learning theory*. Englewood Cliffs, NJ: Prentice-Hall.

Beck, A., Rush, A. J., Shaw, B., & Emery, G. (1979). *Cognitive therapy of depression*. New York: Guilford.

Blackburn, I., Bishop, S., Glen, A. I. M., Whalley, L. J., & Christie, J. E. (1981). The efficacy of cognitive therapy in depression: A treatment using cognitive therapy and pharmacotherapy, each alone and in combination. *British Journal of Psychiatry, 139,* 181–189.

Freeman, A. (1986). Cognitive therapy: An overview. In A. Freeman & V. Greenwood (Eds.), *Cognitive therapy: Applications in psychiatric and medical settings* (pp. 19–35). New York: Human Sciences Press.

Freeman, A., & Davis, D. D. (1990). Cognitive therapy of depression. In A. S. Bellack, M. Hersen, & A. E. Kazdin, *International handbook of behavior modification and therapy*. New York: Plenum.

Freeman, A., Pretzer, J., Fleming, B., & Simon, K. M. (1990). *Clinical applications of cognitive therapy*. New York: Plenum.

Goisman, R. (1988). Resistances to learning behavior therapy. *American Journal of Psychotherapy, 42*(18), 67–76.

Mahoney, M. J., & Freeman, A. (Eds.). (1985). *Cognition and psychotherapy*. New York: Plenum.

Murphy, G. E., Simons, A. D., Wetzel, R. D., & Lustman, P. J. (1984). Cognitive therapy versus tricyclic antidepressants in major depression. *Archives of General Psychiatry, 41,* 33–41.

Norcross, J., Prochaska, & Gallagher. (1989). Clinical psychologists in the 1980s: Theory, research, and practice. *The Clinical Psychologist, 42*(3), 45–53.

Peale, N. V. (1954). Power of positive thinking. Englewood Cliffs, NJ: Prentice-Hall.

Rush, A. J., Beck, A. T., Kovacs, M., & Hollon, S. (1977). Comparative efficacy of cognitive therapy and imipramine in the treatment of depressed outpatients. *Cognitive Therapy and Research, 1,* 17–37.

Safran, J. D., & Segal, Z. V. (1990). *Interpersonal process in cognitive therapy*. New York: Basic Books.

Sullivan, H. S. (1953). *The interpersonal theory of psychiatry*. New York: Norton.

About the Editors

Arthur Freeman, Ed.D., ABPP, ABBP, is Director of the Cognitive Therapy Program at Cooper Hospital/University Medical Center and Clinical Professor of Psychiatry at the University of Medicine and Dentistry of New Jersey, Adjunct Professor of Psychology at LaSalle University, and Visiting Professor of Medical Psychology at Shanghai Second Medical University, People's Republic of China. He is a licensed psychologist and holds diplomates from the American Board of Professional Psychology (Clinical Psychology) and the American Board of Behavioral Psychology (Cognitive Behavior Therapy). He also serves as a senior consultant at the Center for Cognitive Therapy at the University of Pennsylvania.

In addition to his teaching responsibilities, Freeman is a widely published author and editor. His published works include *Cognitive Therapy with Couples and Groups* (1983); *Cognition and Psychotherapy* (1985); *Depression and the Family* (1986); *Cognitive Therapy: Applications in Psychiatric and Medical Settings* (1987); *The Practice of Cognitive Therapy* (1989); *Comprehensive Handbook of Cognitive Therapy* (1989); *Woulda, Coulda, Shoulda* (1989); *Clinical Applications of Cognitive Therapy* (1990); *Cognitive Therapy of Personality Disorders* (1990); and *Cognitive Therapy of Suicidal Behavior: A Treatment Manual* (in press).

Freeman is well known nationally and internationally for his seminars and has presented at a variety of local, regional, national, and international conferences. He has lectured in 15 countries over the past 5 years.

Frank M. Dattilio, Ph.D., ABBP, is clinical associate in psychiatry at the Center for Cognitive Therapy, University of Pennsylvania School of Medicine, and is in private practice with Behavior Therapy Associates in Allentown, Pennsylvania, and Phillipsburg, New Jersey. He is a licensed psychologist and is listed in the National Register of Health Service Providers in Psychology. He is also a diplomate in behavioral psychology with the American Board of Behavioral Psychology and serves as an adjunct faculty member to Lehigh University and the Medical College of Pennsylvania.

Dattilio trained in behavior therapy through the Department of Psychiatry at Temple University School of Medicine under the direction of Joseph Wolpe, M.D., and received his postdoctoral training through the Center for Cognitive Therapy, University of Pennsylvania School of Medicine under the direction of Aaron T. Beck, M.D. He has more than 50 professional publications in the areas of anxiety disorders, behavioral problems, and marital discord and has also presented extensively throughout the United States and Canada, and Europe on the treatment of anxiety disorders and marital discord. Among his many publications, Dattilio is coauthor of *Cognitive Therapy with Couples* (1990), coauthor of *Private Mental Health Practice: A Psychology Practitioner Guidebook* (in preparation) and co-editor of "Cognitive-Behavior Therapy in Crises Intervention" (in preparation). He is also on the editorial board of several professional journals.

About the Contributors

Aaron T. Beck, M.D., is University Professor of Psychiatry at the University of Pennsylvania School of Medicine and director of the Center for Cognitive Therapy. He is the author of over 260 scientific and scholarly articles and monographs and has published eight books on depression, anxiety, personality disorders, suicide, and cognitive therapy.

Robert E. Becker, Ph.D., is in his own practice, Psychological Resources Group of Fort Washington, Pennsylvania. He has authored or coauthored papers on the treatment of social phobia as well as dysthymic disorder. He has published a book about social skills training as a treatment for dysthymia. In addition, he has served as principal or coprincipal investigator on National Institute of Mental Health grants investigating social phobia as well as dysthymia.

Robert J. Berchick, Ph.D., is clinical associate professor of psychology in psychiatry at the University of Pennsylvania School of Medicine, where he served as clinical director of the Center for Cognitive Therapy for over seven years. He is a licensed psychologist in a private practice, specializing in the treatment of depression, anxiety disorders, and marital discord.

Thomas D. Borkovec, Ph.D., is a professor of psychology at Pennsylvania State University and codirector of the Stress and Anxiety Disorders Institute. He is a licensed psychologist, has served on several editorial boards, and was a member of the Treatment Development and Assessment Study Section at NIMH.

Donald A. Bux, Jr., M.S.Ed., is currently a research instructor with the Division of Addiction Research and Treatment, Division of Mental Health Sciences, Hahnemann University. He has previously worked as intake coordinator of the Center for Cognitive Therapy in Philadelphia, where he also received his practicum training in cognitive therapy. He was copresenter with Fred Wright of "Cognitive Therapy of Substance Abuse" at the International Training Institute and Update on Cognitive Therapy Conference, Philadelphia, October 5–7, 1990.

Ellen Costello, Ph.D., is a licensed psychologist who practices at Butler Hospital in Providence, R.I. Her clinical interests include depression, anxiety, eating disorders, and incest.

Constance V. Dancu, Ph.D., is assistant professor in psychiatry at the Medical College of Pennsylvania. She is also a licensed psychologist and coinvestigator of a research project that is investigating the development and treatment of post-traumatic stress disorder in rape and nonsexual crime victims. Her areas of expertise are anxiety disorders, stress management, and crisis intervention.

Mary Helen Davis, M.D., is assistant professor of psychiatry and behavioral sciences at the University of Louisville School of Medicine and director of adult psychiatry at Norton Psychiatric Clinic in Louisville, Kentucky. Her areas of expertise include inpatient psychiatry and affective and personality disorders.

Esther Deblinger, Ph.D., is assistant professor of clinical psychiatry and clinical director of the Center for Children's Support at the University of Medicine and Dentistry of New Jersey—School of Osteopathic Medicine. Her areas of expertise are child sexual abuse and post-traumatic stress disorder; she has published and presented research on these and related topics nationwide.

E. Thomas Dowd, Ph.D., ABPP, is professor and director of counseling psychology at Kent State University. He is a Diplomate in Counseling Psychology of the American Board of Professional Psychology. His areas of interest are in cognitive-behavioral therapy, attributional processes in counseling, paradoxical interventions, and hypnotherapy.

Bruce N. Eimer, Ph.D., is a licensed psychologist and director of the Behavior Therapy Center in Jenkintown, Pennsylvania. He is also president of Senior-PsychCare, Inc., a company that provides mental health consultation services to senior citizens in long-term care facilities. His areas of expertise are biobehavioral treatments for psychophysiologic disorders, including chronic pain and neuropsychological assessment.

Norman Epstein, Ph.D., is an associate professor in the Department of Family and Community Development at the University of Maryland. He also is a licensed psychologist. His areas of expertise are cognitive-behavioral assessment and treatment of couples and families, as well as cognitive therapy for depression. His recent research has focused on the development of instruments for assessing cognitive factors in marital discord.

Catherine G. Fine, Ph.D., is a clinical psychologist in private practice in Philadelphia and in Blue Bell, Pennsylvania. She is a faculty member in psychiatry at Temple University and is program coordinator of the Dissociative Disorders Unit at the Institute of Pennsylvania Hospital. She is president (1990–91) of the International Society for the Study of Multiple Personality and Dissociation.

Edna B. Foa, Ph.D., is a professor in psychiatry and director of the Center for the Treatment and Study of Psychiatry at the Medical College of Pennsylvania. She is also a licensed psychologist and the author of four books and over 100 chapters and articles. Her area of expertise is anxiety disorders, including obsessive–compulsive disorder, post-traumatic stress disorder, and the processing of anxiety-related information.

Michael B. Frisch, Ph.D., is associate professor in the Ph.D. Program in Clinical Psychology at Baylor University. His clinical and research interests focus on depression and subjective well-being, cognitive therapy, relationship skills, and marital therapy. He is currently developing an integrative approach to the treatment of depression called Quality of Life Therapy, which integrates cognitive theories with the literature on subjective well-being, happiness, and life satisfaction.

Dolores Gallagher-Thompson, Ph.D., is currently a visiting associate professor in the Counseling Psychology Program at Stanford University's School of Education. She is also codirector of the Older Adult and Family Center, which is part of the Palo Alto Veterans Affairs Medical Center and the Division of Gerontology, Stanford University School of Medicine. She is licensed psychologist with a private practice specializing in depression, anxiety disorders, and assessment and treatment of problems of later life, including family issues around caregiving for an impaired elder relative.

Frank E. Gantz, Ph.D., is currently a geropsychologist at the Veterans Affairs Medical Center in Salisbury, North Carolina. He is formerly the coordinator of the Older Adult and Family Center in the Division of Gerontology, Stanford University School of Medicine, and the Palo Alto Veterans Affairs Medical Center.

David M. Garner, Ph.D., is professor and director of research in the Eating Disorder Program in the Department of Psychiatry at Michigan State University.

Mark Gilson, Ph.D., is director of the Atlanta Center for Cognitive Therapy and adjunct faculty with the Emory University School of Medicine Department of Psychiatry, and the Georgia State University Department of Psychology. He and Arthur Freeman are cofounders of Cognitive Therapy Consultants, providing training certification that is approved by the American Psychological Association (with consultants retaining program responsibility) and inpatient consultation to hospitals and institutions across the country.

Wayne A. Gordon, Ph.D., is chief psychologist and associate professor of rehabilitation medicine and psychiatry in the Department of Rehabilitation Medicine, Mount Sinai Medical Center, New York. His areas of expertise involve rehabilitation research, neuropsychological assessment, and cognitive intervention with various brain-injured populations.

Ruth L. Greenberg, Ph.D., is a senior consultant at the Center for Cognitive Therapy University of Pennsylvania School of Medicine, Philadelphia. She is also a licensed psychologist in private practice in Philadelphia, specializing in the treatment of depression and anxiety disorders.

Dennis Greenberger, Ph.D., is program director of the Depression Treatment Program, a hospital-based cognitive therapy program at CPC Santa Ana Hospital. He is a licensed psychologist, and his areas of expertise include suicide, depressive disorders, and psychotherapy with patients who are psychiatrically hospitalized.

Susan E. Grober, Ph.D., is currently a rehabilitation psychologist in the Division of Rehabilitation Medicine of Norwalk Hospital, Connecticut. Her area of expertise is rehabilitation psychology.

Mary R. Hibbard, Ph.D., is an assistant professor of rehabilitation medicine and psychiatry and supervisor of psychology in the Department of Rehabilitation, Mount Sinai Medical Center, New York. Her areas of expertise are neuropsychological assessment, cognitive remediation, and cognitive psychotherapy with both brain-injured and nonbrain- injured patients.

Andrea Karfgin, Ph.D., is a clinical psychologist at Sheppard Pratt Hospital, Towson, Maryland, where she is an eating disorders specialist and coordinator of the Obesity Program. Her interest in eating disorders has led to a subspeciality in multiple personality disorders, and she is a staff member in the Dissociative Disorders Clinic at Sheppard Pratt.

Kevin T. Kuehlwein, Psy.D., is a postdoctoral fellow at the Center for Cognitive Therapy at the University of Pennsylvania School of Medicine . He is also an adjunct assistant professor in the Mental Health Sciences Department at Hahnemann University in Philadelphia.

Cory F. Newman, Ph.D., is clinical director of the Center for Cognitive Therapy and assistant professor of psychology and psychiatry at the University of Pennsylvania School of Medicine Philadelphia. Currently, he is collaborating in the writing of two new books on cognitive therapy—working with Aaron T. Beck and Fred D. Wright on *Cognitive Therapy of Substance Abuse Disorders*, and with Susan Byers, Mary Ann Layden, and Arthur Freeman on *Cognitive Therapy of the Borderline Patient*.

Gullan Nordström is a nurse therapist at the Ersboda Treatment Center in Umeå, Sweden.

Carlo Perris, M.D., is professor and chairman in the Department of Psychiatry at the University of Umeå, Sweden, and is affiliated with the World Health Organization Collaborating Center for Research and Training in Mental Health.

Jacqueline B. Persons, Ph.D., is assistant clinical professor in the Department of Psychiatry, University of California, San Francisco, and a licensed psychologist in private practice in Oakland. Her areas of expertise are depression and anxiety. She recently authored *Cognitive Therapy in Practice: A Case Formulation Approach*.

Mark A. Reinecke, Ph.D., is assistant professor of clinical psychiatry and director of the Center for Cognitive Therapy at the University of Chicago School of Medicine. He is also a licensed psychologist and is on the faculty of the School of Social Service Administration and the Program in Mental Health Research at the University of Chicago. His areas of interest center on childhood depression and suicide, anxiety disorders, and cognitive mediation of adjustment to chronic illness.

John L. Rodman, Ph.D., L.C.P., is a staff psychologist at St. Paul Ramsey Medical Center in St. Paul, Minnesota, where he coordinates psychological assessment services for the Department of Psychiatry and provides therapy to depressed and bereaved individuals, with a focus on older adults. He has published papers addressing treatment issues with depressed and bereaved patients, the treatment of affective disorders in older adults, and how to intervene effectively with older adults who present with chronic medical problems.

David Roth, Ph.D., is a clinical psychologist and director of the Inpatient and Outpatient Eating Disorders Program at Sheppard Pratt Hospital, Towson, Maryland. He is chairman of the Governor's Task Force on Eating Disorders in Maryland. He is also interested in treatment for depression and is director of the outpatient depression program at Sheppard Pratt.

Paul G. Salmon, Ph.D., is an associate professor of clinical psychology at the University of Louisville, and director of clinical research for the Arts in Medicine Program of the Department of Psychiatry and Behavioral Sciences. A licensed clinical psychologist, his primary interests concern musical performance skills and the treatment of performance anxiety.

G. Randolph Schrodt, Jr., M.D., is associate professor of psychiatry and behavioral sciences at the University of Louisville School of Medicine. He is also associate clinical director at Norton Psychiatric Clinic in Louisville, Kentucky. His areas of expertise are adolescent psychiatry, affective disorders, and behavioral medicine.

Paula N. Stein, Ph.D., is instructor of rehabilitation medicine and psychiatry, Mount Sinai Medical School, New York. Her area of expertise is cognitive psychotherapy with both brain-injured and nonbrain-injured patients.

Yona Teichman, Ph.D., is professor of clinical psychology at Tel-Aviv University and a senior clinical psychologist in private practice. She specializes in family therapy and is involved in research on depression from an interpersonal point of view.

Larry W. Thompson, Ph.D., is professor of medicine (research) and codirector of the Older Adult and Family Center, Palo Alto Veterans Affairs Medical Center and Division of Gerontology, Stanford University School of Medicine. He is a licensed psychologist who spends considerable time training predoctoral interns and postdoctoral fellows in geropsychology. His private practice focuses on neuropsychological assessment, with particular emphasis on Alzheimer's disease and other disorders of aging.

Louise Troeng is a nurse therapist at the Ersboda Treatment Center in Umeå, Sweden.

Ralph M. Turner, Ph.D., FIAEP, is a licensed psychologist and professor of psychiatry and psychology at Temple University School of Medicine. He is on the editorial board of the *Journal of Consulting and Clinical Psychology and Integrative and Eclectic Psychotherapy*, among others. He has published extensively on anxiety, schizophrenia, and borderline disorders.

Adrian Wells is a Chartered Clinical Psychologist supported by the Medical Research Council at the University of Oxford, Department of Psychiatry. He received his training in cognitive therapy at the Center for Cognitive Therapy University of Pennsylvania School of Medicine in Philadelphia. Among his publications are works on cognitive-attentional aspects of anxiety, self-consciousness, and cognitive therapy.

Janet L. Wolfe, Ph.D., is executive director of the Institute for Rational-Emotive Therapy in New York City, where she conducts therapy and trains interns and postgraduate fellows. She is also a consultant to the Department of Veterans Affairs. She has written extensively and conducted numerous workshops in women's and sex-role issues in therapy, relationship problems, and group therapy.

Fred D. Wright, Ed.D., is assistant professor in counseling psychology and psychiatry at the University of Pennsylvania School of Medicine. He is a licensed psychologist and also director of education at the Center for Cognitive Therapy, University of Pennsylvania School of Medicine. His areas of expertise are cognitive therapy of substance abuse and anxiety disorders.

Jesse H. Wright, M.D., Ph.D., is a professor in the Department of Psychiatry and Behavioral Sciences, University of Louisville School of Medicine. He also serves as medical director of the Norton Psychiatric Clinic, Louisville, Kentucky. He has performed basic research and has written extensively in the areas of psychopharmacology, cognitive therapy, and the interface between these treatments.

M. Jane Yates, R.N., Ph.D., is codirector of the Atlanta Center for Cognitive Therapy and works with both children and adults in private practice. She is a psychological consultant to the Aware Treatment Program for survivors of sexual abuse and is a psychotherapist on the Dissociative Disorders Unit at Ridgeview Institute, a private psychiatric treatment center in Atlanta. She is currently involved with the development of a cognitive therapy inpatient program at Georgia Baptist Medical Center, also in Atlanta.

Index